INFECTIVE ENDOCARDITIS

Collected Reprints (1961-2014)

By
William C. Roberts, MD
and
Colleagues

ISBN: 979-8-88680-076-0
Printed in the United States of America on acid-free paper.

Preface

Infective endocarditis (IE) was always fatal until effective antibiotics were introduced in the early 1940s. Surgical excision of cardiac valves with vegetations, or only the vegetations themselves, started in the late 1960s. In its early years, the stethoscope was important in its diagnosis along with blood cultures. Today, the echocardiogram is key to the diagnosis of IE.

Although I have seen either the heart or excised heart valves in several hundred patients with active and healed IE, I avoid giving talks on the topic because of its complexity. Infection of a right-sided cardiac valve produces a clinical picture much different from IE involving a left-sided cardiac valve. Most patients with IE today are treated with antibiotics before cardiac valve surgery, and this pretreatment changes considerably the histologic features of the excised vegetation. The clinical features of patients with IE involving one or more mechanical or bioprosthetic valves is quite different from IE involving one or more native cardiac valves. Patients with recognized complications of active IE are quite different from those without those complications (ring abscess, heart block emboli, etc.). The varying organisms causing the IE can readily produce differing scenarios. For all these reasons IE is a challenging condition.

—William C. Roberts, MD

Table of Contents

*Articles are numbered based on WCR's CV.

Postoperative endocarditis due to Candida: clinical observations and the experimental production of the lesion

THEODORE COOPER, M.D., PH.D.
ANDREW G. MORROW, M.D.
WILLIAM C. ROBERTS, M.D.
LLOYD G. HERMAN, PH.D.
BETHESDA, MD.
From the Clinic of Surgery, National Heart Institute, The Department of Pathologic Anatomy and the Sanitary Engineering Branch, The National Institutes of Health

Postoperative endocarditis is an infrequent but dreaded complication of operations for the correction of congenital or acquired heart disease.[2, 3] The rarity of the disease is somewhat surprising since all intracardiac procedures result in some damage to the endocardium and foreign bodies in the form of sutures or prosthetic materials are usually inserted. Although a certain number of microorganisms are probably introduced into the circulation in the course of every cardiac operation, the size of this inoculum can be minimized by vigilant asepsis and the defense mechanisms of the patient will ordinarily prevent the development of infection. Also, in many clinics, antibiotics are routinely administered during the early postoperative period, although the role of such prophylaxis in preventing postoperative endocarditis has not been established.

The most lethal form of postoperative endocarditis is that in which the responsible organism is a fungus.[7] Only 2 patients who developed postoperative fungal endocarditis have been described in the surgical literature[4, 6] and in each the disease was recognized only at autopsy. Three patients in this clinic have developed mycotic endocarditis after operations for rheumatic heart disease. Although the infections were recognized and treatment was undertaken, each patient died.

Received for publication Oct. 3, 1960.

This experience prompted an investigation of methods for the production of fungal endocarditis in experimental animals and of the factors which influence the development of the disease. In the present report, the results of these studies are presented as well as brief clinical descriptions of the patients in whom endocarditis occurred.

CASE REPORTS

Case 1. G. V., a 45-year-old man, had acute rheumatic fever at the age of 25 and symptoms of dyspnea and easy fatigability had been noted for several years before his admission. The clinical findings indicated the presence of mitral stenosis. This diagnosis was confirmed at cardiac catheterization when he was found to have a mean left atrial pressure of 22 mm. Hg and an end diastolic gradient of 15 mm. Hg across the mitral valve. In April, 1958, a closed mitral commissurotomy was performed. The valve leaflets were mobile and a satisfactory valve opening was accomplished by digital fracture of the commissures. The patient tolerated the operation well and the postoperative course was uneventful except for the development of atrial fibrillation which could not be converted with quinidine. He was given 1.0 Gm. of streptomycin and 1.2 million units of penicillin daily for 8 days postoperatively and penicillin orally for an additional week. The patient was discharged from the hospital 20 days after operation. Two weeks later he developed fever, sweating, and weakness which persisted in spite of treatment by his physician. When readmitted 9 weeks after operation he was found to have low grade fever and enlargement of the spleen. An apical systolic murmur, not present at the time of his discharge, was audible. Blood cultures revealed a heavy growth of *Candida parakrusei*. In spite of intensive treatment with amphotericin B, the patient died 5 weeks after the presence of the infection had been proved. At autopsy active endocarditis which involved the mitral valve and left atrium was evident and *Candida* was cultured from the vegetations present. Microscopic sections of a vegetation on the anterior mitral leaflet demonstrated the presence of abundant moniliform organisms. Infarcts in the spleen, kidney, liver, lung, and hilar lymph nodes all contained the organism.

Case 2. M. S., a 39-year-old housewife, had had chorea at the age of 9 and an attack of acute rheumatic fever at the age of 29. Since the age of 34 she had experienced increasing cardiac disability. On clinical examination she was in evident cardiac failure and the murmurs of mitral stenosis and regurgitation were audible. At left-heart catheterization the mean left atrial pressure was 34 mm. Hg, an end diastolic gradient of 11 mm. Hg was recorded across the mitral valve, and the contour of the left atrial pressure pulse indicated gross mitral regurgitation. In November, 1958, an open surgical repair of the mitral valve was undertaken. During complete cardiopulmonary bypass, for a period of 1 hour, a posterior annuloplasty was performed and the anterior commissure opened. After operation the patient's course was smooth but her convalescence was slow. She was given 1.0 Gm. of streptomycin daily for 5 days, 1.2 million units of penicillin daily for 14 days and penicillin orally for an addi- oxygenator at the end of the perfusion grew only tional 16 days. A culture of blood taken from the a Flavobacterium which was thought to be a laboratory contaminant. The patient was discharged 4 weeks after operation. Three and one-half months after operation the patient was readmitted because of progressive cardiac failure and fever. *Candida guilliermondi* was grown from the blood in pure culture. Therapy with amphotericin B was initiated, but the patient died 2 weeks after treatment was begun. At autopsy 2 vegetations were present on the mitral valve and one on the right coronary cusp of the aortic valve. Cultures and microscopic sections of these vegetations showed them to be *Candida guilliermondi*. Embolic abscesses were found in the spleen, kidney, brain, and spinal cord.

Case 3. H. D., a 48-year-old dentist, presented with a history of rheumatic fever and the physical findings of aortic stenosis. Left-heart catheterization showed an elevated left atrial pressure, a left ventricular pressure of 250/40 mm. Hg, a brachial artery pressure of 130/70 mm. Hg, and a cardiac output of 6.4 L. per minute. The peak systolic gradient of 120 mm. Hg across the aortic valve indicated severe stenosis. Aortic valvulotomy under direct vision was performed in June, 1959. During the course of the operation cardiopulmonary bypass was employed for 25 minutes. All 3 commissures of a densely calcified valve were opened and a gratifying fall in the pressure gradient was apparent in the operative pressure records. Cultures of blood taken from the heart-lung machine after the operation grew *Candida guilliermondi*. Postoperatively the patient's course was apparently uncomplicated. He was given 1.0 Gm. of streptomycin daily for 5 days and 1.2 million units of penicillin daily for 13 days. He was discharged 16 days after operation. About 2 weeks later the patient experienced spiking fever which persisted in spite of antibiotics given by his physician. He was readmitted 6 weeks after operation. At this time numerous blood cultures showed *Staphylococcus aureus* and *Candida guilliermondi*. Antibiotic therapy was initiated promptly and the antifungal agent, amphotericin B, was also employed. Subsequent blood cultures became negative for *Staphylococcus aureus* but continued to show growth of the Candida. Since maximal doses of amphotericin were ineffective, another antifungal agent, designated RO-2, was employed separately and in conjunction with amphotericin and antibiotic agents. The progress of the infection was essentially unaltered, however, and the patient died 4 months after treatment was begun. Three vegetations, the largest of which was 2.5 cm. in diameter, were found on the aortic valve at autopsy (Fig. 1, *A* and *B*). *Candida guilliermondi* was cultured from the blood and the organisms were visible in microscopic sections (Fig. 1, *C* and *D*). Infected infarcts were found in the spleen and brain.

A more complete description of the clinical courses of these patients and the details of their therapy will be reported elsewhere.[1]

EXPERIMENTAL METHODS

In 14 mongrel dogs which weighed 11 to 24 kilograms, aortic regurgitation was created by the technique previously described by Roshe and Morrow.[8] After induction of anesthesia with thiopental sodium and endotracheal intubation, the right thorax was entered through the fourth intercostal space. During inflow occlusion, the ascending aorta was opened and a disc of tissue 3.9 mm. in diameter was excised from the base of the right coronary aortic leaflet. Circulation was restored and the aortotomy was closed. Four to 6 weeks after operation 12 of the animals were utilized for fungal inoculation and the 2 remaining ones served as uninoculated controls.

Initial studies in normal dogs were carried out to determine the magnitude of inoculum which would maintain a blood level of organisms for several minutes. After the intravenous injection of 32 million cells of *Candida guilliermondi* into normal dogs, it could be grown from blood sampled 5 to 10 minutes later. Consequently, all inoculations into the experimental animals consisted of 32 million or more organisms. Saline suspensions of cultures grown from the blood of patient H. D. were used as the source of *Candida guilliermondi*.

Three controls dogs which had not been operated on and 12 with aortic regurgitation were inoculated. The controls and 3 of those with aortic regurgitation were given no drugs. Of the remaining 9 dogs with aortic lesions, 5 were given 800,000 U. of penicillin and 0.5 Gm. of streptomycin intramuscularly on each of 8 days and 4 received 100 mg. of tetracycline intramuscularly daily for this period. In all animals venous blood cultures were drawn at weekly or biweekly intervals for a period of 3 months. At death, autopsy was performed immediately, and cultures of heart blood, of vegetations if present, and of apparently involved organs were obtained. Tissue was then placed in formalin and prepared for microscopic study.

RESULTS

The results of the study are summarized in Table I.

Inoculated controls with normal aortic valve. Negative blood cultures were obtained

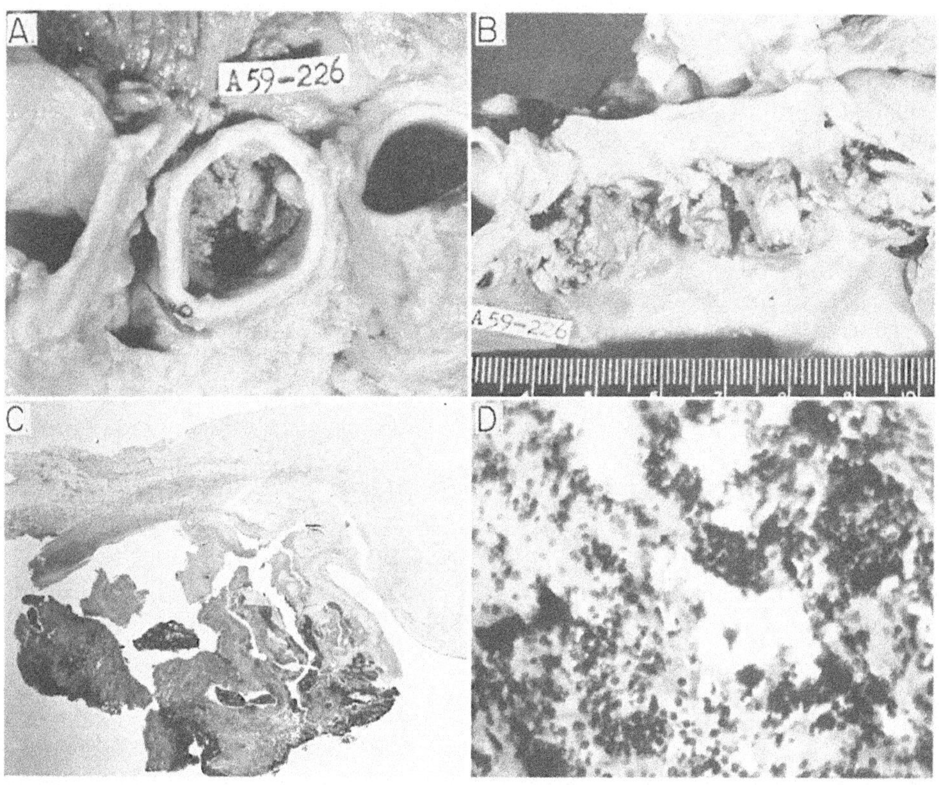

Fig. 1. Gross and microscopic photographs of the heart of patient H. D. *A*, The aortic valve as seen from above. Large fungating vegetations nearly occlude the valve orifice. *B*, The left ventricular outflow tract, aortic valve, and aorta have been opened. Vegetations nearly fill each aortic sinus of Valsalva. *C*, Microscopic section through one of the vegetations (PAS; ×10). The darker areas are colonies of Candida. The ventricular surface of the aortic cusp is free of vegetation. *D*, High power view of one of the colonies of Candida shown in C. (PAS; ×495). Only spore forms are present and hyphae are absent.

Table I. *Results of intravenous inoculation of Candida guilliermondi in dogs*

Group	*No. of dogs*	*During life*		*At autopsy*	
		Positive blood cultures	*Signs of illness*	*Positive blood or tissue culture*	*Valvular vegetations*
Inoculated controls, normal aortic valve	3	None	None	None	None
Inoculation, aortic regurgitation, no antibiotics	3	None	None	None	None
Inoculation, aortic regurgitation, penicillin and streptomycin	5	4	2	3	3
Inoculation, aortic regurgitation, tetracycline	4	1	1	1	1
Aortic regurgitation, no inoculation, no antibiotics	2	None	None	None	None

in all animals over the entire period of observation. The dogs gained weight, were active, and showed no signs of being ill. At postmortem examination none had evidence of endocarditis or other diseases attributable to the inoculation of the organisms.

Inoculation, aortic regurgitation, and no antibiotics. These 3 animals showed no positive blood cultures over 7 test periods. They gained weight and showed no evidence of being ill. At sacrifice no evidence of active endocarditis was present. The right coronary leaflets were scarred and thickened. The holes in them were rimmed by fibrous tissue. In one animal the perforation in the valve was healed. The viscera were free of signs of emboli.

Inoculation, aortic regurgitation, and administration of penicillin and streptomycin. Four of these 5 animals evidenced at least 1 positive blood culture during 6 sampling periods. Two showed repeatedly positive cultures. One dog died 6 days after inoculation, apparently in heart failure. At postmortem examination pleural fluid was present and the heart was dilated. A small (6 mm.) vegetation was present around the regurgitant orifice in the right coronary cusp. The spleen contained septic emboli. Cultures of heart blood and of the spleen were positive for *Candida guilliermondi*. A second animal died 1 month after inoculation in severe heart failure with passive congestion. An ulcerative vegetation 1 cm. in diameter was present on the aortic valve. Infarcts were grossly evident in the spleen. Cultures of the vegetation on the right coronary cusp yielded *Candida guilliermondi* and a gram-negative bacterium. A third animal at sacrifice demonstrated a 2.4 cm. vegetation on the right coronary cusp which extended through the ventricular septum into the right ventricle, probably through a tract inadvertently made by the punch during operation (Fig. 2, *A* and *B*). There were infarcts in the kidneys and spleen. Cultures of the vegetation were positive for *Candida guilliermondi* and moniliform organisms were seen on microscopic section of the valve (Fig. 2, *C* and *D*). In the remaining animals the hearts were normal except for the regurgitant lesions in the aortic leaflets.

Inoculation, aortic regurgitation, and tetracycline administration. One of 4 animals showed a positive culture during the observation period. This animal did not gain weight but otherwise did not appear ill. At sacrifice a vegetation 0.5 cm. in diameter was present on the right coronary cusp. Culture of the vegetation was positive for *Candida guilliermondi* although no organisms were seen on microscopic section of the valve. In the remaining animals the hearts were normal except for the regurgitant lesions in the aortic leaflets.

Aortic regurgitation, no inoculation, and no antibiotics given. The hearts of these 2 animals showed no evidence of endocarditis.

The regurgitant orifices were patent and minimally scarred.

DISCUSSION

The experimental study described demonstrates that fungal endocarditis can be produced in the dog when a site for its localization is provided by damage to an aortic leaflet. Although the number of experimental animals in the study was not large the results imply that antibiotic administration after inoculation with *Candida guilliermondi* facilitated the development of the lesion. This finding was not a surprising one, since it is commonly observed that long-term antibiotic therapy increases susceptibility to fungal infection in other areas of the body.[9] The selection of penicillin, streptomycin, and tetracycline in the investigation was based solely on the fact that postoperative patients commonly receive these drugs. The dosage employed was arbitrary. It is possible that other antibiotics or dosage schedules might alter or enhance the experimental occurrence of the lesion.

All 3 patients whose cases are reported had been treated prophylactically with penicillin and streptomycin and again one must speculate as to the role of these agents in the development of the infections. It has recently been advocated that antibiotics not be given routinely after cardiovascular oper-

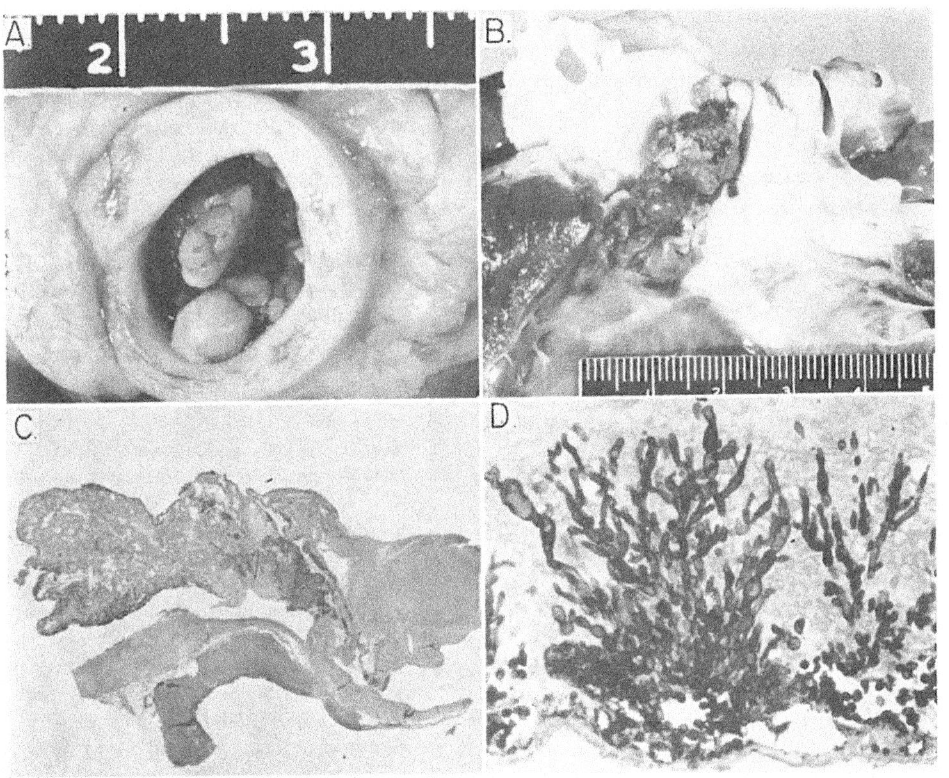

Fig. 2. Gross and microscopic photographs of the heart of a dog in which mycotic endocarditis was experimentally produced. *A,* The aortic valve as seen from above. A large vegetation obstructs the valve orifice. *B,* View taken after the left ventricle, aortic valve, and aorta were opened. The vegetation arises in the right coronary aortic cusp, which had previously ben perforated, and protrudes into the ascending aorta. *C,* Microscopic section through the vegetation demonstrated in *B.* (Hematoxylin and eosin; ×4). The darker areas are colonies of Candida. *D,* High power photomicrograph of Candida organisms (Methenamine silver; ×515). The hyphae forms are predominant here as contrasted to the spore forms shown in Fig. 1.

ations,[5] but until wider experience has validated this suggestion it is unlikely that the practice will be widely embraced. Prevention of endocarditis, therefore, depends upon minimizing the opportunity for inoculation, particularly at operation. In one of the 3 patients described, *Candida guilliermondi* was obtained from culture of the pump-oxygenator blood at the termination of operation and suggested a source of contamination in the operating room. An extensive bacteriologic survey, however, yielded no positive cultures for Candida from any furnishings, supplies, equipment, or instruments. Each patient had had cardiac catheterization shortly before operation and it was thought that the organism might have been introduced at this time and that the infections were already established at the time of operation. The organism was never found during a detailed survey in the catheterization laboratory, however, and the source of the organisms remains obscure.

Recognition of fungal endocarditis before death in these patients was possible because of awareness of its occurrence and of the practice of routinely inoculating blood cultures into media suitable for the growth of fungi as well as bacteria. Although success in treating Candida endocarditis has not been reported, early recognition of the disease will certainly permit a study of its natural history and provide opportunity for the trial of more effective agents as they become available.

SUMMARY

Three patients are described in whom endocarditis due to a "nonpathogenic" Candida occurred after operations for acquired heart disease. In each the disease was recognized in life but therapeutic measures were in vain. This experience suggested an experimental study in which fungal endocarditis was produced in dogs rendered vulnerable to infection by the previous production of aortic regurgitation. Endocarditis due to Candida only occurred in animals which were given antibiotics after inoculation with the organism, which suggests a relationship between the use of these agents and the occurrence of the disease. This method for the experimental production of fungal endocarditis may provide a useful preparation for studies of new chemotherapeutic agents developed for the treatment of this presently universally fatal infection.

REFERENCES

1. Andriole, V. T., Kravetz, H. M., Roberts, W. C., and Utz, J. P.: Candida endocarditis: clinical and pathological observations. In press.
2. Heins, H. L., Jr., and Linde, L. M.: Bacterial endocarditis after surgery for congenital heart disease, Circulation **20:** 712, 1959.
3. Hoffman, F. G., Zimmerman, S. L., Bradley, E. A., and Lapidus, B.: Bacterial endocarditis after surgery for acquired heart disease: report of two cases and review of the literature, New England J. Med. **260:** 152, 1959.
4. Hyun, B. H., Dawson, E. A., and Pence, R. E.: Bacterial and mycotic endocarditis following cardiac surgery, J. Thoracic Surg. **35:** 298, 1958.
5. Kittle, C. F., and Reed, W. A.: Antibiotics and extracorporeal circulation, J. Thoracic Surg. **41:** 34, 1961.
6. Koelle, W. A., and Pastor, B. H.: *Candida albicans* endocarditis after aortic valvulotomy, New England J. Med. **255:** 997, 1956.
7. Merchant, R. K., Louria, D. B., Geisler, P. H., Edgcomb, J. H., and Utz, J. P.: Fungal endocarditis: review of the literature and report of three cases, Ann. Int. Med. **48:** 242, 1958.
8. Roshe, J., and Morrow, A. G.: Experimental production of graded aortic insufficiency, Surg. Gynec. & Obst. **101:** 305, 1955.
9. Zimmerman, L. E.: Candida and Aspergillus endocarditis, with comments on the role of antibiotics in dissemination of fungus disease, Arch. Path. **50:** 591, 1950.

Candida Endocarditis*

Clinical and Pathologic Studies

VINCENT T. ANDRIOLE, M.D.,† HOWARD M. KRAVETZ, M.D.,‡ WILLIAM C. ROBERTS, M.D. *and* JOHN P. UTZ, M.D.

Bethesda, Maryland

THE prevalence of mycotic endocarditis, once considered an uncommon clinical and pathologic entity, seems to have increased during the past decade. Wider use of cultural methods, an improved system of classification, and a greater clinical awareness suggest that this increase may be more apparent than real. Nevertheless, the development of many cases in the course of intensive antibiotic and steroid therapy [*9,15,79–81,88–93,101–103,118*] and its occurrence as a complication of cardiac surgery [*16,19*] provide evidence of a real increase in the frequency of the illness.

One must differentiate between endocarditis caused by "higher bacteria," which belong (in addition to the common bacteria) to the class schizomycetes, and endocarditis caused by the true fungi, or eumycetes. Present methods of classification [*1,2*] place the following etiologic agents of endocarditis in the class schizomycetes: Actinomyces bovis, A. graminis, A. septicus, Nocardia asteroides, leptothrix, Streptobacillus monilliformis, Erysipelothrix rhusiopathiae, diphtheroids, Listeria monocytogenes, and Actinobacillus lignieresi, whereas the following agents are considered eumycetes: Aspergillus flavus, A. fumigatus, Blastomyces dermatitidis, Candida albicans, C. guilliermondii, C. krusei, C. parapsilosis (parakrusei), C. tropicalis, Coccidioides immitis, Cryptococcus neoformans, Histoplasma capsulatum and mucor species.

Candida can be isolated so frequently from the stools, vagina, and throats of apparently healthy persons that their pathogenicity and relation to diseases has been difficult to establish. The isolation of a species of candida from the bloodstream implies systemic infection, but cannot be considered to establish a diagnosis of candida endocarditis. A clinical picture consistent with endocarditis and blood cultures positive for candida species (in the absence of the isolation of a more common etiologic agent), or a pathologic description of valvular vegetations containing forms characteristic of candida are acceptable evidence of candida endocarditis.

Adequately documented, published cases of fungal endocarditis now total thirty-nine [*4,6–39*], thirty-four of which have been previously reviewed by Merchant et al. [*20*]. Fifteen of these thirty-nine cases (38 per cent) [*6–19*] were caused by a species of candida. Of these, C. albicans was responsible for six [*9,12–14,16,18,19*], C. parapsilosis for three [*6–8*], C. guilliermondii for two [*10,13,14*], C. krusei [*11*], C. tropicalis [*17*] for one each, and in two cases [*15,18*] the species was not identified. We have chosen to omit from this list of cases of candida endocarditis several reports [*40–47*] of probable candida septicemia because of inadequate diagnostic information (Table I). The case in which C. parapsilosis was cultured from the surface of a left atrial myxoma, reported by Dick and Mullin [*48*], and of hyphal fragments microscopically appearing to be a species of candida, in a thrombus around a portion of the circumferential suture used to effect reduction in the size of the mitral annulus (hav-

* From the National Institute of Allergy and Infectious Diseases, Laboratory of Clinical Investigation, National Institutes of Health, and the National Cancer Institute, Pathologic Anatomy Branch, National Institutes of Health, Bethesda, Maryland. Manuscript received January 16, 1961.

† Present address: U. S. Public Health Service Research Fellow, Department of Internal Medicine, Yale University School of Medicine, New Haven, Connecticut.

‡ Present address: Clinical and Research Fellow in Medicine, Allergy Unit, Massachusetts General Hospital, Boston, Massachusetts.

TABLE I

PREVIOUSLY REPORTED CASES LACKING SUFFICIENT EVIDENCE OF CANDIDA ENDOCARDITIS FOR INCLUSION IN PRESENT REVIEW

Author	Organism	Reason for Exclusion
Friedman, Donaldson [40]	Yeast (Candida?)	Microscopic description of fungus inadequate for identification; no culture
Sacks, Ata [41]	Candida albicans	Microscopic appearance of vegetation not reported
Cassels, Steiner [42]	Candida	Culture and microscopic description inadequate for identification
Luttgens [43]	Candida	Microscopic description of fungus inadequate for identification; no culture
Peeler, Riley [44]	Candida albicans	Fungi not seen in vegetation microscopically
Paplanus, Cate [45]	Candida	Report not published; case mentioned briefly by Peeler and Riley [44]
Harrell, Thompson [46]	Candida albicans	Autopsy not performed; positive blood urine and pharyngeal cultures
Kushner, Szanto [47]	Candida ?	Inadequate description and identification of the fungus; no culture

ing been misplaced at the time of surgery) reported by Hyun, Dawson and Pence [49] were not considered examples of endocarditis.

To the fifteen cases of candida endocarditis previously noted the present report adds six: three due to C. parapsilosis, two due to C. guilliermondii, and one due to C. albicans. Certain aspects of four of these cases have been mentioned in previous reports [113,192]. These six cases are presented in detail and all twenty-one cases are listed in Table II.

HISTORICAL SURVEY

In 1939 Friedman and Donaldson [40] reported as a case of candida endocarditis the finding of fungi in a heart valve at autopsy. However, no cultures were obtained and the description of the fungus is inadequate for identification. Before this, in 1915, Hurley [21] had described one patient, and Baker and Brian [22], in 1937, two patients who had Blastomyces dermatitides in the right atrium. Epstein [25], in 1938, described a patient with C. immitis endocarditis.

In 1940 Joachim and Polayes [6] reported the first documented case of candida endocarditis. It occurred in an addict who was injecting narcotics intravenously. This and two additional patients described by Wikler et al. [7] and Pasternack [8] in 1942 were infected with C. parapsilosis (parakrusei). Geiger et al. [9], in 1946, recorded a case of endocarditis and meningitis due to C. albicans. Zimmerman [10], in 1950, reported Dr. T. M. Peery's case of C. guilliermondii endocarditis, which also occurred in a narcotic addict. In 1951 Wolfe and Henderson [11] reported C. krusei endocarditis in a patient with diabetes. Kunstadter et al. [12], in 1952, reported the second case and Niel and Köhlmeier [13,14], in 1943, the third case of endocarditis caused by C. albicans. In the same report Niel and Köhlmeier [13,14] recorded a case of C. guilliermondii endocarditis in a fifty-nine year old woman with hypertension. Caplan [15], in 1955, reported candida endocarditis following antibiotic treatment in a patient with a perforated peptic ulcer, but the species was not identified. Koelle and Pastor [16], in 1956, recovered C. albicans from a patient in whom endocarditis developed after an aortic valvulotomy. The only documented case of endocarditis due to C. tropicalis was reported by Conn, Crean, MacCabe and MacLean [17] in 1959. Recently, Pearl and Sidransky [18] reported two additional cases of candida endocarditis, one caused by C. albicans and one in which the species was not identified. Louria and Dineen [19] described clinical aspects of a case of C. albicans endocarditis after mitral valvulotomy. Permission to perform an autopsy could not be obtained.

MYCOLOGY

Members of the genus candida are yeasts, and yeasts belong to a larger group of organisms known as fungi. These species are asporogenous, i.e., neither conjugation or spore formation has been observed, and therefore are placed within the class fungi imperfecti or deuteromycetes [50].

History. Berkhout created the genus "candida" in 1923 to include those yeast-like fungi previously classified as the genus monilia. The Third International Microbiological Congress in New York in 1939 agreed to this taxonomic classification [*50*]. The term "monilia" has since been reserved for the conidial stage of representatives of the genus scleratinia, and for the species belonging to the genus neurospora, and does not now properly serve as a synonym for candida [*50*].

Species. The genus candida includes thirty species and the type species is C. albicans, first described and named Oidium albicans by Robin in 1853 [*50*]. Of the thirty species, seven are known to cause infection in man; five previously listed as causes of endocarditis and, in addition, C. stellatoidea and C. pseudotropicalis [*51*].

Identification. Morphologically, the five species of candida implicated in endocarditis are budding yeasts, 2 to 4 μ. in diameter which, under certain conditions, form mycelia. They are readily isolated and grow on many media. When grown on media other than blood agar, they produce a yeast-like odor. C. albicans and occasionally C. tropicalis and C. stellatoidea produce chlamydospores on cornmeal or rice tween-80 agar. The fermentation and carbon assimilation tests are listed in Table III [*50*].

Animal Pathogenicity. Animal pathogenicity studies of candida species have been confined, for the most part, to the experimental infection of rabbits and mice. The rabbit is readily susceptible to the intravenous inoculation of C. albicans, as shown by Benham [*51*] in 1931, and recent studies [*52–54,200*] have demonstrated that the mouse also is susceptible to the intravenous injection of C. albicans. Rabbits usually succumb to infection during the first eight to nine days after inoculation, but rarely thereafter. Mice, however, may succumb at any time during the first thirty-five to forty days after inoculation. The kidneys are the organs most heavily infected and the site where organisms are readily seen. A dose of 10 million organisms of C. albicans, regardless of strain, will kill all mice. In addition, recent studies by Hasenclever [*54,200*] have shown that C. tropicalis has significant pathogenicity for mice, but not for rabbits; C. parapsilosis does not produce death in mice or rabbits; and C. guilliermondii and C. krusei have no lethal effects on mice. The latter two species were not studied in rabbits [*54,200*]. Both the mouse and rabbit are relatively resistant, however, to infection by intraperitoneal inoculation.

Types of Infection in Man. Candidiasis is an acute or subacute infection which may produce local lesions in the mouth, vagina, skin, nails, bronchi, lung, or occasionally disseminated disease (septicemia, endocarditis, or meningitis). Involvement of the oral cavity, vulvovaginitis, bronchopulmonary, pulmonary, and cutaneous candidiasis has been well described [*55–62*]. The latter may present in the form of onychia, paronychia, intertrigo, perianal or generalized cutaneous candidiasis [*1*]. Involvement of the central nervous system (in the form of meningitis [*9,63,64,77,78*] or brain abscess [*65*]), corneal ulcers [*66,67*], septic retinitis [*76*], and isolated cases of candida infections of the peritoneum [*68*], pleural cavity [*69*], and esophagus [*70*] have been reported. In addition, a syndrome in adults of acute disseminated candidiasis characterized by coma, shock, gastrointestinal bleeding, and death with mycotic abscesses of the kidneys, heart, and brain has been described [*71–75*].

CASE REPORTS

CASE 16. H. R., a twenty-six year old Puerto Rican male narcotic addict, was transferred to the Clinical Center on December 22, 1959, from the Federal Penitentiary at Atlanta, Georgia, with a diagnosis of C. parapsilosis endocarditis. The patient had been a known addict for eight years, and during the past two years had been taking fifteen to twenty daily intravenous injections of heroin. The last injection had been on March 12, 1959.

Splenomegaly and fever were noted during the first week of June 1959. On June 25 a systolic murmur was heard for the first time, and eighteen days later conjunctival petechiae and subungual splinter hemorrhages appeared. Serial blood cultures were positive for C. parapsilosis and hemolytic Staphylococcus aureus, coagulase-negative.

On July 25, a one-month course of intravenously administered penicillin and intramuscularly administered streptomycin was begun. The patient remained febrile while receiving therapy, and progressive weight loss and marked weakness continued. The cardiac murmur remained unchanged. Because of the continued progression of illness an exploratory laparotomy was performed on September 11. Hepatosplenomegaly and schistosome ova in the liver were the only abnormal findings. The patient was given a course of Fuadin® postoperatively but showed no improvement. A progressive anemia was now associated with a marked hyperglobulinemia, and the

Table II
CANDIDA ENDOCARDITIS

Case No.	Author	Organism	Age (yr.) and Sex	Presenting Manifestation	Physical Findings: Heart Murmur	Fever	Petechiae	Splenomegaly	Hepatomegaly	Evidence of Major Emboli to	Other	Associated Disease	Therapy Prior to Diagnosis	Surgical Procedure	Total Duration (from probable onset)	Clinical Diagnosis	Therapy for Endocarditis
Clinical Manifestations																	
1	Joachim, Polayes [6]	C. parakrusei	48,M	Abdominal pain	+	+	+	+	+	Skin	...	Narcotic addiction	None	None	5 mo.(?)	Candida endocarditis	Symptomatic
2	Wikler, Williams, Douglass, Emmons [7]	C. parakrusei	49,M	Hemiplegia	+	+	+	+	...	Brain	...	Narcotic addiction	None	None	3 mo.	Candida endocarditis	...
3	Pasternack [8]	C. parakrusei	45,M	Abdominal pain, fever	+	+	+	+	+	Ileum	...	None	None	None	36 days	Candida endocarditis	...
4	Geiger, Wenner, Axilrod, Durlacher [9]	C. albicans	18,F	Meningeal signs, fever, Osler's node	+	+	+	...	...	Skin, brain, spleen, kidney	Meningeal	Previous bacterial endocarditis	Penicillin (intravenous)	None	16 days	Candida endocarditis	Penicillin sulfa, potassium iodide
5	Zimmerman, Case 1 [10]	C. guilliermondi	38,F	Abdominal pain, fever	+	+	+	...	...	Mesenteric artery	...	Narcotic addiction	None	None	1 mo.	Not stated	...
6	Wolfe, Henderson [11]	C. krusei	57,F	Fever, cough	+	+	+	+	+	Leg	...	Diabetes	None (?)	None	3 mo.	Pyelonephritis, chronic	Penicillin, streptomycin, chloratetracycline, sulfa
7	Kunstadter, MacLean, Greengard [12]	C. albicans	7/12M	Fever	...	+	+	+	+	...	Pneumonitis, thrush	Chronic respiratory illness	Sulfonamides (?)	None	1–2½ mo.	Candida fungemia	Sulfonamides
8	Niel, Kohlmeier, Case 1 [13–14]	C. albicans	41,M	Increasing heart failure	+	+	...	+	+	...	...	None	None	None	2 mo.	Candida endocarditis	Streptomycin, penicillin
9	Neil, Kohlmeier, Case 2 [13–14]	C. quilliermondi	59,F	Fever, heart failure	+	+	...	+	+	...	...	Hypertension	None	None	3 mo.	Candida endocarditis	...
10	Caplan [15]	Candida	43,M	Embolus to leg	+	+	+	...	...	Brain, leg	...	Perforated peptic ulcer	Antibiotics	Subtotal gastrectomy	1 mo. (?)	Not stated	None
11	Koelle, Pastor [16]	C. albicans	40,M	Fever, chest and abdominal pain	+	+	+	+	+	Brain, leg, skin, kidney, mesenteric artery	...	Rheumatic heart disease, aortic stenosis	Penicillin, streptomycin	Aortic valvulotomy	12+ days	Candida endocarditis	Penicillin, streptomycin
12	Conn, Crean, MacCabe, MacLean [17]	C. tropicalis	61,F	Abdominal pain	...	+	...	...	...	...	...	Rheumatoid arthritis, gastric and duodenal ulcer	None	Subtotal gastrectomy, exploratory laparotomy	2¾ mo.	Not stated	Penicillin, streptomycin, tetracycline, sulfonamides, steroids
13	Pearl, Sidransky, Case 1 [18]	Candida	38,M	Perirectal abscess	+	+	+	...	...	Skin	Pleural effusion	Rheumatic heart disease perirectal abscess	Penicillin, streptomycin, erythromycin	None	3 mo.	Enterococcal endocarditis	Penicillin, streptomycin, erythromycin

TABLE II (*Continued*)

CANDIDA ENDOCARDITIS

Case No.	Author	Organism	Age (yr.) and Sex	Presenting Manifestation	Physical Findings							Associated Disease	Therapy Prior to Diagnosis	Surgical Procedure	Total Duration (from probable onset)	Clinical Diagnosis	Therapy for Endocarditis
					Heart Murmur	Fever	Petechiae	Splenomegaly	Hepatomegaly	Evidence of Major Emboli to	Other						
14	Pearl, Sidransky, Case 2 [18]	C. albicans	9,M	Fever, dyspnea	+	+	+	+	+	Skin, fundi	Ascites	Rheumatic heart disease	Prednisone, penicillin, streptomycin	...	3+ mo.	Candida endocarditis	Penicillin, chloramphenicol, steroids, amphotericin B
15	Louria, Dineen [19]	C. albicans	36,F	+	+	+	+	+	...	Right upper and lower extremity	...	Rheumatic heart disease	Penicillin	Mitral valvulotomy	16 mo.	Candida endocarditis	Amphotericin B
16	Present authors	C. parakrusei	26,M	Abdominal pain, fever	+	+	+	+	+	Skin, brain, coronary artery, femoral artery, kidney, spleen, liver	...	Narcotic addiction	None	Exploratory laparotomy	11+ mo.	Candida	Penicillin, streptomycin, amphotericin B, X-5079C U-0178
17	Present authors	C. guilliermondi	48,M	Fever	+	+	...	...	...	...	...	Rheumatic heart disease, calcific aortic stenosis	Penicillin (intramuscular), streptomycin, chloramphenicol, erythromycin	Aortic valvulotomy	6+ mo.	Candida endocarditis	Penicillin, erythromycin, chloramphenicol, amphotericin B, X-5079C ristocetin
18	Present authors	C. parakrusei	45,M	Fever	+	+	+	+	+	...	...	Rheumatic heart disease, mitral stenosis	Penicillin (intramuscular), streptomycin	Mitral valvulotomy	3½ mo.	Candida endocarditis	Amphotericin B
19	Present authors	C. parakrusei	39,M	Fever	+	+	+	+	+	Skin	...	Rheumatic heart disease, mitral insufficiency, minimal aortic stenosis	Penicillin (intramuscular)	Mitral valvuloplasty	3½ mo.	Candida endocarditis	Amphotericin B
20	Present authors	C. albicans	40,M	Fever	+	+	...	...	...	Left iliac and femoral artery	...	Rheumatic heart disease, mitral stenosis and insufficiency	Penicillin (intramuscular), streptomycin	Mitral valvulotomy, pericardiocentesis, femoral and common iliac arteriotomies	5 mo.	Candida endocarditis	Amphotericin B
21	Present authors	C. guilliermondi	68,M	Fever, weight loss	+	+	+	+	...	Right femoral artery	XII cranial nerve palsy	Pulmonary emphysema	Penicillin (intramuscular)	None	3 mo.	Candida endocarditis	Amphotericin B, thymol

Table II *(Continued)*

CANDIDA ENDOCARDITIS

Case No.	Author	Urine	Total Leukocyte Count (per cu. mm.)	Anemia	Previous Valvular Damage	Location and No. of Vegetations	Longest Diameter of Largest Vegetation (cm.)	Fungal Culture of Vegetation	Other Cardiac Pathology	Other Disease	Emboli to:
Clinical and Anatomical Pathology in Candida Endocarditis											
1	Joachim, Polayes [6]	Protein, RBC, WBC, casts	6,800–10,000	Yes	Probable	A (1)	4.0	+	Acute myocarditis, pericarditis, abscess right atrium	Acute hepatitis, meningitis, chronic pyelonephritis	Artery: splenic, renal; brain, spleen, kidney
2	Wikler, Williams, Douglass, Emmons [7]	Protein, RBC, "yeast"	7,000–26,700	Yes	RHD	M (1)	3.0	...	Acute myocarditis	Acute meningitis	Brain, spleen, kidney
3	Pasternack [8]	...	4,500–7,700	Yes	Probable	A (1)	2.8	+	Granulomatous myocarditis	Chronic meningitis, focal embolic glomerulonephritis	Ileum, spleen, kidney
4	Geiger, Wenner, Axelrod, Dorlacher [9]	"Yeast"	13,200	...	RHD	M (2), left atrium, (1)	2.0	+	Focal myocardial necrosis	Granulomatous meningitis	Artery: middle cerebral, left renal
5	Zimmerman [10]	...	...	...	RHD	M (1)	5.0	...	...	...	Artery: mesenteric; ileum, spleen, kidneys
6	Wolfe, Henderson [11]	Protein, RBC, WBC, "yeast"	"Normal"	Yes	...	M (3)	6.0	...	Myocarditis	Chronic pyelonephritis	Spleen
7	Kunstadter, MacLean, Greengard [12]	Protein, WBC, casts	15,000–56,000	Yes	...	"Multiple small nodules"	<1.0	+	Myocarditis, focal myocardial abscess (ventricular septum)	Thrush, jaundice liver abscesses	Liver, myocardium
8	Niel, Kohlmeier, Case, 1 [13–14]	Protein, RBC, WBC, casts	4,100	Yes	RHD	Multiple "glass pin-head sized deposits"	Approx. 0.2	+	Myocarditis, "thrombus—right side of heart"	Uremia, focal "embolic" glomerulonephritis, perforated duodenal ulcer	Spleen, kidneys, meninges
9	Niel, Kohlmeier Case 2 [13, 14]	Protein WBC	12,900	No	RHD	"Poppy seed size"	Approx. 0.1	+	Coronary atherosclerosis	Focal "embolic" glomerulonephritis	Spleen
10	Caplan [15]	RBC	...	...	RHD	M (1)	2.5	...	...	Perforated duodenal ulcer	Artery: external iliac; brain
11	Koelle, Pastor [16]	...	...	...	RHD	A (2)	...	+	...	...	Left external iliac, brain, myocardium, kidney, liver, small intestine, pancreas; artery: middle cerebral
12	Conn, Crean, MacCabe, MacLean [12]	WBC	5,600–12,000	No	None	Pulmonary artery, right atrium, left ventricle, (multiple); no valvular	...	+	Myocarditis, focal myocardial abscesses	Rheumatoid arthritis, subtotal gastrectomy, pyelonephritis	Kidneys
13	Pearl, Sidransky, Case 1 [18]	...	14,800	Yes	RHD	A (several)	...	...	Aortic valve calcification	Hepatic necrosis, acute enterocolitis	...

TABLE II (*Continued*)
CANDIDA ENDOCARDITIS

Case No.	Author	Urine	Total Leukocyte Count (per cu. mm.)	Anemia	Previous Valvular Damage	Location and No. of Vegetations	Longest Diameter of Largest Vegetation (cm.)	Fungal Culture of Vegetation	Other Cardiac Pathology	Other Disease	Emboli to:
14	Pearl, Sidransky, Case 2 [18]	Protein	...	Yes	RHD	M (1) Chordae tendineae (1)	0.4	+	Tricuspid valve deformity	...	...
15	Louria, Dineen [19]	...	3,700–6,600	Yes	RHD	No postmortem examination	...	...	...	...	...
16	Present authors Case 16	Protein	2,300	Yes	None	A (3)	2.0	+	Myocardial infarction, left ventricular aneurysm, granulomatous myocarditis	Uremia, focal "embolic" glomerulonephritis, myocarditis	Artery: left coronary, left exterior iliac, left femoral, splenic; brain, conjunctivas, fundi, skin, digits, spleen, kidney
17	Present authors, Case 17	WBC	730–6,600	Yes	RHD	A (3)	2.5	+	Myocarditis, pericarditis	Uremia, chronic pyelonephritis, jaundice	Brain, spleen
18	Present authors, Case 18	RBC, WBC, casts	8,700–22,500	Yes	RHD	M (1), left atrium (1)	8.0	+	Pericarditis, myocarditis (focal)	Right kidney (marked caseation), chronic pyelonephritis	Spleen, kidneys, liver, hilar lymph nodes
19	Present authors, Case 19	Protein	5,000–6,700	No	RHD	M (2), A (1)	2.0	+	Active rheumatic myocarditis, pericarditis	...	Brain, spinal cord, spleen, kidney
20	Present authors, Case 20	Protein, RBC, WBC, casts	5,600–42,800	Yes	RHD	M (1), left atrial, appendage (1)	4.0	+	Myocarditis focal, acute pericarditis	...	Artery: left common iliac, right and left femoral
21	Present authors, Case 21	Protein, RBC, WBC, casts	1,800–3,700	Yes	RHD	M (1)	2.7	+	Myocarditis	Laennec's cirrhosis, focal "embolic" glomerulonephritis, massive intracerebral hemorrhage	Artery: right iliac, right femoral, left radial, left anterior descending, coronary; brain, spleen

NOTE: WBC, white blood count; RBC, red blood count; RHD, rheumatic heart disease; . . ., no data available; A, aortic; M, mitral.

Table III

FERMENTATION REACTIONS OF CANDIDA SPECIES

Fermentation	Albicans	Parapsilosis	Krusei	Tropicalis	Guilliermondii
Glucose	+	+	+	+	+
Maltose	+	−	−	+	− (+)
Galactose	+	+ weak	−	+	− (+)
Lactose	−	−	−	−	−
Saccharose	−	− (+)	−	+	+
Raffinose	...	...	...	+ −	+ (⅓)
Carbon assimilation	...	...	...	...	...
Glucose	+	+	+	+	+
Maltose	+	+	−	+	+
Galactose	+	+	−	+	+
Lactose	−	−	−	−	−
Saccharose	+	+	−	+	+

presence of marked hematuria, pyuria, and cylindruria. Blood and bone marrow cultures remained positive for C. parapsilosis.

Physical examination on admission to the Clinical Center revealed a pale, chronically ill, young white man. The temperature was 38.6°c., heart rate 132 per minute, regular sinus rhythm, respirations 30 per minute, blood pressure 98/58 mm. Hg. Old needle puncture sites were noted in both antecubital fossae. There were numerous petechiae in both lower conjunctival sacs. The fundi appeared normal. The lungs were clear to percussion and auscultation. The heart was not enlarged. The second pulmonic sound was greater than the second aortic sound. A long, loud, high-pitched, blowing pansystolic murmur was heard best in the fourth intercostal space to the left of the sternum, but was not transmitted. No rubs, thrills, or gallop were present. The liver was enlarged 1 cm. below the right and the spleen 5 cm. below the left costal margins. Both organs were tender to palpation. A loud rub was audible and palpable over the surface of the liver during both phases of respiration. No lymphadenopathy was present. There was marked clubbing of all digits.

Laboratory examinations revealed a hemoglobin of 8.9 gm. per 100 ml. and a leukocyte count of 4,300 per cu. mm., with 38 per cent polymorphonuclear leukocytes, 56 per cent lymphocytes, and 6 per cent monocytes. The erythrocyte sedimentation rate (Westergren method) was 120 mm. per hour, blood urea nitrogen 58 mg., creatinine 3 mg., calcium 8.6 mg. per 100 ml., and the alkaline phosphatase 20 King-Armstrong units. The serum albumin was 2.1 gm. and serum globulin 6.5 gm. per 100 ml.; thymol turbidity was 13 units. Sulfobromophthalein retention in the blood was 10 per cent at forty-five minutes. A reaction to a cephalin flocculation test was 4 plus. Serum electrolytes and other blood chemistry values were within normal limits. Urinalysis revealed innumerable erythrocytes, leukocytes, casts, and albumin. Phenolsulphonphthalein dye test showed 12 per cent total excretion at the end of two hours. Maximal value for the Fishberg concentration test was 1.010. Stools were persistently positive for hookworm ova. Results of tuberculin and fungal skin tests were negative. Thirty-one blood cultures and one bone marrow culture were positive for C. parapsilosis. The result of the agglutination titer for C. parapsilosis was 1:1280. The fungus was susceptible to 0.05 μg. per ml. of amphotericin B, *in vitro.*

On December 24, Osler nodes appeared at the tip of the right thumb and fourth finger. The following day the patient had the sudden onset of excruciating precordial pain accompanied by changes in the electrocardiogram indicative of a massive, acute anterior wall myocardial infarct. Embolization to the left femoral artery occurred later, and new showers of petechiae were noted in both lower conjunctival sacs and the antecubital fossae at the same time. The systolic murmur remained unchanged, however, and there was no evidence of cardiac decompensation. During the next seven days new petechiae were noted over the face, thorax, feet, and mucous membranes. During the following month the patient continued febrile, and multiple Osler's nodes appeared in the phalanges. An intermittent diastolic gallop was noted during this time. Blood and bone marrow cultures remained persistently positive, with colony counts ranging from 25 to 250 colonies per ml.

A marked personality change, ptosis of upper left lid, progressive generalized weakness, and slurring of speech were noted early in January 1960, and an electroencephalogram at that time was interpreted as grossly abnormal. The hemoglobin fell to 6.2 gm. per 100 ml.; the patient was given a transfusion with little improvement. The spleen was now 8 cm. below the left costal margin.

On January 28 large hemorrhagic areas were noted for the first time in the left conjunctival sac. A diastolic murmur was now present. The patient became progressively weaker, and on February 15 marked dyspnea and severe precordial pain were noted. Electrocardiograms revealed evidence of extension of the recent anterior wall myocardial infarct. Serial chest roentgenograms throughout the patient's course were non-contributory. The patient died on February 16, following an episode of ventricular fibrillation.

Antifungal therapy given to this patient consisted of solubilized amphotericin B, given orally for a ten-day period, and two other antifungal agents currently undergoing clinical investigation [*202*]. There was no significant change in the patient's course at any time during therapy.

At autopsy, the body weighed 119 pounds and measured 67 inches in length. Numerous petechiae were present in the skin. The digits were clubbed. Ascites (925 ml.), pleural effusions (420 ml. and 150 ml.), and a pericardial effusion (70 ml.) were present. The heart weighed 400 gm. The right atrium, right ventricle, tricuspid and pulmonic valves, left atrium, and mitral valve were normal. In the apical portion of the anterior wall of the left ventricle there was a 5 by 3.5 by 0.2 cm. infarct. There was aneurysmal dilatation of this myocardial infarct. The infarct was soft, and its epicardial and endocardial surfaces were grey. Ten centimeters from the ostium of the left coronary artery, the left anterior descending coronary artery was occluded for a distance of 2 to 3 cm. The occlusion was immediately proximal to the myocardial infarct. That portion of the left ventricle not infarcted measured 1.3 cm. in thickness. A soft, friable, fungating, grey vegetation was present on the ventricular aspect of each of the three cusps of the aortic valve. (Fig. 1A and 1B.) The largest vegetation was located on the right anterior cusp and measured 2 cm. in largest diameter. The vegetation located on the left anterior cusp protruded slightly into the ostia of the left coronary artery, partially occluding this vessel. C. parapsilosis was cultured from the vegetations. The sinuses of Valsalva were free of vegetations.

The spleen weighed 1,000 gm., and in it were approximately ten firm infarcts. The left internal iliac and left femoral arteries were occluded by soft yellow emboli. The liver weighed 3,650 gm. and, on section, had a "nutmeg" appearance. There was generalized lymphadenopathy, some nodes being 5 cm. in diameter. The left kidney weighed 190 gm., the right 180 gm. The surface had a mottled black and tan appearance. The lungs were heavy and congested. Gross examinations of the remaining organs, including the brain, revealed no abnormalities. Cultures were taken of the spleen, liver, hilar lymph node, and the embolus in the left femoral artery; all were positive for C. parapsilosis.

Microscopically, candida organisms were identified in the aortic valve vegetations, left anterior descending coronary artery, myocardial infarct, left femoral artery and brain. The vegetations consisted of eosinophilic debris, fibrin, and large colonies of candida organisms. (Fig. 1C.) Both yeast and hyphal forms were present. The yeast forms predominated in the more dense colonies. Organisms were present in the depths and on the surfaces of the vegetations. They were most readily identified with the periodic acid-Schiff and Gomori's methenamine silver stains. (Fig. 1D.) Numerous histiocytes and a few lymphocytes were present in the vegetations at the margins adjacent to the "ring" of the aortic valve. Focal areas of necrosis were seen in the valve leaflets. The left anterior descending coronary artery was occluded by a collection of eosinophilic debris. (Fig. 1E.) There was proliferation of intimal tissue around this debris, and candida organisms were identified in the lumens of channels in this intimal stroma. Numerous plasma cells, lymphocytes and macrophages were present in the wall of this vessel and in surrounding epicardial adipose tissue.

In sections of the myocardial infarct there was replacement of myocardium by fibrous tissue, which contained macrophages, lymphocytes, plasma cells, fibroblasts, and foreign body giant cells. Candida organisms were present in and near the giant cells. Chronic inflammatory cells were also noted in the myocardium of the right ventricle.

In sections of kidneys, there were foci of fibrinoid degeneration in many glomeruli. The fibrinoid degeneration was usually present in only one or two glomerular capillaries, but occasionally the entire glomerulus was involved. Many foci of fibrinoid necrosis were adherent to Bowman's capsules. Endothelial or epithelial cells adjacent to these foci were swollen and basophilic. Some glomeruli were hyalinized. (Fig. 1F.) In some glomeruli free of hyaline or fibrinoid material there was occasional thickening of the basement membranes. Scattered throughout the renal interstitial tissue were lymphocytes and plasma cells. Hemosiderin was present in the cytoplasm of many tubular cells. Numerous hyaline casts and small amounts of hemosiderin were present in the lumens of the tubules. No fungi were identified in the kidneys.

Large numbers of plasma cells were present in the sections of lymph nodes. In the lymph nodes, spleen, or liver, no candida organisms were seen, although cultures from these sites were positive. There was severe passive congestion and centrolobular necrosis of the liver. No stainable glycogen was present in the liver. There was erythroid hyperplasia of the bone marrow. Numerous candida organisms were present in the brain, mainly in the perivascular areas. In addition, a few foci of chronic inflammatory cells were noted in the brain and leptomeninges.

The *final anatomic pathologic diagnoses* were: C. parapsilosis endocarditis, aortic valve; candidiasis involving the left anterior descending coronary artery; infarct in left ventricle and brain; mycotic emboli to the left anterior descending coronary artery, left femoral and iliac arteries, small

1A 1B 1C 1D 1E 1F

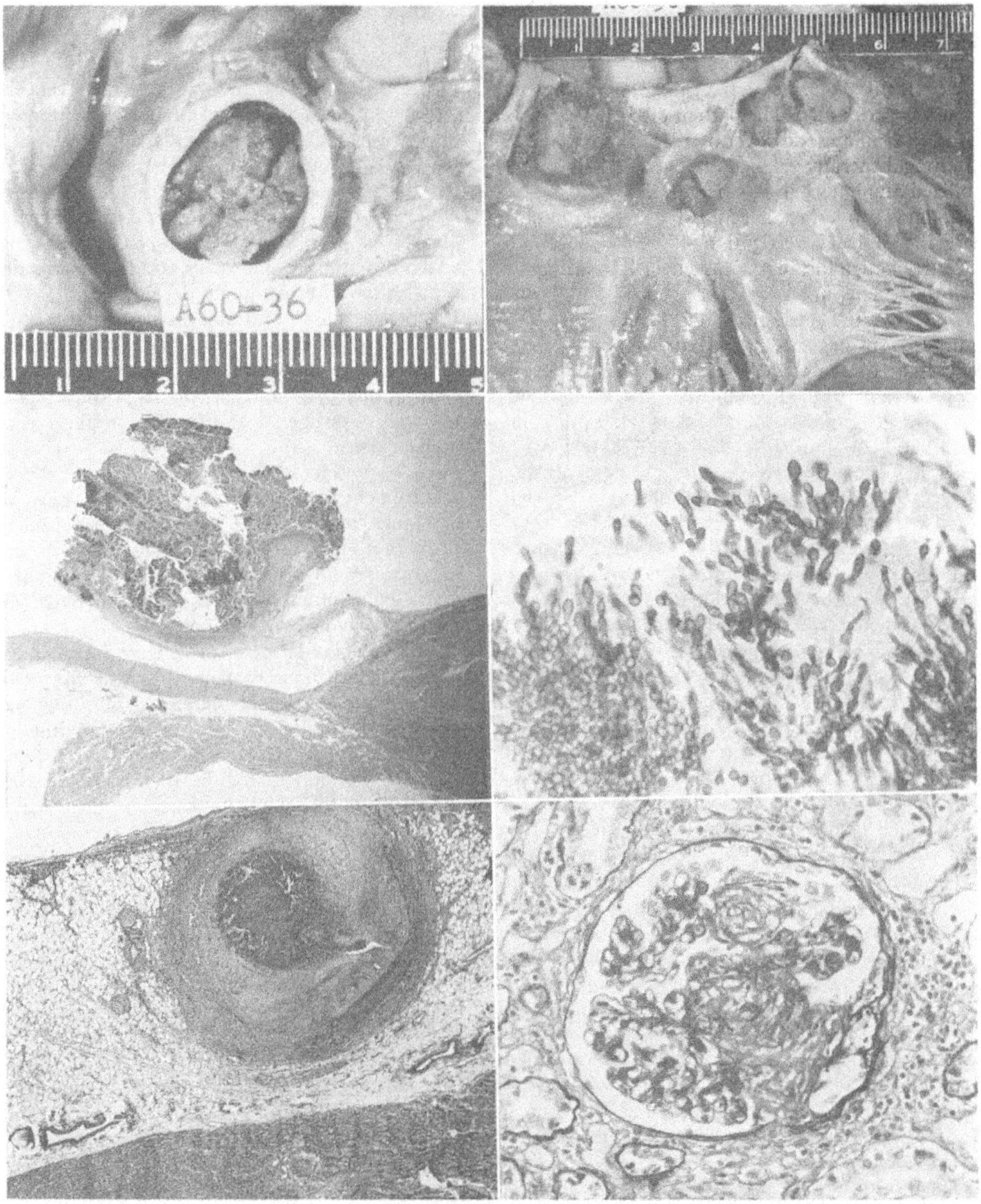

Fig. 1. Case 16. A, aortic valve viewed from above. The large vegetations almost totally occludes the aortic valve orifice. B, aortic valve opened. Note the vegetation on the ventricular aspect of each of the cusps of the aortic valve. The arrow designates the ostium of the left coronary artery which contains a small protrusion from vegetation on the left anterior cusp. C, section through the largest vegetation illustrated in Figure 1B. The darker areas in the vegetation represent collections of candida organisms. Note that the sinus of Valsalva is free of vegetation. Gomori's methenamine silver stain, original magnification × 10. D, close-up of candida organisms present in vegetation shown in Figure 1C. Gomori's methenamine silver, original magnification × 775. E, left anterior descending coronary artery occluded by an organizing mycotic embolus. Candida organisms are present in the organizing channels. Elastic van Gieson stain, original magnification × 21. F, renal glomerulus, focal "embolic" glomerulonephritis. Some Malpighian tufts are hyalinized; other tufts are normal. Periodic acid-Schiff stain, original magnification × 310.

branch of splenic artery, spleen and kidney; multiple foci of necrosis with chronic and granulomatous inflammation, myocardium; aneurysmal dilatation of anterior wall of left ventricle; congestive heart failure; generalized lymphadenopathy; focal endocarditic glomerulonephritis and chronic pyelonephritis; erythroid hyperplasia, bone marrow.

CASE 17. H. D., a forty-eight year old white male dentist, was admitted to the Clinical Center on May 17, 1959, with a diagnosis of inactive rheumatic heart disease and far advanced aortic stenosis. Aortic valvulotomy was performed on June 3, with an uneventful postoperative course. The stenosis was relieved by instrumentation, utilizing complete cardiopulmonary bypass. C. guilliermondii was cultured from the pump postoperatively. One month following operation the patient noted chills and fever, and on July 20 was readmitted to the Clinical Center with the diagnosis of subacute bacterial endocarditis.

Physical examination revealed a well developed, well nourished white man in no distress. The temperature was 39.2°c.; heart rate 122 per minute, regular; respirations 22 per minute; and blood pressure 124/60 mm. Hg. A well healed median sternotomy scar was present. The lungs were clear. There was marked cardiomegaly with the point of maximum impulse in the fifth intercostal space in the anterior axillary line. The second pulmonic sound was greater than the second aortic sound. A grade 4 aortic pansystolic murmur was present over the entire precordium and an early, soft, blowing, low-pitched diastolic murmur was heard, only at the aortic area and not transmitted. No thrill or gallop was noted. There was no hepatosplenomegaly, lymphadenopathy, petechiae, clubbing of the fingers, splinter hemorrhages, or Osler's nodes.

Laboratory examinations revealed a hemoglobin of 10.2 gm. per 100 ml. and a leukocyte count of 5,800 per cu. mm., with 62 per cent polymorphonuclear leukocytes, 28 per cent lymphocytes, 8 per cent monocytes, and 2 per cent eosinophils. The erythrocyte sedimentation rate (Westergren method) was 68 mm. per hour; blood urea nitrogen 17 mg., serum albumin 2.7 gm., and globulin 4.3 gm. per 100 ml. Results of serum electrolyte determinations and the remainder of the liver function tests were within normal limits with the exception of 15 per cent sulfobromophthalein retention in the blood at forty-five minutes. Urinalysis revealed an occasional leukocyte and rare erythrocyte, but otherwise gave normal results. Forty-six of a total of fifty-three blood cultures were positive for C. guilliermondii, and those of July 21 and July 22 were positive for Staph. aureus, coagulase-negative, in addition. Urine and stool cultures were negative for bacteria and fungi. Serial electrocardiograms revealed only left ventricular hypertrophy with no evidence of infarction. Serial chest roentgenograms were non-contributory.

On July 25 the patient was given ristocetin, 1 gm. intravenously, twice daily. This therapy was continued until August 10. On July 31, amphotericin B therapy was begun and continued by the intravenous route until September 4, the patient receiving a total of 1644 mg. The patient continued febrile throughout this course of therapy, with only an occasional negative blood culture. The blood urea nitrogen rose to 68 mg. per 100 ml. during the latter part of this course of therapy. The findings on serial roentgenograms remained unchanged. No change in the cardiac murmurs was noted during treatment. On September 22 therapy with an antifungal agent (X-5079C) [*202*] was started, but did not produce any change in the cultural or clinical status of the patient. Poor response to this therapy prompted the use of X-5079C combined with amphotericin B. Sporadic negative cultures were noted during this period, with some decrease in colony count, but without eradication of the C. guilliermondii. The spiking fever pattern continued. Progressive congestive failure, followed by rapid renal decompensation, was associated with a progressive downhill course, and the patient died on the 114th hospital day (November 10).

At autopsy, the body weighed 122 pounds and measured 67 inches in length. The skin was jaundiced. There was 350 ml. of bile-stained fluid in the peritoneal cavity. There were fibrinous pleural and pericardial adhesions. The heart weighed 600 gm. Except for moderate right ventricular hypertrophy, the chambers and valves of the right side of the heart appeared normal. The left atrium and mitral valve were within normal limits. The thickness of the ventricle was 1.8 cm. The cusps of the aortic valve were thickened. Soft, friable, grey vegetations filled each sinus of Valsalva. (Fig. 2A and 2B.) The largest vegetation measured 2.5 cm. in greatest diameter. C. guilliermondii was cultured. Infarcts were present in the spleen and brain. The spleen weighed 560 gm. and was congested. Pseudomonas species were cultured from the spleen. The liver weighed 2,360 gm. and had a "nutmeg" appearance on cut section. Numerous minute stones were present in the gallbladder; the extrahepatic ducts were patent. The kidneys weighed 180 and 190 gm. and contained no infarcts. The lungs were congested. The adrenal glands weighed 11 and 12 gm., respectively, and were diffusely hypertrophied. A 1 by 1 cm. hemorrhagic infarct was present in the left temporal lobe of the cerebrum. The postmortem heart blood culture grew out pseudomonas species.

Microscopically, the vegetations on the aortic valve consisted of acellular eosinophilic debris and large numbers of candida organisms. (Fig. 2C and 2D.) At the proximal margins of the cusps and at the base of the aortic valve were numerous lymphocytes, fibroblasts, histiocytes, hemosiderophages, capillaries, and proliferative fibrous tissue. There was diffuse interstitial fibrosis of the left ventricular myocardium;

2A 2B 2C 2D

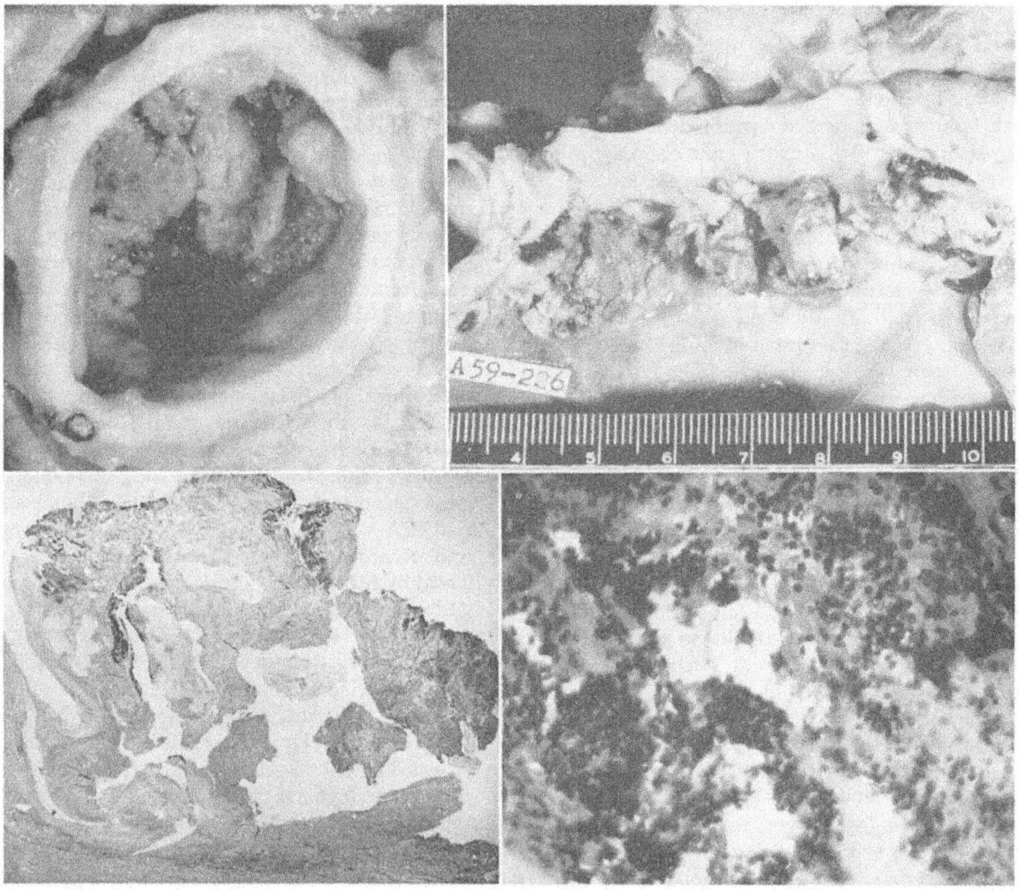

FIG. 2. Case 17. A, aortic valve as viewed from above. Large vegetations partially occlude orifice of aortic valve. B, aortic valve opened. A vegetation is present within each of the three sinuses of Valsalva. C, section through one of the vegetations illustrated in Figure 2B. Note that the vegetation occupies the sinus of Valsalva only. The ventricular aspect of the remnant of the cusp is free of vegetation. The darker areas in the vegetation are colonies of candida organisms. Periodic acid-Schiff stain, original magnification × 10. D, close-up of candida organisms present in vegetation shown in Figure 2C. Note that yeast forms predominate. Only a rare hyphal form is present. Periodic acid-Schiff stain, original magnification × 495.

in these fibrous tissues were foci of acute and chronic inflammation. The myocardial fibers were hypertrophied. There was fibrous proliferation of the intima of myocardial and epicardial coronary arteries. In sections of liver there was passive congestion and centrilobular necrosis. A moderate amount of iron was present in the liver, mainly in the Kupffer cells. Bile plugs were present in centrilobular areas. Organisms were not seen in the liver, spleen, kidney, and brain infarcts. Numerous chronic inflammatory cells were present in the interstitial tissue of the kidneys. The glomeruli were normal. The sections of the adrenal glands showed diffuse hyperplasia. The bone marrow was normocellular.

The *final anatomic pathologic diagnoses* were: C. guilliermondii endocarditis, aortic valve; rheumatic heart disease with aortic stenosis; transaortic valvulotomy, four months prior to death; chronic myocarditis; infarcts, spleen and brain; cardiomegaly with passive congestion, viscera; chronic pyelonephritis; hyperplasia, adrenal glands; jaundice; and chronic cholecystitis with cholelithiasis.

CASE 18. G. V., a forty-five year old white man, was admitted to the Clinical Center on March 23, 1958, with a past history of acute rheumatic fever and polyarthritis at age twenty-five. A cardiac murmur was first noted at age thirty-four but there was no evidence of cardiac decompensation. On December 29, 1957, the patient had a generalized tonic-clonic convulsion and because of a second episode the following day was admitted to the hospital. Cardiac examination at that time revealed an enlarged heart and the murmur of mitral stenosis. The patient was asymptomatic at this time, but was referred to the Clinical Center for possible mitral valvulotomy.

Physical examination revealed a healthy appearing white man in no distress. The temperature was 36.7°c., pulse 100 per minute, respirations 18 per minute, blood pressure 130/70 mm. Hg. The neck veins were flat. The chest showed an increase in anteroposterior diameter, but was clear to percussion and auscultation. The heart was not enlarged, but a right ventricular lift was present. The second pulmonary sound and the first sound at the mitral area were accentuated, and an opening snap was heard. There was a grade 3 apical diastolic rumble with presystolic accentuation. No thrill was noted. There was no organomegaly, lymphadenopathy, petechiae, splinter hemorrhages, Osler's nodes, or clubbing of the fingers.

Laboratory examinations revealed a hemoglobin of 16.8 gm. per 100 ml., hematocrit 52 per cent, and a leukocyte count of 9,200 per cu. mm., with 60 per cent polymorphonuclear leukocytes, 21 per cent lymphocytes, 8 per cent monocytes, and 11 per cent eosinophils. The erythrocyte sedimentation rate (Westergren method) was 2 mm. per hour; blood urea nitrogen 26 mg. per 100 ml.; antistreptolysin-O titer 125 units; C-reactive protein negative. Serum electrolytes and other blood chemistry values were normal. Urinalysis revealed albuminuria and glucosuria with occasional erythrocytes, leukocytes, and hyaline casts. Roentgenograms of the chest revealed minimal enlargement of the left atrium, but no pulmonary disease. An electrocardiogram showed normal sinus rhythm with left atrial enlargement and delayed right ventricular conduction. Cardiac catheterization revealed mitral stenosis with a diastolic gradient across the mitral valve of 15 to 20 mm. Hg. On April 1 the patient underwent mitral commissurotomy, at which time the mitral valve was found to be calcified, with a valve opening of 0.5 cm. No evidence of regurgitation was noted. The anterior commissure was opened to 1½-fingerbreadths diameter. The patient tolerated the operation without incident. The postoperative course was uneventful except for the onset of atrial fibrillation three days postoperatively. Three separate courses of quinidine were given without success to convert the atrial fibrillation to normal sinus rhythm. The patient continued to improve and was discharged to his home on April 20.

Two weeks after discharge the patient noted weakness, diaphoresis, and a temperature of 101°F. He was admitted to another hospital and treated with aspirin, digitalis, and a low sodium diet for a period of two weeks. On this therapy he improved slightly, but continued to have a low grade fever and evidence of congestive heart failure. He was admitted to the Clinical Center for the second time on June 6, 1958, for further evaluation.

Physical examination on admission revealed a temperature of 36.7°c., pulse 100 per minute and irregular, respirations 18 per minute, blood pressure 135/90 mm. Hg. A well healed left, posterolateral thoracotomy scar was seen. The neck veins were flat. Inspiratory and expiratory wheezing was present in both lung fields, but no rales. The heart was not enlarged. A high-pitched grade 3 apical systolic murmur was present, accompanying the previously heard grade 3 apical diastolic rumble that was now without presystolic accentuation. An opening snap was audible, and atrial fibrillation was present. The liver was enlarged 2 cm. below the right costal margin and was not tender. There was no splenomegaly or lymphadenopathy. Minimal bilateral pretibial edema was present, but no cyanosis or clubbing.

The laboratory data were not significantly changed from the first admission except for a fall in hemoglobin to 13.1 gm. per 100 ml. and hematocrit to 48.5 per cent. The leukocyte count was 12,300 per cu. mm., with 74 per cent polymorphonuclear leukocytes, 11 per cent lymphocytes, 11 per cent monocytes, and 4 per cent eosinophils. The erythrocyte sedimentation rate (Westergren method) was now elevated to 20 mm. per hour. Results of urinalysis, blood chemical studies and serum electrolytes were essentially unchanged, except for a C-reactive protein of 4 plus, serum albumin 2.6 gm., globulin 3.5 gm. per 100 ml., and decreased phenolsulfonphthalein excretion in the urine. Results of histoplasmin, blastomyces, and coccidioidin complement fixation tests were negative. All blood cultures during the patient's hospitalization were positive for C. parapsilosis. Throat and urine cultures were negative for this fungus. Serial chest films and electrocardiograms were non-contributory.

The patient was started on amphotericin B therapy on June 21, a total of 821 mg. being given intravenously over a twenty-four-day period.

On the seventh hospital day, splenomegaly was noted for the first time, and on the thirty-eighth hospital day a splinter hemorrhage was noted in the lower right bulbar conjunctiva. The patient remained febrile, and at no time was the bloodstream free of C. parapsilosis despite the amphotericin B therapy. Pulmonary edema and atrial fibrillation developed just prior to death, which occurred on July 18 from intractable cardiac failure.

At autopsy, the body weighed 129 pounds and measured 66 inches in length. Ecchymotic areas were present in the skin. The pleural and pericardial cavities were obliterated by fibrous adhesions. The heart weighed 500 gm. The chambers and valves of the right side of the heart appeared normal. The left atrium was dilated. Two large, white, organizing vegetations, each of which measured 4 cm. in greatest diameter, covered the greater portion of the endocardium of the left atrium. (Fig. 3A.) One was located on the interatrial septum and the other on the posterior wall. The latter vegetation was connected by a narrow isthmus to another 4 cm. vegetation located on the posterior leaflet of the mitral valve. The pulmonary veins at their entrance into the left atrium were partially occluded by these vegetations.

3A 3B 3C

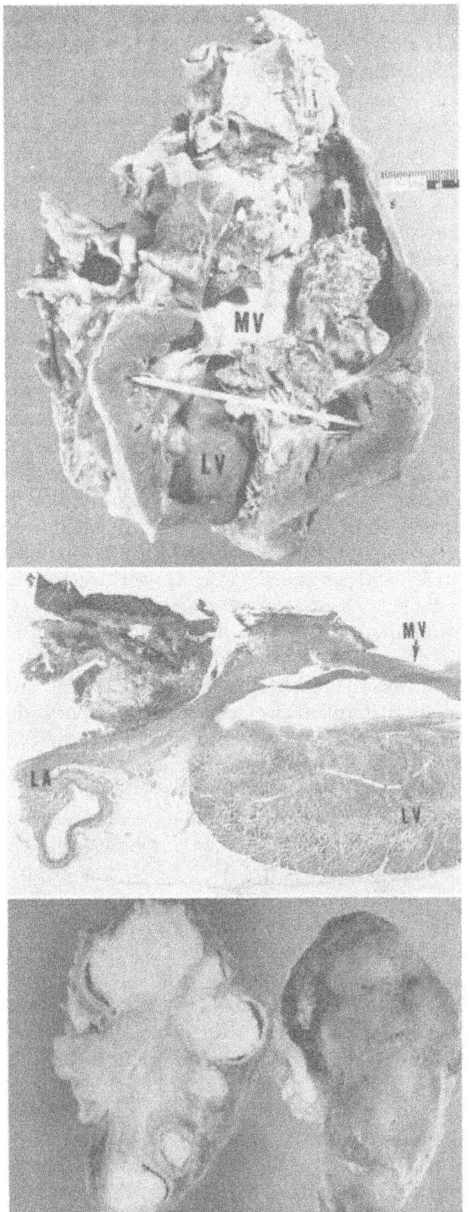

FIG. 3. Case 18. A, the left atrium (LA), mitral valve (MV), and left ventricle (LV) are opened. Large vegetations are present on the endocardium of the left atrium and mitral valve. B, section through mitral valve (MV) and portion of the left atrium (LA) and left ventricle (LV), demonstrating large vegetation on the endocardial surface of the left atrium and mitral valve. Hematoxylin and eosin stain, original magnification × 10. C, right kidney, showing large focal areas filled with caseous necrotic material. The cortex is extremely thin. Candida organisms were seen in the areas of caseation necrosis, but special stains for bacteria and acid-fast organisms were negative. This kidney weighed only 50 cm.

C. parapsilosis was cultured from the vegetations in the left atrium and on the mitral valve. The chordae tendineae of the mitral valve were shortened and thickened. Small, hard, calcified nodules covered by smooth endocardium were present at the margins of the mitral leaflets, the mitral ring was 8 cm. in circumference. The thickness of the left ventricular myocardium was 1.2 cm. The aortic cusps were thickened, the commissures were partially fused, and no verrucae were present on the aortic valve. The coronary arteries were moderately atherosclerotic.

The lungs were congested. There were focal areas of bronchopneumonia. The liver weighed 1,650 gm., and appeared normal. In the left kidney, which weighed 250 gm., there was an infarct 4.5 cm. in size. The right kidney weighed only 50 gm. Its calyceal system was greatly dilated and filled with caseous necrotic material. (Fig. 3C.) The cortex was only 0.1 to 0.3 cm. thick. The cortical surface was coarsely irregular. The calyceal mucosa surrounding the deposits of caseous material was thickened. The ureters were within normal limits. The spleen weighed 530 gm. There was generalized lymphadenopathy; one hilar lymph node was caseous and calcified.

Microscopically, the vegetations in the left atrium and mitral valve were composed primarily of necrotic debris with organization of the deeper portions. (Fig. 3B.) Numerous candida organisms and colonies were present on the more superficial portions of the vegetations. The mitral valve leaflets were thickened, vascularized, and contained foci of fibrinoid degeneration. Many histiocytes were present in the mitral valve. The aortic valve cusps were thickened. In the left ventricle there was moderate interstitial fibrosis. Minute focal, usually perivascular, collections of lymphocytes and plasma cells were noted in the interstitial fibrous tissue. There was intimal fibrous thickening of the intramural coronary arteries.

In the left kidney there was diffuse chronic interstitial inflammation. This infiltrate was greatest at the margins of the large cortical infarct. Some of the glomeruli were partly hyalinized. Rarely, fibrin was seen in a capillary tuft of a glomerulus located near the large infarct. The right kidney consisted of a thin fibrotic parenchyma surrounding a dilated pelvis filled with faintly basophilic necrotic debris. A thick fibrous membrane separated the necrotic pelvic contents from the parenchyma. The tubular epithelium was atrophic, and many tubules contained proteinaceous material and polymorphonuclear leukocytes. The interstitial tissues were infiltrated by numerous lymphocytes, plasma cells, and polymorphonuclear leukocytes. A few candida organisms were seen in the caseous debris. Special stains for bacteria and acid-fast organisms were negative. There was intimal proliferation of the small and large arteries of this kidney.

There was reticuloendothelial hyperplasia and

plasmacytosis of the lymph nodes. The caseocalcific hilar lymph node contained many candida organisms. C. parapsilosis was cultured from this lymph node. A few single candida organisms were present in the hepatic and splenic sinusoids. There was minimal passive congestion of the liver. The bone marrow was normocellular. The other organs were within the limits of normal. E. coli was grown from the postmortem blood culture.

The *final anatomic pathologic diagnoses* were: C. parapsilosis endocarditis, mitral valve, left atrium; rheumatic heart disease with mitral stenosis; candidiasis involving spleen, liver, right kidney, lymph nodes; interstitial myocardial fibrosis, diffuse; caseation, right kidney and hilar lymph node; acute pyelonephritis; infarct, left kidney; generalized lymphadenopathy; bronchopneumonia; and passive congestion, lungs, liver, spleen.

Case 19. M. S., a thirty-seven year old white housewife, was admitted to the Clinical Center on July 14, 1957, because of progressive cardiac decompensation, secondary to mitral stenosis and insufficiency. She had had chorea without rheumatic fever at age nine and an episode of rheumatic polyarthritis at age twenty-one. Exertional and paroxysmal nocturnal dyspnea, recurrent hemoptysis, and left ventricular failure occurred at age thirty-four.

Physical examination revealed a chronically ill woman with evidence of recent weight loss. Her temperature was 36.8°c.; heart rate 80 per minute, irregular; respirations 20 per minute; blood pressure 110/80 mm. Hg. There was internal strabismus and decreased visual acuity of the left eye. The chest was clear to percussion and auscultation. The heart was enlarged with the point of maximal impulse in the sixth intercostal space 1 cm. outside of the midclavicular line. Atrial fibrillation was present. The second pulmonic sound was greater than the second aortic sound. There was a grade 3 apical systolic murmur transmitted to the left axilla and the back. A grade 3 diastolic rumble was present at the apex, as was an opening snap. The liver was enlarged 5 cm. below the right costal margin and was tender. There was no splenomegaly, lymphadenopathy, petechiae or clubbing of the fingers.

Laboratory examinations revealed a hemoglobin of 13.6 gm. per 100 ml., hematocrit 41 per cent, and a total leukocyte count of 4,800 per cu. mm. The erythrocyte sedimentation rate (Westergren method) was 14 mm. per hour. Urinalysis was within normal limits. Blood urea nitrogen was 14 mg. per 100 ml. Serum electrolytes and results of all liver function tests were within normal limits. Serial electrocardiograms were consistent with atrial fibrillation, digitalis effect, and right axis deviation. Cardiac fluoroscopy and routine chest roentgenograms revealed left atrial, and right and left ventricular enlargement. The mitral annulus was calcified. Right and left cardiac catheterization indicated severe mitral stenosis and insufficiency. The remainder of the patient's examination was non-contributory. She was discharged on July 20 to return in October for mitral valvulotomy employing the extracorporeal heart-lung machine.

On readmission to the Clinical Center on October 14 the patient gave an interim history of increasing cardiac decompensation associated with hemoptysis. Results of the physical examination were unchanged from the first admission except for the appearance of a palpable spleen and bilateral pitting pretibial edema. Laboratory data were within normal limits except for a shift of the electrical axis of the heart to the vertical position and increase in the generalized cardiomegaly.

Repeat cardiac catheterization revealed progression of the double mitral lesion and also the presence of minimal aortic stenosis. On November 6 the patient underwent mitral valvulotomy, utilizing cardiopulmonary bypass. The mitral valve was grossly incompetent and stenotic. The stenosis was corrected, but the degree of regurgitation was only moderately diminished. A total of four mattress sutures was placed in the mitral valve. Postoperative culture of blood used in the pump was positive for C. guilliermondii. The patient had an uneventful postoperative course, but repeat catheterization indicated significant residual mitral stenosis.

The patient was discharged on December 6. During the next two months progressive intractable cardiac failure, splenomegaly, and a low grade fever developed. She was admitted to the Clinical Center for the third time on February 18, 1959.

Physical examination at this time revealed the patient to be afebrile and normotensive. Atrial fibrillation was still present. There was dullness to percussion at the base of the right lung posteriorly, with decreased breath sounds and bilateral moist basal rales. The cardiac murmurs were unchanged and the heart was still enlarged. The liver was approximately 24 cm. below the right costal margin, and the spleen tip was palpable. Both organs were tender to palpation. Ascites and 2-plus bilateral pitting pretibial edema were present.

Laboratory examinations were within normal limits except for a fall in hemoglobin to 11.1 gm. per 100 ml. Pyuria was now noted. Results of blood chemical tests and serial electrocardiograms remained unchanged. A chest roentgenogram revealed a right pleural effusion.

Low grade fever developed shortly after admission, and serial blood cultures were positive for C. guilliermondii. No skin manifestations of endocarditis were noted. Antifungal therapy for the candida endocarditis was started on the third hospital day, and a total of 140 mg. of amphotericin B was given intravenously. The patient died in severe congestive failure on February 24, the seventh hospital day.

At autopsy, the body weighed 109 pounds and measured 61 inches in length. Fibrous adhesions obliterated the pleural and pericardial spaces. A loculated empyema, measuring 3.5 cm. in diameter, was present in the right pleural space. The heart weighed 600 gm. The right atrium was dilated. There was slight thickening of the leaflets and chordae tendineae of the tricuspid valve. The thickness of the right ventricle was 0.8 cm. The pulmonic valve appeared normal. The left atrium was dilated. The endocardium of the left atrium was thickened, focally corrugated, and contained an irregular, partly calcified plaque 1 cm. in diameter. There were black silk sutures at the junctions of the anterior and posterior leaflets of the stenotic mitral valve, which measured approximately 4 cm. in diameter. The mitral cusps were greatly thickened, and their margins contained small calcified nodules covered by endocardium. The chordae tendineae were thickened and shortened. Solitary friable 0.5 cm. verrucae were present at the margins of both mitral leaflets. One vegetation surrounded suture material. Culture of the vegetations yielded C. guilliermondii. Postmortem heart blood culture was negative. The left ventricle was dilated and hypertrophied (1.8 cm. thick). The cusps of the aortic valve were thickened, but the commissures were not fused. The aortic valve measured 8.5 cm. in circumference. A 0.3 cm. verruca was present on the ventricular surface of the right anterior cusp. The coronary arteries and aorta were slightly atherosclerotic.

Infarcts were present in the spleen and right kidney. The spleen weighed 350 gm. The liver weighed 2,250 gm. and, on section, had a "nutmeg" appearance. The right kidney weighed 150 gm.; the left kidney 180 gm. The lungs were heavy and congested; there was bronchopneumonia in the upper lobe of the right lung. The remaining organs, including the brain and spinal cord, were normal in appearance.

Microscopically, candida organisms were observed in the small verrucae of the mitral and aortic valves and in the spleen. Several microabscesses were seen in the brain and spinal cord, and in sections of the vegetations from the mitral and aortic valves there were numerous candida organisms interspersed among fibrous tissue.

The mitral valve was thickened, vascularized, and contained numerous Anitschkow's cells, lymphocytes, and macrophages. Areas of fibrinoid necrosis surrounded by fibrous tissue were present in the mitral valve and in the right anterior leaflet of the aortic valve. Numerous Aschoff's nodules and discrete areas of necrosis were seen in both atria and both ventricles. Foreign body giant cells were noted in apposition to the suture material in the mitral valve, but no fungi were seen in the giant cells. A small branch of coronary artery near the apex of the left ventricle was occluded by a recent thrombus. The myocardial fibers were hypertrophied.

In sections of the right kidney, there were several small infarcts. There was no degeneration of the glomeruli and no inflammatory infiltrate in the interstitial tissues. Histologic study of the liver revealed passive congestion and minimal to moderate perilobular fatty change. In the spleen there were several organizing infarcts. Candida organisms were found in wet mount preparations of the spleen. Numerous hemosiderin-laden macrophages were present in the sections of the lungs. An area of acute bronchopneumonia was noted in the lower lobe of the right lung. The bone marrow was hypercellular.

The *final anatomic pathologic diagnoses* were: C. guilliermondii endocarditis, mitral and aortic valves; active rheumatic heart disease involving mitral, tricuspid, and aortic valves, with clinical mitral insufficiency and mitral stenosis; infarcts in spleen, containing C. guilliermondii and rhodotorula; sterile infarct, kidney; microabscesses, cervical spinal cord and cerebrum; acute bronchopneumonia; and congestion, lungs and liver.

Case 20. A. W. was a forty year old Air Force officer in whom a heart murmur was first heard in 1943. He was on active flight duty and asymptomatic until 1951, but had two episodes of pneumonia that year without any evidence of cardiac decompensation. In 1956 progressive dyspnea on exertion was noted for the first time. In September 1957 malaise, fever and increasing severe dyspnea developed. A routine chest roentgenogram at this time revealed an anterior, left-sided, calcified pleural plaque and an enlarged left atrium. Because of fever, elevated erythrocyte sedimentation rate, and an antistreptolysin-O titer of 1:1280, he was observed for active rheumatic fever. He was treated with penicillin and salicylates over a five-day period and transferred to the Walter Reed Army General Hospital on November 11.

Physical examination on admission revealed a healthy appearing white man in no distress. The patient was afebrile, pulse 80 per minute, regular; respirations 20 per minute; blood pressure 124/75 mm. Hg. No petechial lesions or splinter hemorrhages were seen on examination of the skin, mucous membranes, nailbeds or ocular fundi. The lungs were clear to percussion and auscultation. The heart was enlarged, with the point of maximal impulse in the fifth intercostal space 2 cm. to the left of the mid-clavicular line. There was normal sinus rhythm. The second pulmonic sound was split. There was a low-pitched apical diastolic rumble and diastolic thrill. There was no hepatosplenomegaly, clubbing of the digits, edema, or cyanosis.

Laboratory examinations revealed a persistent eosinophilia, elevated erythrocyte sedimentation rate, and C-reactive protein. Urinalysis results and blood chemical findings were within normal limits. Thirteen blood cultures were sterile. On May 22, 1958, a mitral commissurotomy was performed. The mitral valve was found to be stenotic, with a 1 cm. orifice, and was opened by finger-fracture to a diameter of 3.5 cm.

Following surgery he had an uneventful course except for a left pleural effusion, which gradually resolved. Exercise tolerance increased progressively, and he remained afebrile until one month postoperatively when low grade afternoon fever, fatigue, myalgias, and arthralgias were noted. Bedrest was accompanied by disappearance of all symptoms except the fever. On July 3 blood cultures became positive for C. albicans. Thirteen positive blood cultures were obtained from July 3 to August 8. Sputum cultures were negative for C. albicans. On July 30, nine weeks after commissurotomy, intravenous amphotericin B therapy was started. From July 30 to October 10, he received a total of 2,605 mg. of amphotericin B.

Despite therapy, the blood cultures continued to be positive for C. albicans, and the patient remained febrile. The site of fungal multiplication was believed to be a vegetation on the mitral valve or the denuded area of calcified pleural thickening which was decorticated at surgery. The sensitivity of the organism at twenty-four hours was 0.07 μg. per ml. On August 4 a fungicidal test on the serum was performed. The patient's serum diluted 1:3 prevented growth in twenty-four hours. On August 14 the concentration of amphotericin in the serum was 0.48 μg. per ml.

A pericardial aspiration was attempted on August 16 in an attempt to isolate the candida from a small pericardial effusion. Several hours following pericardiocentesis, tachycardia, progressive abdominal distention, a falling hematocrit, and complete loss of pulses in the lower left extremity developed. Emergency exploratory laparotomy revealed a small laceration in the dome of the liver. Hemorrhage was controlled without difficulty. A left femoral arteriotomy was also performed, with removal of a fragment of fresh blood clot, but the limb remained pulseless.

On August 27 a left thoracotomy was performed, with amputation of the suture line of the left atrial appendage. Microscopic examination of the atrial appendage revealed yeast organisms, but these could not be grown in culture.

On September 15 a bypass graft was performed, anastomosing the lower aorta to the left femoral artery, but the next day the right leg was found to be cold and pulseless, and an arteriogram showed a block in the right femoral artery. An embolectomy was performed, with restoration of the pulses in the right leg. Microscopic examination of this clot revealed C. albicans pseudohyphae and blastospores.

One week later the patient's temperature rose to 39°c. Erythromycin, chloramphenicol and penicillin were added to the amphotericin B therapy. On September 26 the fungus was found to be sensitive to methenamine mandelate, and this agent was added to the regimen. On October 6 signs of increasing congestive failure and mental confusion developed. Examination of the spinal fluid revealed no abnormalities, but the patient's mental condition deteriorated. He became comatose, and after several right-sided convulsive seizures he died on October 13.

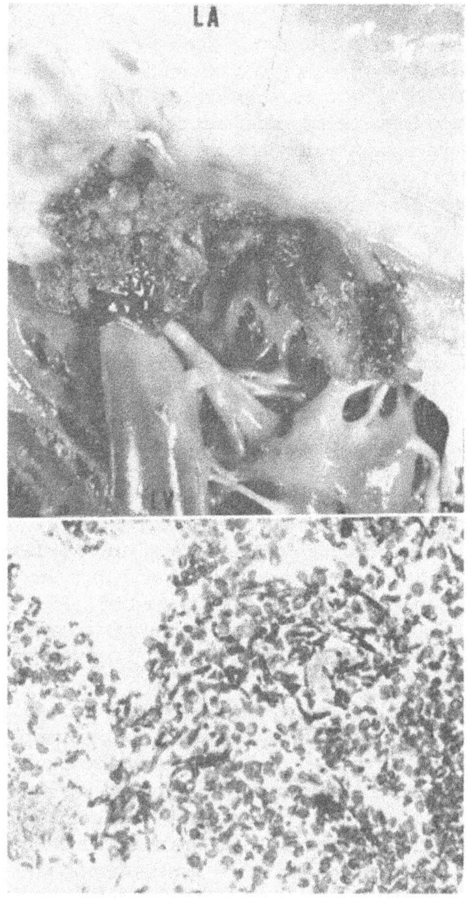

4A

4B

Fig. 4. Case 20. A, the left atrium (LA), left ventricle (LV), and mitral valve are opened. Two vegetations are present on the thickened, contracted mitral valve. The chordae tendineae are thickened and shortened. B, close-up of candida organisms present in vegetations shown in Figure 4A.

At autopsy, the body was that of an emaciated white man weighing 127 pounds and measuring 73 inches in length. The peritoneal cavity contained 250 ml. of clear serous fluid. There were multiple dense fibrous adhesions in the peritoneal cavity, right pleural space, and the pericardial sac. The heart weighed 365 gm. Numerous epicardial petechial hemorrhages were present. The chambers and valves of the right side of the heart were normal. The endocardium of the left atrium was smooth and glistening except for the site of excision of the left atrial appendage; here there was a small, irregular, reddish white vegetation. There was a 4 by 1.4 by 1 cm. red vegetation involving both leaflets of the mitral valve. (Fig. 4A.) The mitral valve leaflets were thickened, and a portion of the valve beneath the vegetation was eroded. The chordae tendineae of the mitral valve were fused, thickened, and shortened. The left ventricle and aortic valve were normal.

The left iliac artery was occluded by an adherent, pinkish white thrombus. A knitted Dacron® graft extended from the lower abdominal aorta to the left femoral artery immediately distal to the inguinal ring. The graft was widely patent.

The spleen weighed 475 gm.; no infarcts were present. The liver weighed 2,750 gm. A healed linear tear covered by fibrous tissue was present on the anterior surface of the left lobe of the liver. (This laceration was attributed to the attempted pericardiocentesis.) On section, the liver had a "nutmeg" appearance. The wall of the gallbladder was thickened; the gallbladder contained no stones. The right kidney weighed 260 gm.; the left kidney 250 gm. The surface of each kidney was smooth except for a depressed stellate scar on the cortical surface of the left kidney. There was mild to moderate generalized lymphadenopathy. The lungs were firm, congested, heavy, and contained focal areas of bronchopneumonia. The pleural surfaces were thickened and white. Mucopurulent material was seen in the bronchi. The brain weighed 1,360 gm. Focal subarachnoid hemorrhages were present on both cerebellar hemispheres and on the occipital poles of the cerebrum.

Microscopically, the mitral valve and left atrial vegetations consisted for the most part of eosinophilic debris in a network of fibrous tissue. Many candida organisms, mostly hyphal forms, were present in the vegetations. (Fig. 4B.) C. albicans was cultured from each vegetation. There was swelling and edema of the ground substance of the mitral leaflets, proliferation of capillaries, collagen fibers, and mononuclear cells. Focal calcium deposits were seen on the mitral valve. The left atrial endocardium was thickened. Chronic inflammatory cells were present in the subendocardial region of the left atrium. The collagen fibers of the subendocardial areas were markedly eosinophilic, edematous and fragmented. Focal collections of chronic inflammatory cells were seen in the myocardium of the left atrium, left ventricle, and ventricular septum. Focal hemorrhages were noted in the left atrial and left ventricular myocardium. The myocardial fibers were hypertrophied. There were minimal atherosclerotic changes in the coronary arteries. Layers of hyalin material and acute inflammatory cells were present on the epicardial surface of the heart. No Aschoff's bodies were seen in the heart.

The left common iliac artery was occluded by an organizing thrombus. Chronic inflammatory cells and fibrous tissue were present in the arterial wall and in the surrounding tissue, but no fungi were seen.

Several abscesses containing candida organisms were present in each kidney. Many polymorphonuclear cells were present in the interstitial areas of the kidneys. There were a few focal interstitial hemorrhages. The proximal convoluted tubules were necrotic. Hyaline casts were present in the lumen of many tubules. Organizing thrombi were found in some of the smaller arteries, and an infarct was seen in the left kidney. No organisms were identified in the renal infarct. There was mild to moderate arterionephrosclerosis. The glomeruli were unremarkable.

In the spleen there was reticuloendothelial hyperplasis of the white pulp and congestion of the red pulp. A few inflammatory cells were present in the periphery of some lobules of the liver, and the central areas were congested. The wall of the gallbladder was thickened by fibrous tissue.

The *final anatomic pathologic diagnoses* were: C. albicans endocarditis, mitral valve and stump of left atrial appendage; chronic rheumatic heart disease with mitral valvulitis; emboli to left kidney, left common iliac, and left and right femoral arteries; acute fibrinous pericarditis, postoperative; chronic focal interstitial myocarditis; focal suppurative pyelonephritis (candida species); congestion of liver and spleen with hepatosplenomegaly; focal hemorrhages, acute bronchopneumonia, acute pulmonary edema, and fibrous adhesions, right pleura, lungs; subarachnoid hemorrhages, cerebral hemispheres and occipital lobes; gangrene, left toes, secondary to embolus in left common iliac artery; ascites.

Case 21. A. L., a sixty-eight year old white male clothing presser, was admitted to the Clinical Center on May 17, 1960, with a diagnosis of C. tropicalis endocarditis. In August 1959 the patient had gradual onset of fever, anemia, an apical systolic murmur, and multiple petechiae in his conjunctivas. There was no past history suggestive of rheumatic fever. In October the patient was admitted to a New York hospital where a diagnosis was made of subacute bacterial endocarditis due to microaerophilic streptococci, and he was given a six-week course of intravenous antibiotic therapy. Gradual defervescence occurred, and the patient was discharged with sterile blood cultures on December 23, 1959.

On March 3, 1960, the patient was admitted to a Veterans Administration hospital because of recurrence of fever, anorexia, and weight loss. The cardiac murmur was unchanged, but petechiae were noted in the fundi. No hepatosplenomegaly was present. Laboratory data were non-contributory except for electrocardiographic evidence of an old posterior wall myocardial infarction. A diagnosis of candida endocarditis was made on the basis of serial blood cultures, positive for C. tropicalis. Intravenous therapy with amphotericin B was begun, but only 105 mg. of the drug was given because of a sudden rise in the blood urea nitrogen to 63 mg. per 100 ml. On April 18 occlusion of the right femoral artery was noted, but the involved extremity responded to conservative treatment at this time. Anemia of undetermined etiology was noted, which did not respond to blood replacement. All blood and bone marrow cultures remained positive throughout the patient's hospital course, and he was transferred to the Clinical Center for further treatment.

On admission, he was disoriented and could give no coherent history. Physical examination revealed an extremely ill, elderly white man with considerable muscle wasting. The temperature was 38.3°c.; heart rate 98 per minute; respirations 22 per minute; blood pressure 100/62 mm. Hg. Multiple petechiae were present in both lower conjunctival sacs. The chest was emphysematous in configuration and hyperresonant to percussion. No rales were heard. The heart was enlarged 3 cm. to the left of the midclavicular line. The first mitral sound was greater than the second mitral sound. A grade 3 systolic murmur was heard at the apex and transmitted over the entire precordium. A diastolic gallop was present. The liver was not enlarged. The spleen was enlarged 3 cm. below the left costal margin and was not tender. There was marked clubbing of all the fingers. No pulses were palpable in the right lower extremity, but no degenerative changes were noted in the skin or muscle. Neurologic examination disclosed twelfth nerve palsy on the right. There was no lymphadenopathy.

Laboratory examinations revealed a hemoglobin of 10.4 gm. per 100 ml. and a leukocyte count of 1,900 per cu. mm., with 80 per cent polymorphonuclear leukocytes, 15 per cent lymphocytes, and 5 per cent monocytes. The erythrocyte sedimentation rate (Westergren method) was 100 mm. per hour, blood urea nitrogen 102 mg., creatinine 3 mg., calcium 8.1 mg., phosphorus 4.6 mg. per 100 ml., and alkaline phosphatase 46 King-Armstrong units. The serum albumin was 2.6 gm. and the globulin 4 gm. per 100 ml. The serum glutamic oxaloacetic acid transaminase was 93 units, cephalin flocculation 3 plus; thymol turbidity 21 units. The bilirubin and serum electrocytes were within normal limits. The results of urinalysis were non-contributory. A chest roentgenogram revealed left ventricular prominence, but no significant pulmonary disease. An electrocardiogram indicated a normal sinus rhythm with periods of bigemini compatible with digitalis toxicity. Forty consecutive blood cultures were all positive for C. parapsilosis.* Cultures of the sputum and urine were negative for the fungus.

Azotemia precluded the use of amphotericin B in this patient, and on the eleventh hospital day oral thymol therapy was started. A total of 4.4 gm. was given, but without significant change in the colony count of candida in the blood. No other antifungal therapy was used in the treatment of this patient, nor were steroids given. On the fourteenth hospital day there was vascular occlusion of the upper left extremity, and the patient lapsed into intractable congestive cardiac failure. He died on June 2, the seventeenth hospital day.

At autopsy, the body weighed 108 pounds and measured 63 inches in length. The scleras were icteric. Bilateral conjunctival hemorrhages were present. There were several petechiae on the right shoulder. No other cutaneous hemorrhages were noted. The fingers and toes were slightly clubbed. The extremities were not edematous, and no fluid was present in the body cavities. The heart weighed 480 gm. The right atrium was dilated. The leaflets of the tricuspid valve were slightly thickened, but the chordae tendineae were neither thickened nor shortened. The thickness of the right ventricle was 0.5 cm. The pulmonary valve was normal. The left atrium was dilated. Two friable, fungating grey vegetations, 2.3 cm. and 2.7 cm. in greatest diameter, were present on the atrial aspects of the leaflets of the mitral valve. (Fig. 5A and 5B.) These leaflets were otherwise normal, and the chordae tendineae were neither shortened nor thickened. The thickness of the left ventricle was 1.4 cm. The posterior papillary muscle was calcified. (Fig. 5B.) A fibrous scar occupied the posterior wall of the apex of the left ventricle. The aortic valve was normal. The coronary arteries were tortuous and sclerotic. The aorta was severely atherosclerotic. The right common iliac artery was partly occluded by an organizing thrombus. The right femoral artery was also completely occluded over a distance of about 15 cm. by a soft yellow embolus.

The spleen weighed 800 gm. and contained several firm infarcts. The liver weighed 1,840 gm. and, on section, had a "nutmeg" appearance. The right kidney weighed 230 gm., the left 210 gm. The surface of each was finely granular and contained numerous petechial hemorrhages. On section, the renal parenchyma was congested. The urinary bladder contained several milliliters of bloody fluid. The vesical epithelium was markedly hemorrhagic and edematous. The lungs were congested. The brain weighed 1,180 gm. and appeared normal.

C. parapsilosis was cultured from heart blood, mitral valve vegetations, liver, lung, brain, spleen, and a supraclavicular lymph node. In addition, proteus was cultured from the mitral valve vegetations and from an atherosclerotic ulcer of the aorta. Alcaligenes faecalis was grown from the heart blood.

Microscopically, candida organisms were identified in the mitral valve vegetations, spleen, right common iliac, and right femoral arteries. The mitral valve vegetations consisted for the most part of large, dense colonies of candida organisms arranged in a "cloud-like" fashion. (Fig. 5C.) The surface of the vegetations was covered by a thin layer of fibrin which also intermingled with the network of the vegetations between the colonies of fungal organisms. Both hyphae and yeast organisms were present. Yeasts were more numerous in the more dense colonies; the hyphal forms in the less dense colonies. The organisms

* These cultures have been reviewed by Dr. Chester Emmons and Dr. Herbert Hasenclever of the National Institutes of Allergy and Infectious Diseases and identified as C. parapsilosis.

5A 5B 5C 5D 5E

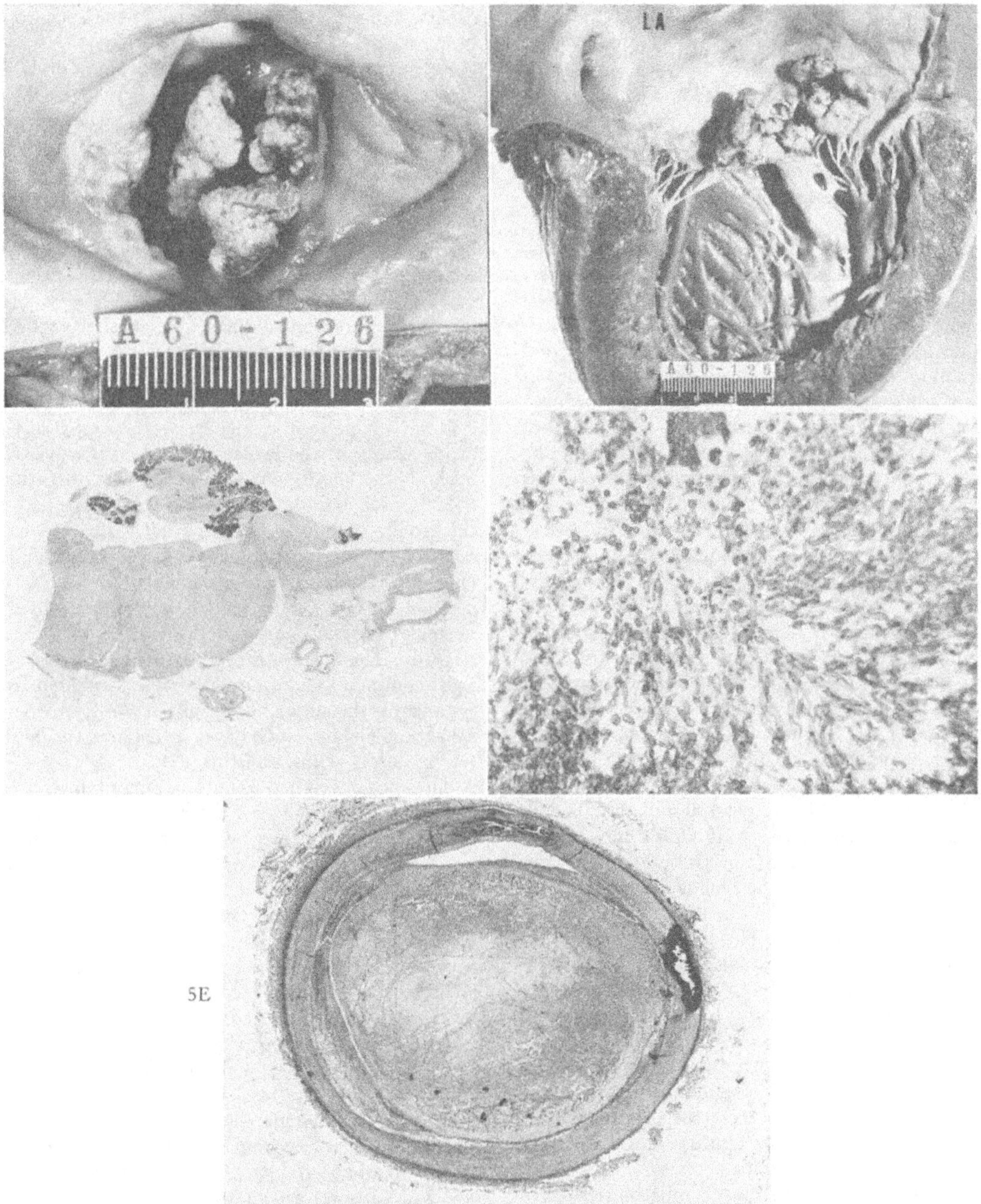

FIG. 5. Case 21. A, mitral valve as seen from the left atrium. Note the two large vegetations involving both the anterior and posterior cusps of this valve. B, the left atrium (LA), mitral valve, and left ventricle (LV) have been opened. The two vegetations are located on the atrial aspect of the mitral valve cusps. The chordae tendineae of the mitral valve are neither shortened nor thickened. The posterior papillary muscle, which is located in close proximity of the vegetations, is completely calcified. C, section through vegetation on posterior cusp of mitral valve. The dark areas of the vegetation are colonies of candida organisms. Note their location on the periphery of the vegetation. Gomori's methenamine silver stain, original magnification × 3.5. D, close-up of candida organisms present in vegetation shown in Fig. 5C. Numerous hyphal as well as yeast forms are present. E, section through right femoral artery, which is almost totally occluded by a fresh mycotic embolus. Numerous candida organisms were present in the embolus. The focal black area in the media of this vessel represents an area of calcification (Mönckeberg's medial calcinosis). Elastic van Gieson stain, original magnification × 12.

were easily seen in sections stained by periodic acid-Schiff and methenamine silver technics. (Fig. 5D.) No bacteria were seen in the vegetations. The valve leaflets were thickened by fibrous tissue. Occasionally, focal areas of necrosis were seen in the leaflets, and adjacent to these were small collections of acute inflammatory cells. The valve ring consisted of edematous fibrous tissue and contained many capillaries, numerous histiocytes, hemosiderin-laden macrophages, lymphocytes, a few plasma cells, "cholesterol" clefts, and minute foci of calcification. In interstitial areas of the myocardium of all chambers, and on the epicardium, were small focal areas containing acute and chronic inflammatory cells. The posterior papillary muscle of the left ventricle was calcified. The posterior wall of the left ventricle, extending from the apex almost to the mitral valve ring, was diffusely replaced by fibrous tissue. In addition, focal areas of interstitial myocardial fibrosis were seen in all chambers of the heart. The left posterior coronary artery was partly occluded by intimal fibrous tissue. The left anterior descending coronary artery was partly occluded by intimal fibrous proliferation and calcific deposits. Some of the myocardial fibers of the left ventricle were hypertrophied.

Sections through the right femoral artery disclosed complete occlusion of this vessel, distally, by organizing thrombi and, proximally, by large colonies of Candida organisms arranged in a "cloud-like" fashion similar to the mitral valve vegetations. (Fig. 5E.) There was a marked calcinosis of the media of the femoral arteries. The wall of the right femoral artery, containing the mycotic embolus, and the immediate perivascular area were infiltrated by numerous plasma cells, lymphocytes, fibroblasts, and occasionally by foreign body giant cells and hemosiderin-laden macrophages. Focal areas of necrosis were also noted in the wall of this vessel. A large myoctic embolus partially occluded the right common iliac artery. This vessel was microscopically similar to the right femoral artery except that the wall of the right common iliac artery was invaded by candida organisms.

Sections of the kidneys revealed severe arterionephrosclerosis. An occasional medium-sized intrarenal artery was totally occluded by atherosclerotic plaques. Hemorrhages were present in Bowman's space of many glomeruli and in the lumen of numerous tubules. Iron pigment was frequently noted in the tubular cells. Red blood cell casts and hyaline casts were seen in the lumen of many tubules. A rare focal area of acute necrosis, involving both the interstitial and tubular areas, was present. No fungal or bacterial organisms were seen in these areas of necrosis or elsewhere in the kidneys.

Histologic study of the spleen disclosed many organizing infarcts, some of which contained candida organisms. The spleen was congested. A few megakaryocytes were present in the spleen, and the plasma cells were increased. The vertebral, sternal, and rib bone marrow was hypercellular. It contained numerous plasma cells, but the megakaryocytes were of normal configuration and number. There was definite erythroid hyperplasia of the bone marrow. The lymph nodes also contained an excessive number of plasma cells. Sections of the liver showed mild chronic passive congestion with mild centrolobular necrosis. A few lymphocytes, plasma cells and, occasionally, polymorphonuclear cells were present in the periportal areas, which also contained a slightly increased amount of fibrous tissue and some fat vacuoles. A rare bile plug was noted. Periodic acid-Schiff stain was negative for fungal organisms, but showed perilobular deposits of glycogen.

Sections of the cerebrum, brain stem, cerebellum, and spinal cord disclosed focal areas of gliosis. The lungs were acutely and chronically congested. Focal infiltrations of lymphocytes and a few plasma cells were seen in the adrenal gland and surrounding adipose tissue. There was increased fibrous tissue in the periductal and intralobular areas of the pancreas. The lower esophagus was ulcerated and infiltrated by acute and chronic inflammatory cells. The testes were atrophic and contained focal collections of acute and chronic inflammatory cells. The lumen of many ducts of the prostate gland were filled with acute inflammatory cells.

The *final anatomic pathologic diagnoses* were: C. parapsilosis endocarditis, mitral valve; mycotic emboli to spleen, right common iliac and right femoral arteries; acute and chronic myocarditis, focal; cachexia; generalized atherosclerosis, severe, with old posterior myocardial infarct; arterionephrosclerosis; acute focal pyelonephritis; infarcts, spleen; congestion, lungs and viscera; jaundice; acute and chronic cholangitis; extramedullary hematopoiesis, spleen; hyperplasmacytosis, bone marrow, lymph nodes, and spleen; and acute prostatitis and orchitis.

CLINICAL MANIFESTATIONS

The clinical manifestations of mycotic endocarditis do not differ from those of bacterial endocarditis. Fever, chills, anorexia, nausea, vomiting, abdominal pain, and heart failure in patients who may have had previous rheumatic heart disease or who manifest recent cardiac murmurs, hepatosplenomegaly, petechiae, splinter hemorrhages, Osler's nodes, or large vessel embolism represent the most common clinical features of the disease.

History. Fever, present in all twenty-one cases, was the most common chief complaint and in five cases it was the only presenting symptom. Fever was accompanied at the onset of the illness (Table IV) by abdominal pain in six patients, heart failure in six, cough in three, and hemiplegia in one.

TABLE IV
CHIEF COMPLAINT IN TWENTY-ONE CASES OF CANDIDA ENDOCARDITIS

Complaint	No. of Cases
Abdominal pain, fever	6
Heart failure, fever	6
Fever only	5
Cough, fever	3
Hemiplegia, fever	1

Shortly after onset of the illness or during the later stages of the disease (Table v) there were associated symptoms of anorexia in eight cases; nausea, vomiting, and chills in five; weakness and mental confusion in three; weight loss, leg pain, malaise, headache, aphasia, and hemiplegia in two each; and chest pain, precordial pain, insomnia, and syncope in one case.

The youngest patient was a seven month old male infant (Case 7), the oldest a sixty-eight year old male clothes presser (Case 21). Although the age range covers seven decades, nearly half of the patients were in the fifth decade of life. (Table VI.) There was a 2:1 ratio of male to female patients. No predominance of occupation was apparent.

Physical Findings. A significant cardiac murmur was audible in nineteen of twenty-one patients (90 per cent). More than half (twelve of twenty-one) had a history of previous rheumatic heart disease. One patient had signs of aortic stenosis later proved to be secondary to atherosclerotic changes of the aortic valve. Six of the patients with murmurs and the two patients without murmurs had no evidence of previous heart disease. Seven of the twelve patients with rheumatic heart disease had pure mitral stenosis,

TABLE VI
AGE RANGE IN DECADES

Age (yr.)	No. of Cases
0–9	2
10–19	1
20–29	1
30–39	4
40–49	9
50–59	2
60–69	2

TABLE V
ASSOCIATED SYMPTOMS

Symptoms	No. of Cases
Anorexia	8
Nausea	5
Vomiting	5
Chills	5
Weakness	3
Mental confusion	3
Weight loss	2
Leg pain	2
Chest and precordial pain	2
Malaise	2
Headache	2
Aphasia	2
Hemiplegia	2
Insomnia	1
Syncope	1

one had predominately mitral insufficiency, two had pure aortic stenosis, one had predominate aortic insufficiency, and one had stenosis and insufficiency of both aortic and mitral valves. Congestive heart failure developed in fourteen of twenty-one patients. There was no evidence for failure in four cases, and in the remaining three patients it was not mentioned. Ten of the fourteen patients in whom congestive heart failure developed had previous heart disease. Only one of these had angina, and none had clinical evidence of myocardial infarction. However, two patients in congestive heart failure without rheumatic heart disease had evidence of myocardial infarctions (Case 16) due to a mycotic embolus and (Case 21) due to a non-mycotic thrombosis. (Table VII.)

Hepatomegaly was a physical finding in fifteen cases, attributable in a few cases to the concomitant development of congestive heart failure. Splenomegaly was present in all eighteen patients in whom the size of the spleen was mentioned. Petechiae occurred in sixteen patients, were absent in three, and not mentioned in the remaining two cases. (Table VIII.) Petechiae were reported most commonly on the conjunctiva, especially the lower palpebrum, and were frequently observed on the trunk and extremities and, in isolated instances, in the retina, the face, neck, and soft palate. (Table IX.) Osler's nodes and splinter hemorrhages were seen in only five and three patients, respectively. (Table VIII.)

TABLE VII
COEXISTENT CARDIAC DISEASE

Case No.	Heart Disease	Congestive Failure	Murmur	Myocardial Infarct
16	–	+	+	+
21	–	+	+	+
19	RHD,MI,MS AI,AS	+	+	–
13	RHD-AI,AS	+	+	–
14	RHD-MI,MS	+	+	–
11	RHD-AS	+	+	–
17	RHD-AS	+	+	–
2	RHD-MS	+	+	–
4	RHD-MS	+	+	–
18	RHD-MS	+	+	–
20	RHD-MS	+	+	–
15	RHD-MS	+	+	–
10	RHD-MS	–	+	–
5	RHD-MS	...	+	–
3	Scl.	...	+	–
6	–	...	+	...
1	–	–	+	–
8	–	+	+	–
9	–	+	+	–
7	–	–	–	–
12	–	–	–	–
21	13	14	19	2

NOTE: ..., no data available; RHD, rheumatic heart disease; MI, mitral insufficiency; MS, mitral stenosis; AI, aortic insufficiency; AS, aortic stenosis; Scl., arteriosclerosis.

TABLE IX
SITE OF PETECHIAE

Site	No. of Cases	
Conjunctivas		9
Palpebral		
Lower	7	
Upper	0	
Bulbar	2	
Trunk		8
Chest	2	
Abdomen	4	
Back	2	
Extremities		8
Upper	4	
Lower	4	
Other		10
Retina	4	
Soft palate	3	
Face	2	
Neck	1	

TABLE VIII
OTHER PHYSICAL FINDINGS

Findings	No. of Cases
Fever	21
Arterial emboli	19
Splenomegaly	18
Hepatomegaly	15
Petechiae	16
Osler's nodes	5
Splinter hemorrhages	3

A clinical feature that occurred with impressive frequency (eight of twenty-one cases) was embolism to the large arteries, indicating the large size of the mycotic vegetations. The large arteries of the extremities were the most common site of embolization. The usual picture of sudden pain, absence of peripheral pulsations, discoloration and change in temperature in the affected extremity were noted. In one case (Case 20) surgical removal of clot and bypass did not alter the over-all prognosis.

Involvement of the arteries to the spleen, kidneys, and intestines was accompanied by sudden, severe abdominal pain; involvement of the brain and spinal cord by headache, mental confusion, syncope and, on occasion, specific localizing motor or sensory neurologic signs. In three cases asymptomatic embolization to the liver occurred. Emboli to the smaller arteries were frequently seen at autopsy but were usually not clinically evident. Organ involvement by arterial emboli is listed in Table x.

TABLE X
ARTERIAL EMBOLIZATION IN TWENTY POSTMORTEM EXAMINATIONS

Site	No. of Cases
Spleen	13
Kidney	13
Brain	9
Lower extremity	5
Small intestine	3
Liver	3
Lung	2
Coronary	1
Colon	1
Pancreas	1
Spinal cord	1
Upper extremity	1

TABLE XI
LABORATORY DATA

Data	Present	Absent	% Present
Blood			
Elevated erythrocyte sedimentation rate	11	1	91
Anemia	15	2	89
Leukocytosis	8	9	47
Leukopenia	6	11	34
Urine			
Microscopic pyuria	12	2	85
Proteinuria	11	4	74
Microscopic hematuria	10	4	71
Casts	9	5	64

Laboratory Data. Numerous laboratory tests were performed in almost all cases, with significant results observed in the blood counts, erythrocyte sedimentation rate, routine urinalysis, and blood cultures for fungi.

Anemia was present in fifteen of seventeen cases in which the hematocrit, hemoglobin, or red blood count was recorded. Similarly, the erythrocyte sedimentation rate was accelerated in all but one case in which this determination was obtained. The white blood cell count was recorded in seventeen cases and ranged from 780 to 56,300 per cu. mm., being elevated in eight cases, low in six, and normal throughout the course of illness in three. (Table XI.)

Review of reported urinalyses revealed hematuria, pyuria, proteinuria, and granular casts (Table XI). In addition, yeast cells were occasionally seen in the sediment (three cases) and in two instances were recovered from the urine on culture.

The five species of candida identified in the twenty-one reported cases were repeatedly recovered from the bloodstream on culture in all but one patient (Case 10). No cultures were obtained in this case but the organism was identified by its morphologic features as belonging to the genus candida. In addition, C. parapsilosis was recovered from cultures of the bone marrow of two patients (Cases 16 and 21). The diagnosis of endocarditis was suspected antemortem in twelve of the twenty-one patients.

PREDISPOSING FACTORS

Predisposing factors in systemic fungal diseases, particularly fungal endocarditis, fall into two general groups: associated drug therapy and debilitating illnesses. (Table XII.)

TABLE XII
PREDISPOSING FACTORS IN TWENTY-ONE CASES OF CANDIDA ENDOCARDITIS

Predisposing Factors		No. of Cases	%
Antibiotic therapy		14	67
Rheumatic heart disease		12	57
Steroid therapy		2	10
Bone marrow depressant		0	0
Roentgen radiation		0	0
Debilitating illnesses		10	48
Subacute bacterial endocarditis	4		
Peptic ulcer	2		
Diabetes mellitus	1		
Chronic pulmonary disease	1		
Syphilis of central nervous system	1		
Hypertension	1		
Narcotic addiction		4	19
Surgery		9	43

Drug Therapy. Antibiotic therapy: The use of intensive antibiotic therapy for prolonged periods is frequently complicated by super-infection with C. albicans or other fungi [*9,10,12,15,16,46,49,61,74,79–101,115–117*]. Clinical evidence of vaginitis [*85*], oral and intestinal lesions [*86,96,100*], generalized peritonitis [*95*], pneumonia [*87,99*], acute anuria [*98*], and disseminated candidiasis [*71–75,106*] has been observed following treatment with oxytetracycline [*91–95*], chlortetetracycline [*85–90,95–100,106*], chloramphenicol [*84–89,96,98*], penicillin [*84,86,106*], streptomycin [*106*], and sulfadiazine [*100*]. How antibiotics affect the pathogenicity of fungi is not known. A number of mechanisms have been invoked to explain their mode of action: (1) direct stimulation of growth [*46*]; (2) suppression of bacteria, allowing use of environmental food supply by fungi and thus indirectly supporting multiplication [*108*]; and (3) host hypersensitivity to a specific antibiotic [*109*] or decreased bacterial production of certain essential nutritive requirements, e.g., an unspecified B vitamin [*80*], causes an alteration in the integrity of the intestinal mucous membranes.

Chlortetracycline has been shown to exert a direct stimulatory effect on the growth of C. albicans in Sabouraud's media [*80,90,97*] and to enhance the virulence of C. albicans in mice [*93*]. Streptomycin enhanced the growth of Sporotrichum schenckii, C. immitis, Phialophora verrucosa, Trichophyton mentagrophytes, and H. capsulatum that had not been previously exposed to this antibiotic [*87*]. Contrariwise, it has been demonstrated in one study that penicillin, chloramphenicol, streptomycin, and oxytetracycline [*80*], and in a second study penicillin, chloramphenicol, chlortetracycline, and oxytetracycline [*61,79*] failed to enhance the growth of C. albicans *in vitro*.

Candida species, which may be cultured from the mouth, intestinal tract, and vagina in 35 to 40 per cent of normal persons [*1,11,107*], are known to multiply excessively in the bowel or mouth when the normal bacterial flora is suppressed by antibiotic therapy [*61,74,79,86,88,89,91*]. However, Kligman reported no adverse influence of various antibiotics on the course of experimental C. albicans infection in mice [*61,79*].

Some studies have shown that antibiotics decrease production of certain essential nutritive requirements, e.g., vitamin B, which when deficient causes an alteration in the integrity of the mucous membranes, thus affording more ready access of fungi [*80*]. A single injection of penicillin on the chorio-allantoic membrane of chick embryos increased the mortality rate resulting from infection with C. albicans [*83*]. However, Meenan [*105*] concluded that vitamin B administration did not influence the incidence of C. albicans infection in patients receiving antibiotic therapy.

Fourteen of the twenty-one patients in this report had received antibiotic therapy before onset of their endocarditis.

Steroids, Roentgen Radiation, and Bone Marrow Depressants. Seligmann [*103*], Bratlund [*101*], and Louria [*112*] reported that cortisone shortens the survival time of mice infected with C. albicans and increases the severity of such infections. Kligman et al. [*110*] observed that cortisone enhanced cutaneous T. mentagrophytes infection. Friedman et al. [*111*] postulate that roentgen radiation or cortisone, alone, or in combination, enhanced the pathogenicity of B. dermatitidis. Mankowski and Littleton [*102*] showed that cortisone-treated mice infected with C. albicans, aspergillus species, penicillium species, H. capsulatum, and C. neoformans exhibited shorter survival times than similar controls. Craig and Farber [*106*] allude to the clinical association of systemic candidiasis with acute leukemia in eleven children who had been treated with antifolic acid compounds, the triethylmelamines, cortisone, or adrenocorticotropic hormone. All had received long-term antibiotic therapy. Levy and Cohen [*118*] reported the development of systemic candidiasis in a patient receiving corticotropin therapy.

One patient (Case 14) received prolonged therapy and another (Case 12) minimal corticosteroid therapy for rheumatic carditis and rheumatoid arthritis, respectively [*17,18*]. No patient in this series received bone marrow depressants or significant roentgen radiation.

Debilitating Disease. Twelve of the twenty-one patients had previous rheumatic heart disease. Ten of the twelve patients received prolonged antibiotic therapy and two were narcotic addicts. Eight of the twelve patients underwent major surgery.

Diabetes mellitus has been considered a predisposing factor in candidiasis of the skin and genitalia [*10,11*]. Experimental diabetes enhances infection with C. albicans in the mouse [*120*]. It is not known if this is due to hyperglycemia or other metabolic abnormalities. Wolfe and Henderson [*11*] suggest that diabetes was a predisposing factor in their case of candida endocarditis.

Hypocalcemia is another factor of possible significance in lowering host resistance to infection with candida organisms [*74*]. A relationship of hypocalcemia to candidiasis in children with hypoparathyroidism has been observed and it is thought to be related to the epidermal changes that accompany this metabolic disorder [*121*]. An excessive growth of candida organisms from the bowel of patients with sprue, another disease with chronic hypocalcemia, has been reported [*122*].

The reported cases of meningitis, endocarditis, or systemic candidiasis have occurred in patients in a poor state of general health [*71*], possibly in negative nitrogen balance. This latter factor has been reported to enhance the mortality of rats experimentally infected with C. albicans [*123,124*].

PORTAL OF ENTRY

A striking feature in the history of patients in whom candida endocarditis developed is the frequency of vascular trauma or intravenous medication which may have served as portals of entry of the fungus. Six patients (Cases 11, 15, 17, 18, 19, and 20) had had prior cardiac valvulotomies (two aortic and four mitral). In two of these patients (Cases 17 and 19) the organism was cultured postoperatively from the heart-lung oxygenator.

An additional five patients (Cases 4, 13, 15, 16, and 21) had received long-term intravenous medication for antecedent bacterial endocarditis. In four patients (Cases 1, 2, 5, and 16) self-administered intravenous narcotics may have served as the site or means of fungal infection. In Case 1 culture of the drug container employed yielded the same organism as that obtained from the patient's blood [6]. Although Wikler et al. [7] raised the possibility that the infecting organism in their patient might be a common contaminant of heroin or one of its adulterants, Emmons [7] was unable to culture candida from eleven samples of diacetylmorphine (heroin).

Two additional patients (Cases 10 and 12) had prior surgery for peptic ulcer and one patient (Case 7) had antecedent bronchoscopy; vascular and mucosal trauma was implicated in these three cases. In one patient (Case 6) it was speculated that the portal of entry had been a contaminated needle or syringe used by a diabetic patient.

PATHOLOGY

On microscopic examination, candida organisms were seen in the endocardial vegetations in the twenty autopsies. No bacteria were noted in the vegetations of the six patients we observed. Both hyphal and yeast forms of candida organisms were seen in the vegetations. In some of the twenty cases, yeast forms predominated, in others hyphal forms were abundant and yeast forms rare. The morphologic variability was not related to the species of candida present. In several instances the organisms were located only in the superficial portions of the vegetations, in others the fungi were present in the interior as well as on the surface. In five of the twenty patients there was only one vegetation. Of the fifteen patients with more than one vegetation, six had two vegetations, five had three, and four patients had more than three (usually millimeter-sized) vegetations. The size of the vegetations was described for sixteen of the twenty patients. It varied from "poppyseed sized" (Case 9) to a largest diameter of 8 cm. (Case 17). In ten of the sixteen patients the diameters of vegetations ranged from 2 to 4 cm. All vegetations but one (Case 12) were located in the left side of the heart. The mitral valve was the site of involvement in thirteen of the twenty patients. Only the aortic valve was involved in six patients; both the aortic and mitral valves were involved in five patients.

The left atrium contained vegetations in three patients, and in each they were also present on the mitral valve. These vegetations were located on the atrial surface in all instances. Vegetations were usually located on the ventricular surface of the aortic valve, but on rare occasion only in the sinuses of Valsalva. There were vegetations of the right atrium, pulmonary artery, and the outflow tract of the left ventricle (without valvulitis) in the only patient with right-sided cardiac lesions (Case 12). Previous valvular damage was common; it was definitely present in twelve patients, probably present in four, and absent in two. In all instances the valvular damage was attributed to chronic rheumatic disease. There is no record of the presence or absence of previous valvular damage in two patients.

Myocarditis was described in thirteen of fourteen patients; no information is available in six cases. In the myocardium there were focal or diffuse collections of acute or chronic inflammatory cells. Abscesses were rare. Granulomas with foreign body giant cells were found in two hearts. One patient had active rheumatic myocarditis with Aschoff's bodies. An acute myocardial infarct was found in one heart (Case 15); it resulted from mycotic embolus to the anterior descending coronary artery. In one patient (Case 21) there was a healed calcified myocardial infarct of the posterior papillary muscle of the left ventricle. The fungal vegetation on the mitral valve of this patient was located close to this infarct. The heart was enlarged in fourteen of the twenty patients. Cardiac weights were recorded in twelve adult patients, and averaged 443 gm. with a range from 250 to 600 gm. The heart was reported as "not enlarged" or "normal-sized" in three patients, and no information was available in two.

Pericarditis was present in five of twenty patients. Three of the five had had recent cardiac surgery.

Emboli to large arteries were noted in eight of twenty patients. The femoral and iliac arteries were involved in five patients, the renal and splenic arteries in two, the cerebral, mesenteric, and axillary arteries in one each. The embolus to the cerebral artery was associated with a mycotic aneurysm which ruptured. The embolus to the mesenteric artery was followed by fatal, massive infarction of the ileum. The reported incidence of emboli to large arteries (especially the femoral, axillary and radial) might have been greater had these arteries been removed more frequently at autopsy. On the valves of patients with emboli to large arteries there were vegetations 2 cm. or larger in diameter. Emboli to the spleen occurred in fourteen patients, to the kidneys in thirteen, and to the brain or meninges in ten. The weight of the spleen was recorded in eleven patients, and noted to be "enlarged" in three, and "normal-sized" in one. The weights of the spleen ranged from 300 to 1,080 gm.; the average weight was 670 gm., which is more than three times the normal. Congestion accounted for the splenic enlargement in most instances. Candida organisms were identified, usually in infarcts, in the spleens of seven patients.

The weight of the kidneys was recorded in nine patients. The weight of the right kidney averaged 187 gm., the left 205 gm., and the range was from 50 to 260 gm. The kidneys were described as "not enlarged" in three other protocols. The most common renal lesions were infarcts (twelve patients). Focal "embolic" glomerulonephritis was noted in five patients. Candida organisms were seen in sections from the kidneys of two of these five patients. Diffuse glomerulonephritis was not described. Pyelonephritis or interstitial nephritis was present in six patients. Renal infarcts, pyelonephritis, and focal "embolic" glomerulonephritis were sometimes present in the same kidney. Examination of the urinary sediment was not helpful in distinguishing one type of renal lesion from another. The presence of a few candida organisms seems insufficient to account for the caseation necrosis of the right kidney in Case 18, and an etiology was not determined.

Hepatic weights were recorded in nine instances. Their average was 2,332 gm., ranging from 1,650 to 3,650 gm. The liver was mentioned as "enlarged" in two other patients, and as "markedly enlarged" and "swollen and congested" once each. The increased weight was related in most cases to passive congestion. Candida organisms were seen in the liver of only two patients.

TREATMENT

Many chemotherapeutic agents and antibiotics possessing fungistatic properties have been tested by the disk method against candida species [*134*]. These include acids, esters, alcohols, aldehydes, antibiotics, antihistamines, detergents, dyes, halogens, heavy metals, oxidizing agents, phenols, sulfonamides, and dermatologic preparations [*191*]. Of these, sodium caprylate, boric acid, methylrosaniline chloride, and metacresylacetate (cresatin) were significantly fungistatic [*191*]. In addition, an inhibitory action against C. albicans *in vitro* has been demonstrated with esters of p-hydroxybenzoic acid [*136*], Nepara 1968 [*139*], candicidin [*140, 141*], stilbamidine, 2-hydroxystilbamidine [*143*], and the nitrostyrenes [*144*]. In experimental infections, Nepara 1968 suppressed mortality in mice infected with C. albicans [*138*], whereas stilbamidine and 2-hydroxystilbamidine were reportedly ineffective [*143*].

Esters of p-hydroxybenzoic acid [*135*], oral undecylenic acid [*142*], local administration of the nitrostyrenes [*144*], and brilliant green and methyl blue aerosol inhalations [*145–147*] have been used in clinical candida infections with reportedly favorable results [*191*], as have potassium [*1*] and ethyl [*184*] iodide inhalations. Methylrosaniline chloride was effectively used for treating candida infections prior to the advent of nystatin [*1*]. Candicidin is too toxic for use in man [*191*].

Nystatin, an antibiotic derived from a culture of Str. noursei, is highly effective against C. albicans in *in vitro* studies [*131,132,148–151*] and in experimental infections of mice and rabbits [*149,152–157*]. In man, superficial infections of skin, whether local, generalized, or ulcerative [*149,161–170*] (particularly around colostomies) [*171*]; and of mucous membranes of mouth and vagina [*150,159–162*] (vulvovaginitis) [*160,161, 172–176*] responded to local or oral nystatin therapy [*191*]. The earlier treatment was begun, the greater was the response to nystatin therapy. Nystatin has also been used to prevent the multiplication of candida organisms in the gastrointestinal tract during therapy with broad-spectrum antibiotics [*179*].

Pulmonary [*177,178*] and disseminated candidiasis [*133,149,170*] have been reported to respond to nystatin therapy, but not as well as cutaneous infections [*191*] because of the poor absorption of the drug from the gastrointestinal tract. Parenteral administration seemed effective in two cases of disseminated candidiasis [*46,149*], but of no value in one case (Case 15) of C. albicans endocarditis [*79*]. Parenterally

TABLE XIII
TREATMENT WITH AMPHOTERICIN B

Case No.	Maximal Daily Dose (mg.)	Duration of Rx (days)	Total Dose (mg.)	Peak Serum Level (µg./ml.)	Sensitivity Inhibition of Fungus (µg./ml.)
11	Few doses (oral)	1	?	. . .	. . .
16	5000 (oral)	10	50,000	1.44	0.05
19	50 (I.V.)	4	140	. . .	. . .
21	45 (I.V.)	3	105	. . .	0.03
14	12 (I.V.)	20	184	. . .	. . .
	20 (I.M.)	50	965	. . .	. . .
15	60 (I.V.)	230*	7,840	1.4–2.4	0.03–0.06
17	75 (I.V.)	46	1,644	0.36	0.09
18	50 (I.V.)	24	821	0.36	0.07
20	60 (I.V.)	72	2,370	0.48	0.07

NOTE: . . ., no data; I.V., intravenous; I.M., intramuscular.
* Three separate courses.

administered nystatin has produced severe toxicity and is no longer available for clinical administration [*19,192*].

Amphotericin B, introduced in 1956 by Gold et al. [*186*], was isolated from an unidentified species of streptomyces. Its tentative empirical formula is $C_{46}H_{73}NO_{20}$ [*198*]. Amphotericin B inhibits a wide variety of pathogenic and nonpathogenic fungi [*194*] and is highly inhibitory to the candida species *in vitro* [*186*] and by tissue culture tests [*141*]. C. albicans-infected animals responded to treatment with amphotericin B by the intraperitoneal or oral routes [*185,187,188*]. Studies in man indicate that when amphotericin is orally administered it is poorly absorbed, resulting in low blood and spinal fluid levels [*193*]. Intramuscular administration in therapeutic amounts resulted in low serum levels and produced local irritation and often abscesses [*194*]. Intravenous administration of amphotericin B produced better blood levels, which were maintained, since excretion was slow, for prolonged periods after the medication was discontinued [*193,196*]. For favorable results in fungal meningitides, intrathecal therapy has been used because of the high blood-brain barrier for this drug [*113,196,197*].

Oral amphotericin B will eliminate C. albicans from the fecal flora in man [*181,189*], and topical administration of this drug is effective against candidiasis involving the skin [*195*] and cornea [*197*]. The intrathoracic injection of amphotericin B was successful in treating C. albicans empyema [*69*], and amphotericin B has been injected into the bladder with reported benefit in candida infections of the urinary tract [*199*].

Intravenous therapy with amphotericin B has been reported effective in reducing the colony count and clearing candida organisms, within a few days, from the bloodstream of patients with systemic candidiasis [*191,195*]. Apparent recoveries following therapy with intravenous amphotericin B have been reported in three patients with C. albicans septicemia [*19,192*]. Similar therapy was not effective, however, in four additional cases of disseminated candidiasis [*113,192,196,197*]. An accurate estimate of the value of amphotericin B for the treatment of systemic candidiasis is difficult unless definite tissue invasion can be demonstrated. Positive blood and urine cultures have been observed during prolonged antibacterial therapy, but in these patients blood and urine cultures became negative following discontinuation of these antibiotics even though no antifungal therapy was administered [*196*].

Nine patients with candida endocarditis were treated with amphotericin B. Two patients (Cases 11 and 16) received short courses of oral therapy, and two patients (Cases 19 and 21) four and three days of intravenous therapy, respectively, prior to death. Five patients (Cases 14, 15, 17, 18, and 20), however, received prolonged therapy with good dosage of amphotericin B. (Table XIII.) Treatment transiently modified the course and blood cultures became negative in four of five patients (Cases 14, 15, 17, and 20), and a decrease in the colony count occurred in the fifth (Case 18) during therapy. Therapy, however, did not completely eradicate the microorganism, and the patients eventually died of their disease. The serum levels of amphotericin in three of the five patients (Cases 15, 18, and 20) are on record, as is the least concentration of amphotericin B which inhibited *in vitro* the infecting organism in four of the five patients (Cases 15, 17, 18, and 20). (Table XIII.) In each instance the serum level of amphotericin B was greater than the level of amphotericin B necessary to inhibit the growth of the respective species of candida. It is possible that larger daily doses of amphotericin B for longer periods of uninterrupted therapy might produce more beneficial results.

PROGNOSIS

The approximate duration of illness in twenty-one patients ranged from two weeks (Cases 4 and 11) to seventy-one weeks (Case 15), with a median of thirteen weeks and a mean of seventeen weeks. (Table xiv.)

C. albicans was the responsible organism in the two cases of shortest duration. Only three of seven patients with this species survived longer than eleven weeks, and these three received significant antifungal therapy. Only two of twelve patients (species not identified in two cases) with endocarditis caused by other species of candida (parapsilosis, guilliermondii, tropicalis, and krusei), however, lived less than thirteen weeks. The relative pathogenicity of these species may be a partial explanation of this difference. In addition, five of the seven patients (Cases 15, 17, 18, 19, and 20) with the longest duration of illness (fifteen to seventy-one weeks) received significant antifungal therapy.

The observed clinical course was distinguished by one of steady progression manifested by persistent fever, increasing weakness, general deterioration, and heart failure. Dissemination occurred, with showers of petechiae, lethargy, confusion, coma, and death. Candida endocarditis, despite suggested prolongation of life with antifungal therapy, must be considered, as of now, to be a uniformly fatal disease.

TABLE XIV
DURATION OF ILLNESSES IN TWENTY-ONE CASES

Weeks	No.
2	2
4	2
5	1
9	1
11	1
13	7
15	2
22	2
26	1
48	1
71	1
Total	21

Median . . . . 13 weeks
Mean . . . . 17 weeks

CONCLUSIONS

The adequately documented cases of candida endocarditis now total twenty-one. Of these, C. albicans was responsible for seven, C. parapsilosis (parakrusei) for six, C. guilliermondii for four, C. krusei and C. tropicalis for one each; in two cases the species was not identified. A clinical picture consistent with endocarditis, with blood cultures positive for candida (in the absence of the isolation of a more common etiologic agent) or an adequate description of the valvular vegetations and fungus, are accepted as evidence of candida endocarditis. Several case reports which do not fulfill these criteria have been omitted.

Associated drug therapy and specific debilitating illnesses are predisposing factors to candida endocarditis. Prolonged antibiotic, steroid, roentgen radiation, and bone marrow depressant therapy are known to enhance candida infections; hypocalcemia and negative nitrogen balance may also be adverse factors. Insulin administration (in diabetic subjects), surgery (in patients with rheumatic heart disease), intravenous antibiotic therapy, and self-administration of narcotics seem to have served as the specific portals of entry in candida endocarditis.

Fever, chills, anorexia, nausea, vomiting, abdominal pain, and heart failure (in patients who may have had previous rheumatic heart disease or in whom recent cardiac murmurs have developed), hepatosplenomegaly, petechiae, splinter hemorrhages, Osler's nodes, or large vessel embolism represent the most common clinical features of the disease. The principal clinical difference between candida endocarditis and bacterial endocarditis is the occurrence of large vessel embolism, a reflection of the large size of mycotic vegetations. An elevated erythrocyte sedimentation rate, anemia, leukocytosis or leukopenia, hematuria, pyuria, proteinuria, and cylindruria were frequent laboratory observations. Fungemia was repeatedly demonstrated.

The approximate duration of illness ranged from two to seventy-one weeks with a median of thirteen and a mean of seventeen weeks. The patients receiving intense antifungal therapy survived longer than the untreated regardless of the known relative pathogenicity of the species of candida.

Treatment with intravenously administered amphotericin B, which is effective in reducing the colony count and clearing the bloodstream of candida organisms, transiently modified the course of candida endocarditis. Serum concentrations of amphotericin B, which exceed those necessary to inhibit the growth of candida, can be attained by intravenous administration of the drug. The use of larger doses of amphotericin B for longer periods of uninterrupted therapy is suggested until more effective therapy is discovered. The prognosis of candida endocarditis must presently be considered to be uniformly fatal.

ADDENDUM

Since the submission of this manuscript other cases of Candida endocarditis continue to be reported [*201–207*] the most notable of which is that of Kay and others [*206*] who describe the first case in which the patient was ever cured, in this instance by the surgical removal of the infected portion of the tricuspid valve.

Acknowledgment: We are indebted to Captain Melvin D. Cheitlin, M.C., U.S.A. and Captain Edward Kamin, M.C., U.S.A., for their assistance in the study of one of the patients described, and to Miss Margaret Huber for her technical assistance.

REFERENCES

1. Conant, N. F., Smith, D. T., Baker, R. D., Callaway, J. L. and Martin, D. S. Manual of Clinical Mycology, 2nd ed., p. 381. Philadelphia, 1954. W. B. Saunders Co.
2. Simons, R. D. Medical Mycology, p. 11. Amsterdam, 1954. Alsevier Publishing Co.
3. Jones, M. Subacute bacterial endocarditis of non-streptococcal etiology. *Am. Heart J.*, 40: 106, 1950.
4. Beamer, P. R., Reinhard, E. H. and Goodof, I. I. Vegetative endocarditis caused by higher bacteria and fungi. *Am. Heart J.*, 29: 99, 1945.
5. Hoeprich, P. D. and Chernoff, H. M. Subacute bacterial endocarditis due to Listeria monocytogenes. *Am. Heart J.*, 19: 488, 1955.
6. Joachim, H. and Polayes, S. H. Subacute endocarditis and systemic mycosis (monilia). *J. A. M. A.*, 115: 205, 1940.
7. Wikler, A., Williams, E. G., Douglass, E. D., Emmons, C. W. and Dunn, R. C. Mycotic endocarditis: report of a case. *J. A. M. A.*, 119: 333, 1942.
8. Pasternack, J. G. Subacute monilia endocarditis: new clinical and pathological entity. *Am. J. Clin. Path.*, 12: 496, 1942.
9. Geiger, A. J., Wenner, H. A., Axilrod, H. D. and Durlacher, S. H. Mycotic endocarditis and meningitis: report of a case due to Monilia albicans. *Yale J. Biol. & Med.*, 18: 259, 1946.
10. Zimmerman, L. E. Candida and aspergillus endocarditis, with comments on the role of antibiotics in dissemination of fungus disease. *Arch. Path.*, 50: 591, 1950.
11. Wolfe, E. I. and Henderson, F. W. Mycotic endocarditis: report of a case. *J. A. M. A.*, 147: 1344, 1951.
12. Kunstadter, R. H., MacLean, H. and Greengard, J. Mycotic endocarditis due to C. albicans. *J. A. M. A.*, 149: 829, 1952.
13. Niel, K. Zur Klinik der Candidainfektionen. *Klin. Med.*, 8: 49, 1953.
14. Kohlmeier, W. Zur Kenntnis der Candidainfektionen. *Klin. Med.*, 8: 54, 1953.
15. Caplan, H. Monilia (candida) endocarditis following treatment with antibiotics. *Lancet*, 2: 957, 1955.
16. Koelle, W. A. and Pastor, B. H. Candida albicans endocarditis after aortic valvulotomy. *New England J. Med.*, 255: 997, 1956.
17. Conn, N. K., Crean, G. P., MacCabe, A. F. and MacLean, N. Systemic candidiasis and endocarditis due to Candida tropicalis. *Brit. M. J.*, 5127: 944, 1959.
18. Pearl, M. A. and Sidransky, H. Candida endocarditis. Two new cases with a review of twelve cases previously reported. *Am. Heart J.*, 60: 345, 1960.
19. Louria, D. B. and Dineen, P. Amphotericin B in the treatment of disseminated moniliasis. *J. A. M. A.*, 174: 273, 1960.
20. Merchant, R. K., Louria, D. B., Geisler, P. H., Edgcomb, J. H. and Utz, J. P. Fungal endocarditis: review of the literature and report of three cases. *Ann. Int. Med.*, 48: 242, 1958.
21. Hurley, T. D. A unique lesion of the heart in systemic blastomycosis. *J. M. Res.*, 33: 499, 1915.
22. Baker, R. D. and Brian, E. W. Blastomycosis of the heart. *Am. J. Path.*, 13: 139, 1937.
23. Martin, D. S. and Smith, D. T. Blastomycosis. *Am. Rev. Tuber.*, 39: 488, 1939.
24. Pond, N. E. and Humphreys, R. J. Blastomycosis with cardiac involvement and peripheral embolization. *Am. Heart J.*, 43: 615, 1952.
25. Epstein, E. Prognostic significance of cutaneous lesions in coccidioidal granuloma. *Arch. Dermat. & Syph.*, 38: 752, 1938.
26. Cawley, E. P. Aspergillosis and the aspergilli: report of a unique case of the disease. *Arch. Int. Med.*, 80: 423, 1947.
27. Welsh, R. A. and Buchness, J. M. Aspergillus endocarditis, myocarditis, and lung abscess: Report of a case. *Am. J. Clin. Path.*, 25: 782, 1955.
28. Kirschstein, R. L. and Sidransky, H. Mycotic endocarditis of the tricuspid valve due to Aspergillus flavus: report of a case. *Arch. Path.*, 62: 103, 1956.
29. Lombardo, T. A., Rabson, A. S. and Dodge, H. T. Mycotic endocarditis: report of a case due to Cryptococcus neoformans. *Am. J. Med.*, 22: 664, 1957.
30. Broders, A. C., Dochat, G. R., Herrell, W. E. and Vaughn, L. D. Histoplasmosis producing vegetative endocarditis. *J. A. M. A.*, 122: 489, 1943.
31. Kemper, J. W. and Bloom, H. J. Histoplasmosis: report of a case. *J. Oral Surg.*, 2: 167, 1944.
32. Parsons, R. J. and Zarafonetis, C. J. D. Histoplasmosis in man. *Arch. Int. Med.*, 75: 1, 1945.
33. Fawell, W. N., Browns, H. L. and Ernstene,

A. C. Vegetative endocarditis due to Histoplasma capsulatum. *Cleveland Clin. Quart.*, 18: 305, 1951.

34. Binford, C. H. Histoplasmosis: tissue reactions and morphologic variations of the fungus. *Am. J. Clin. Path.*, 25: 25, 1955.
35. Zimmerman, L. E. Some contributions of the histopathological method to the study of fungus disease. *Tr. New York Acad. Sc.*, 19: 358, 1957.
36. Sulack, M. H. In: Clinicopathologic Conference. *U. S. Armed Forces M. J.*, 8: 70, 1957.
37. Moore, M. Morphologic variation in tissue of organisms of the blastomycoses and of histoplasmosis. *Am. J. Path.*, 31: 1049, 1955. Quoting unpublished case of Dominguez, R. and Golden, A.
38. Torack, R. M. Fungus infections associated with antibiotic and steroid therapy. *Am. J. Med.*, 22: 872, 1957.
39. Nicolaides, N. J. Fungal endocarditis complicating staphylococcal endocarditis. *M. J. Australia*, 1: 793, 1957.
40. Friedman, N. B. and Donaldson, L. Systemic mycosis with mycotic endocarditis. *Arch. Path.*, 27: 394, 1939.
41. Sacks, I. and Ata, G. Subacute bacterial endocarditis from infection by Monilia albicans. *South African M. J.*, 15: 456, 1941.
42. Cassels, D., and Steiner, P. Mycotic endocarditis: report of a case with necropsy: review of the literature. *Am. J. Dis. Child.*, 67: 128, 1944.
43. Luttgens, W. F. Endocarditis in "main line" opium addicts: report of eleven cases. *Arch. Int. Med.*, 83: 653, 1949.
44. Peeler, M. B. and Riley, H. D. Cardiac tamponade due to swallowed foreign body. *Am. J. Dis. Child.*, 93: 308, 1957.
45. Paplanus, S. and Cate, W. R. Monilia endocarditis due to foreign body in heart. Unpublished, as referred to by Peeler and Riley [*44*].
46. Harrell, E. R. and Thompson, G. R. Systemic candidiasis (moniliasis) complicating treatment of bacterial endocarditis with review of literature and report of apparent cure of one case with parenteral mycostatin. *Ann. Int. Med.*, 49: 208, 1958.
47. Kushner, D. S. and Szanto, P. B. Heart failure, fever, and splenomegaly in a morphine addict. *J. A. M. A.*, 166: 2162, 1958.
48. Dick, H. J. and Mullin, E. W. Myxoma of heart complicated by bloodstream infection of Staphylococcus aureus and Candida parapsilosis. *New York State J. Med.*, 56: 856, 1956.
49. Hyun, B. K., Dawson, E. A. and Pence, R. F. Bacterial and mycotic endocarditis following cardiac surgery. *J. Thoracic Surg.*, 35: 298, 1958.
50. Lodder, J. and Kreger-Van Rij, N. J. W. The Yeasts. A Taxonomic Study, pp. 67–69, 459–594. Amsterdam, 1952. Worth Holland Publishing Co.
51. Benham, R. W. Certain monilias parasitic on man. Their identification by morphology and by agglutination. *J. Infect. Dis.*, 49: 183, 1931.
52. Solotorovsky, M., Ironson, E. J., Gregory, F. S. and Winsten, S. Activity of certain diamidines against blastomycosis and candida infection in mice. *Antibiotics & Chemotherap.*, 4: 165, 1954.
53. Mankowski, Z. T. The experimental pathogenicity of various species of candida in Swiss mice. *Tr. New York Acad. Sc.*, 19: 548, 1957.
54. Hasenclever, H. F. Comparative pathogenicity of Candida albicans for mice and rabbits. *J. Bact.*, 78: 105, 1959.
55. Orlath, R. W., Donath, D. H., Johnstone, H. G. and Kerr, W. J. Pulmonary moniliasis. *Ann. Int. Med.*, 35: 97, 1951.
56. Hiatt, J. S. and Martin, D. S. Recovery from pulmonary moniliasis following serum therapy. *J. A. M. A.*, 130: 205, 1946.
57. Hurwitz, A. and Yesner, R. A report of case of localized bronchopulmonary moniliasis successfully treated by surgery. *J. Thoracic Surg.*, 17: 826, 1948.
58. Jones, C. P., Carter, B., Thomas, W. L., Ross, R. A. and Creodick, R. N. Mycotic vulvovaginitis and the vaginal fungi. *Am. J. Obst. & Gynec.*, 54: 738, 1947.
59. Robinson, S. S. and Tasker, S. Chronic latent oral moniliasis. *Arch. Dermat. & Syph.*, 55: 85, 1947.
60. Keeney, E. L. Sodium capylate. A new and effective treatment for moniliasis of skin and mucous membranes. *Bull. Johns Hopkins Hosp.*, 78: 333, 1946.
61. Lipnik, M. J., Kligman, A. M. and Strauss, R. Antibiotics and fungus infections. *J. Invest. Dermat.*, 18: 247, 1952.
62. Seale, E. R. and Clark, W. A. Treatment of intertriginous moniliasis. *South. M. J.*, 41: 926, 1948.
63. Halpert, B. and Wilkins, H. Mycotic meningitis due to candida. *J. A. M. A.*, 130: 932, 1946.
64. Morris, A. A., Kalz, G. G. and Lotspeich, E. S. Ependymitis and meningitis due to Candida albicans. Report of a fatal case of meningitis with comment on its clinical, bacteriologic, and pathologic aspects. *Arch. Neurol. & Psychiat.*, 54: 361, 1945.
65. Craig, W. McK. and Gates, E. M. Metastatic mycotic abscesses of the brain. *Arch. Neurol. & Psychiat.*, 62: 314, 1949.
66. Mendelblatt, D. L. Moniliasis. A review and a report of the first case demonstrating the Candida albicans in the cornea. *Am. J. Ophth.*, 36: 379, 1953.
67. Manchester, P. T. and Georg, L. K. Corneal ulcer due to Candida parapsilosis. *J. A. M. A.*, 171: 1339, 1959.
68. Ohwiler, D. A. and Bricker, E. M. Candida albicans peritonitis successfully treated with amphotericin B. *New England J. Med.*, 260: 488, 1959.
69. Sarot, I. A., Littman, M. L. and Cerruti, M. M. Intrathoracic injections of amphotericin B in the treatment of monilial empyema. *Sea View Hosp. Bull.*, 17: 95, 1959.
70. Marsh, A. P. Esophageal moniliasis. *Am. J. Roent.*, 82: 1063, 1959.
71. Schaberg, A., Hildes, J. A. and Wilt, J. C. Disseminated candidiasis. *Arch. Int. Med.*, 95: 112, 1955.
72. Davis, J. B., Whitakar, J. D., Ding, L. K. and Kiefer, J. H. Disseminated fatal postpartum candidiasis with renal suppuration: case report. *J. Urol.*, 75: 930, 1956.

73. Barrett, B., Volwiler, W., Kirby, W. M. M. and Jensen, C. R. Fatal systemic moniliasis following pancreatitis. *Arch. Int. Med.*, 99: 209, 1957.
74. Braude, A. I. and Rock, J. A. The syndrome of acute disseminated moniliasis in adults. *Arch. Int. Med.*, 104: 91, 1959.
75. Richart, R. and Dammin, G. J. Candida tropicalis as a pathogen for man. *New England J. Med.*, 263: 474, 1960.
76. Van Buren, J. M. Septic retinitis due to Candida albicans. *Arch. Path.*, 65: 137, 1958.
77. Miale, J. B. Candida albicans infection confused with tuberculosis. *Arch. Path.*, 35: 427, 1943.
78. Smith, L. W. and Sane, M. E. Moniliasis with meningeal involvement. *J. Infect. Dis.*, 53: 187, 1933.
79. Kligman, A. M. Are fungus infections increasing as a result of antibiotic therapy? *J. A. M. A.*, 149: 979, 1952.
80. Huppert, M., MacPherson, D. A. and Cazin, J. Pathogenesis of Candida albicans infection following antibiotic therapy. *J. Bact.*, 65: 171, 1953.
81. Campbell, C. C. and Saslaw, S. Enhancement of growth of certain fungi by streptomycin. *Proc. Soc. Exper. Biol. & Med.*, 70: 562, 1949.
82. Grekin, R. H., Cawley, E. P. and Zheutlin, B. Generalized aspergillosis. *Arch. Path.*, 49: 387, 1950.
83. Foley, G. E. and Winter, W. D. Increased mortality following penicillin therapy of chick embryos infected with Candida albicans var. stellatoidea. *J. Infect. Dis.*, 85: 26, 1949.
84. Gausewitz, P. L., Jones, F. S. and Worley, G. Fatal generalized moniliasis: case. *Am. J. Clin. Path.*, 21: 41, 1951.
85. Harris, H. J. Aureomycin and chloramphenicol in brucellosis, with special reference to side effects. *J. A. M. A.*, 142: 161, 1950.
86. Woods, J. W., Manning, I. H. and Patterson, C. N. Monilial infections complicating the therapeutic use of antibiotics. *J. A. M. A.*, 145: 207, 1951.
87. Ormerod, F. C. and Friedmann, I. Case of moniliasis. *Brit. M. J.*, 2: 1439, 1951.
88. McGovern, J. J., Parrott, R. H., Emmons, C. W., Ross, S., Burke, F. G. and Rice, E. C. The effect of aureomycin and chloramphenicol on the fungal and bacterial flora of children. *New England J. Med.*, 248: 397, 1953.
89. Tomaszewski, T. and Poznan, M. D. Side-effects of chloramphenicol and aureomycin, with special reference to oral lesions. *Brit. M. J.*, 1: 388, 1951.
90. Pappenfort, R. B. and Schnall, E. S. Moniliasis in patients treated with aureomycin. *Arch. Int. Med.*, 88: 729, 1951.
91. Sharp, J. L. The growth of Candida albicans during antibiotic therapy. *Lancet*, 1: 390, 1954.
92. Robinson, H. M. Moniliasis complicating antibiotic therapy. *Arch. Dermat. & Syph.*, 70: 640, 1954.
93. Seligmann, E. Virulence enhancing activities of aureomycin on Candida albicans. *Proc. Soc. Exper. Biol. & Med.*, 79: 481, 1952.
94. Merliss, R. R. and Hoffman, A. Steatorrhea following the use of antibiotics. *New England J. Med.*, 245: 328, 1951.
95. Reynell, P. C., Martin, E. A. and Beard, A. W. Monilia peritonitis. *Brit. M. J.*, 1: 919, 1953.
96. Hewitt, W. L. and Williams, B. Chloromycetin (chloramphenicol) in the treatment of infections. *New England J. Med.*, 242: 119, 1950.
97. Moore, M. *In vivo* and *in vitro* effect of aureomycin hydrochloride on syringospora (Monilia, Candida) alibicans. *J. Lab. & Clin. Med.*, 37: 703, 1951.
98. Taylor, H. and Runolf, J. A. Acute moniliasis of the urinary tract. *Lancet*, 1: 1236, 1952.
99. Wolfe, F. W. Moniliasis pneumonia following aureomycin therapy. *Lancet*, 1: 1236, 1952.
100. Beemer, A. M., Pryce, D. M. and Ridell, R. W. Candida albicans infection of the gut. *J. Path. Bact.*, 68: 359, 1954.
101. Bratlund, H. and Holten, C. Moniliasis of mucous membranes and lungs as a complication of treatment with antibiotics, corticotropin and cortisone. *Danish M. Bull.*, 1: 79, 1954.
102. Mankowski, Z. T. and Littleton, B. J. Action of cortisone and ACTH on experimental fungus infections. *Antibiotics & Chemotherap.*, 4: 253, 1954.
103. Seligmann, E. Virulence enhancement of C. albicans by antibiotics and cortisone. *Proc. Soc. Exper. Biol. & Med.*, 83: 778, 1953.
104. Duhig, J. V. and Mead, M. Systemic mycosis due to Monilia albicans. *M. J. Australia*, 1: 179, 1951.
105. Meenan, F. O. C. The incidence of Candida albicans after antibiotic therapy. *Irish J. M. Sc.*, 6: 265, 1957.
106. Craig, J. M. and Farber, S. The development of disseminated visceral mycosis during therapy for acute leukemia. *Am. J. Path.*, 29: 601, 1953.
107. Benham, R. W. and Hopkins, A. M. Yeastlike fungi found on the skin and in the intestines of normal subjects: survey of 100 persons. *Arch. Dermat. & Syph.*, 28: 532, 1933.
108. Miller, C. P. New problems in the treatment of infectious diseases. *Ann. Int. Med.*, 35: 763, 1951.
109. Reiches, A. J. Antibiotic sensitivity and moniliasis. *Arch. Dermat. & Syph.*, 64: 604, 1951.
110. Kligman, A. M., Baldridge, G. D., Schell, G. and Pillsbury, D. M. The effect of cortisone on the pathogenic responses of guinea pigs injected intravenously with fungi, viruses and bacteria. *J. Lab. & Clin. Med.*, 57: 615, 1951.
111. Friedman, J., Roth, F. J., Werder, A. A. and Syverton, J. T. Fulminant experimental blastomycosis produced by employment of roentgen radiation and cortisone. *Fed. Proc.*, 11: 415, 1952.
112. Louria, D. B. and Brown, H. G. The effects of cortisone on experimental fungus infections. *Ann. New York Acad. Sc.*, 89: 39, 1960.
113. Utz, J. P. and Andriole, V. T. Analysis of amphotericin treatment failures in systemic fungal disease. *Ann. New York Acad. Sc.*, 89: 277, 1960.
114. Benham, R. W. Species of candida most frequently isolated from man: methods and criteria for their identification. *J. Chronic Dis.*, 5: 460, 1957.
115. Wessler, S. and Browne, H. R. Candida albicans infection with bloodstream invasion: report of a case with strain clinically resistant to sulfonamide drugs and to penicillin *in vitro*. *Ann. Int. Med.*, 22: 886, 1945.
116. Brown, C., Jr., Propp, S., Guest, C. M., Beebe,

R. T. and Early, L. Fatal fungus infections complicating antibiotic therapy. *J. A. M. A.*, 152: 206, 1953.

117. Matthias, J. Q. and Rees, E. G. Candida septicemia complicating antibiotic therapy. *J. Path. & Bact.*, 71: 512, 1956.

118. Levy, E. S. and Cohen, D. B. Systemic moniliasis and aspergillosis complicating corticotropin therapy. *Arch. Int. Med.*, 95: 118, 1955.

119. Lutembacher, R. Endocardite infectieuse secondaire des cardiaques. *Presse méd.*, 26: 546, 1918.

120. Andriole, V. T. and Hasenclever, H. F. Factors influencing experimental fungus infections. I. Alloxan diabetes. To be published.

121. O'Donovan, D. K. Hypoparathyroidism and moniliasis. *Irish J. M. Sc.*, 6: 255, 1957.

122. Ashford, B. K. Sprue. In: Practice of Medicine, vol. 4, p. 173. Edited by Sloan, L. H. Hagerstown, Md., 1957. W. F. Prior.

123. Graciansky, P. de and Delaporte, J. Yeast Accidents Upon Antibiotic Treatment, vol. 1., Paris, 1956. Masson et Cie.

124. Richet, G., Drouhet, E., Ducrot, H. and Jungers, P. Guérison de deux cas de septicémie à Candida albicans compliquant une anurie grave. Action de l'amphotericine B. *Bull. et mém. soc. méd. d. hôp. de Paris*, 75: 22, 1959.

125. Syverton, J. T., Werder, A. A., Friedman, J., Roth, F. J., Jr., Graham, A. B. and Mira, O. J. Cortisone and roentgen radiation in combination as synergistic agents for production of lethal infections. *Proc. Soc. Exper. Biol. & Med.*, 80: 123, 1952.

126. Loh, W-P. and Baker, E. E. Fecal flora of man after oral administration of chlortetracycline or oxytetracycline. *Arch. Int. Med.*, 95: 74, 1955.

127. Chapman, M. G. Fatal disseminated moniliasis during prolonged antibiotic therapy. *California Med.*, 86: 120, 1957.

128. Scherr, G. H. The effect of cortisone on the course of systemic moniliasis in mice. I. The efficacious effect of cortisone for severe infections. II. An attempt to reverse the toxic effect of cortisone with lowered environmental temperature or somatotrophic hormone (STH). *Mycopathology*, 6: 325, 1953.

129. Roth, F. J., Jr., Friedman, J. and Syverton, J. T. Effects of roentgen radiation and cortisone on susceptibility of mice to Candida albicans. *J. Immunol.*, 78: 122, 1957.

130. Roth, F. J., Jr., Syverton, J. T. and Friedman, J. The effects of roentgen radiation and cortisone upon experimental moniliasis. *Bact. Proc.*, 52: 87, 1952.

131. Hazen, E. L. and Brown, R. Fungicidin, an antibiotic produced by a soil actinomycete. *Proc. Soc. Exper. Biol. & Med.*, 76: 93, 1951.

132. Brown, R. and Hazen, E. L. Nystatin and actidione: two antifungal agents produced by Streptomyces noursei. In: Therapy of Fungus Diseases: An International Symposium. Edited by Sternberg, T. H. and Newcomer, V. D. Boston, 1955. Little, Brown, & Co.

133. Smith, D. T. Therapy for pulmonary and systemic fungus diseases. *Postgrad. Med.*, 20: 18, 1956.

134. Carpenter, A. Studies on candida. In: Therapy of Fungus Diseases: An International Symposium, p. 119. Edited by Sternberg T. H. and Newcomer, V. D. Boston, 1955. Little, Brown & Co.

135. McVay, L. V. and Sprunt, D. H. A study of moniliasis in aureomycin therapy. *Proc. Soc. Exper. Biol. & Med.*, 78: 759, 1951.

136. Metzger, W. I., Wright, L. T. and Di Lorenzo, J. C. Effect of esters of parahydroxybenzoic acid on candida and yeast-like fungi. *J. A. M. A.*, 155: 352, 1954.

137. Lamb, J. H. Combined therapy in histoplasmosis and coccidioidomycosis: methylestosterone and meth-dia-mer-sulfonamides. *Arch. Dermat. & Syph.*, 70: 695, 1954.

138. Campbell, C. C., Hill, G. B. and Brooks, B. E. Therapeutic activity of a new antibiotic, 1968, in mice with experimental histoplasmosis, sporotrichosis and moniliasis. In: Antibiotics Annual 1955–1956, p. 240. Edited by Welch, H. and Marti-Ibanez, F. New York, 1956. Medical Encyclopedia, Inc.

139. Oswald, E. J., Reedy, R. J. and Randall, W. A. An antifungal agent, 1968, produced by a new streptomyces species. In: Antibiotics Annual 1955–1956, p. 236. Edited by Welch, H. and Marti-Ibanez, F. New York, 1956. Medical Encyclopedia, Inc.

140. Lechevalier, H., Acker, R. F., Corke, C. T., Haenseler, C. M. and Waksman, S. A. Candicidin, a new antifungal antibiotic. *Mycologia*, 45: 155, 1953.

141. Larsh, H. W., Silberg, S. L. and Hinton, A. Use of the tissue culture method in evaluating antifungal agents. In: Antibiotics Annual 1956-1957, p. 918. Edited by Welch, H. and Marti-Ibanez, F. New York, 1957. Medical Encyclopedia, Inc.

142. Mountain, D. C. and Krumenacher, F. P. Oral undecylenic acid in the prevention of the so-called monilial complications secondary to the use of aureomycin, chloramphenicol and terramycin. *Am. J. M. Sc.*, 225: 274, 1953.

143. Solotorovsky, M., Ironson, E. J., Gregory, F. J. and Winsten, S. Activity of certain diamidines against blastomycosis and candida infection in mice. *Antibiotics & Chemotherap.*, 4: 165, 1954.

144. Curtis, A. C. The aromatic diamidines, cinnamic acids and nitrostyrenes in the treatment of fungus diseases. In: Therapy of Fungus Diseases: An International Symposium, p. 136. Edited by Sternberg, T. H. and Newcomer, V. D. Boston, 1955. Little, Brown & Co.

145. Kass, I., Sasano, K. T. and Klein, W. S. Treatment of bronchopulmonary moniliasis by dye inhalation. *Dis. Chest*, 21: 205, 1952.

146. Smith, G. M. and Armen, R. N. Pulmonary moniliasis treated by brilliant green aerosol: report of a case. *Ann. Int. Med.*, 43: 1302, 1955.

147. Winston, R. B. and Webster, J. S. A fatal case of pulmonary moniliasis treated with brilliant green aerosol. *Guthrie Clin. Bull.*, 26: 77, 1956.

148. Donovick, R., Pansy, F. E., Stout, H. A., Stander, H., Weinstein, M. J. and Gold, W. Some *in vitro* characteristics of nystatin (mycostatin). In: Therapy of Fungus Diseases: An International Symposium, p. 176. Edited by Sternberg, T. H.

and Newcomer, V. D. Boston, 1955. Little, Brown & Co.

149. Drouhet, E. Therapeutic activity of nystatin (mycostatin) in candida infections. In: Therapy of Fungus Diseases: An International Symposium, p. 211. Edited by Sternberg, T. H. and Newcomer, V. D. Boston, 1955. Little, Brown & Co.

150. Stewart, G. T. Laboratory and clinical studies with nystatin in post antibiotic mycotic infections. *Brit. M. J.*, 1: 658, 1956.

151. Jennison, R. F. and Stenton, P. Sensitivity of candida strains to nystatin. *J. Clin. Path.*, 10: 219, 1957.

152. Campbell, C. C. Therapeutic activity of mycostatin in mice infected with Histoplasma capsulatum, Coccidioides immitis, Cryptococcus neoformans, Candida albicans, or Sporotrichum schenkii. In: Therapy of Fungus Diseases: An International Symposium, p. 255. Edited by Sternberg, T. H. and Newcomer, V. D. Boston, 1955. Little, Brown & Co.

153. Brown, R., Hazen, E. L. and Mason, A. Effect of fungicidin (nystatin) in mice injected with lethal mixtures of aureomycin and Candida albicans. *Science*, 117: 609, 1953.

154. Hazen, E. L., Brown, R. and Mason, A. Protective action of fungicidin (nystatin) in mice against virulence enhancing activity of oxytetracycline on Candida albicans. *Antibiotics & Chemotherap.*, 3: 1125, 1953.

155. Sternberg, T. H., Tarbet, J. E., Newcomer, V. D., Huddleson, H. G., Weir, R. H., Wright, E. T. and Egeberg, R. O. Antifungal effects of nystatin on the fecal flora of animals and man. In: Antibiotics Annual 1953–1954, p. 199. Edited by Welch, H. and Marti-Ibanez, F. New York, 1954. Medical Encyclopedia, Inc.

156. Steinberg, B. A. and Jambor, W. P. The effect of nystatin (mycostatin) on experimental candidiasis in mice and embryonated eggs. In: Therapy of Fungus Diseases: An International Symposium, p. 195. Edited by Sternberg, T. H. and Newcomer, V. D. Boston, 1955. Little, Brown & Co.

157. Hazen, E. L., Brown, R. and Little, G. N. Moniliasis in experimental animals: prophylaxis and therapy with nystatin. In: Therapy of Fungus Diseases: An International Symposium, p. 199. Edited by Sternberg, T. H. and Newcomer, V. D. Boston, 1955. Little, Brown & Co.

158. Eisenberg, G. M., Weiss, W. and Flippin, H. F. Microbiological studies and preliminary clinical experiences with nystatin. I. In vitro susceptibility of Candida albicans. In: Antibiotics Annual 1955–1956, p. 837. Edited by Welch, H. and Marti-Ibanez, F. New York, 1956. Medical Encyclopedia, Inc.

159. Sloane, M. B. A new antifungal antibiotic mycostatin (nystatin), for the treatment of moniliasis: a preliminary report. *J. Invest. Dermat.*, 24: 569, 1955.

160. Huang, N. N., Kendall, N., Lamberti, A. J. and High, R. H. Effects of nystatin on oral moniliasis in infants. In: Antibiotics Annual 1955–1956, p. 711. Edited by Welch, H. and Marti-Ibanez, F. New York, 1956. Medical Encyclopedia, Inc.

161. Robinson, R. C. V. Candida albicans infection of skin and mucous membranes treated with nystatin. In: Antibiotics Annual 1955–1956, p. 851. Edited by Welch, H. and Marti-Ibanez, F. New York, 1956. Medical Encyclopedia, Inc.

162. Dobias, B. Moniliasis in pediatrics. *J. Dis. Child.*, 94: 234, 1957.

163. Graham, J. H., Wright, E. T., Newcomer, V. D. and Sternberg, T. H. The use of nystatin as a topical antifungal agent. In: Therapy of Fungus Diseases: An International Symposium, p. 220. Edited by Sternberg, T. H. and Newcomer, V. D. Boston, 1955. Little, Brown & Co.

164. Dobias, B. Cutaneous moniliasis in pediatrics: diagnosis and treatment with nystatin. In: Therapy of Fungus Diseases: An International Symposium, p. 205. Edited by Sternberg, T. H. and Newcomer, V. D. Boston, 1955. Little, Brown & Co.

165. Wright, E. T., Graham, J. H., Newcomer, V. D. and Sternberg, T. H. The use of nystatin in the treatment of moniliasis. In: Antibiotics Annual 1955–1956, p. 846. Edited by Welch, H. and Marti-Ibanez, F. New York, 1956. Medical Encyclopedia, Inc.

166. Kozinn, P. J., Taschdjian, C. L., Dragutsky, D. and Minsky, A. Treatment of cutaneous candidiasis in infancy and childhood with nystatin and amphotericin B. In: Antibiotics Annual 1956–1957, p. 128. Edited by Welch H. and Marti-Ibanez, F. New York, 1957. Medical Encyclopedia, Inc.

167. Cabaniss, W. H., Manley, W. F. and Swan, R. E. Cutaneous moniliasis in a premature infant. *J. Pediat.*, 50: 480, 1957.

168. Robinson, R. C. V. Cutaneous moniliasis in infants. *J. Pediat.*, 50: 721, 1957.

169. Kozinn, P. J., Taschdjian, C. L., Dragutsky, D. and Minsky, A. Cutaneous candidiasis in early infancy and childhood. *Pediatrics*, 20: 827, 1957.

170. Robinson, R. C. V. Systemic moniliasis treated with mycostatin: case report. *J. Invest. Dermat.*, 24: 375, 1955.

171. Ochoa, A. G. Two cases of abdominal wall moniliasis, after colostomy, treated with nystatin. In: Therapy of Fungus Diseases: An International Symposium, p. 228. Edited by Sternberg, T. H. and Newcomer, V. D. Boston, 1955. Little, Brown & Co.

172. Perl, G., Gutmacher, A. F. and Jakubowicz, H. Vaginal candidiasis: new method of diagnosis and treatment. *Obst. & Gynec.*, 5: 640, 1955.

173. Sarewitz, A. B. Treatment of genitourinary moniliasis with orally administered nystatin. *Ann. Int. Med.*, 42: 1187, 1955.

174. Pace, H. R. and Schantz, S. I. Nystatin (mycostatin) in the treatment of monilial and nonmonilial vaginitis. *J. A. M. A.*, 162: 268, 1956.

175. Jennison, R. F. and Llywelyn-Jones, J. D. Treatment of monilial vaginitis: a clinical trial of nystatin. *Brit. M. J.*, 1: 145, 1957.

176. Thomas, H. H. Candidal vulvovaginitis: treatment with mycostatin. *Obst. & Gynec.*, 9: 163, 1957.

177. Weiss, W., Eisenberg, G. M., Sass, D. K., Kayser, H. L. and Flippin, H. F. Microbiologic studies and preliminary clinical experiences with nystatin. II. Preliminary clinical experiences with

nystatin. In: Antibiotics Annual 1955–1956, p. 842. Edited by Welch, H. and Marti-Ibanez, F. New York, 1956. Medical Encyclopedia, Inc.

178. Beckmann, A. J. and Navarro, J. E. Pneumonia complicating oral thrush treated with mycostatin, a new antifungal antibiotic. *J. Pediat.*, 46: 587, 1955.

179. Newcomer, V. D., Wright, E. T. and Sternberg, T. H. The effect of nystatin when administered simultaneously with tetracycline upon the yeast flora of the gastrointestinal tract of man. In: Antibiotics Annual 1954–1955, p. 686. Edited by Welch, H. and Marti-Ibanez, F. New York, 1955. Medical Encyclopedia, Inc.

180. Brabander, J. O. W., Blank, F. and Butas, C. A. Intestinal moniliasis in adults. *Canad. M. A. J.*, 77: 478, 1957.

181. Halde, C., Wright, E. T., Pollard, W. H., Newcomer, V. D. and Sternberg, T. H. The effect of amphotericin B upon the yeast flora of the gastrointestinal tract of man. In: Antibiotics Annual 1956–1957, p. 123. Edited by Welch, H. and Marti-Ibanez, F. New York, 1957. Medical Encyclopedia, Inc.

182. Alter, R. L., Jones, C. P. and Carter, B. The treatment of mycotic vulvovaginitis with propionate vaginal jelly. *Am. J. Obst. & Gynec.*, 53: 241, 1947.

183. Hopkins, J. G., Weld, J. T. and Kesten, B. M. The treatment of monilia (Candida albicans) infections with carbowax-sulfur ointment (a preliminary report). *J. Invest. Dermat.*, 18: 419, 1952.

184. Swartz, J. H. in discussion on Halde, C. et al. [*187*].

185. Sternberg, T. H., Wright, E. T. and Oura, M. A new antifungal antibiotic amphotericin B. In: Antibiotics Annual 1955–1956, p. 566. Edited by Welch, H. and Marti-Ibanez, F. New York, 1956. Medical Encyclopedia, Inc.

186. Gold, W., Stout, H. A., Pagano, J. F. and Donovick, R. Amphotericins A and B, antifungal antibiotics produced by a Streptomycete. I. *In vitro* studies. In: Antibiotics Annual 1955–1956, p. 579. Edited by Welch, H. and Marti-Ibanez, F. New York, 1956. Medical Encyclopedia, Inc.

187. Halde, C., Newcomer, V. D., Wright, E. T. and Sternberg, T. H. An evaluation of amphotericin B *in vitro* and *in vivo* in mice against Coccidioides immitis and Candida albicans, and preliminary observations concerning the administration of amphotericin B to man. *J. Invest. Dermat.*, 28: 217, 1957.

188. Steinberg, B. A., Jambor, W. P. and Suydam, L. O. Amphotericins A and B: Two new antifungal antibiotics possessing high activity against deep-seated and superficial mycoses. In: Antibiotics Annual 1955–1956, p. 574. Edited by Welch, H. and Marti-Ibanez, F. New York, 1956. Medical Encyclopedia, Inc.

189. Summary of information for clinical investigators—Fungizone-Squibb-amphotericin B, New York, Medical Division, E. R. Squibb & Sons, March 1957.

190. Fungizone for Infusion: Squibb amphotericin B, Medical Division, E. R. Squibb & Sons, November 1957.

191. Procknow, J. J. and Loosli, C. G. Treatment of the deep mycoses. *Arch. Int. Med.*, 101: 765, 1958.

192. Utz, J. P. and Treger, A. The current status of chemotherapy of systemic fungal disease. *Ann. Int. Med.*, 51: 1220, 1959.

193. Louria, D. B. Some aspects of the absorption, distribution and excretion of amphotericin B in man. *Antibiotic Med. & Clin. Therap.*, 5: 295, 1958.

194. Newcomer, V. D., Sternberg, T. H., Wright, E. T. and Reisner, R. M. Current status of amphotericin B in the treatment of the systemic fungus infections. *J. Chronic Dis.*, 9: 353, 1959.

195. Fraser, W. M. and Knox, J. M. Amphotericin as a topical antifungal antibiotic. *Arch. Dermat.*, 80: 436, 1959.

196. Seabury, J. H. and Dascomb, H. E. Experience with amphotericin B. *Ann. New York Acad. Sc.*, 89: 202, 1960.

197. Newcomer, V. D., Sternberg, T. H., Wright, E. T., Reisner, R. M., McNall, E. G. and Sorensen, L. J. The treatment of systemic fungus infections with amphotericin B. *Ann. New York Acad. Sc.*, 89: 221, 1960.

198. Dutcher, J. D., Young, M. D., Sherman, J. H., Hibbits, W. and Walters, D. J. Chemical studies of amphotericin B. I. Preparation of the hydrogenation product and isolation of mycosamine and acetolysis products. In: Antibiotics Annual 1956–1957, p. 866. Edited by Welch, H. and Marti-Ibanez, F. New York, 1957. Medical Encyclopedia, Inc.

199. Goldman, H. J., Littman, M. L., Oppenheimer, G. D. and Glickman, S. I. Monilial cystitis—effective treatment with instillations of amphotericin B. *J. A. M. A.*, 174: 359, 1960.

200. Hasenclever, H. F. and Mitchell, W. O. Pathogenicity of Candida albicans and Candida tropicalis. *Sabouraudia*, in press.

201. Hyun, B. H. and Collier, F. C. Mycotic endocarditis following intracardiac operations. *New England J. Med.*, 263: 1339, 1960.

202. Utz, J. P., Andriole, V. T. and Emmons, C. W. Chemotherapeutic activity of X-5079C in systemic mycoses of man. *Am. Rev. Resp. Dis.*, 84: 514, 1961.

203. Boldesco, J., Duca, E., Negoïtza, C. and Marco, C. Endocardite mycosique A. Candida guilliermondi. *Sem. hôp. Paris*, 36: 3181, 1960.

204. Persellin, R. H., Haring, O. M. and Lewis, F. J. Fungal endocarditis following cardiac surgery. *Ann. Int. Med.*, 54: 127, 1961.

205. Wilson, R. M. Candida endocarditis *J. A. M. A.*, 177: 332, 1961.

206. Kay, J. H., Bernstein, S., Feinstein, D. and Biddle, M. Surgical cure of Candida albicans endocarditis with open-heart surgery. *New England J. Med.*, 264: 907, 1961.

207. Heineman, H. S., Yunis, E. J., Siemenski, J. and Braude, A. Chlamydospores and dimorphism in Candida albicans endocarditis. *Arch. Int. Med.*, 108: 126, 1961.

Focal Glomerular Lesions in Fungal Endocarditis

WILLIAM C. ROBERTS, M.D., and ALAN S. RABSON, M.D.
Bethesda, Maryland

FOCAL AREAS OF NECROSIS and sclerosis have frequently been seen in the renal glomeruli of autopsied patients with subacute endocarditis due to bacteria. These glomerular lesions have been called "focal embolic (endocarditic) glomerulonephritis," with the implication that they were the result of multiple small emboli, which were dislodged from cardiac vegetations and landed in the glomerular capillaries. Allen (1) summarized the reasons for rejecting the embolic theory of the pathogenesis of these lesions and agreed with Longcope (2) who considered these lesions to be of an allergic nature. Since fungal infections in man are commonly associated with manifestations of hypersensitivity to the organisms, the presence of focal glomerular lesions in some patients with endocarditis caused by fungi might be expected. Focal glomerular lesions have been mentioned in four (3–6) of the 44 autopsy-proven cases of endocarditis caused by the higher fungi (*Eumycetes*) reported in the literature (3, 7, 8), and all four have been in patients with endocarditis caused by organisms of the Candida species. Nine (3, 8) of these 44 patients with fungal endocarditis were studied clinically and at autopsy at the Clinical Center of the National Institutes of Health, and one of the nine showed the typical renal lesion of "focal embolic glomerulonephritis." The latter patient is the subject of this communication.

Received August 14, 1961; accepted for publication November 22, 1961.

From the Pathologic Anatomy Department, Clinical Center, National Institutes of Health, Bethesda, Maryland.

Requests for reprints should be addressed to William C. Roberts, M.D., Pathologic Anatomy Department, Clinical Center, National Institutes of Health, Bethesda 14, Maryland.

CASE REPORT

A 26-year-old Puerto Rican man (C.C. No. 02-78-74), who was a narcotic addict, was transferred to the Clinical Center (National Institute of Allergy and Infectious Diseases) from a federal penitentiary hospital two months prior to death. He gave no history of rheumatic heart disease. He was in good health until 11 months before death, when he experienced acute left upper quadrant abdominal pain, and was believed to have a splenic infarct. Shortly after this episode he had the onset of fever which persisted until his death. A heart murmur and splenomegaly also were noted, and three blood cultures were positive for *Candida parapsilosis*. Hemolytic *Staphylococcus aureus*, coagulase negative, grew in one of the blood cultures. The patient was treated with penicillin, streptomycin, and neoantimosan (Fuadin) without clinical response. Five months before death, anemia and thrombocytopenia were noted. His urine showed hematuria, pyuria, albuminuria, and cylindruria.

On admission to the Clinical Center, his temperature was 38.6 C; heart rate, 132/min; respiratory rate, 30/min; and blood pressure, 100/60 mm Hg. He was chronically ill, thin, and pale. Petechiae were present in the lower conjunctival sac and over the right buttock. The heart was not enlarged. A loud, high-pitched, blowing systolic murmur was heard over the precordium. The liver and spleen were markedly enlarged and tender. There was clubbing of the fingers bilaterally.

During the hospital course, the hemoglobin ranged from 6.9 to 8.9 g/100 ml; platelet count, from 44,000 to 120,000/mm^3; and leukocyte count, from 2,400 to 4,300/mm^3. The leukocyte differential count showed more than 50% lymphocytes on all determinations. The erythrocyte sedimentation rate (Westergren method) was 104 to 140 mm/hr; blood urea nitrogen was 36 to 63 mg/100 ml; uric acid, 6.7 to 9 mg/100 ml; creatinine, 2.6 to 3.5 mg/100 ml; calcium, 8.4 to 9.2 mg/100 ml; alkaline phosphatase, 20 to 53 King-Armstrong units; albumin, 1.6 to 2.1, and globulin, 5.5 to 6.5 g/100 ml; bromsulphalein retention in the blood, 6 to 16% at 45 min; cephalin flocculation test, 3 to 4+; and thymol turbidity, 13 to 20 units. Multiple urinalyses revealed the presence of innumerable erythrocytes and leukocytes with persistent 1 to 3+ albumin, and "occasional" to a "moderate number" of granular casts. Serial Addis counts disclosed persistently abnormal values for erythrocytes, leukocytes, and casts. Nine urine cultures were positive for *Klebsiella* and hemolytic *Staphylococcus albus,* coagulase negative, hemolytic *Staphylococcus aureus,* coagulase positive, or both, but colony counts were less than 50,000 bacteria/ml of urine, except once when the count was greater than 1 million/ml of urine. The phenolsulfonphthalein test showed 12% excretion at the end of two hours, and the Fishberg concentration test showed maximal concentration to be only 1.010. Thirty-one blood cultures and one bone marrow culture were positive for *Candida parapsilosis.* None of the blood cultures were positive for bacteria.

Two days after admission to the Clinical Center, the patient had clinical and electrocardiographic evidence of a massive anterior wall myocardial infarct. His last two months of life were characterized by a progressive downhill course with congestive heart failure, marked personality changes, slurring of speech, ptosis of the left upper lid, increasing weakness, and enlargement of the liver and spleen. The day prior to death he had an extension of the previous myocardial infarct, and he exhibited ventricular fibrillation at death the following day. During the last two months of life, he was treated with amphotericin B via a nasogastric tube and an experimental antifungal drug (RO-2), without apparent benefit.

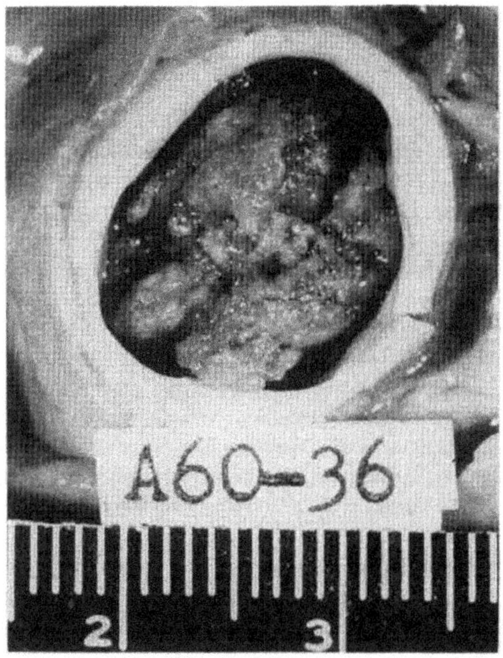

FIGURE 1A. Aortic valve viewed from above. The large vegetations almost totally occlude the aortic valve orifice.

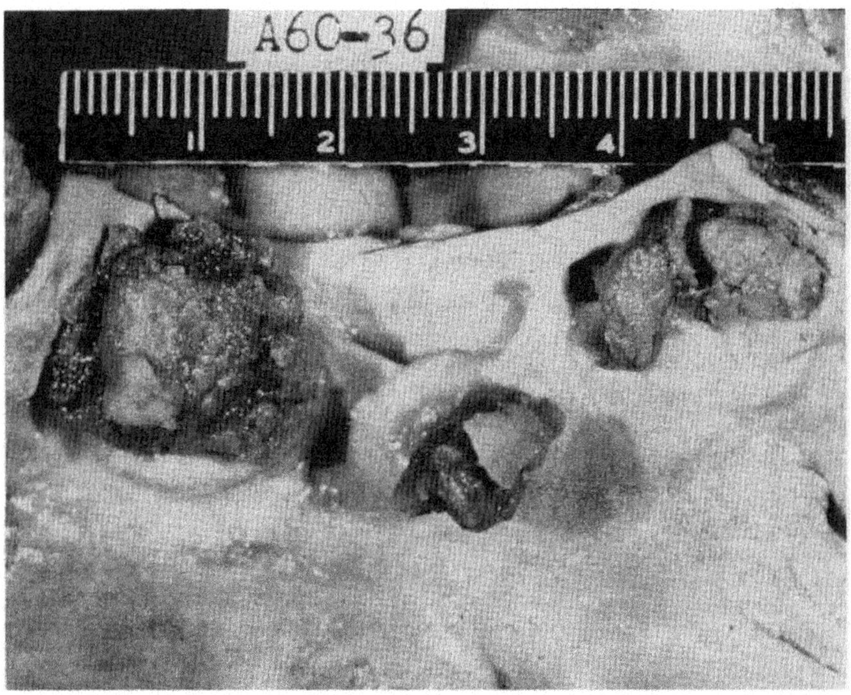

FIGURE 1B. Aortic valve opened. Note the presence of a vegetation on the ventricular aspect of each of the cusps of the aortic valve.

Autopsy Findings

Necropsy was started 15 hours after death. See Figures 1A–1D. Effusions were present in the abdominal cavity (925 milliliters), pleural spaces (420 and 150 milliliters), and pericardial sac (70 milliliters). The heart weighed 400 grams. The right and left atria, tricuspid and mitral valves, right ventricle, and pulmonic valve were unremarkable. There was aneurysmal dilatation of an infarct, 5 by 3.5 by 0.2 centimeters, in the anterior wall of the left ventricle. The left anterior descending coronary artery was totally occluded just proximal to the myocardial infarct. A soft, friable, greyish vegetation was present on the ventricular aspect of each of the three cusps of the aortic valve (Figures 1A and 1B). The largest vegetation measured 2 centimeters in longest diameter.

The kidneys (Figure 2A) were enlarged; the left weighed 190 grams, and the right, 180 grams. The surface of each kidney was glistening, greyish purple, and smooth, except for two focal indentations in the right kidney. No petechiae were noted on the surfaces. On section, the corticomedullary junctions were well delineated. The ureters were widely patent. The

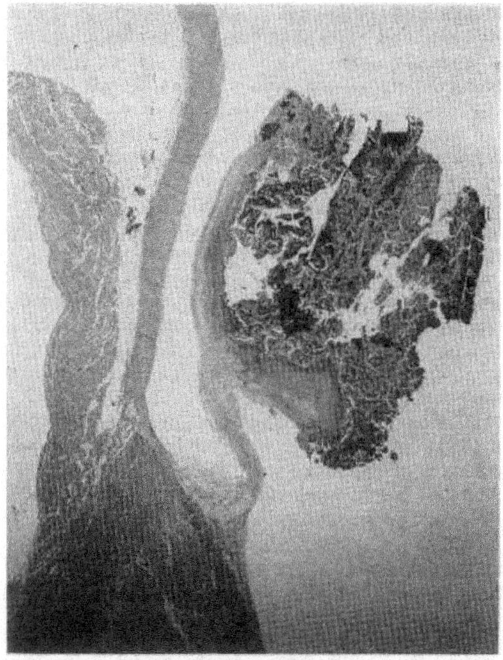

Figure 1C. Photomicrograph of section through the largest vegetation illustrated in Figure 1B. The darker areas in the vegetation represent collections of candida organisms. Note that the sinus of Valsalva is free of vegetation. Gomori's methenamine silver stain, × 10.

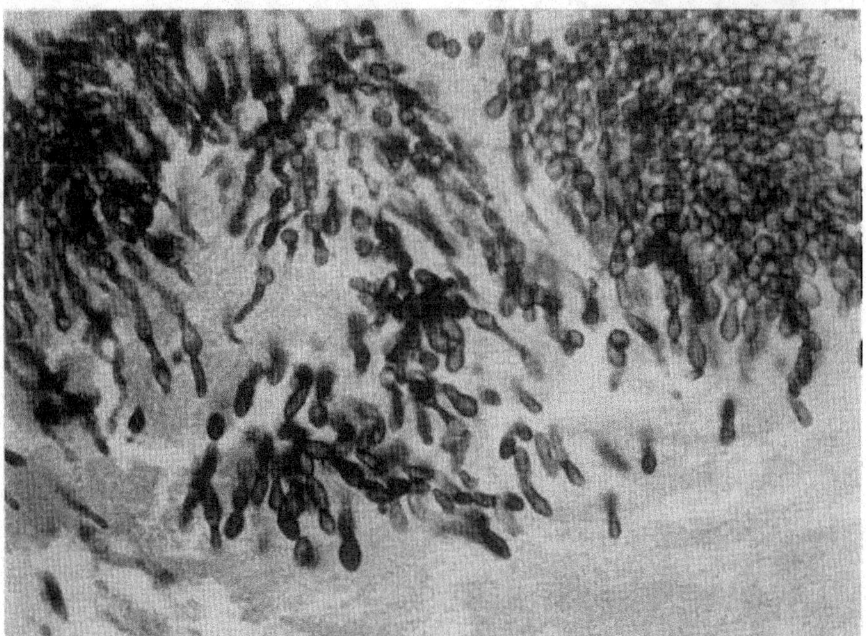

Figure 1D. Photomicrograph (high power) of candida organisms present in vegetation shown in Figure 1C. Gomori's methenamine silver, × 495.

large renal arteries and veins were free of atheromata and of emboli.

The spleen weighed 1,000 grams and contained several infarcts. The liver weighed 3,650 grams and, on section, had a nutmeg appearance. There was marked generalized lymphadenopathy. The left internal iliac and left femoral arteries were occluded by soft yellow emboli. Cultures were taken of the aortic valve vegetation, spleen, liver, hilar lymph node, and left femoral artery and all grew *C. parapsilosis.*

Microscopically, candida organisms were identified in the aortic valve vegetations, left anterior descending coronary artery, myocardial infarct, left femoral artery, and brain. The vegetations consisted of eosinophilic and basophilic debris, fibrous tissue, and large colonies of candida organisms (Figures 1C and 1D). The left anterior descending coronary artery was totally occluded except for a small organizing channel which contained candida organisms. Sections of the myocardial infarct disclosed that the myocardial fibers were largely replaced by fibrous tissue, which contained macrophages, lymphocytes, plasma cells, fibroblasts, Langhans type giant cells, and a few candida organisms.

In the sections from the kidneys, there were focal areas of fibrinoid necrosis and fibrosis in numerous glomeruli (Figures 2B–2D). Some of the glomeruli were completely hyalinized. Approximately 90% of the glomeruli were involved in some manner by the fibrinous and fibrous processes. No abnormalities were noted in the uninvolved glomeruli or in the uninvolved portions of the affected glomeruli. The diseased portions of the glomeruli were frequently adherent to Bowman's capsule. There was no cellular proliferation in the glomerular tufts. Proliferation of the epithelium of Bowman's capsule, however, to form epithelial crescents, occasionally was seen. The basement membrane of involved glomeruli was usually thickened. In some places, it was thickened in the absence of involvement of the glomerular tufts. Heidenhain's azan modification of Mallory's connective tissue stain disclosed that most of the focal glomerular lesions were of the "healed fibrous" type as described by Bell (9, 10). The "fresh hyalin" lesion of Bell was seen only occasionally, and then frequently was associated with a "healed fibrous" lesion in the same glomerulus. Red blood cells were present to a limited extent in Bowman's space and commonly were seen in the lumen of the tubules. The tubules immediately adjacent to some of

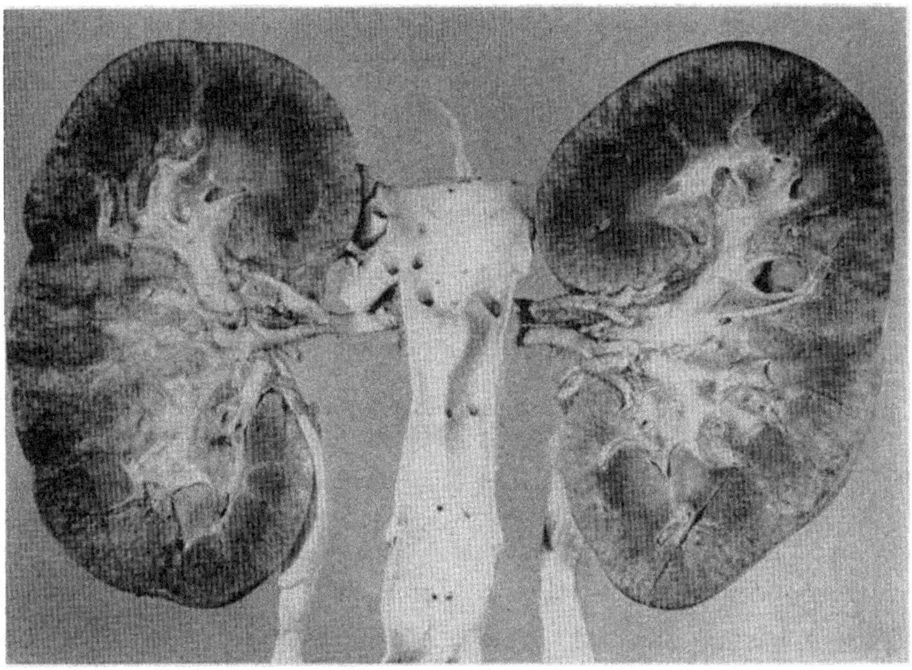

FIGURE 2A. Surface of cut section of each kidney, showing marked congestion.

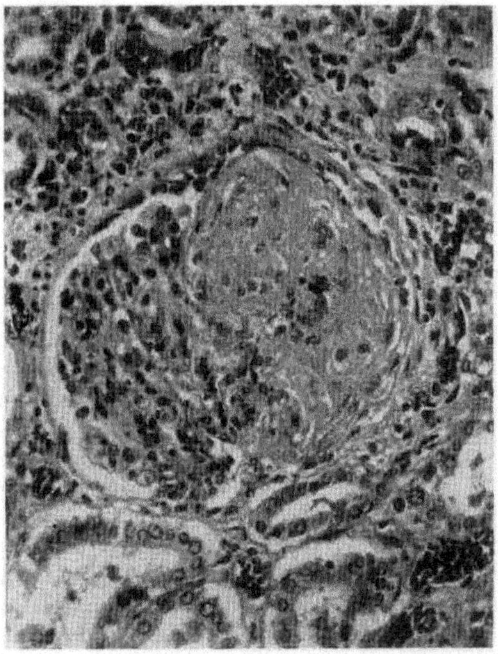

FIGURE 2B. Photomicrograph of kidney showing focal glomerular lesion which is adherent to Bowman's capsule. Hematoxylin and eosin stain, × 310.

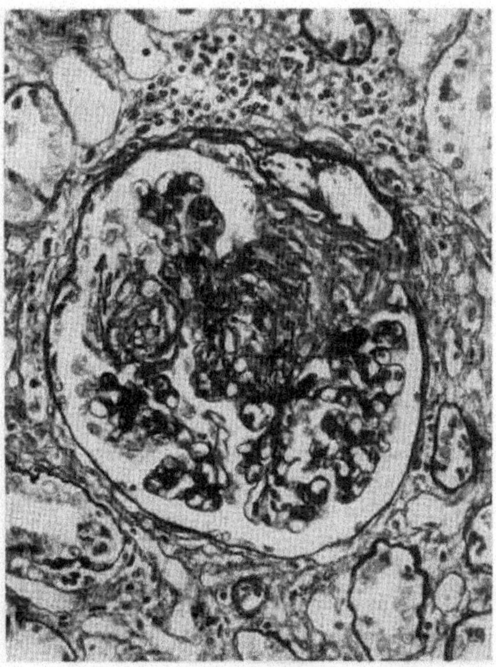

FIGURE 2C. Photomicrograph of renal glomerulus demonstrating "focal embolic glomerulonephritis." Some malpighian tufts are hyalinized; other tufts are normal. Periodic acid-Schiff stain, × 310.

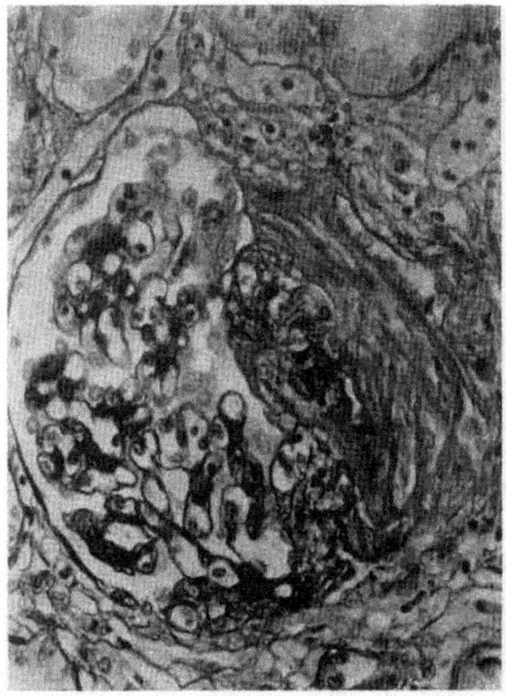

FIGURE 2D. Photomicrograph of glomerulus. Periodic acid-Schiff stain, × 415.

the more severely involved glomeruli were atrophic. Prussian blue stain revealed the presence of iron pigment in numerous tubular cells, and in the lumina of some tubules. Hyaline and granular casts also were present in the lumina of many tubules. The interstitial tissue contained many focal collections of lymphocytes and plasma cells. No fungi or bacteria were identified in the sections from the kidneys.

COMMENT

"Focal embolic glomerulonephritis" at one time was considered to be associated only with subacute streptococcal endocarditis (11, 12). Subsequently, it was seen in endocarditis produced by a number of other bacteria (13). Furthermore, "focal embolic glomerulonephritis" has been reported in septicemia without endocarditis (9, 14), in rheumatic endocarditis (9), in acute bacterial endocarditis—that is, of less than six weeks' duration—(9), and in systemic lupus erythematosus (15, 16). The use of the renal biopsy has disclosed the presence of focal glomerular lesions in a group of patients who heretofore would not have been suspected of having this disorder. Bates, Jennings, and Earle (17) found focal glomerular lesions on renal biopsy in four of ten patients with proteinuria, hematuria, and pharyngitis, without bacterial or immunological evidence of a recent hemolytic streptococcal infection. Heptinstall and Joekes (16) reported "focal glomerulonephritis" in 13 of 100 patients from whom renal biopsies were obtained because of some urinary abnormality (usually proteinuria and hematuria). Four of the patients were believed to have systemic lupus erythematosus or polyarteritis nodosa, three appeared to have Schönlein-Henoch purpura, and the remainder would have been diagnosed clinically as having Ellis type II glomerulonephritis had the renal biopsies not been done.

The cause of "focal embolic glomerulonephritis" has not been definitely determined. Löhlein (18), Baehr (11, 12), Fahr (14), and Bell (9) ascribed the glomerular lesions to the embolization of minute fragments from the vegetations on the heart valves. However, there are several reasons, which Allen (1) has summarized, to doubt this concept. First, bacteria rarely are seen in the involved glomeruli. Second, focal glomerular lesions are rarely found in acute endocarditis, which has even more friable vegetations than does the subacute variety. Third, focal glomerular lesions are seen, although rarely, in the presence of bacteremia alone, without endocarditis, and in certain collagen diseases. In addition, "focal embolic glomerulonephritis" has been seen with endocarditis that involved only valves on the right side of the heart (19). Fourth, it is difficult to accept the idea that hundreds of approximately equal-sized minute emboli are dislodged from a vegetation and seed only one organ, the kidneys, practically to the exclusion of others. Fifth, "focal embolic glomerulonephritis" cannot be produced experimentally by injecting solid particles into the blood stream of an animal. Thus, since these focal glomerular lesions do not appear to result from the implantation of minute emboli in the glomerular capillaries, since they occur in the absence of endocarditis, as well as in its presence, and since there usually is no inflammatory response in the glomeruli, the terms "embolic," "endocarditic," and "-nephritic" should be discarded. We favor, as does Fishberg (13), simply the descriptive term, "focal glomerular lesions." (As pointed out by Heptinstall and Joekes (16), the glomerular lesions are local as well as focal. The "local" refers to the condition in which only a part of an individual glomerulus is involved by the lesion and the "focal," to the condition in which some glomeruli are involved and others are uninvolved, the latter being normal.)

Since the embolic mechanism seems untenable, the immuno-allergic theory has found much favor. Originally suggested by Longcope (2) and advanced later by Allen (1), this idea ascribes the glomerular lesion to sensitization of the glomerular capillaries, to the bacteria themselves, or to the products of the bacteria present in the blood. This hypothesis is consistent with the occurrence of "focal embolic glomerulonephritis" in occasional cases of acute bacterial endocarditis, in bacteremias without endocarditis, and in isolated right-sided endocarditis. Since it is known that candida organisms are good antigens, the immuno-allergic theory also is consistent with the occurrence of "focal embolic glomerulonephritis" in candida endocarditis. Drake (20) has shown that 45% of normal human sera agglutinate *C. albicans*, and that approximately 40 or 50% of adults show a positive skin test to vaccine of *C. albicans*. It seems reasonable to believe that the same mechanisms which produce "focal embolic glomerulonephritis" in bacterial endocarditis also may play a role in the focal glomerulonephritis associated with candida endocarditis.

Of the 44 cases reported of endocarditis caused by the higher fungi and proven at autopsy, 23 were due to candida species (3, 21, 22). The endocarditis in each of the four patients with well-documented "focal embolic glomerulonephritis" was caused by organisms of the candida species. No focal glomerular lesions have been reported in patients with endocarditis due to *Coccidioides immitis*, *Cryptococcus neoformans*, *Blastomyces dermatitidis*, *Histoplasma capsulatum*, *Aspergillus*, or *Mucor*, although several of these fungi appear to be good antigens. "Focal embolic glomerulonephritis" has been mentioned in the protocols of three other patients (22–24) who died of endocarditis due to fungi, probably of candida species, but these cases are omitted from this report because of inadequate diagnostic information. None of the four patients with "focal embolic glomerulonephritis" listed in Table 1 had an associated bacterial endocarditis. The patient reported by Kushner and Szanto (21), with "focal embolic glomerulonephritis" associated with fungal endocarditis, also had bacteria in the cardiac vegetations and is therefore excluded from this report. The incidence of "focal embolic glomerulonephritis" associated with fungal endocarditis may be less than 10%, whereas the incidence of focal glomerulonephritis associated with subacute bacterial endocarditis is in the order of 50 to 90% (9–11). There was no mention of organs other than the heart in several reports of patients with fungal endocarditis; consequently, the former percentage is probably low. Diffuse glomerulonephritis is uncommon in bacterial endocarditis and has not been mentioned in any reports of patients with fungal endocarditis.

Table 1 summarizes the renal findings in the documented cases of "focal embolic glomerulonephritis" associated with fungal endocarditis. Examination of the urinary sediment is of little help in distinguishing "focal embolic glomerulonephritis" from diffuse glomerulonephritis. Although the hematuria associated with focal glomerular lesions is classically microscopic and transient, massive, though intermittent, hematuria does occur (patient 2, Table 1). Leukocytes were described in the urinary sediment of two patients, but pyelonephritis was present histologically in all four patients (Table 1) at autopsy. Bacteria rarely are present in the glomeruli of patients with focal glomerular lesions associated with subacute endocarditis due to bacteria. In contrast, fungi were seen in the kidneys in two of the four patients with "focal embolic glomerulonephritis" associated with endocarditis due to fungi. The fungi were present in the glomeruli as well as in the lumina of the tubules and in the interstitial tissues. In each of the two patients with *C. tropicalis* without endocarditis reported by Richart and Dammin (25), candida organisms were present in the glomeruli, as well as intratubularly and interstitially. In addition, in one of their patients, there was "partial destruction of the glomerular tuft without inflammatory response." The latter finding may represent an example of "focal embolic glomerulonephritis" associated with candidiasis without endocarditis.

Uremia was present in two of the four patients with focal glomerular lesions associated

TABLE 1. Patients with Focal Glomerular Lesions (Focal Embolic Glomerulonephritis) in Fungal Endocarditis

Patients	1	2	3	4
Author	Pasternack	Neil-Kohlmeier	Neil-Kohlmeier	Present Authors
Year	1942	1953	1953	1962
Age (years), sex	45 M	41 M	60 F	26 M
Length of illness (months)	1¼	3	2	11
Location of endocarditis (heart valve)	Aortic	Aortic Mitral	Aortic Mitral	Aortic
Organism causing endocarditis	*C. parapsilosis*	*C. albicans*	*C. guilliermondi*	*C. parapsilosis*
Renal function				
Specific gravity		1.018	1.027	1.010
Pyuria		0	+	+
Hematuria		+	0	+
Cylindruria		+	+	+
Uremia		+		+
Renal morphology				
Pyelonephritis	+	+	+	+
Infarcts	+	0	0	0
Size	↑	Normal	Normal	↑
"Flea-bitten" surface (petechiae)	0	+	0	0
No. of glomeruli involved	"Occasional"	"Severe"	"Slight"	90%

with fungal endocarditis (Table 1). Uremia on the basis of "focal embolic glomerulonephritis" associated with subacute bacterial endocarditis has been considered a rarity. Indeed, Libman is quoted by Fishberg (13) as saying that in 800 cases of subacute bacterial endocarditis he never had seen uremia due to focal glomerular lesions. Boyarsky, Burnett, and Barker (26), however, found reports in the literature of 16 patients with "focal embolic glomerulonephritis" that produced uremia, and they added one of their own. Baehr (11) felt that renal function was rarely altered in the presence of focal glomerular lesions because the uninvolved portions of the damaged glomeruli remained normal, leaving enough healthy glomerular tissue to maintain normal glomerular functions.

Summary

"Focal embolic glomerulonephritis" may occur in patients with endocarditis due to organisms other than bacteria, and indeed may occur occasionally in patients without endocarditis. A young man is presented who had endocarditis due to a fungus (*Candida parapsilosis*) and whose kidneys at autopsy showed the classical lesion of "focal embolic glomerulonephritis." It is mentioned that "focal embolic glomerulonephritis" probably occurs, proportionally, less commonly in fungal than in bacterial endocarditis. This lesion has been described in only four of 44 autopsied patients who died of fungal endocarditis, and in each of the four the endocarditis was caused by organisms of the candida species. The term "focal embolic glomerulonephritis" is considered unsatisfactory, since the process appears not to be "embolic," and there rarely is an inflammatory response in the glomeruli. The descriptive term "focal glomerular lesions" is preferred.

Acknowledgment

The authors wish to thank Doctors Arthur Allen and Paul Kimmelsteil for reviewing the histological sections from the kidneys, and Doctors Louis B. Thomas and Ross C. MacCardle for reviewing the manuscript.

Summario in Interlingua

"Focal glomerulonephritis embolic" pote occurrer in patientes con endocarditis causate per organismos altere que bacterios; de facto, illo pote occurrer in patientes qui ha nulle endocarditis del toto. Es presentate le caso de un juvene homine qui habeva endocarditis causate per un fungo (*Candida parapsilosis*) e in qui le renes revelava al necropsia le lesion classic de "focal glomerulonephritis embolic." Es mentionate que "focal glomerulonephritis embolic" occurre probabilemente in un plus basse procentage del casos in endocarditis fungal que in endocarditis bacterial. Iste lesion esseva notate in solmente quatro de 44 necropsiate patientes morte ab endocarditis fungal, e in omne ille quatro casos le endocarditis esseva causate per organismos del specie Candida. Le termino "focal glomerulonephritis embolic" es considerate como non satisfactori in vista del facto que le processo non pare esser embolic e que il occurre rarmente un responsa inflammatori in le glomerulos. Le termino descriptive "focal lesiones glomerular" es preferite.

References

1. Allen, A. C.: *The Kidney, Medical and Surgical Diseases.* Grune & Stratton, Inc., New York, 1951, pp. 164–170.
2. Longcope, W. T.: The susceptibility of man to foreign proteins. *Amer. J. Med. Sci.* 152: 625, 1916.
3. Andriole, V. T., Kravetz, H. M., Roberts, W. C., Utz, J. P.: Candida endocarditis: clinical and pathological studies. *Amer. J. Med.* 32: 251, 1962.
4. Pasternack, J. G.: Subacute monilia endocarditis: new clinical and pathological entity. *Amer. J. Clin. Path.* 12: 496, 1942.
5. Niel, K.: Zur Klinik der Candidainfektionen. *Klin. Med. (Wien)* 8: 49, 1953.
6. Kohlmeier, W.: Zur Kenntnis der Candidainfektionen. *Klin. Med. (Wien)* 8: 54, 1953.
7. Cooper, T., Morrow, A. G., Roberts, W. C., Herman, L. G.: Postoperative endocarditis due to candida: clinical observations and the experimental production of the lesion. *Surgery* 50: 341, 1961.
8. Merchant, R. K., Louria, D. B., Geisler, P. H., Edgcomb, J. H., Utz, J. P.: Fungal endocarditis: review of the literature and report of three cases. *Ann. Intern. Med.* 48: 242, 1958.
9. Bell, E. T.: Glomerular lesions associated with endocarditis. *Amer. J. Path.* 8: 639, 1932.
10. Bell, E. T.: *Renal Diseases,* Lea & Febiger, Philadelphia, 1950, pp. 165–169.
11. Baehr, G.: Glomerular lesions of subacute bacterial endocarditis. *Amer. J. Med. Sci.* 144: 327, 1912.
12. Baehr, G.: Glomerular lesions of subacute bacterial endocarditis. *J. Exp. Med.* 15: 330, 1912.

13. Fishberg, A. M.: *Hypertension and Nephritis*, 5th ed., Lea & Febiger, Philadelphia, 1954, pp. 665–671.

14. Fahr, T.: In *Handbuch der Speziellen pathologischen Anatomie und Histologie*, vol. 6, pt. 1, ed. by Henke, F., and Lubarsch, O. Springer, Berlin, 1925, pp. 355–362.

15. Klemperer, P., Pollack, A. D., Baehr, G.: Pathology of disseminated lupus erythematosus. *Arch. Path.* 32: 569, 1941.

16. Heptinstall, R. H., Joekes, A. M.: Focal glomerulonephritis. *Quart. J. Med.* (new series) 28: 329, 1959.

17. Bates, R. C., Jennings, R. B., Earle, D. P.: Acute nephritis unrelated to group A hemolytic streptococcus infection: report of ten cases. *Amer. J. Med.* 23: 510, 1957.

18. Löhlein, M.: Ueber hämorrhagische Nierenaffektionen bei; chronischer ulzeröser Endokarditis. (Embolische nichteiterige Herdnephritis.) *Med. Klin.* 6: 375, 1910.

19. Bain, R. C., Edwards, J. E., Scheifley, C. H., Geraci, J. E.: Right-sided bacterial endocarditis and endarteritis. *Amer. J. Med.* 24: 98, 1958.

20. Drake, C. H.: Quoted by Dubos, R. J. in *Bacterial and Mycotic Infections of Man*, 2d ed., J. B. Lippincott Company, Philadelphia, 1952, p. 664.

21. Kushner, D. S., Szanto, P. B.: Heart failure, fever, and splenomegaly in a morphine addict. *J. A. M. A.* 166: 2162, 1958.

22. Cassels, D., Steiner, P.: Mycotic endocarditis: report of a case with necropsy: review of the literature. *Amer. J. Dis. Child.* 67: 128, 1944.

23. Caplan, H.: Monilia (candida) endocarditis following treatment with antibiotics. *Lancet* 2: 957, 1955.

24. Nicolaides, N. J.: Fungal endocarditis complicating staphylococcal endocarditis. *Med. J. Aust.* 1: 793, 1957.

25. Richart, R., Dammin, G. J.: Candida tropicalis as a pathogen for man. *New Engl. J. Med.* 263: 474, 1960.

26. Boyarsky, S., Burnett, J. M., Barker, W. H.: Renal failure in embolic glomerulonephritis as a complication of subacute bacterial endocarditis. *Bull. Johns Hopkins Hosp.* 84: 207, 1949.

Bacterial Endocarditis Following Aortic Valve Replacement

Clinical and Pathologic Correlations

By Lawrence H. Cohn, M.D., William C. Roberts, M.D., S. David Rockoff, M.D., and Andrew G. Morrow, M.D.

In recent years numerous devices for prosthetic replacement of the diseased mitral or aortic valve have been developed. With their application, both stenotic and regurgitant malformations may be effectively corrected, and although most patients derive gratifying clinical and hemodynamic benefit, many complications may alter the postoperative course of a patient with a prosthetic cardiac valve. Among those most feared is the development of infectious endocarditis. In reported experiences, such infections, whether dating from the time of operation or occurring in the late postoperative period, have almost always proved to be fatal.[1-4] At the National Heart Institute, prosthetic mitral or aortic valves, or both, have been utilized in more than 200 patients, and none has developed endocarditis during the early postoperative period. Three patients who had had aortic valve replacement, however, developed bacterial endocarditis a number of months after operation. In each of them the infection resulted in detachment of the prosthetic valve and massive, fatal aortic regurgitation. The clinical and pathologic findings in these patients are described, and the inadvisability of secondary operative treatment in patients with infected prosthetic valves is discussed.

Clinical and Pathologic Findings

H. L. (03-44-81), a 57-year-old man, had calcific aortic stenosis and regurgitation, and in November 1962, the aortic valve was replaced with a flexible Teflon prosthesis. His immediate postoperative course was uneventful, he evidenced marked clinical improvement, and 6 months after operation cardiac catheterization revealed only a trivial pressure gradient across the prosthetic valve. In December 1963, all of his teeth were removed; at this time he was given 600,000 units of procaine penicillin intramuscularly twice daily for 3 days before and for 4 days after the procedure. In May 1964, he was fitted with dentures. He remained well until June 1964, when he experienced the onset of exertional dyspnea, fever, and chills. At another hospital, *beta hemolytic Streptococcus* was grown from several blood cultures. He was treated with intravenous penicillin (20 million units daily) for 4 weeks, but remained febrile, and on July 23, 1964, he was readmitted to the National Heart Institute. He was in acute left- and right-sided heart failure, had loud precordial murmurs characteristic of aortic stenosis and aortic regurgitation, splinter hemorrhages, splenomegaly, and anemia. The blood pressure was 150/50 mm. Hg. Chest roentgenograms revealed that the heart was distinctly larger than it had been previously. Numerous blood cultures were sterile. Despite daily administrations of penicillin (40 million units intravenously), kanamycin (1 Gm. intramuscularly), streptomycin (2 Gm. intramuscularly), and chloramphenicol (4 Gm. intravenously), his condition failed to improve and he died on August 14, 1964.

At autopsy (A64-148), the right and noncoronary leaflets of the Teflon aortic valve were found to be partially detached from the annulus (fig. 1), and two of the suspended commissures of the valve had disrupted. Cultures of the necrotic aortic annulus grew a variety of organisms (*Candida albicans, Escherichia coli,* and *Enterobacter* and *Bacillus* species), but no bacteria or fungi were seen in the histologic sections of this area.

F. H. (03-29-09), a 55-year-old man, who had calcific aortic stenosis and regurgitation, had a partial aortic valve replacement in December 1960. Postoperatively, he did well and was asymptomatic until July 1962, when exertional dyspnea and angina pectoris recurred. These symptoms progressed and, on examination and

From the Clinic of Surgery, National Heart Institute and the Diagnostic X-ray Department, Clinical Center, National Institutes of Health, Bethesda, Maryland.

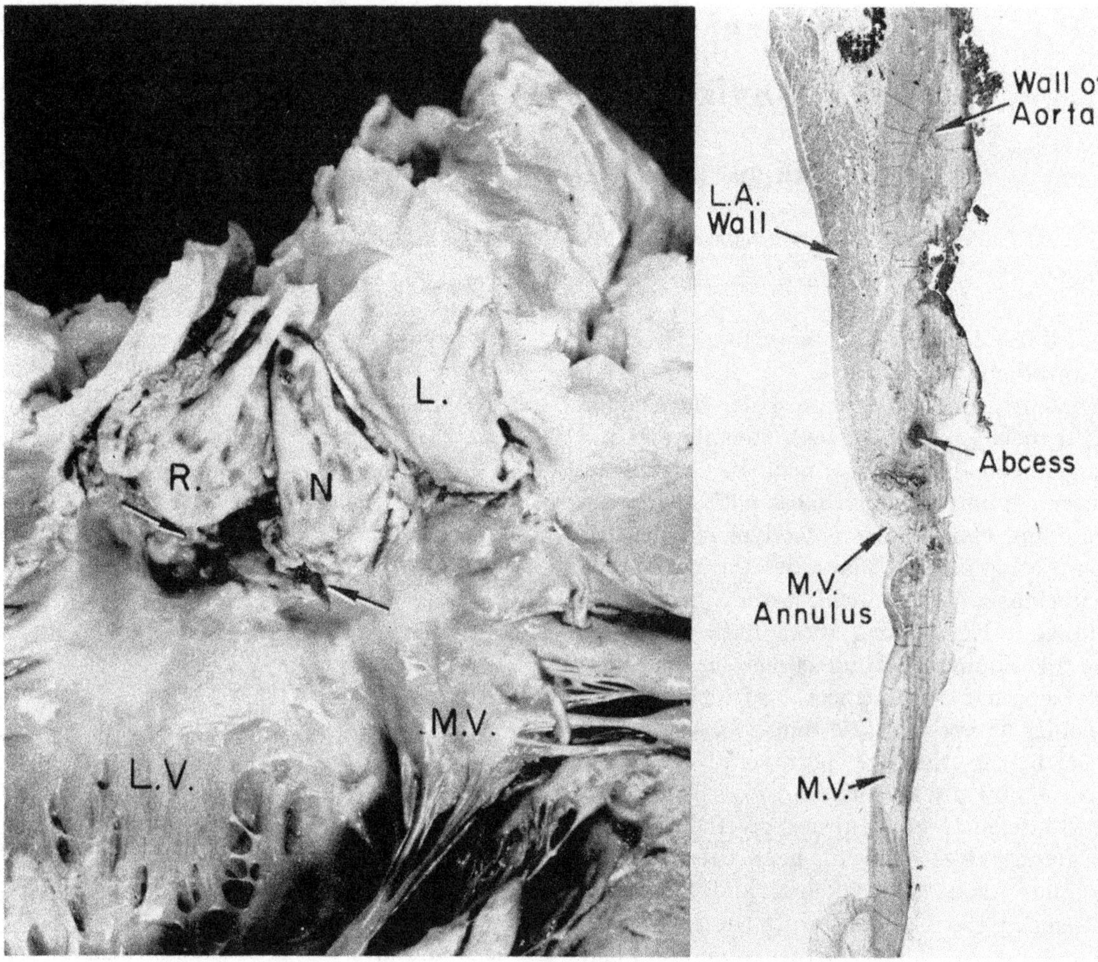

Figure 1

Photograph of the Muller-Teflon aortic valve in patient H. L. (left) *and photomicrograph of the aortic root* (right). Left. *The vertical attachment (not seen) of the right (R.) and non-coronary (N) Teflon cusps is completely separated from the aortic wall, and these cusps are largely detached from the aortic annulus (between the arrows). In addition, the suspended commissure between the right and left (L.) cusps is partially detached.* Right. *Section includes the anterior mitral leaflet (M.V.) and walls of the ascending aorta and left atrium (L.A). The surface of the aorta contains fibrin material but no organisms. A small abscess is located between the aortic valve "annulus" and the mitral valve ring. L.V., left ventricle.*

at cardiac catheterization, he was found to have severe recurrent aortic regurgitation. In February 1963, he was operated upon again and the prosthetic leaflet was found fragmented; the entire valve was replaced with a tricuspid Teflon prosthesis. Postoperatively, the patient again improved, but, in May 1963, he apparently had an acute myocardial infarction and 2 weeks later developed fever and chills. On readmission there was again evidence of aortic regurgitation; dermal petechiae, splenomegaly, and anemia were present. Chest roentgenograms showed the heart to be larger than it had been previously. Nonhemolytic *Staphylococcus albus*, coagulase negative, was grown from each of six blood cultures. In vitro, the organism was sensitive to penicillin and he was treated daily for 6 weeks with 30 million units intravenously. All blood cultures following the initiation of penicillin therapy were sterile, and the clinical manifestations of active infection disappeared. In July 1964, he was operated upon for the third time. The Teflon prosthesis was largely detached from the aortic annulus, which was partially necrotic. The Teflon valve was removed and replaced with a Starr-Edwards ball valve. Cultures of the aortic annulus obtained at the time of operation, however, grew *Staph. albus*. Penicillin (20 million units intravenously daily) was given for 3 weeks after the operation. Three weeks after it was discontinued, and while the patient was still in the hospital, he became febrile once more and *Staph. albus* was again cultured from the peripheral blood. Treatment was instituted with methicillin, 20 Gm. intravenously daily, but there was little apparent response to the drug, and after 1 week he suddenly developed acute pulmonary edema, signs of massive aortic regurgitation, and died.

At autopsy (A63-176), the fixation ring of the Starr-Edwards prosthetic valve was found detached around more than half of its circumference (fig. 2). The cage of the prosthetic valve lay within an infected aneurysm of the aorta (figs. 2 and 3). There were large foci of necrosis and numerous abscesses in the periaortic tissues and, although cultures of this area grew multiple organisms (*Torulopsis glabrata, Pseudomonas aeruginosa, E. coli, hemolytic Staphylococcus aureus*), none was visible in histologic sections.

W. L. (04-00-86), a 51-year-old man, had a flexible Teflon prosthetic valve inserted for the treatment of calcific aortic stenosis in January 1962. Initially, he experienced good symptomatic improvement, but 1 year after operation the signs and symptoms of left-sided heart failure reappeared, and precordial murmurs typical of aortic stenosis and regurgitation again became audible.

The patient's symptoms progressed, and in October 1963 a second operation was performed. There was no evidence of infection, but the Teflon valve was perforated and calcified. It was replaced with a Starr-Edwards valve and the patient made an uneventful recovery. Ten months after operation the patient returned for postoperative study. He was asymptomatic, and there was no clinical or hemodynamic evidence of aortic regurgitation. In September 1964, the patient had several carious teeth extracted, and his physician gave him intramuscular injections of 600,000 units of penicillin on the day before, the day of, and the day after, the procedure. Two days later, however, he developed chills, fever, weakness, and malaise, and during the next 5 weeks lost 6 Kg. in weight and became anemic. On readmission in October 1964 he was acutely ill, febrile, pale, and edematous. The blood pressure was 100/50 mm. Hg, a loud, blowing diastolic murmur was audible along the left sternal border, and the spleen was palpable. Roentgenograms of the chest showed the heart to be much larger than it had been at the time of the last study (fig. 4). At fluoroscopic examination, the metallic ring and cage of the Starr-Edwards valve were seen to move in a strikingly abnormal manner during

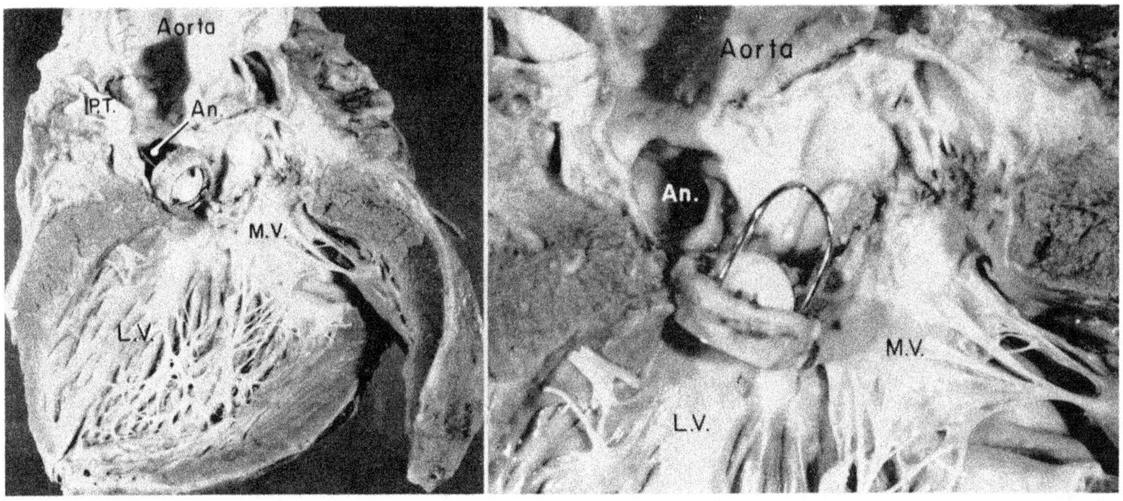

Figure 2

Photographs of the heart of patient F. H. Left. *The left ventricle, aortic valve "ring" and ascending aorta are shown. Only three or four sutures remain to fix the Starr-Edwards prosthesis to the necrotic annulus. The apex of the cage has burrowed into the wall of the ascending aorta forming a saccular aneurysm (An.). The Teflon tape, which was wrapped around the ascending aorta at the time of the operation, has burrowed through the aorta to form a part of the interior lining of this vessel. Thick scar tissue and numerous inflammatory cells are present in the periaortic area.* Right. *A close-up view of the aortic valve region. The prosthetic suture line is necrotic. L.V., left ventricle; M.V., anterior mitral leaflet; and P.T., pulmonary trunk.*

the phases of the cardiac cycle. During systole, the valve tilted sharply forward and to the right, then returned to a normal position during diastole. These motions of the valve were recorded by cineradiography, and also by means of serial biplane x-rays exposed at a rate of 6 per second.

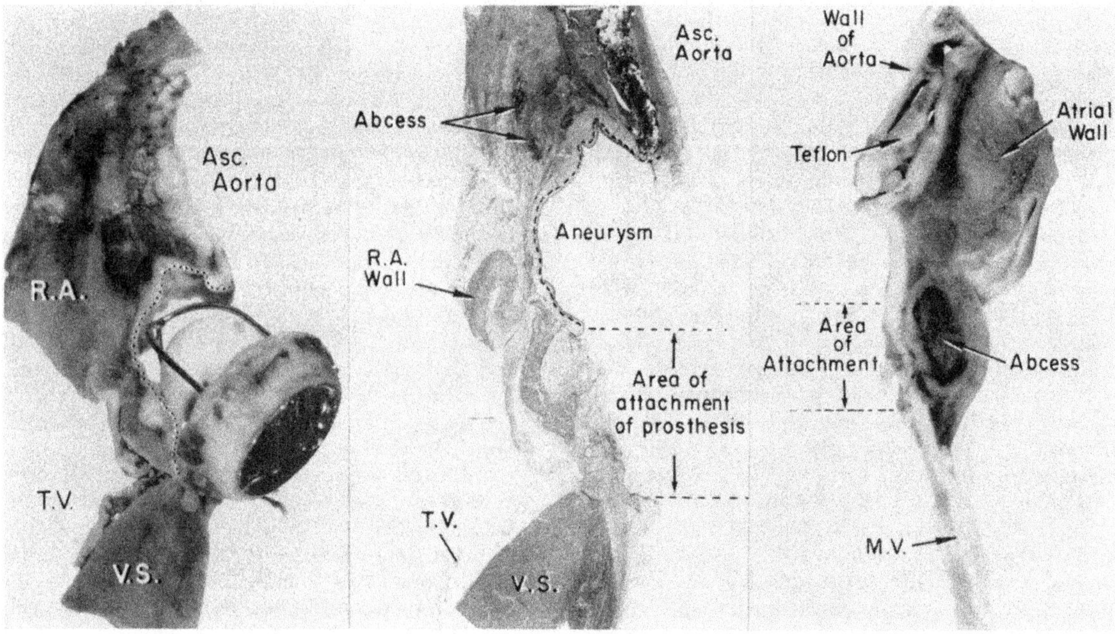

Figure 3

The aortic root in patient F. H. The left *photograph and* middle *photomicrograph are sections through the saccular aortic aneurysm formed by the cage of the Starr-Edwards prosthesis. The dotted line delineates the borders of the aneurysm. The area of attachment of the prosthesis is indicated. No elastic fibers were present in the wall of the saccular aortic aneurysm. Hematoxylin and eosin stain;* × 2.2 (middle). *The* right *photograph is a section through the aortic root, cut to include the anterior leaflet of the mitral valve (M.V.). A large abscess is present between the left atrial wall and the aortic valve ring, immediately beneath the area of attachment of the prosthesis. T.V., tricuspid valve; R.A., right atrium; V.S., ventricular septum.*

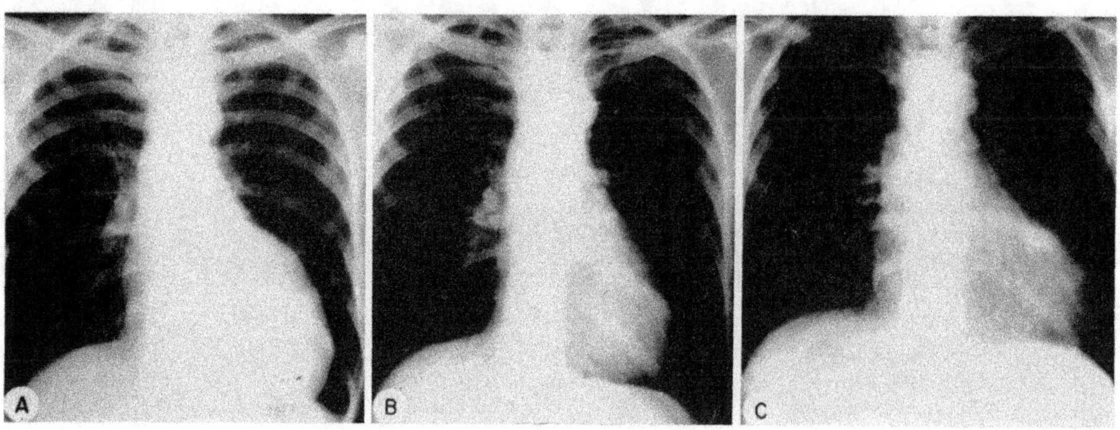

Figure 4

Chest roentgenograms of patient W. L., illustrating changes in heart size before (A) *and 10 months after* (B) *insertion of the Starr-Edwards aortic valve prosthesis. The appearance of the heart following the onset of severe aortic regurgitation secondary to the acute bacterial endocarditis is shown in* C.

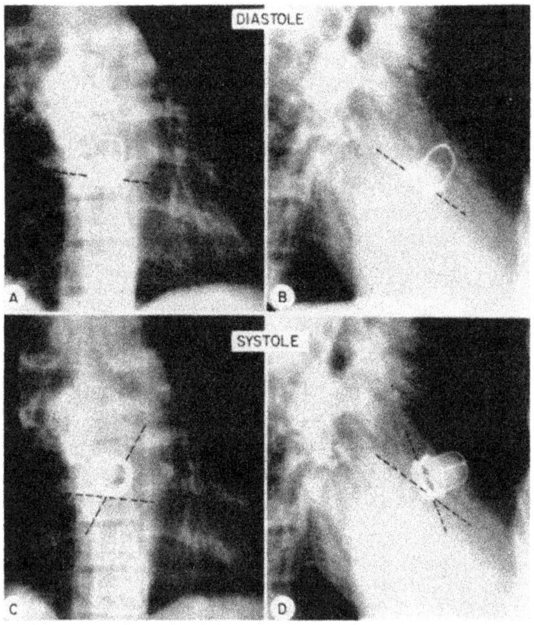

Figure 5

Frontal and lateral roentgenograms exposed during diastole (A and B) and systole (C and D) in patient W. L., when the Starr-Edwards aortic valve prosthesis was partially detached. During systole the cage is seen to tilt sharply forward and to the right, and returns to a more normal position during diastole.

The positions of the valve during systole and diastole are shown in figure 5, and the motions of a normally functioning Starr-Edwards valve, recorded in another patient, are shown for comparison in figure 6.

After blood cultures had been obtained, the patient was empirically treated with total daily doses of penicillin (20 million units intravenously), streptomycin (2 Gm. intramuscularly), methicillin (4 Gm. intravenously), and chloramphenicol (2 Gm. intravenously). Each of five blood cultures subsequently grew *Staph. albus,* and in three of them *Cytophaga anitratum* (*Herellea*) was also found. In vitro, the *Staph. albus* was found sensitive to methicillin, and the *C. anitratum* to both chloramphenicol and streptomycin, and the initial therapeutic regimen was continued. The patient remained febrile, however, and became progressively more dyspneic. On his fifth hospital day, pulmonary edema and hypotension suddenly occurred, and the diastolic murmur, which had been consistently present, was no longer audible. At this time, a pulse was palpable in the right arm, but not in the left arm or legs. The lower half of the body became progressively cyanotic, and the patient died 1 hour later. A chest roentgenogram, obtained immediately after death, showed the prosthetic valve to be lying in the transverse aortic arch (fig. 7).

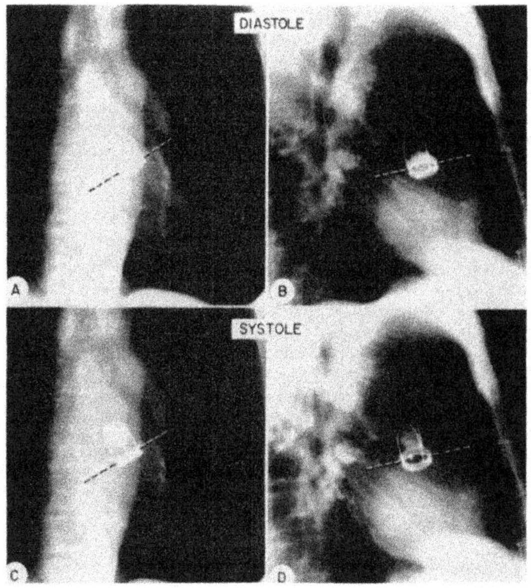

Figure 6

Frontal and lateral roentgenograms exposed during diastole (A and B) and systole (C and D) in a patient with a normally functioning Starr-Edwards aortic ball-valve prosthesis. There is little movement of the prosthesis during the phases of the cardiac cycle.

The appearance of the heart and aorta at autopsy (A64-189) is shown in figure 8. The prosthetic valve was found impacted in the aortic arch, completely occluding it immediately distal to the origin of the left carotid artery. The tissues of the aortic root, to which the valve had been sutured, were still attached to the Teflon ring of the valve. The entire area from which the valve had been dislodged was necrotic and ulcerated, and numerous Gram-positive cocci were evident histologically. An abscess was present in the periaortic area (fig. 9), and cultures of it grew *hemolytic* S. *albus* and *Enterobacter.*

Discussion

The clinical and pathologic findings in the three patients described would indicate that the inevitable consequence of infective endocarditis in a patient with a prosthetic aortic valve will be disruption of the valve from the aortic annulus. In each patient the development of bacterial endocarditis was shortly followed by evidences of progressively severe aortic regurgitation and death from cardiac

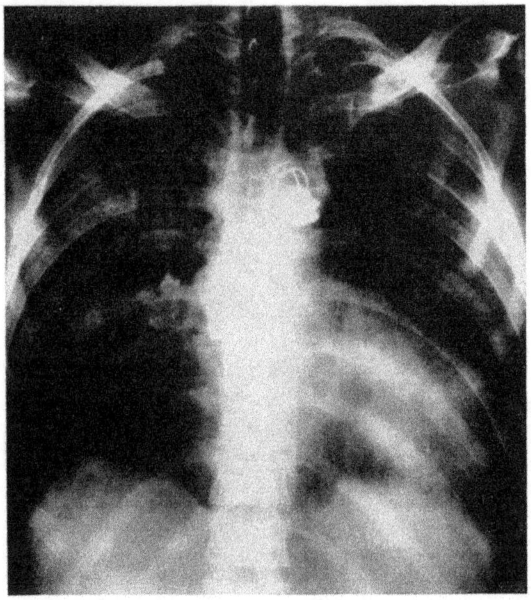

Figure 7

Chest roentgenogram of patient W. L., exposed immediately after death, and following complete detachment of the aortic valve prosthesis, which is located in the arch of the aorta. The base of the valve is now distal to the cage, and the ball is seated in the closed position, completely occluding the aorta.

failure. At necropsy, the primary site of infection was found to be the tissues to which the prosthesis had been attached. The sutures fixing the valve were not broken, but had torn through the necrotic aortic annulus, and the valve was partially or completely detached. Although the wall of the aorta at the site of fixation of the valve was completely disrupted by the acute necrotizing infection, surrounding scar tissue prevented bleeding from the aortic lumen. The infectious process also involved the periaortic tissues, and acute abscesses and foci of necrosis were evident between the aorta and the walls of both right and left atria in each patient. In addition, in patient H. L., the infection extended into the mitral annulus; in patient W. L., to the tricuspid annulus via the membranous ventricular septum.

As noted above, aortic regurgitation and left heart failure, rather than the sequelae of infection, were the immediate causes of death in the patients described. In each of them the ominous progression of aortic regurgitation was appreciated, and replacement or reattachment of the infected prosthesis was considered. Such emergency operations were not undertaken, however, and the subsequent pathologic findings indicated that they would certainly have been fruitless. Dissection of the mediastinum, sufficient to permit cannulation and an aortotomy, would clearly have disseminated the infection in the periaortic tissues, and secure fixation of either the infected valve or a new one would also have proved impossible because of the necrotic tissues in the annulus. Thus, the experience with the present patients and, with one exception,[5] the reports of others indicate that when infection becomes established at the site of a prosthetic aortic valve that it cannot be eradicated by antibiotics presently available. Also, since reoperation in such a patient is considered inadvisable, it would appear that major attention must be directed to prophylactic measures.

The application of meticulous aseptic technics at the time of operation is, of course, the single most important factor in the prevention of postoperative infection, but in operations upon the heart and great vessels prophylactic antibiotics are also of proven value. In this clinic, daily doses of penicillin (2.4 million units) and streptomycin (1.0 Gm.) are given on the day before operation and for 1 week thereafter. With this regimen, and within the surgical environment of the Clinical Center, early postoperative endocarditis has not occurred in any of the more than 200 patients in whom prosthetic valves have been inserted. Accordingly, methicillin or other antibiotics are not given prophylactically, principally because of the increased risk of superinfection associated with their administration.[6] Also, because of similar considerations, long-term penicillin administration, usually indicated in patients with rheumatic heart disease, is not given to patients with prosthetic valves.

In one of the present patients, W. L., staphylococcal endocarditis clearly resulted from dental extractions, even though he was

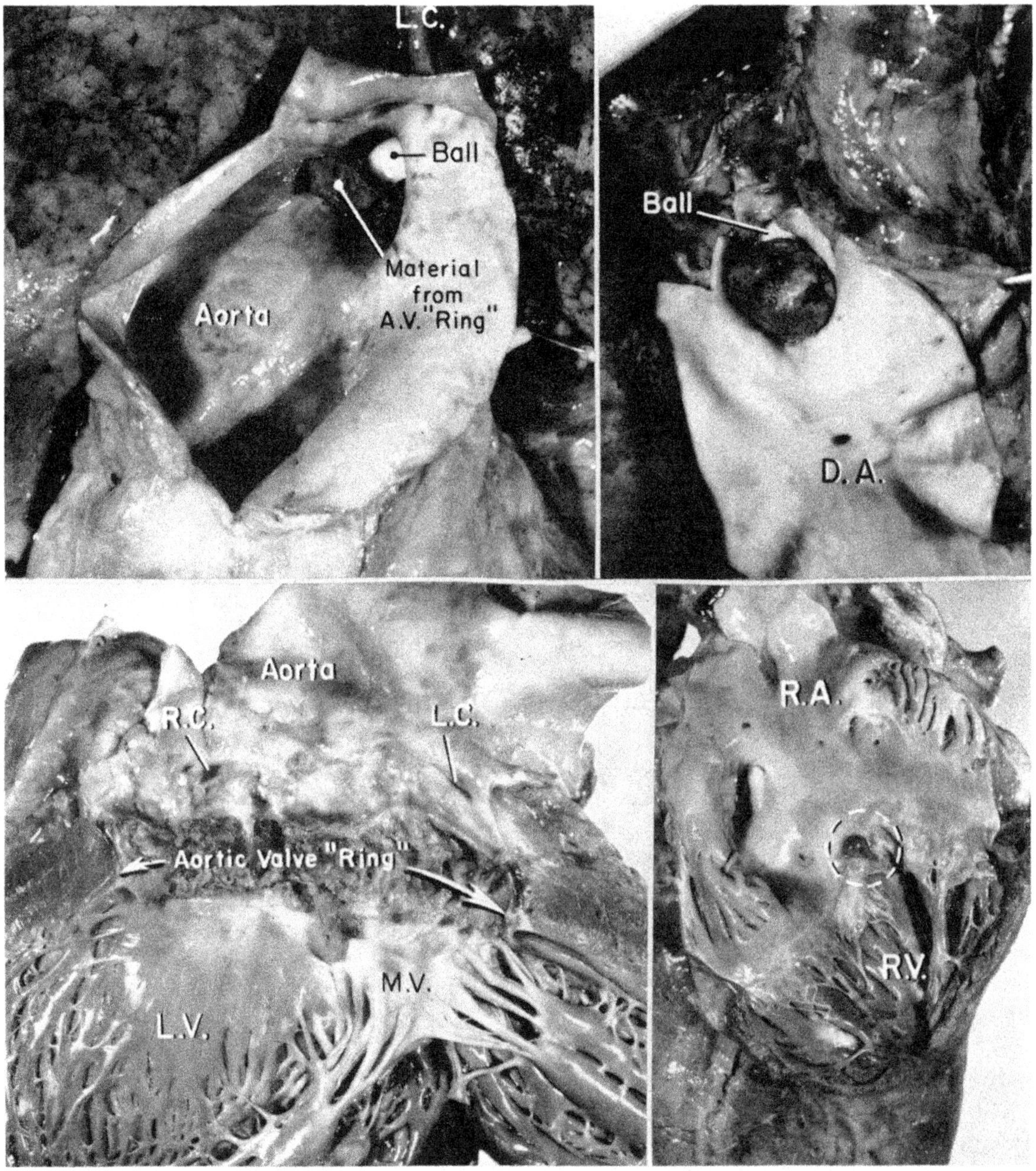

Figure 8

Photographs of the aorta and heart of patient W. L. Upper left. *The ascending aorta is opened and the Starr-Edwards valve is lodged in the aortic arch. Tissue from the aortic valve "ring" is attached to the Teflon ring of the prosthesis. L.C., left carotid artery.* Upper right. *The detached prosthesis is viewed from the descending thoracic aorta (D.A.). Necrotic tissue is attached to the Teflon ring of the prosthesis.* Lower left. *The ascending aorta, aortic valve "ring," and left ventricle are opened. The site of the previous attachment of the prosthesis to the aortic root is totally necrotic. R.C., ostium of right coronary artery; L.C., ostium of left coronary artery. M.V., anterior mitral leaflet; L.V., left ventricle.* Lower right. *The right atrium (R.A.), tricuspid valve, and right ventricle (R.V.) are opened. The bulging membranous ventricular septum, which has become inflamed by direct extension of the infection from the aortic valve, is indicated by the dashed circle.*

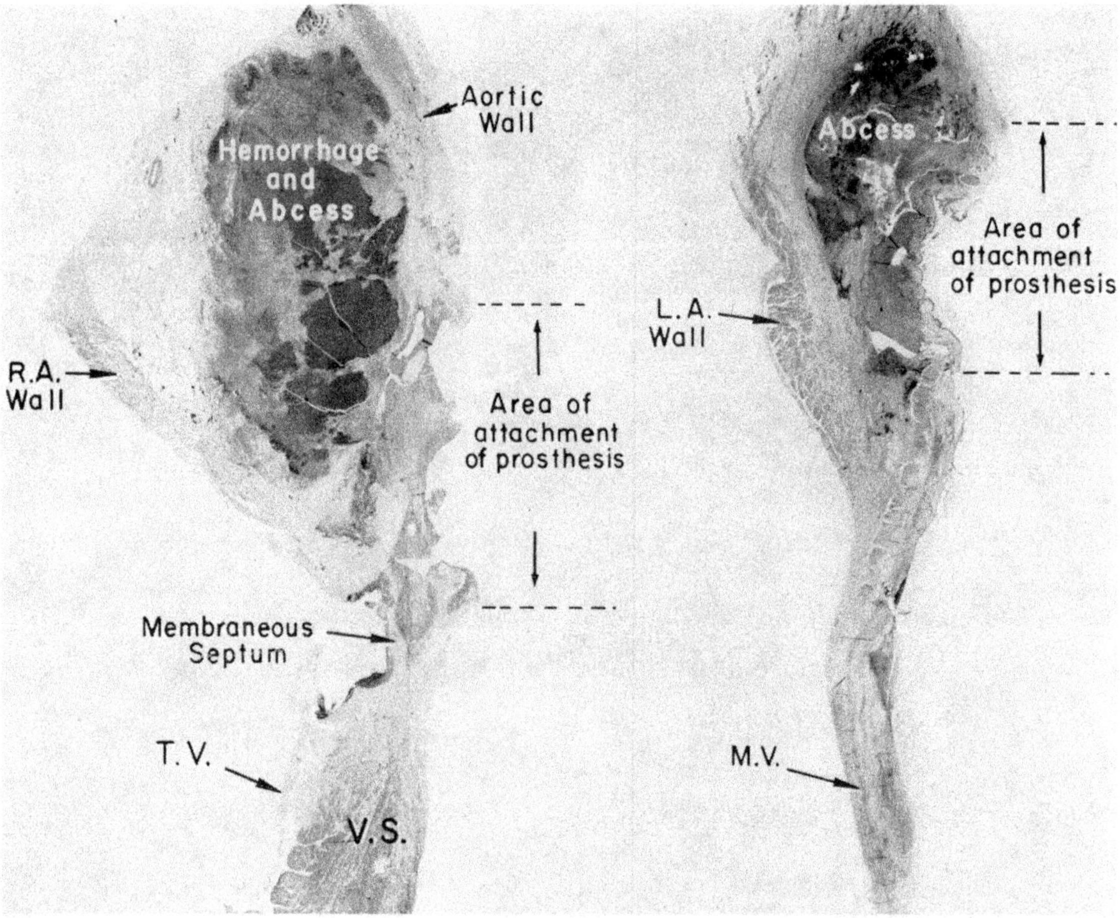

Figure 9

Photomicrographs of the aortic valve "ring" in patient W. L., showing the acute abscesses in the area between the aortic wall and the atria. The membranous septum (left) *is inflamed and appears to be nearing perforation. The left section includes the aortic wall, right atrial (R.A.) wall, tricuspid valve (T.V.), and ventricular septum (V.S.). The right section includes the anterior leaflet of the mitral valve (M.V.) and the left atrial (L.A.) wall. There is considerable fibrous thickening of the mitral valve. Hematoxylin and eosin stains; × 2.2 in each.*

given prophylactic penicillin in doses similar to those recommended by the American Heart Association for patients with rheumatic heart disease.[7]* Patient H. L. also received penicillin before and after dental extractions but did not contract endocarditis at that time. Six months later, however, when he was edentulous and shortly after he had been fitted with dentures, he developed an ultimately fatal infection caused by *beta hemolytic Streptococcus.* It is known that bacteremia can result from gingival ulcers caused by ill-fitting dentures,[8] but one may only speculate as to whether this mechanism was responsible for endocarditis in this patient, and whether prophylactic penicillin would have been effective.

In a comprehensive study in this hospital by Rogosa and others,[9] bacteremia was documented in more than 80 per cent of patients in whom either dental extractions or periodon-

*Six hundred thousand units of both aqueous and procaine penicillin intramuscularly 1 hour before the operative procedure, and 600,000 units of procaine penicillin intramuscularly on each of the 2 days following the procedure.

tal procedures were carried out. A wide variety of organisms was recovered and, although Streptococcus strains were frequent, many species and strains of organisms were identified that were presumably resistant to penicillin. Thus study and the course of patient W. L. indicate that the penicillin regimen recommended by the American Heart Association for patients with rheumatic heart disease may be inadequate for patients with prosthetic cardiac valves who must undergo dental prophylaxis or extractions. The following antibiotic regimen is presently employed in such patients in this clinic: (1) broad-spectrum antibiotic troches on each of the 2 days before the procedure. (Such troches will not, of course, sterilize the oral cavity, but will substantially reduce the number of organisms in the mouth, and consequently the number that enter the bloodstream at the time of the dental procedure[10]); (2) procaine penicillin, 600,000 units intramuscularly every 6 hours, and streptomycin 0.5 Gm. every 12 hours the day before, the day of, and for 3 to 5 days following the procedure; (3) methicillin, 5 Gm. intravenously during the day of operation; and (4) oxacillin, 4 Gm. orally for 3 to 5 days following the procedure. For other operations in potentially infected areas, e. g., genitourinary or anorectal regions, a similar regimen is employed.

Summary

The clinical and pathologic findings in three patients with bacterial infection at the sites of prosthetic aortic valves are described. Each presented typical clinical features of acute bacterial endocarditis followed by the sudden development of severe and ultimately fatal aortic regurgitation. Pathologically the infectious process was characterized by extensive necrosis of the aortic annulus, disruption of the aortic wall, and the formation of abscesses in the periaortic tissues. In two patients the prosthetic valve was partially detached from the annulus, whereas in the other it was totally dislodged and impacted in the aortic arch shortly before death. In all, secondary operative intervention would have been fruitless because of the extent of the infection and the character of the tissue at the aortic root. In one patient fatal staphylococcal endocarditis followed dental extractions despite penicillin prophylaxis. A more comprehensive antibiotic regimen for patients with prosthetic cardiac valves is suggested.

References

1. Bjork, V. O.: Aortic valve replacement. Thorax **19:** 369, 1964.
2. Nelson, T. G., and Cooley, D. A.: Prosthetic replacement of the mitral or aortic valves: A preliminary report on 111 cases. Am. J. Cardiol. **14:** 148, 1964.
3. Starr, A., and Edwards, M. L.: Mitral replacement: Clinical experience with ball-valve prosthesis. Ann. Surg. **154:** 726, 1961.
4. Effler, D. B., Favaloro, R., and Groves, L. K.: Heart valve replacement. Ann. Thor. Surg. **1:** 4, 1965.
5. Littlefield, J. B., Muller, W. H., Jr., and Dammann, J. F.: Successful treatment of *Pseudomonas aeruginosa* septicemia following total aortic valve replacement. Circulation **31** (suppl. 1): 103, 1965.
6. Klein, J. O., and Finland, M.: The new penicillins. New England J. Med. **269:** 1019, 1963.
7. Chamberlin, F. L.: Management of medical-dental problems in patients with cardiovascular diseases. Mod. Concepts Cardiovas. Dis. **30:** 697, 1961.
8. Massaro, D., and Katz, S.: Subacute bacterial endocarditis due to *Streptococcus viridans* in an edentulous man. New England J. Med. **263:** 911, 1960.
9. Rogosa, M., Hampp, E. G., Nevin, T. A., Wagner, H. N., Driscoll, E. J., and Baer, P. N.: Blood sampling and cultural studies in the detection of postoperative bacteremias. J. Am. Dent. A. **60:** 43, 1960.
10. Hook, E. W., and Kaye, D.: Prophylaxis of bacterial endocarditis. J. Chronic Dis. **15:** 635, 1962.

Bacterial endocarditis after dental procedures in patients with aortic valve prostheses

Howell O. Archard, DDS,
William C. Roberts, MD, Bethesda, Md.

Bacterial endocarditis and death followed dental treatment in two patients with prosthetic cardiac valves. They had received what was considered adequate prophylactic doses of antibiotics, but irreparable damage developed in the vulnerable tissues underlying the prosthesis. Since antibiotics and operative intervention are of little effect once infection is established, prevention becomes most important — via preoperative oral evaluations, control of periodontal disease, and a more aggressive antibiotic approach.

The importance of prophylactic antibiotics for patients who have rheumatic or congenital heart disease and who undergo dental procedures is well established and, in general, appreciated.[1,2] In recent years, advanced surgical technics for correction of these cardiac lesions have been developed and, consequently, an increasing number of patients with cardiac prostheses are being seen by dentists.

Many of the mitral and aortic valve lesions can be corrected by total removal of the valve and replacement with a prosthesis. This report describes two patients with prosthetic aortic valves who developed bacterial endocarditis—one immediately after a dental procedure and the other several months after the dental procedure. Each died as a result of infection around the cardiac prosthesis. The patients had received what was considered adequate doses of prophylactic antibiotics at the time of the dental operations. Although dental manipulation cannot be definitely implicated as a causal factor in the second patient, discussion of these patients together appears appropriate.

Report of cases

▪ *Patient 1* . . . A 48-year-old man with known aortic valve stenosis and regurgitation, had this valve replaced with a Teflon prosthesis on January 31, 1962. He was improved for some months by this procedure but, in July, 1963, he developed severe aortic regurgitation, necessitating replacement of the Teflon prosthesis, which had developed several perforations, with a caged-ball (Starr-Edwards) prosthesis. The second operation was carried out in September, 1963; before being discharged, he was seen in the dental clinic for

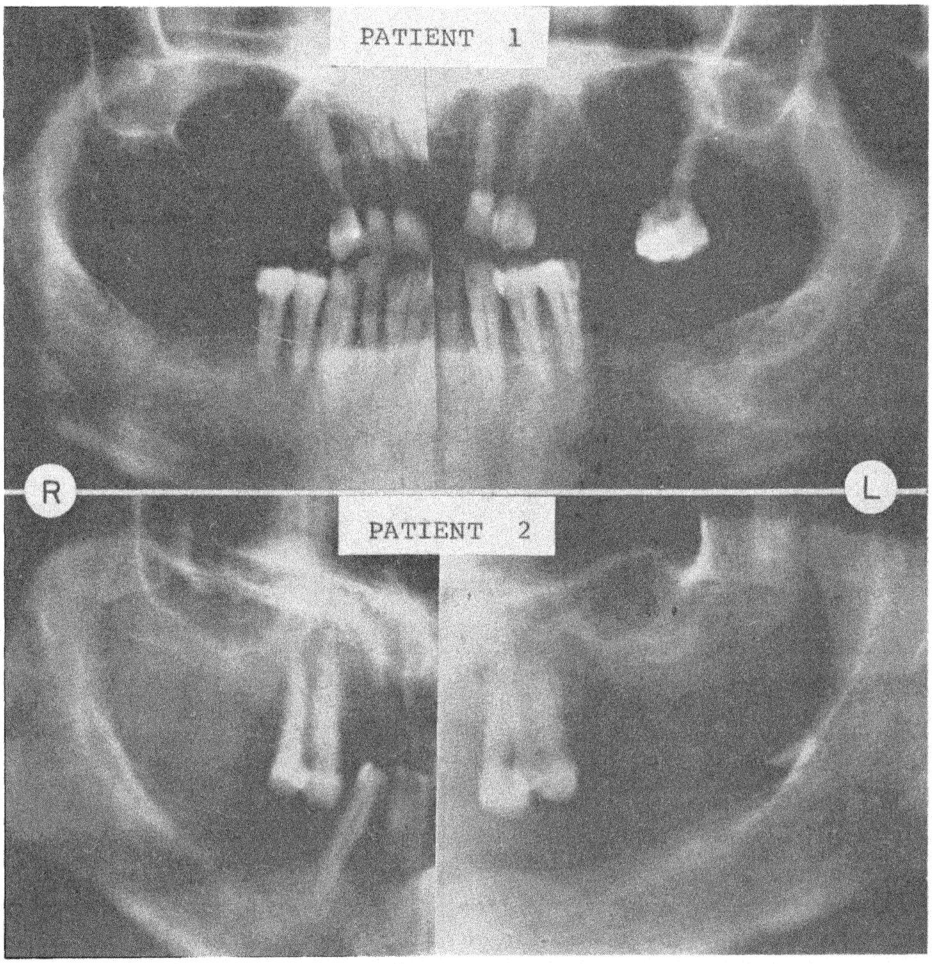

Fig. 1 Top: Patient 1 —Panoramic radiograph shows 16 remaining permanent teeth, all with advanced periodontal disease and one with periapical involvement. Clinically, caries, stain, calculus, and mobility were noted. Bottom: Patient 2 —Panoramic radiograph reveals 8 remaining permanent teeth, including roots of lower left third molar. Extensive periodontal disease and caries rendered these teeth useless for restorative measures

the first time. His mouth had been neglected, and only half of the permanent dentition remained (Fig. 1). He wanted complete upper and lower dentures rather than extensive restorative procedures; however, no therapy was undertaken since he was soon to be discharged.

During the next several months, the patient was virtually asymptomatic and, when seen in August, 1964, he appeared healthy. A repeat dental examination showed similar findings and, since he was eager to return home, it was decided that the extractions would be carried out by an oral surgeon near his home. At the time of these extractions, he received penicillin, 600,000 units intramuscularly, the day before, the day of, and the day after the procedure. Despite this medication, he developed chills, fever, pedal edema, anorexia, weight loss, and severe weakness several days later. On October 15, 1964, he was readmitted to the Clinical Center. Hemolytic *Staphylococcus albus* and *Cytophaga anitrata* were grown from several blood cultures, and he was treated daily with penicillin (20 million units intravenously), streptomycin (2 Gm. intramuscularly), methicillin (4 Gm. intravenously), and chloramphenicol (2 Gm. intravenously). In spite of receiving these antibiotics, his condition deteriorated and, approximately an hour before death, the prosthetic aortic valve became totally detached and migrated to the aortic arch as was seen on radiographs.

At autopsy, the prosthetic valve was located in the aortic arch (Fig. 2, left), and its previous site of attachment at the aortic root was necrotic, inflamed, and surrounded by abscesses and foci of hemorrhage (Fig. 2, right and Fig. 3, left). Massive aortic regurgitation obviously was the result of the detachment of the aortic valve prosthesis.

▪ *Patient 2* . . . A 54-year-old man with rheumatic valvular aortic stenosis and insufficiency, had this valve replaced with a Teflon prosthesis in November, 1962. He was greatly improved by

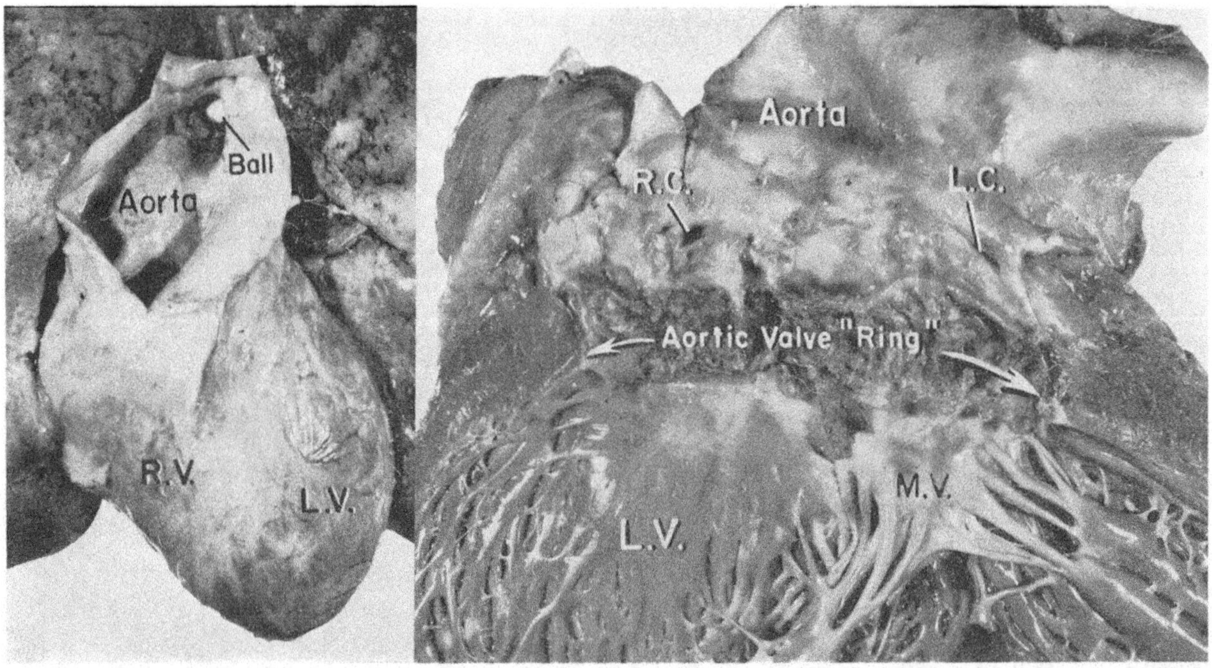

Fig. 2 Patient 1—Left: Heart and aorta as seen anteriorly. Caged-ball prosthesis is located in arch of the aorta, having migrated to this position after complete detachment from aortic valve "ring." R.V. = right ventricle; L.V. = left ventricle. Right: Aorta, aortic valve "ring," and left ventricle (L.V.) open. Previous site of attachment of prosthesis of the aortic valve "ring" is necrotic, inflamed, and perforated. R.C. = ostium, right coronary artery; L.C. = ostium, left coronary artery; M.V. = anterior leaflet of mitral valve

the operation. During a follow-up visit in December, 1963, he was seen for the first time in the dental clinic of the National Institutes of Health. Examination by panoramic radiograph revealed periodontal involvement of the remaining 8 teeth and several periapically involved teeth (Fig. 1, bottom). Full-mouth extractions and appropriate alveolectomies were performed at this time. The patient received intramuscularly 600,000 units of procaine penicillin, twice daily, for several days before, the day of, and for 5 days after the procedure. The postoperative course was uncomplicated, and he was discharged from the hospital 2 weeks later. During another admission in April, 1964, complete upper and lower dentures were constructed without difficulty. His cardiac condition remained satisfactory.

The patient did reasonably well until June, 1964, when he noticed the sudden onset of dyspnea on exertion, orthopnea, and fever; he was hospitalized in his hometown. Beta hemolytic *Streptococcus* was isolated from each of 2 blood cultures. The patient was given aqueous penicillin (40 million units intravenously daily) and streptomycin (1 Gm. intramuscularly daily) and immediately transferred to the Clinical Center where this regimen was continued. He failed to improve, however, and died 20 days later.

At autopsy, the Teflon aortic valve prosthesis was found to be about 60 per cent detached (Fig. 4). The cause of the partial detachment was infection at the site of fixation of the prosthesis. The tissues surrounding the prosthesis were necrotic and inflamed but free of stainable organisms (Fig. 3, right). Severe aortic regurgitation was the result of the detachment.

Discussion

The onset of bacterial endocarditis in patient 1 is clearly related to the dental procedure. The relationship of the dental work and the onset of bacterial endocarditis in patient 2, on the other hand, is not definite. In the latter, there was a 6-month interval between the time of the dental extractions and the onset of signs and symptoms of bacterial endocarditis. Perhaps the establishment of a bacterial focus on the valve at the time of the dental surgery smoldered until clinical manifestation of the disease. Or, since there was only a 2-month interval from the time of the denture insertion until death, it is possible that mucosal irritation attendant to

Fig. 3 Photomicrographs of sections through the aortic valve ring areas in patients 1 (left) and 2 (right). Previous site of attachment of prosthesis is designated in left view. Infectious process extends from site of attachment through membranous septum and to the surrounding periaortic tissues. R.A. = right atrium; T.V. = tricuspid valve leaflet; V.S. = ventricular septum. Right: This section includes anterior leaflet of the mitral valve (M.V.), site of prosthetic attachment (in vicinity of abscess), aortic and left atrial (L.A.) walls. Again, note that infectious process extends into the periaortic tissues. The mitral valve leaflet is considerably thickened as a result of rheumatic disease

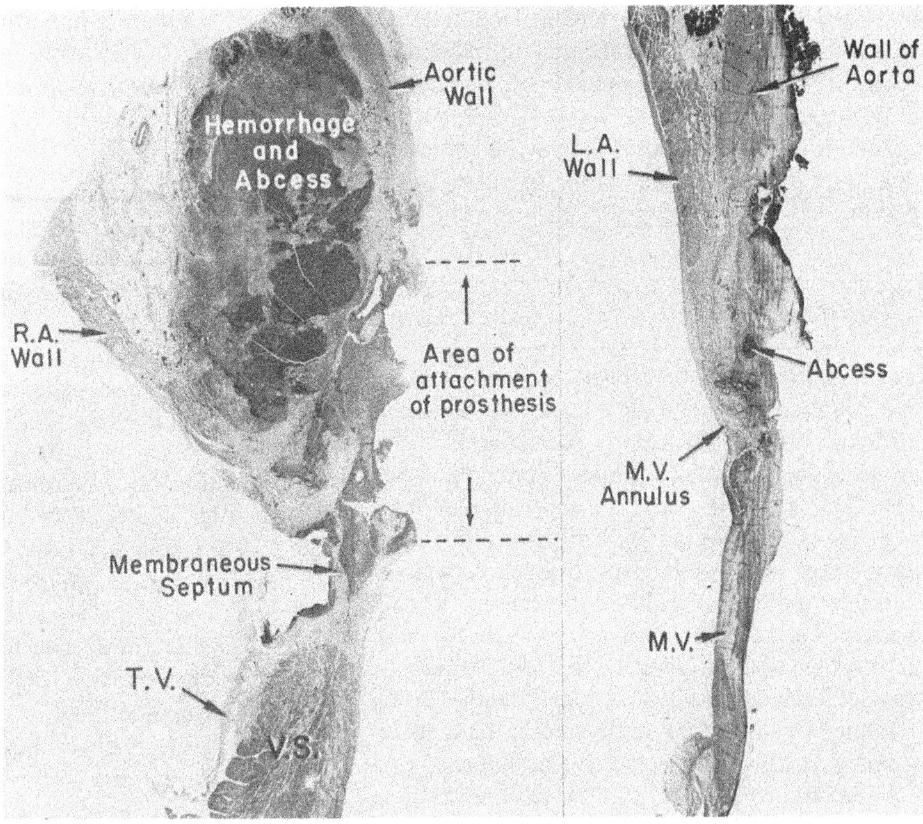

Fig. 4 Opened aortic valve Teflon prosthesis and left ventricle (L.V.) in patient 2. Bases of right (R.) and noncoronary cusps (N) have been detached (between the arrows), as has vertical support of these cusps, by the underlying infection. There is no ingrowth of tissue into these Teflon cusps. L = left Teflon cusp, and M.V. = anterior leaflet of mitral valve

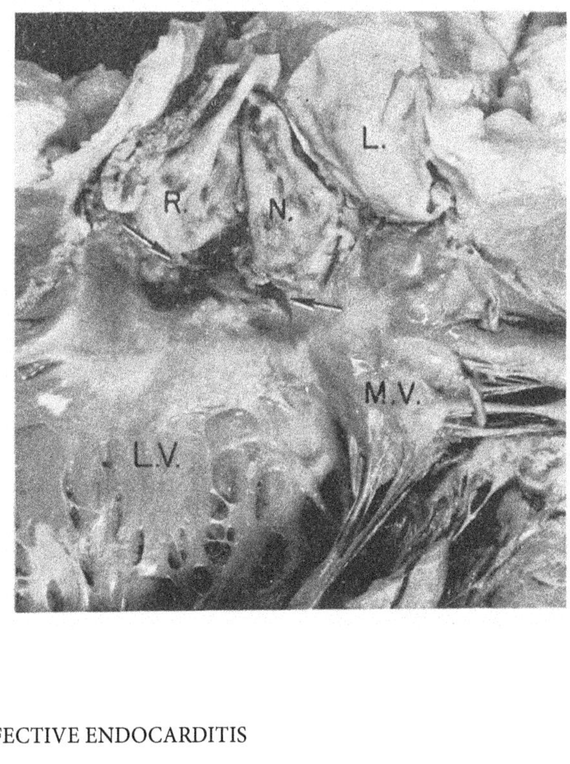

denture conditioning or some unrecognized residual infection provided a source for the microorganisms. Whatever the origin, the patient demonstrated the fatal outcome of infection around such prosthetic valves.

Prevention—most important factor

Since there is no appreciable ingrowth of tissue, the cardiac valvular prostheses are held in position almost solely by sutures. The tissues underlying the prosthesis seem particularly vulnerable to attack by microorganisms. Any disease, such as dental infection, or operative procedure that is capable of producing bacteremia or fungemia takes on considerable importance in patients with prosthetic cardiac valves.

Infections developing at the sites of prosthetic cardiac valves are almost always fatal because the underlying tissues are destroyed, and irreparable valvular regurgitation develops. Since antibiotics and operative intervention are of little benefit once the infection has become established, prevention is the most important factor. Thus, it is now the policy at the National Institutes of Health for all patients scheduled for a cardiac valve replacement to have thorough dental and oral evaluations preoperatively. If oral surgery or other dental procedures are at all indicated, this work is carried out before the cardiac operation.

Periodontal disease hazard

The majority of patients who undergo cardiac valve replacement are middle-aged. The incidence of dental disease, particularly periodontal, in this group is high, and it is chronic periodontal disease that frequently has been the cause of transient bacteremia. Periodontal treatments,[3] simple massage of inflamed gingiva,[4] or even rocking of a single tooth[5] are well-known causes of bacteremia. Periodontal conditions, particularly those in which it is doubtful that the condition can be arrested, should be given serious attention when planning treatment for such cardiac patients; it seems wise to be most aggressive in removing any possible future sites of focal infection in these patients.

The prophylactic antibiotic regimen routinely employed for patients with rheumatic or congenital heart disease, who have not had heart surgery, and who are undergoing dental procedures is completely inadequate for patients with prosthetic cardiac valves undergoing similar procedures. A more aggressive antibiotic approach is now being used at the Clinical Center for all patients with prosthetic cardiac valves who must receive dental treatment, and the regimen is outlined in the table. Since intravenous antibiotics are required over a period of several days, dental work on patients with prosthetic cardiac valves must be performed in a hospital. Good oral hygiene and maintenance of a healthy tissue state is of paramount importance in these patients, and planned dental care must be instituted before the cardiac operation in order to provide this ideal care.

Table Prophylaxis for dental procedures in patients with prosthetic cardiac valves

1. Procaine penicillin—600,000 units intramuscularly every 6 hours, day before, day of, and 3 to 5 days after dental procedure.
2. Streptomycin—0.5 Gm. intramuscularly every 12 hours, day before, day of, and 3 to 5 days after dental procedure.
3. Aqueous penicillin—1,000,000 units intramuscularly 1 hour before dental procedure.
4. Methicillin—4 Gm. intramuscularly or intravenously every 6 hours, day of and 3 to 5 days after dental procedure.
5. Broad-spectrum antibiotic troches on each of 2 days before dental procedure.

Summary

Patients with cardiac valve prostheses require extensive antibiotic therapy for any dental operation. This article reports on the clinical and pathological features of two patients with aortic valve prostheses who were given what were considered adequate doses of prophylactic antibiotics for the operation, but who contracted bacterial endocarditis after dental procedures.

The more aggressive antibiotic approach and the regimen employed at the clinical center are described; since some of these antibiotics are administered intravenously, the dental work must be performed while the patient is in the hospital.

Preventive care is the most important factor. It is, therefore, absolutely necessary that candidates for cardiac valve operations undergo thorough dental examinations and completion of all possible dental procedures *before* heart surgery in order to eliminate any possible sites of focal infection in the oral cavity.

Doctor Archard is with the Department of Health, Education, and Welfare, Public Health Service, National Institutes of Health, and he is senior oral surgeon of the oral medicine and surgery branch, National Institute of Dental Research, Bethesda, Md.

Doctor Roberts is with HEW, National Institutes of Health, and he is chief of the National Heart Institute, laboratory of pathology, clinic of surgery, Bethesda, Md.

1. Management of dental problems in patients with cardiovascular disease. Report of a Working Conference jointly sponsored by the American Dental Association and American Heart Association. JADA 68:333 March, 1964.

2. Burch, G. E., and DePasquale, N. P. Relationship of dentistry to cardiology. Amer. Heart J. 67:99 Jan., 1964.

3. Cobe, H. M. Transitory bacteremia. Oral Surg., Oral Med. & Oral Path. 7:609 June, 1954.

4. Richards, J. H. Bacteremia following irritation of foci of infection. JAMA 99:1496 Oct. 29, 1932.

5. Elliott, S. D. Bacteremia and oral sepsis. Proc. Roy. Soc. Med. 32: 747 May, 1939.

Bacterial Endocarditis Involving Prosthetic Mitral Valves

Clinical and Pathologic Observations

WILLIAM C. ROBERTS, MD, AND ANDREW G. MORROW, MD, BETHESDA, MD

The clinical and necropsy findings are described in two patients who developed staphylococcal endocarditis following replacement of the mitral valve with Starr-Edwards prostheses. In each, death resulted from large thrombi which formed on the prostheses, causing them to become both stenotic and incompetent. The character and extent of the infection in the mitral annulus would have made secondary operative intervention fruitless.

BACTERIAL or fungal endocarditis is an infrequent but dreaded complication of cardiac valve replacement. At the National Heart Institute, more than 150 patients have undergone mitral valve replacement with Starr-Edwards prostheses. None of these patients developed endocarditis as an immediate consequence of the operation, but fatal infections have occurred in two patients in the late postoperative period. Previous reports concerning endocarditis in patients with prosthetic valves [1-3] generally have emphasized the clinical features of the disease, and have suggested prophylactic measures to prevent its occurrence.[4] The present report focuses attention on the pathologic features of this cardiac infection, as demonstrated by the findings in the two patients who developed infective endocarditis after mitral valve replacement.

Accepted for publication April 22, 1966.

From the Clinic of Surgery, National Heart Institute, National Institutes of Health, Bethesda, Md.

Reprint requests to Laboratory of Pathology, Clinic of Surgery, National Heart Institute, National Institutes of Health, Bethesda, Md 20014 (Dr. Roberts).

Report of Cases

CASE 1 (06-11-64).—A man 47 years of age had his calcified stenotic mitral valve replaced with a Starr-Edwards prosthesis on April 29, 1965. On the day before, the day of, and on each of the seven days after the cardiac operation he received erythromycin ethylsuccinate (1.0 gm intramuscularly), streptomycin (1.0 gm intramuscularly) and sodium methicillin (12 gm intramuscularly). This prophylactic regimen was utilized because the patient had had allergic manifestations when he had been given penicillin on other occasions. The patient's postoperative course was uneventful, but some weeks after discharge he developed a superficial ulcer on his left lower leg. On July 21, at his local hospital, a split-thickness skin graft was applied to the ulcerated area. No local or systemic antibiotics were administered before or immediately after the procedure. Eight hours following the grafting operation, the patient had a chill, vomited, and became disoriented. On the following day he was semicomatose, incontinent of urine and feces, his temperature was 105.8 F. (41 C); later that day signs of left hemiparesis became evident. Chloramphenicol, streptomycin, and kanamycin sulfate were then administered, and a blood culture obtained two days later remained sterile. On August 5, penicillin (15 million units intravenously) and methicillin (4 gm intravenously) daily were substituted for the other antibiotics. On August 15, all antibiotics were discontinued, since no improvement had occurred, and three blood cultures obtained on August 19 grew *Staphylococcus aureus*, coagulase positive. The patient died on August 20.

The heart (A65-186) was returned to us for examination. The orifice of the prosthetic mitral valve was occluded by a large vegetation (Fig 1) which, on microscopic examination, contained numerous clumps of gram-positive cocci. The infected thrombotic material also was present on the ventricular aspect of the prosthesis, attached to both the Teflon and metallic rings and to the base of each of the four metallic struts (Fig 2). About

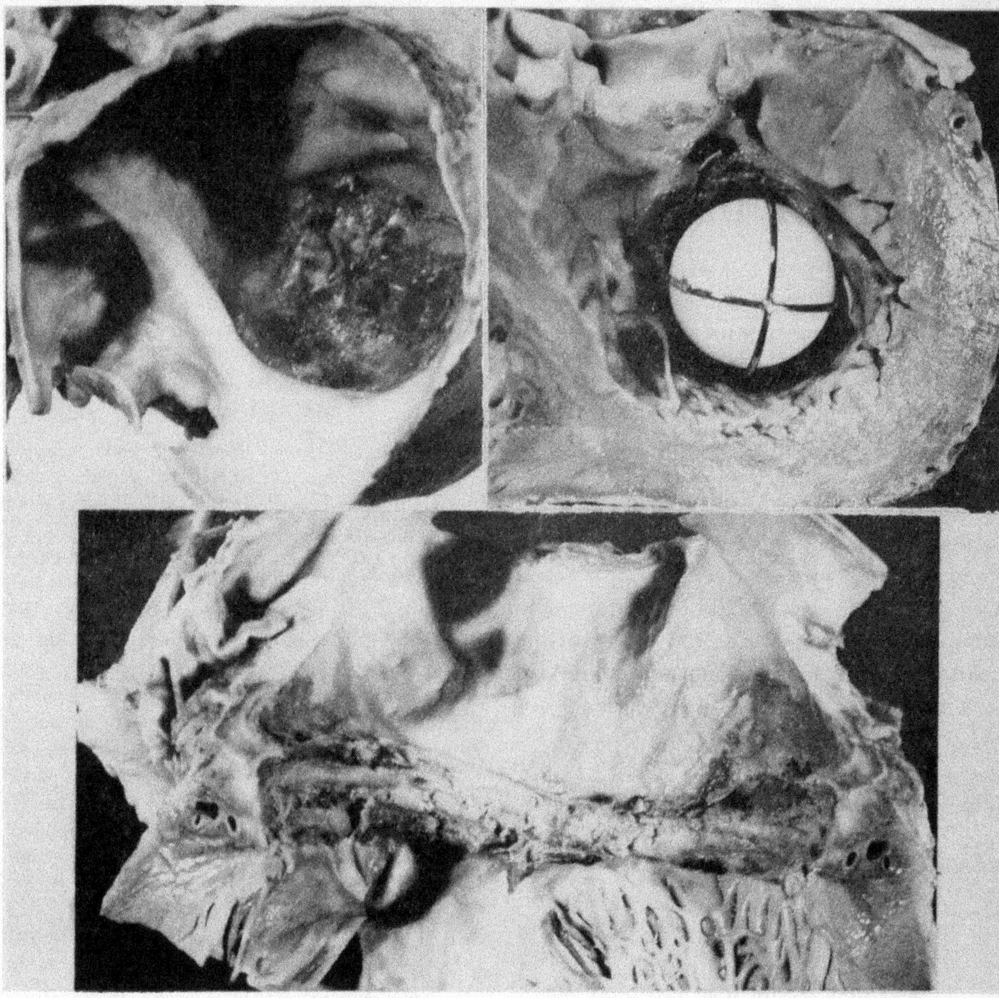

Fig 1.—Heart of patient 1. *Top left,* Opened left atrium, showing the prosthetic mitral orifice completely obscured by a large thrombus. *Top right,* Opened left ventricular cavity disclosing vegetative material about the metallic base of the prosthesis. *Bottom,* Opened left atrium, mitral annulus, and left ventricle. The entire mitral annulus is necrotic. Acute necrotizing inflammation also is present in the adjacent myocardium, and in the atrioventricular sulcus surrounding the coronary vessels.

30% of the circumference of the Teflon fixation ring of the prosthesis was not attached to the mitral annulus, but since the unattached portion of the fixation ring was covered by infected thrombus, which also was adherent to the left atrial wall, no peribasilar communications were present. Following removal of the prosthesis, the entire mitral annulus was found to be necrotic, and the inflammatory process also was present in the subepicardial tissue of the artrioventricular sulcus, and in the adjacent myocardium (Fig 3). Histologic sections of the myocardial walls disclosed acute and subacute abscesses and infarcts. Many intramural coronary arteries contained infected emboli, and had acutely inflamed walls (Fig 4). Focal infarcts also were present in the spleen (240 gm), kidneys and brain.

Case 2 (05-68-27).—A 46-year-old man had a stenotic and incompetent mitral valve replaced with a Starr-Edwards prosthesis on July 23, 1964. Cardiac catheterization eight months later (March 1965) disclosed that the left atrial pressure and cardiac output had returned to normal, and he was asymptomatic. He continued to be well until Nov 5, 1965, when he suddenly fainted, and during the next 24 hours he vomited several times, became listless and anorexic. On November 19 he noted fever (102 F [39.9 C]), and consulted his physician who administered an antibiotic, which was probably erythromycin. He was readmitted to the National Heart Institute on November 24 and was lethargic and disoriented. His temperature rose daily to 102 F (39.9 C). On auscultation the sounds of the prosthetic mitral valve were normal, and no murmur suggesting mitral regurgitation was audible. Dental examination revealed his teeth to be in excellent condition, except for two small cavities. The white blood cell count was 41,000/cu mm, and the hematocrit, 41%. On November 28 cultures of blood drawn during the previous four days grew *Staphylococcus albus,* and daily doses of penicillin (100 million units intravenously) and streptomycin (2 gm intramuscularly) were initiated. The patient became hypotensive, evidenced progressively decreasing cardiac output, and died on Nov 30, 1965.

At autopsy (A65-221), the orifice of the prosthetic mitral valve was almost totally occluded by a thrombus, and thrombus was also present on the ventricular aspect of the mitral prosthesis (Fig 5). Cultures of left ventricular blood at autopsy were sterile, but cultures of the thrombus on the valve grew *S albus.* The movement of the ball in the cage of the Starr-Edwards prosthesis was severely limited by the mass of infected thrombus, and the ball was neither able to extend to the apex of the cage nor to seat completely (Fig 6). The entire mitral annulus was necrotic, and the inflammatory process was present in the adjacent myocardium, and in the subepicardial fat of the atrioventricular sulcus (Fig 7). A histologic section of the mitral annulus is shown in Fig 3. Gram-positive organisms in clumps were identified in the mitral vegetations. Several organizing microinfarcts were present in the left ventricular wall near its base, but no acute microinfarcts, abscesses, or coronary arterial emboli were found. Multiple cerebral and splenic infarcts were present.

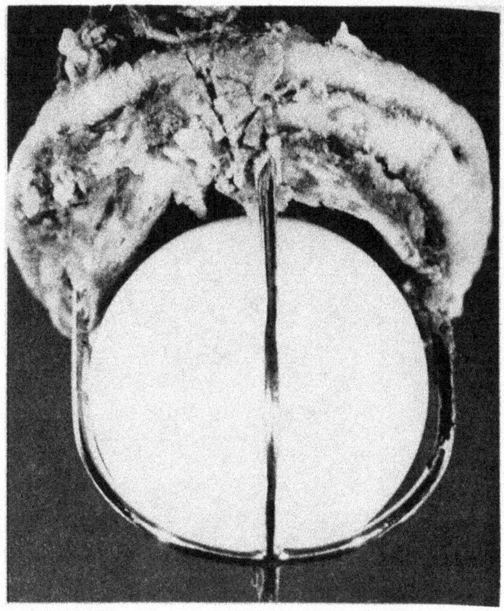

Fig 2.—The Starr-Edwards mitral valve removed from the heart of patient 1. The infected thrombus restricts the motion of the ball, and prevents it from seating completely. As a result, the prosthetic valve is both stenotic and incompetent.

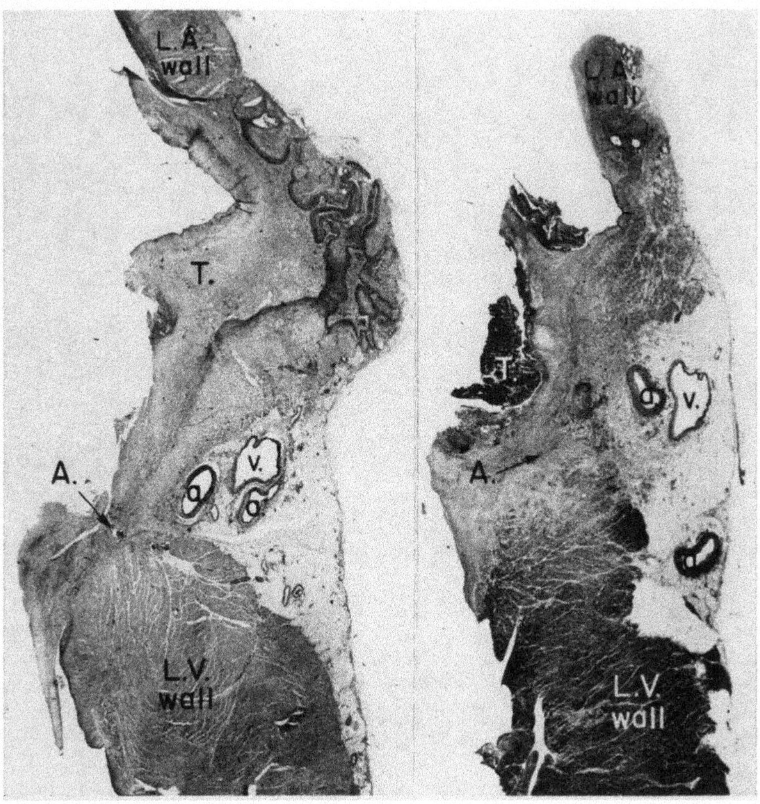

Fig 3.—Section of left atrial (*L.A.*) and left ventricular (*L.V.*) walls and mitral annulus (*A., arrow*) in patients 1 (at left) and 2 (at right). The infected thrombus (*T.*) covers a considerable portion of the left atrial endocardium, and extends into the adjacent myocardium and into the atrioventricular sulcus. (*a.*) indicates coronary artery and (*v.*) coronary sinus (hematoxylin and eosin; × 3, reduced about 15%).

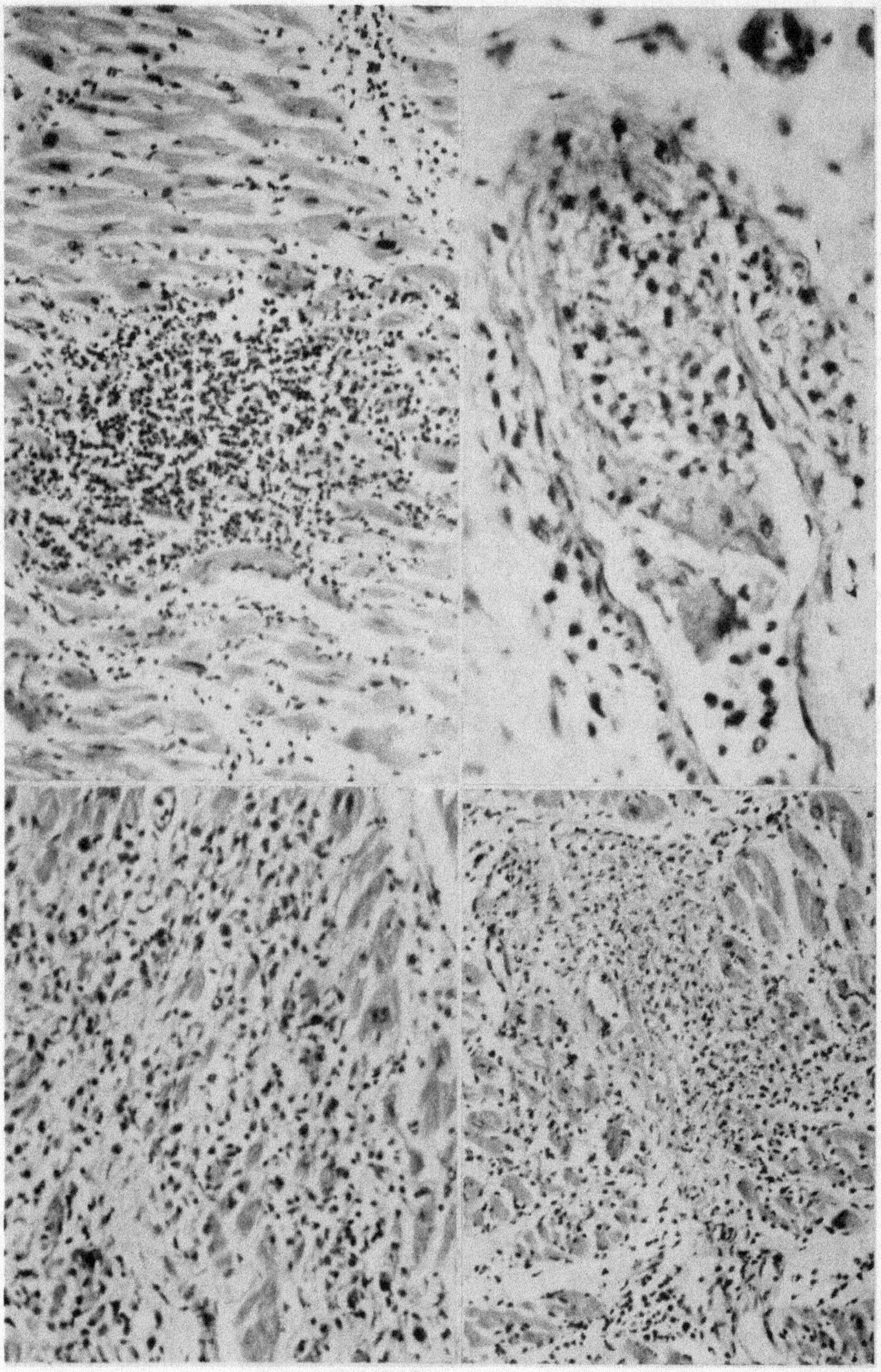

Fig 4.—Lesions in the left ventricular wall in patient 1. *Top left,* Acute abscess (hematoxylin and eosin, × 160). *Top right,* Intramural coronary artery containing infected embolus. The inflamed embolus appears to burrow into the vessel wall producing an acute arteritis (hematoxylin and eosin, × 400). *Bottom left,* Organizing abscess. Other areas disclosed both acute and healed microinfarcts. The lesion illustrated probably represents a transitional stage between acute abscess or acute infarct, and healed microinfarct (hematoxylin and eosin, × 186). *Bottom right,* Acute vasculitis probably resulting from an infected embolus penetrating its wall (hematoxylin and eosin, × 186).

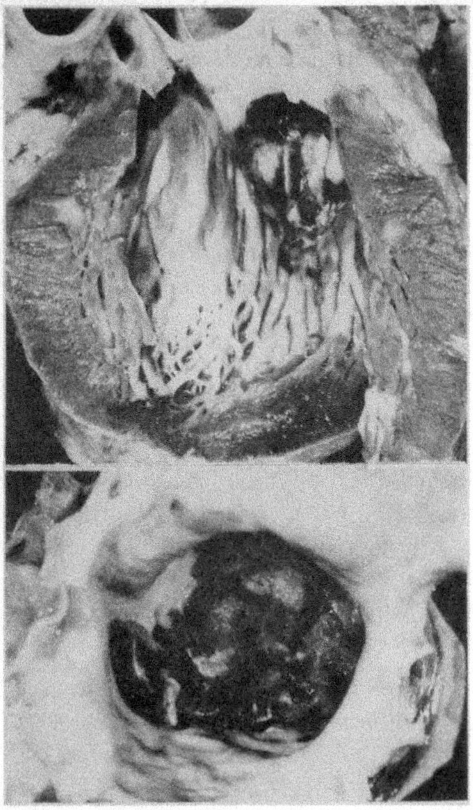

Fig 5.—Opened left ventricle and aortic valve (*top*) and opened left atrium (*bottom*) in patient 2. The infected thrombus is located on both the atrial and ventricular aspects of the Starr-Edwards mitral prosthesis, and from the atrial aspect the prosthetic orifice is seen to be obliterated. The thickened left ventricular endocardium appears to result primarily from healing of the stumps of the amputated papillary muscles.

Comment

The courses of the two patients described above, and the reported experiences of others,[1-3] indicate that infection at the site of a prosthetic cardiac valve is almost always fatal, and that death usually occurs within a month following the onset of signs and symptoms. Death from endocarditis at the site of a prosthetic aortic valve is usually related to detachment of the valve from the aortic annulus, with resulting severe aortic regurgitation and cardiac failure.[4] In the present two patients, the infected thrombi or vegetations on the mitral prostheses interfered with the motion of the ball in the cage and death resulted from obstruction to flow and to valvular incompetence.[5] Although the fixation ring of the mitral prosthesis was partially detached from the mitral annulus in each of the two patients described, a regurgitant leak between the prosthetic ring and the mitral annulus did not occur since the areas of disruption were covered by thrombi.

Staphylococcus is the organism most often responsible for endocarditis in patients with prosthetic valves. It is well recognized that staphylococci produce an acute destructive endocarditis,[6] and this fact is again emphasized by the two patients described herein. Not only did the infectious process involve the mitral ring in each patient, but it ex-

Fig 6.—The mitral prosthesis removed from the heart of patient 2. The movement of the ball in the cage is severely restricted by the mass of the infected thrombus. Several sutures had torn away from the necrotic annulus. The valve is seen from both its anterior and posterior aspects.

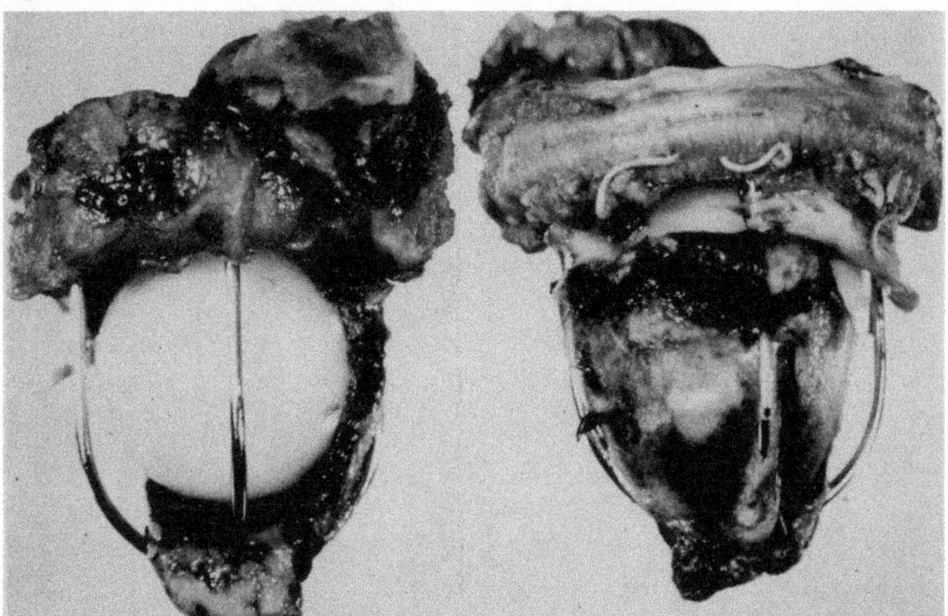

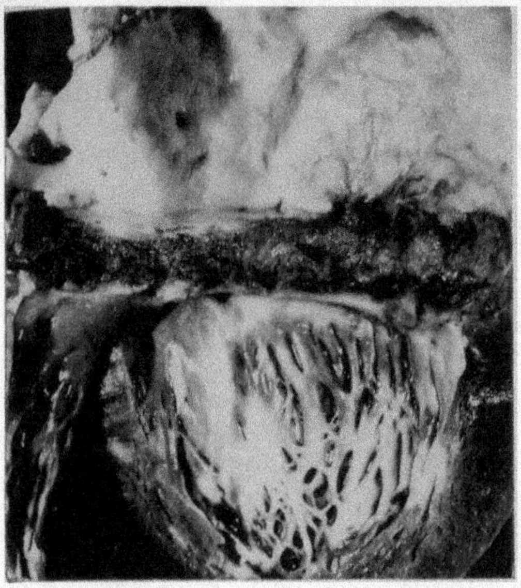

Fig 7.—Opened left atrium, mitral annulus, and left ventricle in patient 2 following removal of the mitral prosthesis. The entire mitral ring is necrotic.

tended into the adjacent myocardium, and into the subepicardial adipose tissue of the left atrioventricular sulcus. The extent of the infection and the character of the tissue of the mitral annulus in these patients clearly indicate that an attempt at secondary operative intervention would have been fruitless. Consequently, since presently available antibiotics are rarely effective in eradicating infection at the site of a prosthetic cardiac valve the infection must be prevented. In patient 1, the infection could, perhaps, have been prevented by prophylactic antibiotics administered before and immediately after the skin grafting operation, but no source of infection was evident in patient 2. The value of prophylactic penicillin in patients with rheumatic heart disease who undergo dental procedures is well established, but the necessity of even more vigorous prophylactic regimens in patients with prosthetic cardiac valves who undergo similar procedures has only recently been emphasized.[4]

Generic and Trade Names of Drugs

Sodium methicillin—*Dimocillin-RT, Staphcillin.*
Kanamycin sulfate—*Kantrex.*
Chloramphenicol—*Chloromycetin.*
Erythromycin ethylsuccinate—*Erythrocin Ethyl Succinate, Pediamycin.*

REFERENCES

1. Amoury, R.A.; Bowman, F.O.; and Malm, J.R.: Endocarditis Associated With Intracardiac Prostheses: Diagnosis, Management and Prophylaxsis, *J Thorac Cardiov Surg* **51**:36, 1966.
2. Stein, P.D.; Harken, D.E.; and Dexter, L.: The Nature and Prevention of Prosthetic Valve Endocarditis, *Amer Heart J* **71**:393, 1966.
3. Herr, R., et al: Special Problems Following Valve Replacement: Embolus, Leak, Infection, Red Cell Damage, *Ann Thorac Surg* **1**:403, 1965.
4. Cohn, L.H., et al: Bacterial Endocarditis Following Aortic Valve Replacement: Clinical and Pathologic Correlations, *Circulation* **33**:209, 1966.
5. Roberts, W.C., and Morrow, A.G.: The Mechanisms of Acute Left Atrial Thrombosis After Mitral Valve Replacement: Pathologic Findings Indicating Obstruction to Left Atrial Emptying, *Amer J Cardiol*, to be published.
6. Sheldon, W.H., and Golden, A.: Abscesses of the Valve Rings of the Heart: A Frequent but Not Well Recognized Complication of Acute Bacterial Endocarditis, *Circulation* **4**:1, 1951.

Valvular Stenosis Produced by Active Infective Endocarditis

By William C. Roberts, M.D., Gordon A. Ewy, M.D., D. Luke Glancy, M.D., and Frank I. Marcus, M.D.

SUMMARY

Two patients with obstructed valve orifices secondary to infective endocarditis are described. In one patient the mitral valve orifice was obstructed by large streptococcal vegetations, and in the second, the aortic valve orifice was obstructed by fungal vegetations. The occurrence of obstructive valvular lesions secondary to infective endocarditis is rare.

Additional Indexing Words:
Mitral stenosis
Aortic stenosis
Fungal vegetations
Streptococcal vegetations

THE DEVELOPMENT of valvular regurgitation is a well-recognized complication of active bacterial or fungal endocarditis. The development of valvular stenosis during active infective endocarditis, on the other hand, has not been described previously. In two patients with such endocarditis whom we have studied, however, valvular stenosis developed.

One, a 21-year-old woman, who had had acute rheumatic fever at the age of 10 years, developed beta hemolytic streptococcal (group B) endocarditis 3 months following a full-term pregnancy with normal delivery, and died a month later. At necropsy, a vegetation was found that nearly filled the mitral orifice (fig. 1). Examination before death had disclosed a short apical diastolic murmur as well as a grade III/VI blowing apical pansystolic one. She died of a large intracerebral hemorrhage.

From the Laboratory of Pathology, Clinic of Surgery, National Heart Institute, National Institutes of Health, U.S. Public Health Service, Bethesda, Maryland, and the Georgetown University Medical Division, District of Columbia General Hospital, Washington, District of Columbia.

The second patient,[1] a 26-year-old narcotic addict, died of *Candida parapsilosis* endocarditis after an 11-month illness. On examination, a loud ejection-type systolic murmur had been audible along the left sternal border, and at necropsy large vegetations partially occluded the aortic valve orifice (fig. 2).

Even though hemodynamic confirmation of valvular stenosis was not obtained in these patients, the degree of valvular obstruction by vegetative material was judged to be severe at necropsy. In neither patient was valvular obstruction by the vegetations suspected clinically. One patient had a mildly scarred but probably functionally normal mitral valve secondary to rheumatic involvement before the appearance of streptococcal endocarditis. Fungal endocardial vegetations tend to grow larger than bacterial endocardial vegetations,[1] and this feature appears to have been important in the second patient. In each of the two patients the vegetations alone were entirely responsible for narrowing the valve orifices.

References

1. Andriole, V. T., Kravetz, H. M., Roberts, W. C., and Utz, J. P.: Candida endocarditis: Clinical and pathologic studies. Amer J Med 32: 251, 1962.

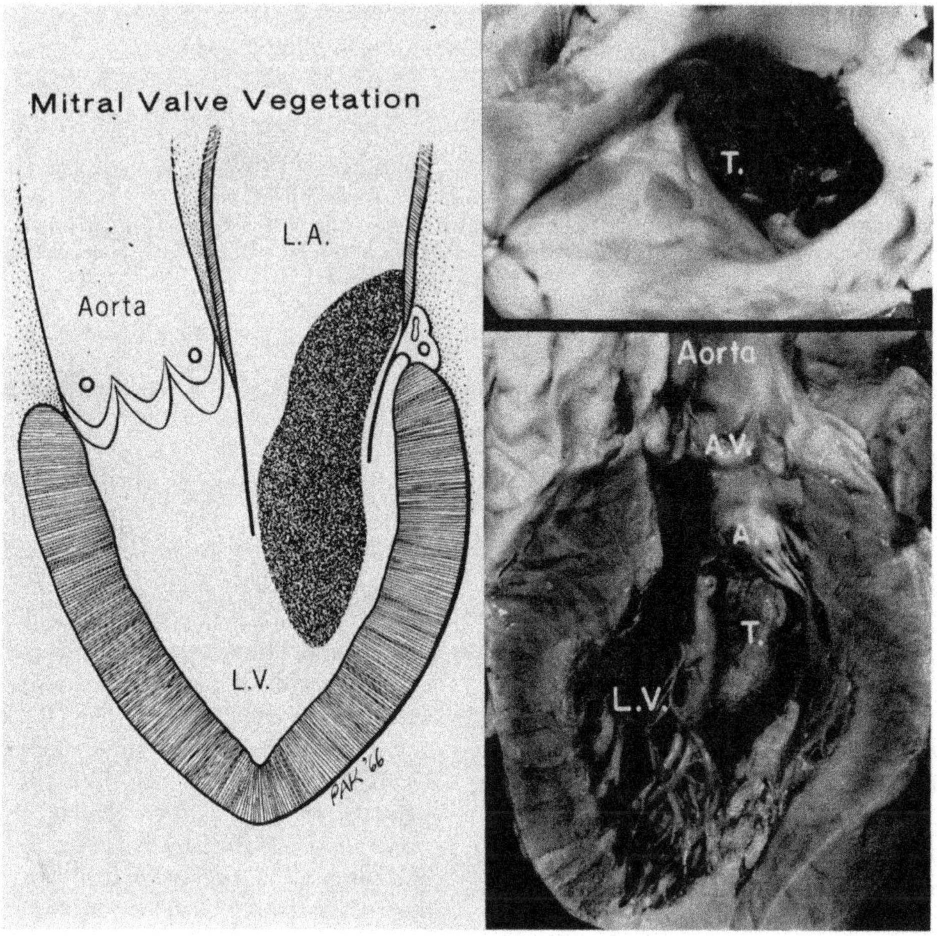

Figure 1

Streptococcal endocarditis of the mitral valve occluding the mitral orifice. (Left) *Diagram demonstrating the size of the vegetation relative to the size of the left atrium (L.A.), mitral orifice, and left ventricle (L.V.).* (Upper right) *Infected thrombotic material (T.) as viewed from the left atrium. The orifice is partially obstructed by the vegetative material which is adherent primarily to the left atrial wall.* (Lower right) *Opened left ventricle (L.V.), aortic valve (A.V.), and aorta in the same patient demonstrating the large infected thrombus (T.) protruding into the left ventricular cavity. The chordae tendineae from the posterior half of the anterior mitral leaflet have been ruptured by the infective process (not shown).*

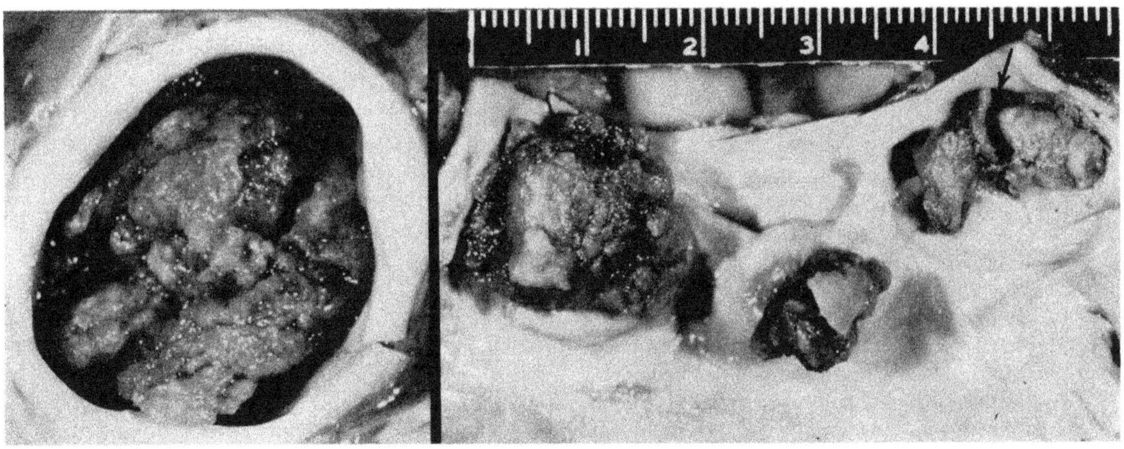

Figure 2

Candida parapsilosis *endocarditis of the aortic valve.* (Left) *Aortic valve as viewed from above. The orifice is obviously obstructed by the large vegetations.* (Right) *The same aortic valve is now opened. Large vegetations are adherent to the ventricular aspects of each of the three aortic valvular cusps. The arrow points to the ostium of the left coronary artery. Vegetative material containing Candida organisms entered this vessel, obstructed the left anterior descending coronary artery, and produced a large myocardial infarct.*

Active Infective Endocarditis Confined to Mural Endocardium

A Study of Six Necropsy Patients

Neil A. Buchbinder, MD, and
William C. Roberts, MD, Bethesda, Md

The clinical and pathologic features pertaining to six patients with infective endocarditis confined to mural endocardium are described. Five patients had leukemia, and one had lymphoma. Although each patient had associated myocarditis, none had clinical evidence of cardiac dysfunction. In each patient the endocarditis represented an extension of a fungal infection which had originated elsewhere: each of the four patients with right ventricular vegetations had underlying myocardial abscesses which had extended into the endocardium; each of the two patients with left atrial vegetations had mycotic pulmonary abscesses which had extended into this cardiac chamber via pulmonary veins. Although it did not cause death in any of our patients, mural endocarditis is not a pathologic curiosity, since it has, as indicated by earlier reports, caused cardiac rupture, aortico-right ventricular fistula, and embolization.

ACTIVE infective endocarditis confined to nonvalvular (mural) endocardium is rare and its clinicopathologic features are poorly understood. This report describes clinical and necropsy findings from six patients with active mural infective endocarditis and attempts to delineate its pathogenesis.

Report of Cases

Data pertaining to the six patients are summarized in Table 1. Five patients had leukemia and one had lymphoma. All were treated with cytotoxic agents. The vegetations were confined to the mural endocardium of the right ventricle (Fig 1) in four patients and to left atrium in two patients (Fig 2 and 3). The causative organism was a fungus in all six patients: *Candida* species in four, *Mucor* species in one, and *Aspergillus* species in 1 patient. *Candida* species were cultured in one of four patients from whom blood was drawn for fungal culture, and each patient was treated with antifungal agents. All six patients had fever. A precordial murmur (grade 2/6, mid-systolic, at left sternal border in each) was present in two patients,

Accepted for publication Oct 15, 1971.

From the Section of Pathology, National Heart and Lung Institute, and the Laboratory of Pathology, National Cancer Institute, National Institutes of Health, Bethesda, Md.

Reprint requests to Section of Pathology, National Heart and Lung Institute, National Institutes of Health, Bethesda, Md 20014 (Dr. Roberts).

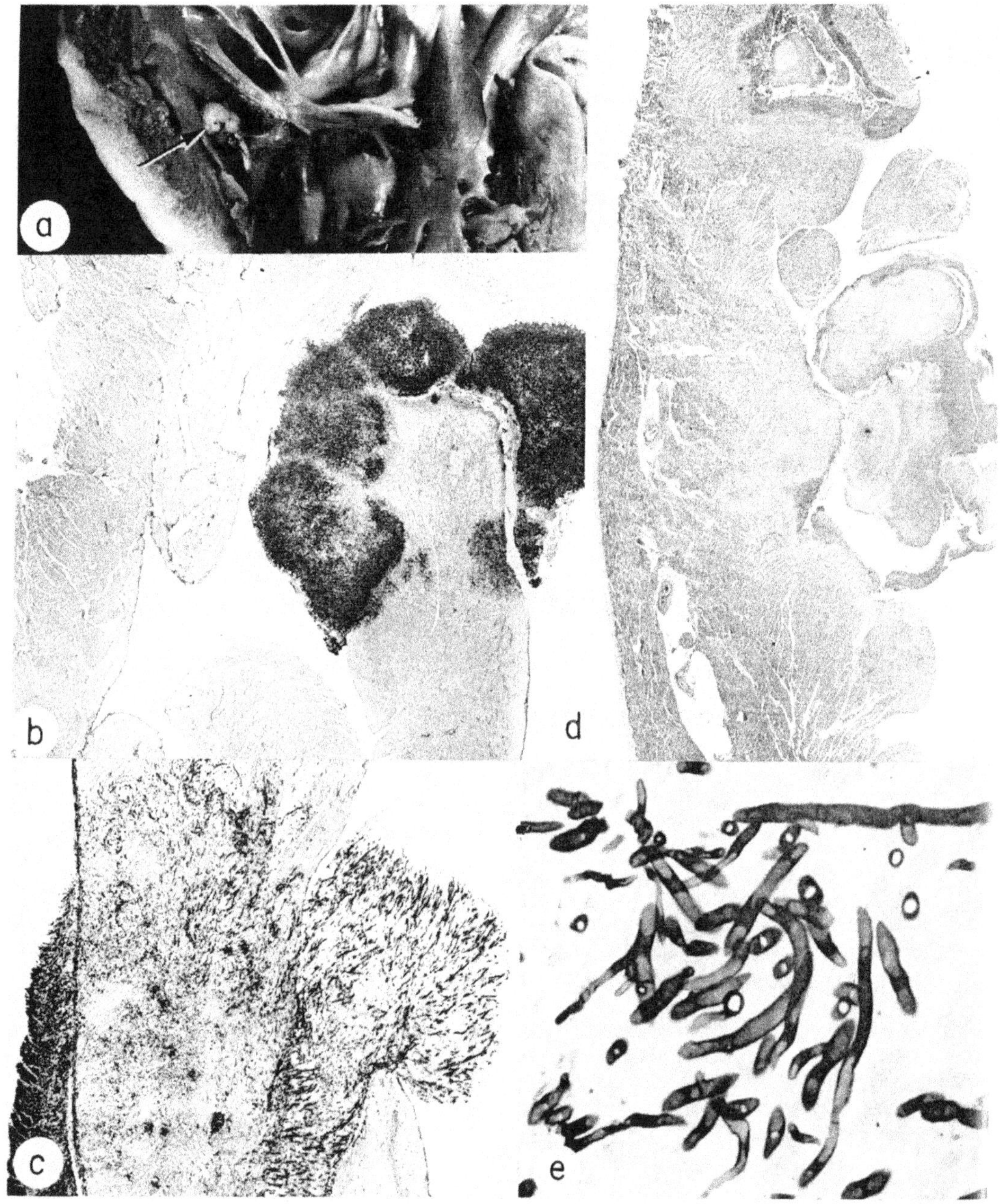

Fig 1.—Mural endocarditis of right ventricle in three different patients. **a** and **b**, Right ventricular endocardial vegetation **(arrow)** in 65-year-old man (A66-180) with chronic myelocytic leukemia for one year. **Candida** species abscesses were present in many body organs including heart. **b**, Right ventricular wall showing endocardial vegetation loaded with **Candida** species organisms (methenamine silver stain, ×14). **c** and **e**, Right ventricular vegetation with organisms extending through whole thickness of wall from epicardium to endocardium in 7-year-old girl (A63-246) with acute lymphocytic leukemia for eight months.[14] Five days before death, **C albicans** was cultured from blood and despite therapy with amphotericin B, death resulted from acute pneumonia. **e**, High-power photomicrograph of portion of endocardial vegetation showing **Candida** species (methenamine silver stain, ×18 [**c**]; ×520 [**e**]). **d**, Right ventricular wall showing myocardial abscess which has extended to form endocardial vegetation in 29-year-old man (A66-159) with chronic myelocytic leukemia for four years. Three months before death, pleural effusion developed from which **Candida** species were cultured. Death resulted from extensive acute pneumonia (hematoxylin-eosin, ×7).

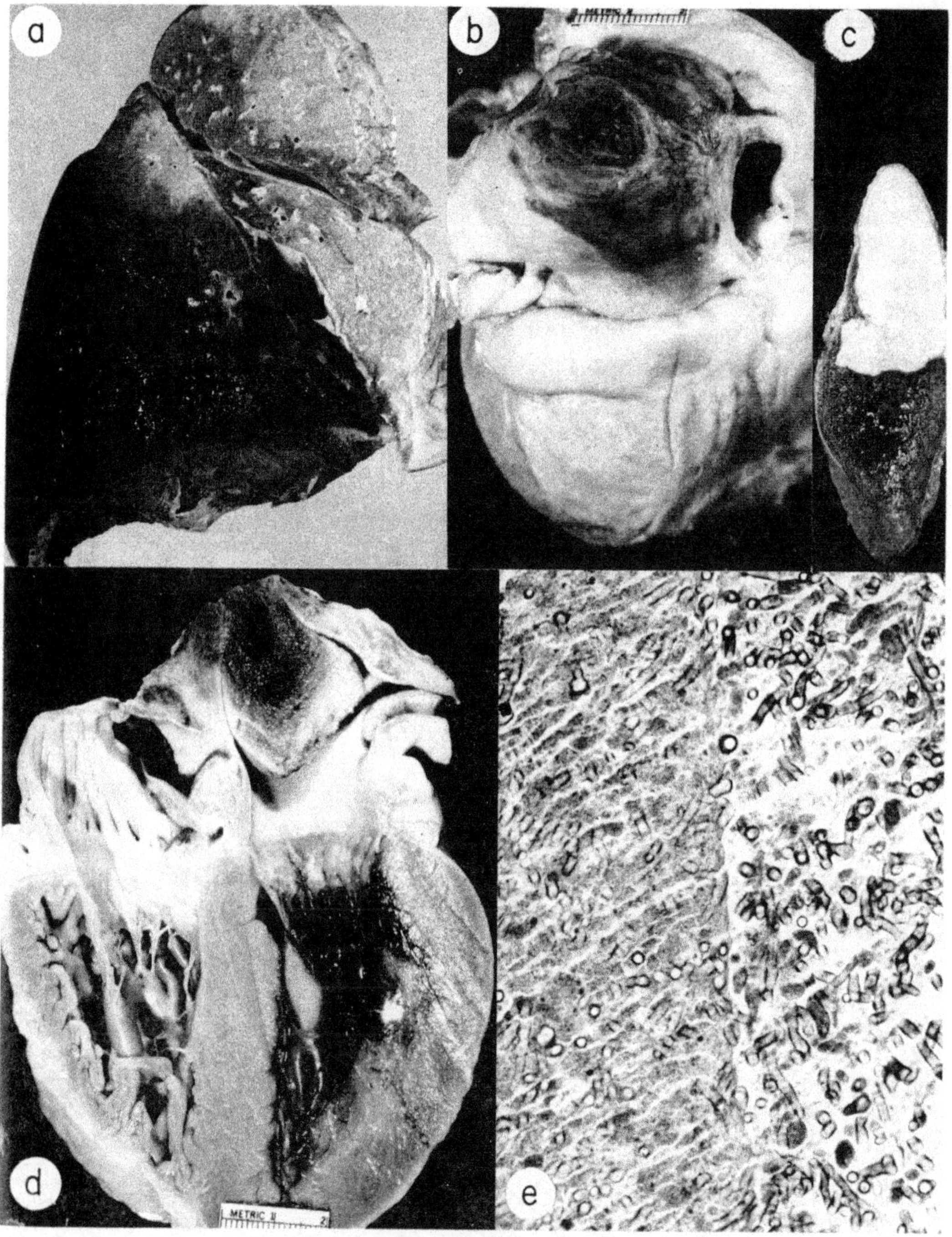

Fig 2.—**Mucor** species endocarditis involving left atrium in 15-year-old boy (A69-104) with acute myelocytic leukemia, six months' duration. One month before death, acute bilateral pneumonia developed. **a**, Section of lung showing hemorrhagic necrotizing pneumonia. **b**, Posterior view of heart showing large area of epicarditis around pulmonary vein occluded by fungal mass. **c**, Transverse section of spleen showing large embolic infarct. **d**, Longitudinal section through both atria and ventricles of heart, showing large fungal mass extending from occluded pulmonary vein onto endocardium of left atrium. **e**, Mass in left atrium showing numerous **Mucor** organisms (hematoxylin-eosin, ×400).

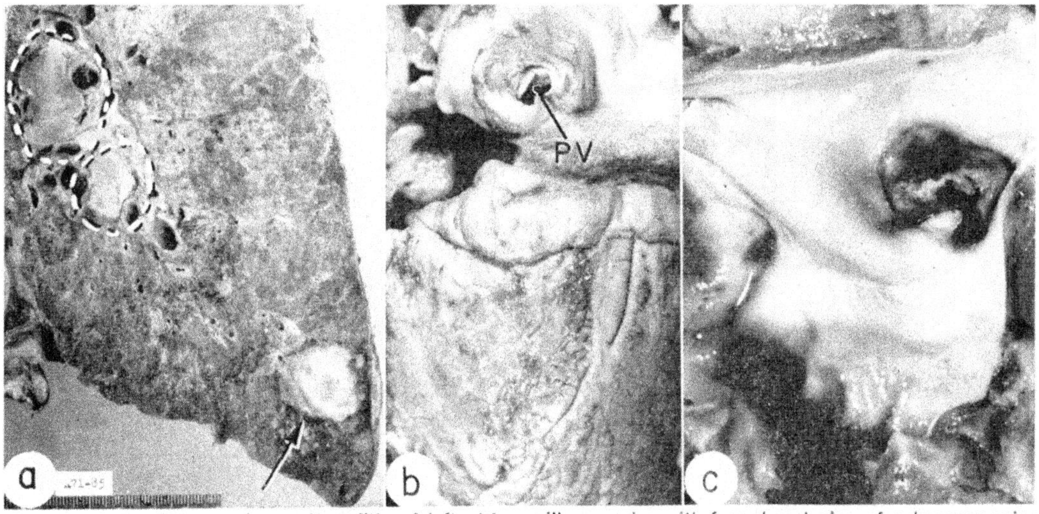

Fig 3.—**Aspergillus** species endocarditis of left atrium in 27-year-old man (A71-85) with lymphosarcoma for five months. Fever, cough, dyspnea, and right-sided pleural effusion appeared nine weeks before death. Blood cultures were negative. Death resulted from extensive acute pneumonia. **a,** Section through left lung showing abscess (**arrow**) caused by **Aspergillus** species with fungal occlusion of pulmonary veins (enclosed by **broken lines**). **b,** Posterolateral view of heart showing epicarditis involving left ventricle and left atrium. Pulmonary vein (**PV**) surrounded by fungal mass. **c,** Opened left atrium showing endocardial vegetation resulting from propagation of infective process from pulmonary vein.

Table 1.—Clinical and Necropsy Data From Six Patients With Mural Infective Endocarditis*

Patient	Age, Sex	Primary Disease	Site of Vegetation	Organism	Blood Culture	Precordial Murmur	Cause of Death
A63-246	7, F	AML	RV	**Candida tropicalis**	+	0	Acute pneumonia
A66-159	29, M	CML	RV	**Candida** sp	0	0	Acute pneumonia
A66-180	65, M	CML	RV	**C albicans**	0	0	Brain abscess
A66-182	30, F	CML	RV	**Candida** sp	0	+	Bleeding
A69-104	15, M	AML	LA	**Mucor** sp	0†	0	Acute pneumonia
A71-85	27, M	Lymphoma	LA	**Aspergillus** sp	0	+	Acute pneumonia

* Acute myelocytic leukemia, AML; chronic myelocytic leukemia, CML; left atrium, LA; right ventricle, RV.
† Blood not cultured specifically for fungus; positive, +; negative, 0.

Table 2.—Data From 14 Previously Reported Cases*

Authors	Age, Sex	Site of Vegetation	Causative Organism	Underlying Disease
Chance, 1846[1]	13, M	LV	...	0
Howitt, 1846[2]	8, M	RV	...	0
Moxon, 1869[3]	11, M	LV, RA	...	0
Moorhouse, 1916[4]	20, M	RV	...	Traumatic hemothorax
Horder, 1920[5]	..., ...	...	...	...
Weiss & Wilkins, 1937[6]	73, M	RV	Gram-positive coccus (**Staphylococcus aureus**)‡	Diabetes mellitus
Trasoff & Meranze, 1944[7]	47, F	LA	**Diplococcus pneumoniae**‡	Pancreatitis
Taniguchi & Murphy, 1950[8]	55, F	LA	**Proteus** SP	0
Gorlin et al, 1950[9]	..., ...	RV	...	...
Cates & Christie, 1951[10]†	..., ...	LA	...	...
Hirsch, 1958[11]	60, F	RA, RV	β-hemolytic streptococcus‡	Thrombophlebitis
Persaud, 1970[12]	13, M	RV, LV	Cytomegalovirus	Burns
Milstoc & Berger, 1971[13]	4, F 65, F	RV LV	Gram-positive coccus Gram-positive coccus	Bronchiectasis Paralysis agitans

* Aortic regurgitation, AR; left atrium, LA; left ventricle, LV; right atrium, RA; right ventricle, RV.
† One patient with isolated mural infective endocarditis was mentioned by authors, but he was not described in detail.
‡ Postmortem culture.

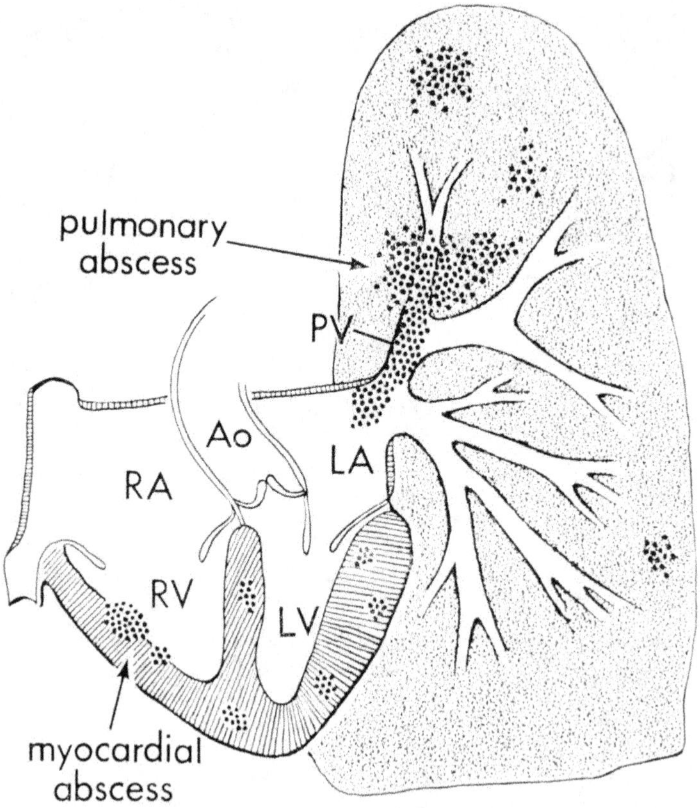

Fig 4.—Schema of pathogenesis of mural infective endocarditis in six patients. Right ventricular (**RV**) endocardial vegetations resulted from extension of myocardial abscesses onto endocardium. Left atrial (**LA**) vegetations resulted from extension of pulmonary abscesses via pulmonary veins (**PV**). Right atrium (**RA**), aorta (**Ao**), and left ventricle (**LV**) also shown.

of Mural Infective Endocarditis*

Precordial Murmur	Pathogenesis	Cause of Death
0	Myocardial abscess	Sepsis
0	Myocardial abscess	Sepsis
0	Myocardial abscess	Sepsis
AR	Myocardial abscess	Heart failure
0	...	...
AR	Myocardial abscess	Cardiac tamponade
0	Myocardial abscess	Sepsis
0	...	Cerebrovascular accident
...	...	...
...	...	...
0	...	Pulmonary embolus
0	...	Acute pneumonia & sepsis
0	...	Acute pneumonia
0	Myocardial abscess	Sepsis

but both had fever, anemia, and tachycardia at the time and, therefore, the murmur was probably hemic in origin. Splenomegaly occurred in all six patients and was attributed to the underlying blood disease. Results from electrocardiograms, recorded in four patients, were normal in two; one patient had nonspecific ST-T wave abnormalities, and another, a 65-year-old man, had right bundle-branch block. Heart disease was not suggested clinically in any patient. All had normal-sized hearts. Death was attributed to acute pneumonia in four patients, brain abscess in one, and generalized bleeding in one.

In all six patients, the endocardial lesions were not primary, but resulted from extension of infections originating at other sites. All four patients with right ventricular vegetations had numerous myocardial abscesses as part of a generalized fungal pyemia. The endocardial vegetations in these four patients resulted from extension of myocardial abscesses onto endocardium. The two patients with left atrial vegetations had massive pulmonary mycosis with fungal thrombi occluding main pulmonary veins and extending onto left atrial endocardium. Myocardial abscesses were not present in either of these two patients, but each had focal acute myocarditis, as well as focal fungal pericarditis involving left atrium.

Comment

Review of the English literature disclosed 14 previously reported cases of patients with infective endocarditis confined to mural endocardium (Table 2).[1-13] Of the total 20 patients, including our 6, the mural endocardium of right ventricle was involved in 11. Eleven of the 14 previously reported cases were described in detail: the causative organism was a bacterium in six, a virus in one, and was unknown in four; an underlying debilitating illness was present in seven; precordial murmurs (aortic regurgitation) occurred in two cases; and in seven cases, the mural endocarditis resulted from extension of a myocardial abscess onto mural endocardium. Myocardial lesions, remote from the endocardial lesions, were common. Our four patients with mural infective endocarditis caused by myocardial abscesses had numerous abscesses throughout myocardium. In eight of 11 previously reported cases, descriptions of myocardium away from the endocardial lesion were given: myocarditis or myocardial "degeneration" was present in five.

The pathogenesis of mural infective endocarditis is diagrammatically depicted in Fig 4. In none of our six patients were the mural vegetations primary, but they resulted from extension of an infective process originating at another site (myocardium or lung).

Mural infective endocarditis itself rarely causes death. In all our six patients, and in at least 6 of the 11 previously reported, well-described cases, death resulted from generalized sepsis or extracardiac foci of infection (brain or lungs). The mural endocarditis or the underlying myocardial abscesses are not, however, always without clinical sequelae. The myocardial abscesses present in the patient described by Moorhouse,[4] and in the patient described by Weiss and Wilkins,[6] not only led to right ventricular endocardial lesions but extended through the ventricular septum and the aortic wall, producing an aortico-right ventricular fistula, in the first patient described, and in the second patient, the abscesses extended into the pericardial space, causing tamponade. Mural vegetations also may dislodge. The sudden cerebrovascular accident which caused death in the patient described by Taniguchi and Murphy[8] was probably embolic in origin. The patient described by Hirsch[11] died from a large septic pulmonary embolus which probably came from vegetations on mural endocardium of right atrium and right ventricle. The patient described by Taniguchi and Murphy[8] also had "focal embolic glomerulonephritis."

Nonproprietary and Trade Names of Drug

Amphotericin B—*Fungizone*.

References

1. Chance EJ: Abscess of the heart. *Lancet* **1**:548-550, 1846.
2. Howitt T: Remarkable case of abscess of the heart. *Lancet* **1**:684-685, 1846.
3. Moxon W: Case of abscess of the heart bursting into the left ventricle. *Trans Path Soc London* **20**:113, 1869.
4. Moorhouse VHK: Abscess of the myocardium resulting in aortic leakage in the right heart. *Lancet* **1**:292-293, 1916.
5. Horder T: Discussion on the clinical significance and course of subacute bacterial endocarditis. *Brit Med J* **2**:301-303, 1920.
6. Weiss S, Wilkins RW: Myocardial abscess with perforation of the heart. *Amer J Med Sci* **194**:199-205, 1937.
7. Trasoff A, Meranze DR: The association of acute interstitial pancreatitis with acute pneumococcic mural endocarditis. *J Lab Clin Med* **29**:590-594, 1944.
8. Taniguchi T, Murphy FD: Mural bacterial endocarditis produced by *Proteus*. *JAMA* **143**:427-428, 1950.
9. Gorlin R, Favour CB, Emery FJ: Long-term follow-up study of penicillin-treated subacute bacterial endocarditis. *New Eng J Med* **242**:995-1001, 1950.
10. Cates JE, Christie RV: Subacute bacterial endocarditis: A review of 442 patients treated in 14 centres appointed by the Penicillin Trials Committee of the Medical Research Council. *Quart J Med* **20**:93-130, 1951.
11. Hirsch EF: Septic thrombophlebitis of the leg with mural endocarditis and pulmonary embolism. *Illinois Med J* **114**:289-292, 1958.
12. Persaud V: Two unusual cases of mural endocarditis, with a review of the literature. *Amer J Clin Path* **53**:832-838, 1970.
13. Milstoc M, Berger HR: True bacterial mural endocarditis. *Chest* **59**:103-105, 1971.
14. Roberts WC, Bodey GP, Wertlake PT: The heart in acute leukemia: A study of 420 autopsy cases. *Amer J Cardiol* **21**:388-412, 1968.

Right-Sided Valvular Infective Endocarditis

A Clinicopathologic Study of Twelve Necropsy Patients

WILLIAM C. ROBERTS, M.D.
NEIL A BUCHBINDER, M.D.
Bethesda, Maryland

Clinical and necropsy features are described in twelve patients with infective endocarditis involving right-sided cardiac valves. In six patients infective endocarditis was limited to the tricuspid valve; in the other six vegetations also were present on one left-sided cardiac valve, but in only one of them was the infective endocarditis definitely primary on the left side of the heart. The tricuspid valve was the site of infective endocarditis in eleven patients and the pulmonic valve in one. The organisms responsible for the infective endocarditis were Staphylococcus aureus in six patients, Diplococcus pneumoniae in four, alpha Streptococcus in one and Aspergillus flavus in one. Five patients were alcoholics, four were heroin addicts, two had blood dyscrasias, and one had congenital cardiac disease (ventricular septal defect). The infective endocarditis in each of the nine patients with alcoholism or heroin addiction and in the one with congenital heart disease was primary in the heart; in the remaining two patients, it was secondary to generalized infection affecting many body organs.

Acute pneumonia was a dominant clinical feature in ten of the twelve patients and appeared to be secondary to dislodgment of material from the right-sided cardiac vegetations. Six patients also had acute meningitis. Although the vegetations caused considerable damage to the right-sided cardiac valves, evidence of cardiac dysfunction was either absent or attributable to acute cor pulmonale secondary to the acute pneumonia. Attention is called to the common tetrad of chronic alcoholism, acute pneumonia, acute meningitis and infective endocarditis. In nine of the twelve patients the right-sided vegetations did not extend to involve the basal attachments of the leaflets to the annuli. Thus, in these nine patients total excision of the valve leaflets would have eradicated their valvular endocarditis.

With the striking increase in heroin addiction in recent years, right-sided infective endocarditis has received considerable attention. Emphasis has been placed on the clinical features of right-sided infective endocarditis, and little attention has been given to the morphologic findings in infective endocarditis involving the tricuspid or pulmonic valves. We attempt to fill in this void by describing cardiac necropsy observations and relating them to clinical findings in twelve fatal cases of infective endocarditis involving right-sided cardiac valves.

From the Section of Pathology, National Heart and Lung Institute, National Institutes of Health, Bethesda, Maryland 20014. Requests for reprints should be addressed to Dr. William C. Roberts, Section of Pathology, National Heart and Lung Institute, Bethesda, Maryland 20014. Manuscript received November 4, 1971; revised January 18, 1972

TABLE I Clinical and Necropsy Data in Twelve Patients with Right-Sided Infective Endocarditis (IE)

Case	Age (yr) and Sex	Valve(s) Involved	Causative Organism	Predisposing Factor	Acute Pneumonia	Acute Meningitis	Systolic Precordial Murmur and Intensity (0–6)	Diagnosis of IE During Life	Valve Dysfunction	Heart Failure Right-sided	Heart Failure Left-sided
1	64,M	TV	Staph. aureus*	Lymphoma	0	0	0	0	0	0	0
2	31,F	TV	Staph. aureus	H	+	0	+ (3/6)	+	TR	+	0
3	65,M	TV	D. pneumoniae	A	+	+	+ (3/6)	+	TR	+	0
4	33,M	TV	Staph. aureus	H	+	0	0	0	0	0	0
5	35,F	TV	Staph. aureus	H	+	+	+ (2/6)	0	?TS	+	0
6	22,F	TV	Staph. aureus	H	+	0	+ (2/6)	+	TR	+	0
7	62,M	AV,TV	D. pneumoniae	A	0	+	+ (2/6)	0	0	0	0
8	10 mo,M	MV,TV	A. flavus*	Thymic dysplasia‖	+	0	0	0	0	0	0
9	55,M	MV,PV	Staph. aureus	A	+	0	+ (1/6)	0	PR	0	0
10	58,M	AV,MV,TV	D. pneumoniae	A	+	+	+ (3/6)¶	0	AR	+	+
11	55,M	AV,TV	D.pneumoniae	A	+	+	+ (3/6)¶	+	TR,AR	+	+
12	5,F	AV,MV,TV	Strep. viridans	0	+	0	+ (5/6)¶	+	AR	+	+

NOTE: A = alcoholism; AR = aortic regurgitation; AV = aortic valve; CA = coronary artery; CHF = congestive heart failure; GN = glomerulonephritis; H = heroin addiction; IE = infective endocarditis; MV = mitral valve; PR = pulmonic regurgitation; PV = pulmonic valve; TR = tricuspid regurgitation; TS = tricuspid stenosis; TV = tricuspid valve.
* IE secondary to generalized sepsis.
† Represent minimum duration.

PATIENTS STUDIED

Among fifty-seven patients with fatal active valvular infective endocarditis studied at necropsy by us, forty-five had vegetations limited to the left side of the heart [1], and twelve had vegetations involving one right-sided cardiac valve. Certain clinical and necropsy observations in the latter twelve patients are summarized in Table I. Their ages ranged from ten months to sixty-five years; eight were male, and four were female. In six, vegetations were confined to the tricuspid valve; in the other six, vegetations involved one left-sided cardiac valve in addition to the tricuspid (five patients) or pulmonic valve (one patient). Blood cultures, obtained in eleven patients, were positive in each: Staph. aureus in six, D. pneumoniae in three, alpha Streptococcus in one and Aspergillus flavus in one. Culture of cerebrospinal fluid in the twelfth patient yielded D. pneumoniae, and histologic study of his vegetations at necropsy showed gram-positive diplococci. Nine patients were either alcoholics (five patients) or heroin addicts (4 patients), two others had altered defense mechanisms (Hodgkin's disease in one and thymic dysplasia in one) and one had congenital cardiac disease (ventricular septal defect). Four of the five alcoholics had pneumococcal endocarditis, and all four heroin addicts had staphylococcal endocarditis. The infective endocarditis in each of the nine patients with alcoholism or heroin addiction and in the patient with congenital heart disease was primary in the heart; in the remaining two patients (Cases 1 and 8), the infective endocarditis appeared secondary to generalized infection affecting many body organs.

The clinical features in all twelve patients were dominated by symptoms clearly attributable to extracardiac foci of infection. In eleven of the twelve patients, either acute pneumonia (six patients), acute meningitis (two patients) or both (four patients) were the major initial presentations and remained the dominant clinical feature in ten. Although evidence of congestive cardiac failure (cardiomegaly, distended neck veins, hepatomegaly or ventricular gallop sounds) developed in seven patients, in four the "failure" could be attributed to acute cor pulmonale from the acute pneumonia; each of the other three patients (Cases 10, 11 and 12) had both right- and left-sided congestive cardiac failure secondary to endocarditis, causing regurgitation of one left-sided cardiac valve in two patients and a left ventricular-right atrial shunt in one (Case 11).

Precordial murmurs were heard in nine of the twelve patients. All nine had systolic murmurs, and three of them (Cases 10, 11 and 12) had diastolic murmurs (from destruction of aortic valves by infection). Four of six patients with endocarditis limited to the tricuspid valve had systolic murmurs, but in only one did the murmur get louder with inspiration. In one patient (Case 11) whose membranous ventricular septum was ruptured by the infective process, a continuous precordial murmur developed several days before his death, and clinically a diagnosis of acquired ventricular septal defect was made. All twelve patients had fever (oral temperature more than 100°F). The spleen was palpated in three patients, fundal hemorrhages were observed in two, and one had dermal petechiae. The diagnosis of infective endocarditis was made during life in only three of the six patients with isolated tricuspid valve endocarditis and in only two of six with

Duration of IE (days)	Principal Causes of Death	Heart Weight (gm)	Ruptured TV Chordae Tendineae	Bacteria in TV or PV	Papillary Muscle Necrosis	Myocarditis: Abscess	Myocarditis: Non-suppurating	Renal Abnormalities	Spleen Weight (gm)
56†	Generalized infection	325	0	+	0	+	0	GN	960‡
35	Renal failure	340	+	+	0	0	0	GN	300
112	Meningitis	450§	+	0	0	0	0	Healed infarcts	350
28	Pneumonia	260	+	+	0	0	0	GN	350
	Meningitis	290	+	+	0	0	0	GN	400
49	Pneumonia	340	+	+	0	0	0	Chronic pyelonephritis	180
35	Meningitis	230	0	0	0	0	0	0	...
42	Generalized infection	40	0	+	+	+	+	Abscesses	35‡
4	Pneumonia + renal failure	410	0	0	+	+	+	Abscesses	200
2	CHF	300	0	+	0	0	0	GN	100
21	CHF	420	+	0	0	0	+	0	...#
120	CHF	150	0	0	+	0	0	Septic infarcts	120

‡ Spleen palpated clinically.
§ Patient had systemic hypertension.
‖ Agammaglobulinemia and lymphocytopenia.
¶ Diastolic murmur of aortic regurgitation present also.
\# Operatively excised in distant past.

combined right- and left-sided endocarditis. Eleven patients received antibiotics: eight received a drug appropriate for the causative organism, three a questionably appropriate antibiotic and one an inappropriate drug

All valves were functionally normal before they became the sites of active infective endocarditis. Infective endocarditis caused valve dysfunction in seven patients regurgitation in six (tricuspid valve three, aortic valve three) and possible tricuspid stenosis in one Each of these seven patients had right- (four patients) or left-sided (three patients) cardiac failure. Congestive heart failure was the principal cause of death, however, in only three patients, and each of them had aortic regurgitation. In the remaining nine patients in whom congestive cardiac failure was either not present (five patients) or of secondary importance (four patients), the principal cause of death was related to extracardiac abnormalities: acute pneumonia, acute meningitis, generalized infection, renal failure or combinations of these. Acute pneumonia was the most common factor, occurring in ten of the twelve patients, and the two without pneumonia had either single or small flat tricuspid valve vegetations.

NECROPSY FINDINGS

Certain necropsy findings are summarized in Table I and illustrated in Figures 1 through 12. Vegetations were present on twenty of the forty-eight cardiac valves of the twelve patients. The tricuspid valve was involved in eleven, pulmonic valve in one, mitral valve in four and aortic valve in four. With the exception of the aortic valve in one patient (Case 12) each of the twenty valves containing vegetations appeared to be anatomically normal at sites not involved by the infection. The aortic valve in this patient (Case 12), who also had a small ventricular septal defect, consisted of three distinctly unequal sized cusps, but none was thickened, and the valve almost certainly functioned normally before it became infected. Thus, the infective endocarditis in eleven of the twelve patients involved previously anatomically normal valves.

Of the eleven patients with infective endocarditis involving the tricuspid valve vegetations were present on twenty-four of the thirty-three tricuspid valve leaflets; five patients had vegetations on all three leaflets, three on two leaflets and three on only one leaflet. Each of the three patients with only one tricuspid valve leaflet involved also had infective endocarditis involving one or both left-sided cardiac valves. Six of the eight patients with vegetations on two or more tricuspid valve cusps had infective endocarditis limited to the right side of the heart; the seventh patient (Case 11) had left-sided involvement only because of extension of the tricuspid valve infection through the membranous ventricular septum to the base of one aortic valve cusp; the eighth patient had vegetations on all three tricuspid valve cusps and only a minute vegetation on one of the three aortic valve cusps. In the latter patient, therefore, the left-sided infection is considered secondary to the

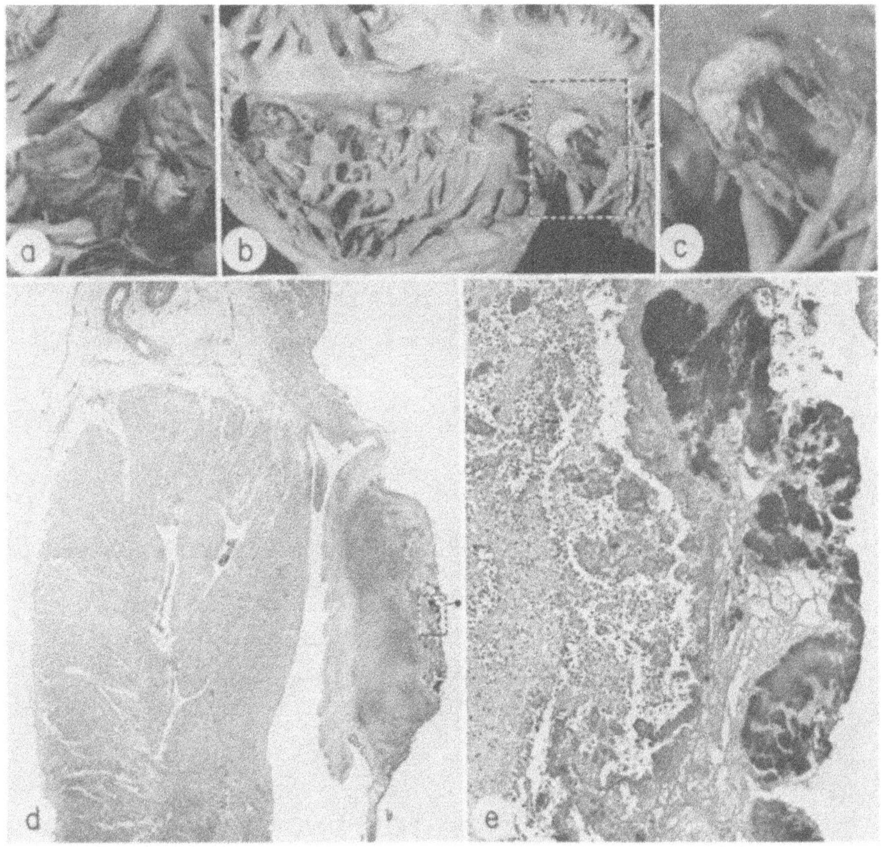

Figure 1. *Case 2. Staphylococcus aureus endocarditis of tricuspid valve in a thirty-one year old female heroin addict (A67-257). Acute pneumonia developed, probably from septic emboli, about thirty-five days before death. Pulmonary abscesses were seen on the chest roentgenogram when she was hospitalized thirteen days before death. A grade 3/6 blowing precordial systolic murmur was audible and the liver was pulsatile. She died of congestive heart failure and renal failure. "Focal embolic" glomerulonephritis was found at necropsy.* ***a,*** *tricuspid valve viewed from right ventricle showing vegetations on each leaflet.* ***b,*** *opened right heart showing vegetations on each tricuspid valve cusp.* ***c,*** *close-up of bracketed area in* ***b*** *showing several ruptured chordae tendineae.* ***d,*** *photomicrograph of section through right atrium, right ventricle and tricuspid valve leaflet. Hematoxylin and eosin stain; original magnification × 5, reduced by 28 per cent.* ***e,*** *high power view of bracketed area in* ***d.*** *Vegetation consists of numerous polymorphonuclear leukocytes enmeshed in a fibrin network. Darkly stained areas are colonies of gram-positive cocci. Hematoxylin and eosin stain; original magnification × 108, reduced by 28 per cent.*

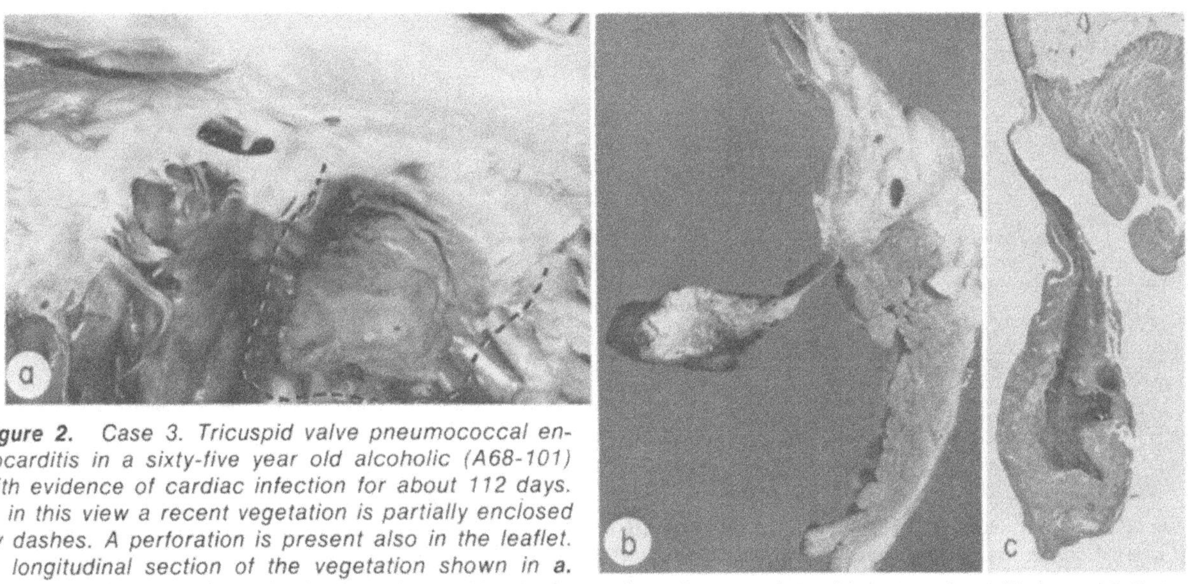

Figure 2. *Case 3. Tricuspid valve pneumococcal endocarditis in a sixty-five year old alcoholic (A68-101) with evidence of cardiac infection for about 112 days.* ***a,*** *in this view a recent vegetation is partially enclosed by dashes. A perforation is present also in the leaflet.* ***b,*** *longitudinal section of the vegetation shown in* ***a.*** *The vegetation contains calcific deposits.* ***c,*** *histologic section of vegetation which contained fibrin and inflammatory cells but no stainable organisms. Elastic van Gieson stain; original magnification × 3, reduced by 25 per cent.*

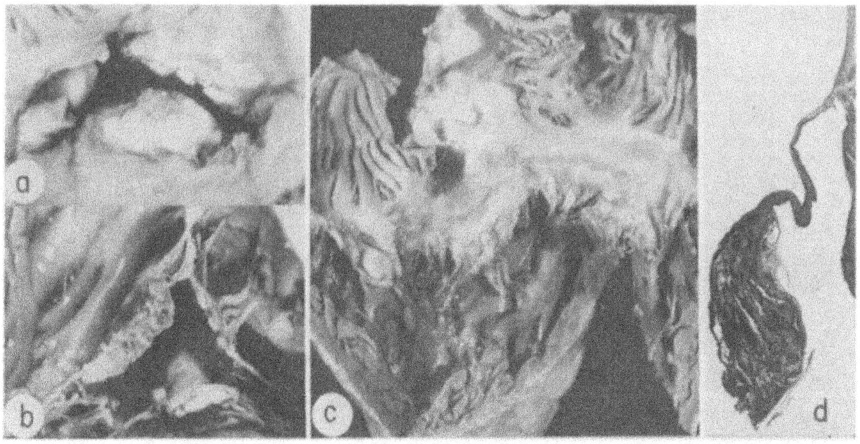

Figure 3. Case 4. Staphylococcus aureus endocarditis of tricuspid valve (A70-140). **a,** tricuspid valve viewed from right atrium. **b,** same valve viewed from right ventricle. **c,** view of opened right atrium, tricuspid valve and right ventricle. **d,** histologic section of vegetation which involves the distal half of the anterior tricuspid leaflet. Movat stain; original magnification × 4, reduced by 30 per cent.

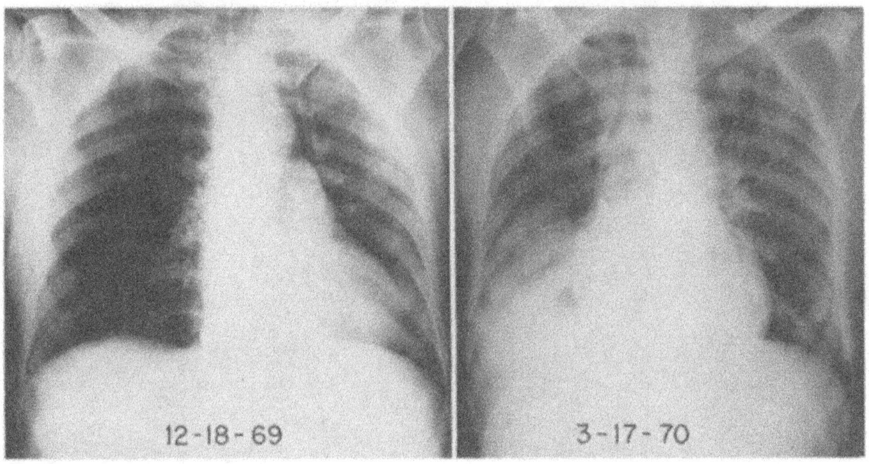

Figure 4. Case 5. Chest roentgenograms taken on dates shown (A70-87). Patient died of pulmonary infection on March 17, 1970.

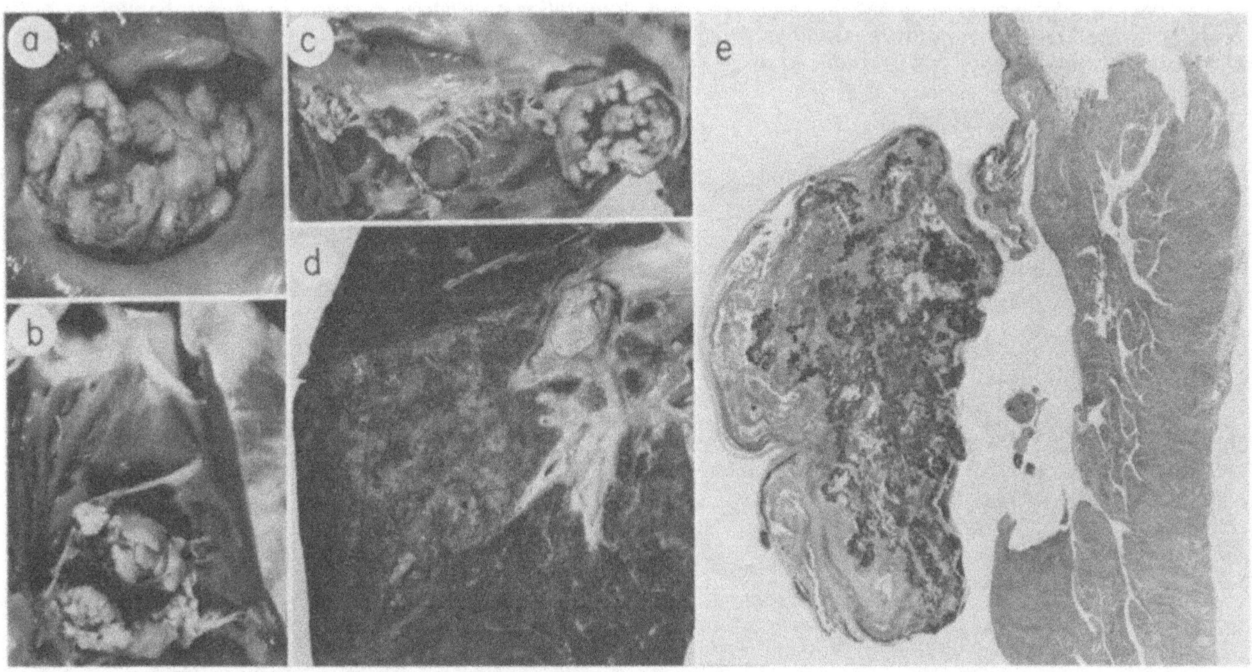

Figure 5. Case 5. Staphylococcus aureus endocarditis of tricuspid valve in a thirty-five year old female heroin addict whose chest roentgenograms are shown in Figure 4. She had been well until about one week before death when "acute pneumonia" developed. About three days before death, she suffered from headache and stiff neck. When hospitalized several hours before death, in addition to evidence of acute pneumonia, probably from septic emboli, and acute meningitis, she had a grade 2/6 precordial systolic murmur, which increased with inspiration, and a pulsatile liver. **a,** tricuspid valve viewed from right atrium. The orifice appears to be narrowed by the vegetation. **b,** tricuspid valve viewed from right ventricle. **c,** view of opened tricuspid valve. **d,** section of right lung showing infarct caused by septic embolus in right pulmonary artery. **e,** photomicrograph of portion of tricuspid valve vegetation. Dark staining areas in the leaflet represent gram-positive cocci. The surface of the vegetation is relatively smooth. Movat stain; original magnification × 5, reduced by 17 per cent.

right-sided one. The number of vegetations on the tricuspid leaflets varied from one (in three patients) to innumerable (in Case 5). The number of vegetations on the tricuspid valve leaflets in the remaining seven patients varied from two to five. The individual vegetations on the tricuspid valve varied from 0.1 to 5 cm in largest diameter. The largest single vegetation occurred in Case 5, and although it appeared to obstruct the valvular orifice it was attached entirely to the anterior leaflet. The next largest occurred in a patient with fungal endocarditis (Case 8). The tricuspid valve vegetations involved the basal attachments of the leaflets, i.e., the annulus, in three patients, but in only one of them (Case 11) did it actually extend into the annulus and cause a ring abscess. Thus, excision of the leaflets would have totally removed the tricuspid valve vegetations in eight of the eleven patients. The shapes of the tricuspid valve vegetations in six patients were relatively flat and in the other five fungating. The surfaces of most vegetations were relatively smooth in seven patients and relatively rough in the other four. The vegetations caused rupture of several chordae tendineae in five patients, all of whom had multiple and usually large vegetations; in the other six without ruptured chordae the vegetations were either single or small. In none of the eleven patients did the vegetations cause gross disappearance of leaflet tissue either by perforation or by dissolution of a portion of tricuspid leaflet.

On histologic examination, organisms were observed in tricuspid valve vegetations in seven of the eleven patients. Polymorphonuclear leukocytes were observed in the vegetations in all eleven patients; in eight abscesses were present. In three patients the inflammatory process and organisms were found in the central portions of the leaflets with preservation of cuspal tissue peripherally. In four other patients, distal portions of leaflet were completely destroyed, being incorporated into the inflammatory process; in three other patients the inflammatory process was superimposed on the surface of the tricuspid leaflets with good preservation of the underlying cusp. Calcific deposits were present in one tricuspid valve (Case 3), but this patient had had clinical evidence of infective endocarditis for at least 112 days.

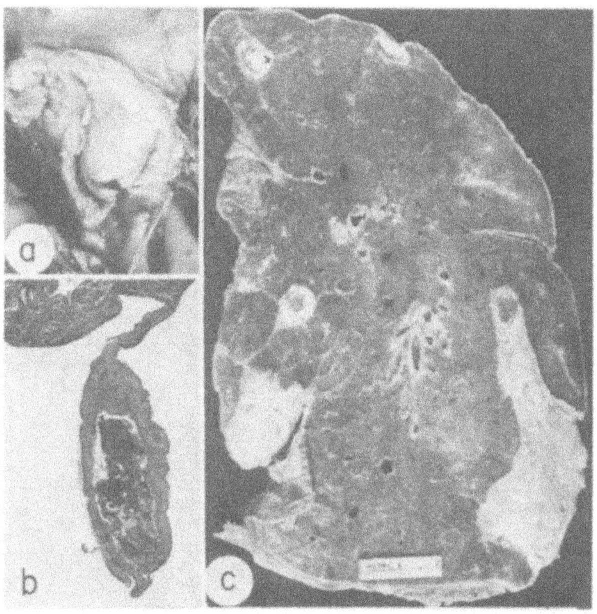

Figure 6. *Case 6. Staphylococcus aureus endocarditis of tricuspid valve with septic pulmonary emboli (A70-42).* ***a,*** *view of portion of friable vegetation on tricuspid valve.* ***b,*** *longitudinal section of vegetation involving distal two thirds of the leaflet. Movat stain; original magnification × 4, reduced by 18 per cent.* ***c,*** *section of lung showing multiple septic infarcts with abscess formation.*

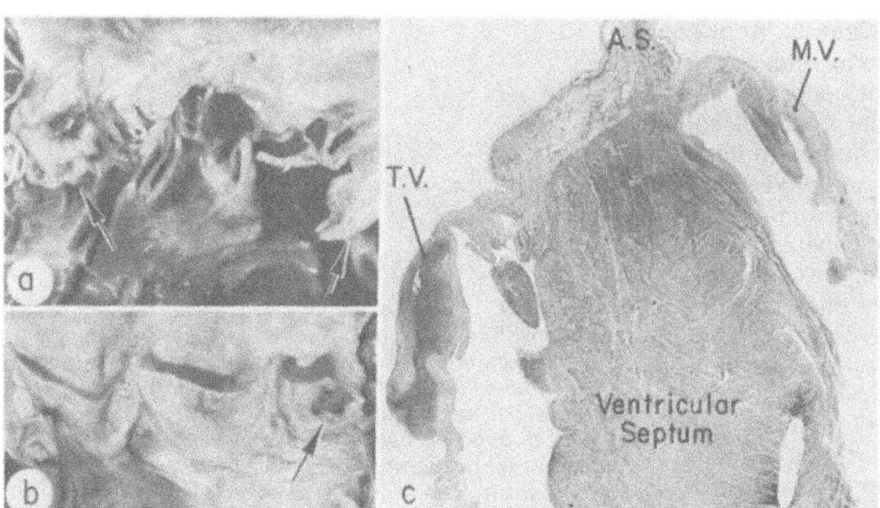

Figure 7. *Case 7. Pneumococcal endocarditis involving tricuspid (****a****) and aortic (****b****) valves (A69-155). That the vegetations are larger and involve all three tricuspid valve cusps as compared to their being smaller and involving only one aortic valve cusp is evidence that the infection originated on the right side of the heart.* ***c,*** *histologic section showing vegetations in middle two thirds of a tricuspid valve (T.V.) cusp. M.V. = mitral valve leaflet; A.S. = atrial septum. Hematoxylin and eosin stain; original magnification × 3, reduced by 24 per cent.*

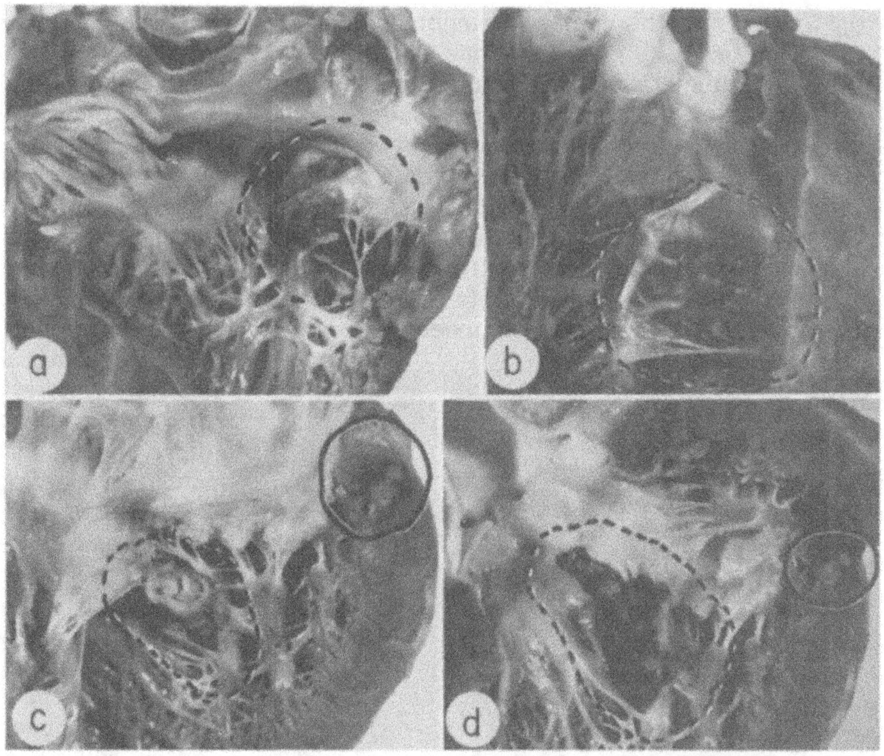

Figure 8. *Case 8. Fungal endocarditis in a ten month old boy with a generalized infection involving many body organs (A70-78). Single large vegetations (dashed circles) were present on the tricuspid (**a** and **b**) and mitral (**c** and **d**) valves. A large myocardial abscess is designated by the closed circle in **c** and **d**.*

The infection involving the pulmonic valve in one patient consisted of a single flat, relatively rough-surfaced vegetation involving two cusps and the intervening commissure. The vegetation produced a large tear in one cusp, almost surely producing pulmonic regurgitation. The infective process extended to the margin of attachment of one cusp. On histologic study, the involved pulmonic cusps contained large collections of polymorphonuclear leukocytes, and both surfaces were covered by fibrin. Organisms were not found in the involved pulmonic cusps.

Mural vegetations were present in three patients. In two they were located on the right ventricular endocardium: in one (Case 3) from contact with the free swinging anterior tricuspid leaflet (since its chordae were ruptured), and in one (Case 12) on a mural jet lesion produced earlier by congenital ventricular septal defect. In the third patient (Case 5) vegetative material was located on the right atrial endocardium and was due to contact of a large tricuspid valve vegetation.

On gross examination, distinct lesions were observed in myocardial walls in only two of the twelve patients: one (Case 8) had well circumscribed abscesses in the left ventricular free wall; the other (Case 9) had extensive, less well circumscribed foci of inflammatory necrosis in both left ventricular papillary muscles and a focus of acellular necrosis in the left ventricular free wall. On examination of 100 separate histologic sec-

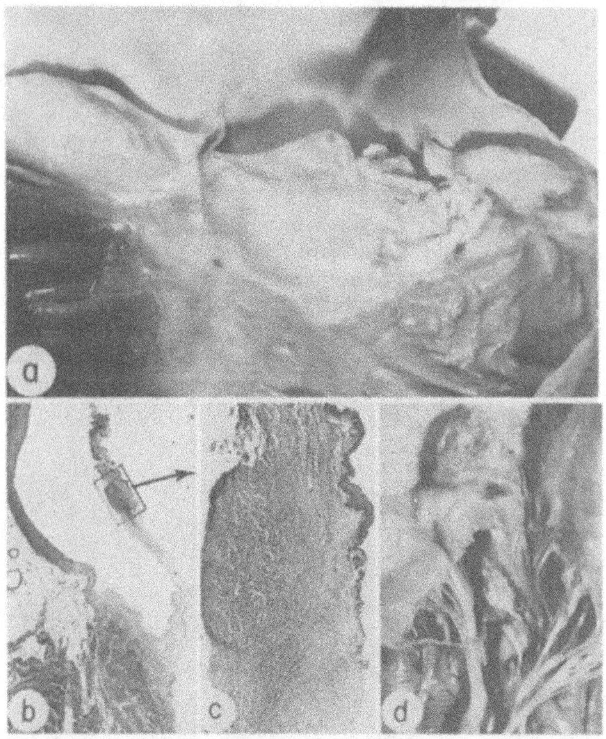

Figure 9. *Case 9. Staphylococcus aureus endocarditis involving pulmonic (**a**, **b** and **c**) and mitral (**d**) valves in a fifty-five year old alcoholic who died of pneumonia (A70-141). The vegetation on the pulmonic valve caused tearing of one leaflet. **b**, histologic section through portion of pulmonic valve cusp. **c**, close-up view of portion of inflamed cusp. Hematoxylin and eosin stain; original magnification × 4 (**b**) and × 27 (**c**), reduced by 33 per cent.*

tions of cardiac wall (five to fourteen per patient [average 9]) including sections of at least two of the three major papillary muscles of each heart, focal myocardial lesions were observed in the hearts of four patients. Three patients (Cases 1, 8 and 9) had myocardial abscesses. In the latter two patients (Cases 8 and 9), as already mentioned, they were large enough to be visible grossly; in the third (Case 1) only one minute myocardial abscess, containing colonies of bacteria, was observed on examination of eight large [2] sections of myocardial wall. Colonies of organisms also were observed in the myocardial abscesses in two patients (Cases 8 and 9), in both of whom septic emboli were observed in one or more coronary arteries (extramural in Case 9, intramural in Case 8). A minute focus of acute inflammatory cells also was observed in one patient (Case 11), but the cells were present in fibrous tissue, not in myocardium, in the distal portion of one papillary muscle. Only three patients had foci of myocardial necrosis, and two of them had coronary arterial emboli. The foci of necrosis in all three were located in both left ventricular papillary muscles, and two also had foci of necrosis in the left ventricular free wall. None of the other nine patients had papillary muscle necrosis, and none of the twelve had necrosis of the anterior papillary muscle of the right ventricle. The necrosis in one patient (Case 8) was associated with extensive dystrophic calcification of individual myocardial fibers. In another patient (Case 11) calcific deposits also were found in several individual myocardial fibers. Except for microscopic-sized foci in the apices of the left ventricular papillary muscles in several patients, no interstitial or replacement myocardial fibrosis was observed.

At necropsy, acute pneumonia with pulmonary infarcts was found in ten of the twelve patients, and seven had pulmonary abscesses. Material similar to that forming the right-sided cardiac vegetations was found in pulmonary arteries in

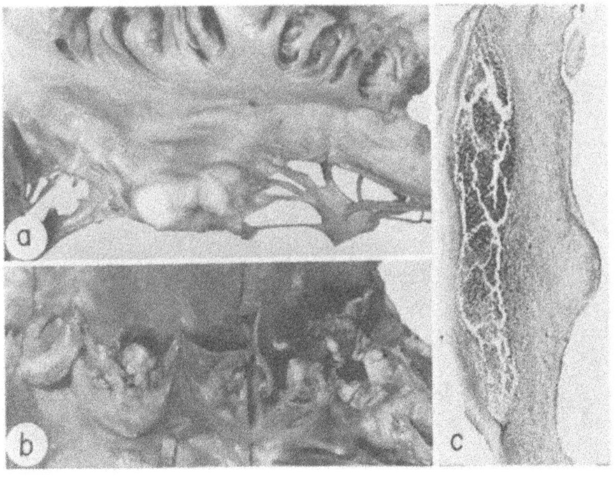

Figure 10. *Case 10. Pneumococcal endocarditis involving tricuspid (**a**) and aortic (**b**) valves in a fifty-eight year old alcoholic (DCGH No. 71A-14). The vegetation on the tricuspid valve is small, whereas the vegetations on the aortic valve are large and cause extensive destruction of the cusps. **c,** histologic section of a portion of tricuspid leaflet showing abscess formation. Hematoxylin and eosin stain; original magnification × 16, reduced by 33 per cent.*

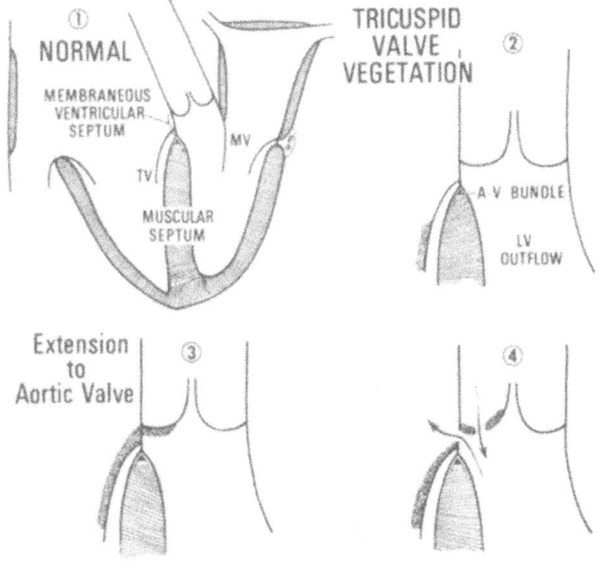

Figure 11. *Diagrammatic representation of development of aortic regurgitation and left to right shunt in a fifty-five year old man (WHC No. A70-155) with pneumococcal endocarditis and alcoholism. He noted fever, cough, and neck and knee pain twenty-six days before death. Overt signs of acute meningitis were present at the time of hospitalization nineteen days before death. Subsequently a murmur and signs of aortic regurgitation developed, and after that a "continuous murmur" due to the aortico-right atrial fistula. Death was due to intractable heart failure. (1) Normal cardiac anatomy. (2) Initial nidus of infection on tricuspid valve leaflet. (3) Extension of tricuspid vegetation through membranous portion of ventricular septum onto one of three aortic valve cusps. (4) Consequent perforation of aortic valve cusp causing aortic regurgitation and rupture of the membranous ventricular septum causing a left ventricular-right atrial fistula.*

seven of the ten patients with pneumonia, strongly suggesting that the pneumonia was secondary to dislodgment of vegetative material into the pulmonary circulation.

COMMENTS

Certain facts regarding right-sided infective endocarditis have emerged from review of previous reports on this subject and from study of our patients: (1) Its frequency is far less than left-sided infective endocarditis. It composes about 10 per cent of all cases of infective endocarditis. (2) It is usually caused by highly virulent or unusual organisms, the Staphylococcus being the most common. (3) The involved right-sided valve is, with rare exception, anatomically and functionally normal before the onset of infective endocarditis. (4) A predisposing factor is nearly always apparent. The most frequent ones are opiate addiction; alcoholism; generalized infections in patients with immunologic deficiencies, particularly lymphoma; congenital cardiac disease and dermal infections, particularly in young children or infants, with subsequent septicemia. (5) Diagnosis is difficult since the predominant clinical features are extracardiac, mainly, acute pneumonia; precordial murmurs are frequently absent or if present are soft and atypically located, and evidences of congestive cardiac failure are absent or if present rarely prominent.

The infrequency of right-sided infective endocarditis compared to the relative frequency of left-sided infective endocarditis has been explained by the lower pressure in the right side of the heart [3]. If the difference in pressure on the two sides of the heart is the major factor, the ratio between the frequency of right-sided to left-sided infective endocarditis might be expected to approximate the ratio between the peak systolic pressure in the right ventricle and that in the left ventricle,

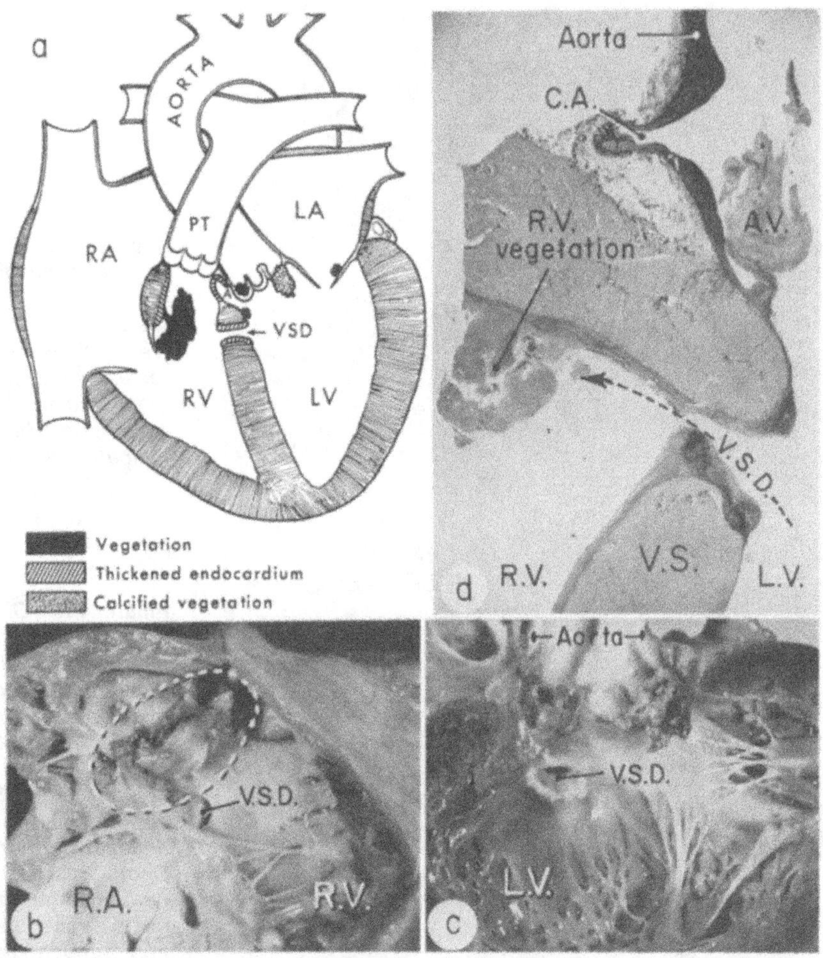

__Figure 12.__ Alpha hemolytic Streptococcus endocarditis in a five year old girl (A68-260) with congenital ventricular septal defect (VSD). Pneumonia and anemia developed four months before death, and two months later a grade 2/6 murmur of aortic regurgitation was noted for the first time. Death resulted from a large brain embolus. Vegetation probably formed initially on the jet lesion in the right ventricular outflow tract. Dislodgment of portions of right ventricular vegetation produced septic pulmonary emboli which presented clinically as "acute pneumonia." The exact mechanism of involvement of the aortic valve by the infective process is uncertain. __a,__ diagrammatic representation of location of vegetative material. Calcific deposits developed in aortic valve vegetation during the four month course. RA = right atrium; RV = right ventricle; PT = pulmonary trunk; LA = left atrium; A = aneurysm with orifice just below aortic valve. __b,__ view of opened right atrium, tricuspid valve and right ventricle showing the large vegetation (enclosed by dashed line) in the right ventricular outflow tract adjacent to the small ventricular septal defect. __c,__ view of opened left ventricle, aortic valve and aorta showing partial but extensive destruction of aortic valve cusps by vegetative material. The borders of the ventricular septal defect are free of vegetation. __d,__ photomicrograph of section through the ventricular septal defect including a portion of aorta, aortic valve (A.V.) cusp and ventricular septum (V.S.). The endocardium bordering the ventricular septal defect and that in the right ventricular outflow tract is very thick. C.A.-coronary artery. Elastic van Gieson stain; original magnification × 8, reduced by 15 per cent.

and indeed this is the case. The peak ventricular systolic pressure normally is about one sixth or 17 per cent of the peak left ventricular systolic pressure, and in at least 10 per cent of all cases of infective endocarditis the right-sided valves are involved. Thus, these figures of 10 and 17 per cent are sufficiently close to one another to allow this pressure explanation to be extremely plausible. Another factor mentioned as explaining the much lower frequency of right-sided infective endocarditis is lack of underlying disease of the right-sided cardiac valves compared to that involving the left-sided valves. In our study [1] of forty-five necropsy patients with active valvular infective endocarditis limited to the left side of the heart, there was evidence that the valve had been anatomically abnormal before the onset of infective endocarditis in 47 per cent whereas there was no evidence of previous right-sided valvular disease in any of our patients with right-sided infective endocarditis. The increased susceptibility of previously abnormal valves to infective endocarditis is well established, and this factor may be the second most important one in explaining the higher frequency of left-sided infective endocarditis. Whether or not the lower oxygen tension of the blood in the right side of the heart is important (by discouraging growth of aerobic bacteria) is uncertain.

Most studies [4–18], including ours, show that right-sided cardiac valves are usually attacked by highly virulent and unusual organisms. Of the twenty-three necropsy patients with right-sided (two had pulmonary arterial endarteritis from patent ductus arteriosus) infective endocarditis observed at the Mayo Clinic from 1910 to 1955 and described by Bain et al. [11] in 1958, the offending organism was identified in nineteen: Staphylococcus was responsible in eleven (58 per cent), Pneumococcus in three (16 per cent), Streptococcus in four (21 per cent) (viridans in two) and Gonococcus in one (5 per cent). In contrast, of Thayer's total 536 cases of infective endocarditis described in 1931 [5], Staph. aureus was responsible in only 7 per cent, Pneumococcus in 15 per cent, Streptococcus in 63 per cent and Gonococcus in 11 per cent. Of 100 patients with infective endocarditis acquired outside the hospital between 1956 and 1965 [19], Staphylococcus was responsible in twenty-three, Streptococcus in fifty-six (viridans in twenty-seven), miscellaneous in seven (but none had Pneumococcus or Gonococcus) and negative in fourteen. Studies in opiate addicts [7–10,13–18] have shown an even greater propensity for the Staphylococcus to be the cause of right-sided infective endocarditis. A review of forty-eight cases (69 per cent fatal) of infective endocarditis in opiate addicts by Louria et al. [14] disclosed that the offending organism was Staphylococcus (aureus in thirteen, epidermidis in two) in fifteen of the sixteen patients with right-sided endocarditis (tricuspid valve in each). Among sixty-two fatal cases of infective endocarditis in opiate addicts reviewed by Sapira [16] in 1968, Staph. aureus was the offending organism in nine of thirteen with isolated right-sided cardiac vegetations, whereas it was responsible in only six of forty-six patients with isolated left-sided infective endocarditis (organism unknown in thirteen). Of sixteen opiate addicts with infective endocarditis described in 1970 by Ramsey et al. [18], Staph. aureus was the cause in three of the four patients with right-sided (tricuspid) infective endocarditis in whom the organism was known but in only one of twelve patients with isolated left-sided infective endocarditis. Staph. aureus also was the cause of the right-sided infective endocarditis in each of four heroin addicts described herein but was responsible for infective endocarditis in only one of the remaining eight patients. Although it usually attacks previously normal right-sided cardiac valves, Staphylococcus is commonly the offending organism in patients with infective endocarditis complicating congenital cardiovascular malformations. Of thirty-eight patients with infective endocarditis and congenital heart disease (twenty-three had ventricular septal defect) described by Vogler and Dorney [20], Staphylococcus was responsible for the infection in thirteen (41 per cent) and alpha Streptococcus in nine (28 per cent) of the thirty-two patients in whom the organism was known.

In none of the multiple papers concerning right- or left-sided infective endocarditis in opiate addicts has Pneumococcus been mentioned as the offending organism. In four of our twelve patients with right-sided infective endocarditis, D. pneumoniae was the offending bacterium. Each of these patients was a chronic alcoholic and three also had meningitis. In the pre-heroin-addiction era, however, Pneumococcus was recognized as a frequent cause of right-sided infective endocarditis. Of twenty cases of infective endocarditis involving the tricuspid valve reported before 1940 [6], nine (45 per cent) were caused by Pneumococcus. Of a total of 584 patients with infective endocarditis subjected to necropsy at the Philadelphia General Hospital from 1920 to 1940, only eleven (2 per cent) had infective endocarditis restricted to the tricuspid valve, but of the sixty-two with pneumococcal endocarditis the tricuspid valve alone was involved in nine (15 per cent) [6]. Even earlier, in 1904, Preble [4] in reviewing 141 cases of pneumococcal endocarditis showed that in 18 per cent there were vegetations on right-sided cardiac valves, whereas infective endocarditis due to organisms other than Pneumococcus caused right-sided vegetations in only 7 per cent of the cases. Preble also mentioned alcoholism, as well as malnutrition, as a predisposing factor to pneumococcal endocarditis, and he also stressed the frequent association of pneumococcal infective endocarditis with meningitis and pneumonia. He found that 60 per cent of patients with pneumococcal endocarditis had meningitis and that 30 per cent of patients with pneumococcal meningitis had endocarditis. Goldburgh et al. [6] found pneumococcal endocarditis in 5 per cent of the patients who died with lobar pneumonia. Although Pneumococcus was the offending organism in 15 per cent of Thayer's 536 patients with infective endocarditis described before 1931 [5], since the introduction of antibiotics it has caused less than 3 per cent of the cases of infective endocarditis [21]. Of fifteen patients (ten fatal) with pneumococcal endocarditis studied at the Cincinnati General Hospital from 1945 to 1965, three had vegetations limited to the tricuspid valve (the other twelve had either mitral or aortic vegetations) [21]. Thirteen of the fifteen patients also had meningitis.

Although heroin addiction is now a well recognized predisposing factor to infective endocarditis on either side of the heart, the frequency of alcoholism as a predisposing factor to right-sided infective endocarditis apparently is not well appreciated. Congenital cardiac disease is a well recognized predisposing factor to infective endocarditis [20,22–24]. In this circumstance the right-sided vegetations are most frequently observed in patients with small ventricular septal defects and left to right shunts through them as in our Case 12. The resulting vegetations, however, most often occur on the thickened right ventricular mural endocardium rather than on valvular (tricuspid) endocardium, but both were involved in our patient. Persistent patent ductus arteriosus also may be complicated by vegetations occurring on the pulmonary arterial side of the left to right shunt. Strictly speaking, however, vegetations involving the ductus or pulmonary artery represent endarteritis and not endocarditis. Infective endocarditis complicating previously stenotic tricuspid or pulmonic valves is uncommon. Rheumatic tricuspid valve disease is always accompanied by rheumatic mitral stenosis and frequently also by aortic valvular involvement [25]. Infective endocarditis involving hearts with previously diseased left- and right-sided valves nearly always attacks only one or both left-sided valves and spares the right-sided valves. Infective endocarditis, however, rarely attacks hearts with previous three- or four-valve involvement anyway, possibly because the left-sided valves in this circumstance are usually heavily calcified and stenotic, and superimposition of infective endocarditis on heavily calcified valves is uncommon. Furthermore, involvement of congenitally malformed, particularly stenotic, pulmonic valves is infrequent, although several patients with congenital pulmonic stenosis and infective endocarditis have been described [20,22–24].

Although the diagnosis of left-sided infective endocarditis is usually established during life, the diagnosis of right-sided infective endocarditis is far more difficult to make and often is not even suspected during life. The major reason is because the latter illness is dominated by extracardiac signs and symptoms. Acute pneumonia is the usual presenting feature of right-sided infective endocarditis, occurring in ten of our twelve patients, and it dominates the clinical course. The pneumonia is usually embolic in origin, resulting from dislodgment of vegetative material from the right-sided cardiac vegetations. Acute meningitis also may occur and be the dominant feature. Signs of right-sided congestive cardiac failure may be absent or minimal or, if present, readily explainable as secondary to acute cor pulmonale from the acute pneumonia. Precordial murmurs may be absent entirely and, if present, may be soft, atypically located and may not increase in intensity with inspiration. Since fever and anemia are common, the precordial murmurs may be dismissed as being "hemic" in origin. Cardiomegaly, distention of jugular veins and pulsation of the liver are often not observed in patients with right-sided infective endocarditis. Death in patients with isolated right-sided infective endocarditis usually can be attributed to the extracardiac manifestations, usually pneumonia. In none of our six patients with isolated right-sided infective endocarditis was congestive cardiac failure an important factor. Furthermore, in only two of the six patients with infective endocarditis involving both right- and left-sided cardiac valves was congestive cardiac failure a major manifestation of the illness, and in both infective endocarditis caused severe aortic regurgitation.

A number of papers have been published on right-sided infective endocarditis, but none have emphasized the cardiac-pathologic features of this condition, and few have even illustrated its morphologic aspects. Of our twelve patients, infective endocarditis was definitely primary on the right side of the heart in nine; in six of these no left-sided vegetations were present, and in the other three the right-sided vegetations were large or extensive, and the left-sided vegetations were minute or smaller. Dislodgment of organisms from the inflamed lungs into the pulmonary veins may be the mechanism responsible for the left-sided vegetations. In two other patients single similar-sized vegetations were located on both tricuspid and mitral valves and therefore which one came first is uncertain; both patients had generalized infection involving several body organs. In one of the twelve patients large vegetations destroyed the aortic valve, and only one small vegetation was present on the right side of the heart. Thus, this patient (Case 10) appears to be the only one in whom the right-sided infective endocarditis was definitely secondary to left-sided infective endocarditis.

Vegetations on the tricuspid valve may be similar in appearance to those involving the mitral valve. Rupture of chordae tendineae is common, occurring in five of our eleven patients with tricuspid valve vegetations. Unlike rupture of chordae tendineae of the mitral valve, which virtually always leads to severe mitral regurgitation [26], rupture of tricuspid valvular chordae may produce no clinical evidence of tricuspid regurgitation since normally the pressures in the right ventricle and right atrium are low and not markedly different. When evidence of tricuspid regurgitation is present in patients with infective endocarditis involving this valve, it is probable that the elevation in right ventricular pressure is a consequence of extensive acute pneumonia and acute cor pulmonale. Perforation or disappearance of tricuspid leaflet tissue occurred in none of our eleven patients despite highly virulent organisms. Again, this difference may be explained by the lower pressure on the right side of the heart which may decrease the rate of valve destruction by the infective process. Another factor may be the duration of illness which is shorter in patients with right-sided infective endocarditis as compared to patients with isolated left-sided infective endocarditis. Possibly the former patients die of widespread pneumonia before the right-sided vegetations have had time to destroy the valves more extensively.

From study of our twelve patients and from reports of others of right-sided infective endocarditis [4–18,20–24,27–30], it appears that the tricuspid valve is far more prone to be the site of vegetations than is the pulmonic valve. Only one of our twelve patients had pulmonic valve vegetations, and he also had mitral valve infective endocarditis. Pulmonic valve vegetations were present in only one of the twelve fatal cases of isolated right-sided infective endocarditis reported by Sapira [16]. In contrast, infective endocarditis on the left side involves the semilunar (aortic) valve more frequently than the atrioventricular (mitral) valve [1]. Fungating vegetations on the pulmonic valve also appear to be infrequent as contrasted to their frequency on the aortic valve. In none of our twelve patients with infective endocarditis were both right-sided cardiac valves involved, whereas involvement of both left-sided cardiac valves by infective endocarditis is common. This difference results from several factors. Although pulmonic regurgitation may result from infective endocarditis involving this valve, the amount of regurgitation is usually small since the valve usually is not extensively damaged and the pulmonary pressure is relatively low. In contrast, vegetations on the aortic valve are usually larger and frequently severely damage the cusps with resultant marked regurgitation. Also, the higher aortic diastolic pressure may dislodge the aortic vegetations and cause them to attach to mitral leaflets or chordae. The pulmonary arterial pressure may not be high enough to dislodge the pulmonic valve vegetations retrogradely. Also, the pulmonic valve is separated from the tricuspid valve by myocardium (crista supraventricularis), whereas the anterior mitral leaflet is continuous with the aortic valve.

Although myocardial lesions are frequent in patients with infective endocarditis involving one or both left-sided cardiac valves, they are usually absent in patients with isolated right-sided infective endocarditis. Only one of our six patients with isolated right-sided infective endocarditis had myocardial lesions and he had widespread abscesses in many body organs. Two of our six patients with combined right- and left-sided infective endocarditis had myocardial foci of inflammation, and in each coronary arterial septic emboli were the explanation.

Recently, total valve excision has been employed as therapy for patients with right-sided infective endocarditis unresponsive to antibiotic therapy [31]. In nine of our eleven patients with tricuspid valve infective endocarditis, the vegetations did not extend to the basal attachments of the leaflets. Therefore, total excision of the tricuspid valves would have eradicated the right-sided infective endocarditis. In only one of the two patients in whom the infective process extended to the level of the basal attachment of a tricuspid leaflet did it actually burrow into the annulus to cause a ring abscess. Even though the infective endocarditis may have extended to the level of the valve annulus, this would not necessarily preclude total valve excision and successful outcome because valve excision may serve simply to eradicate the source of septic emboli to the lungs which cause infarction, pneumonia and abscesses, and the pulmonary infection is the major cause of death in these patients. Although man may tolerate total excision of either the tricuspid or pulmonic valve without symptomatic evidence of cardiac dysfunction, if both valves become incompetent, or if one becomes stenotic and the other incompetent, cardiac decompensation is the result. An ideal way to produce severe congestive heart failure in animals is to incise or excise the tricuspid valve causing incompetency and banding the pulmonary trunk causing stenosis [32].

ACKNOWLEDGMENT

Eight patients described herein were studied clinically at Washington, D.C., hospitals. We are, therefore, indebted to Doctors Frank I. Marcus, Gordon A. Ewy, Ross D. Fletcher, Lucia Gomez, Rashid A. Massumi, Tazewell Banks and Michael Cuadra at the D.C. General Hospital, and to Doctors James Bocus, Sander H. Mendelsohn and Chester Emmonds at the Washington Hospital Center for allowing us to include their patients in this study.

REFERENCES

1. Buchbinder NA, Roberts WC: Left-sided valvular active infective endocarditis A study of 45 necropsy patients. Amer J Med 53: 000 1972
2 Ent LD, Roberts WC: The processing of large blocks of tissue. Amer J Clin Path 50: 726, 1968.
3. Lepeschkin E: On the relation between the site of valvular involvement in endocarditis and the blood pressure resting on the valve Amer J Med Sci 224 318, 1952.
4 Preble HB. Pneumococcus endocarditis. Amer J Med Sci 128: 782, 1904.
5 Thayer WS· Bacterial or infective endocarditis. Edinburgh Med J 38: 237, 307, 1931
6 Goldburgh HL, Baer S, Lieber MM: Acute bacterial endocarditis of the tricuspid valve. Amer J Med Sci 204 319, 1942
7. Hussey HH, Keliher TF, Schaefer BF, Walsh BJ: Septicemia and bacterial endocarditis resulting from heroin addiction. Report of five cases. JAMA 126. 535, 1944
8 Hussey HH, Katz S: Septic pulmonary infarction. Report of 8 cases Ann Intern Med 22 526, 1945.
9 Luttgens WF Endocarditis in "main line" opium addicts Report on eleven cases. Arch Intern Med (Chicago) 83 653, 1949
10 Dowling HF, Lepper M, Caldwell ER, Spies HW: Staphylococcic endocarditis. an analysis of 25 cases treated with antibiotics, together with a review of the recent literature. Medicine 31 155, 1952.
11 Bain RC, Edwards JE, Scheifley CH, Geraci JE· Right-sided bacterial endocarditis and endarteritis Amer J Med 24 98, 1958.
12 Bain RC, Edwards JE, Scheifley CH, Geraci JE· Right-sided bacterial endocarditis and endarteritis. Staff Meet Mayo Clin 33. 182, 1958.
13 Olsson RA, Romansky MJ· Staphylococcal tricuspid endocarditis in heroin addicts Ann Intern Med 57· 755, 1962.
14 Louria DB, Hensle T, Rose J. The major medical complications of heroin addiction. Ann Intern Med 67· 1, 1967
15 Massumi RA, Just H, Twawkkol A: Pulmonary valve regurgitation secondary to bacterial endocarditis in heroin addicts Amer Heart J 73· 308, 1967.
16. Sapira JD: The narcotic addict as a medical patient. Amer J Med 45· 555, 1968
17 Cherubin CE, Baden M, Kavaler F, Lerner S, Cline W. Infective endocarditis in narcotic addicts. Ann Intern Med 69 1091, 1968.
18 Ramsey RG, Gunnar RM, Tobin JR Jr· Endocarditis in the drug addict. Amer J Cardiol 25. 608, 1970.
19. Lerner PI, Weinstein L: Infective endocarditis in the antibiotic era. New Eng J Med 274: 199, 259, 323, 388, 1966.
20. Vogler WR, Dorney ER: Bacterial endocarditis in congenital heart disease. Amer Heart J 64 198, 1962.
21 Straus AL, Hamburger M: Pneumococcal endocarditis in the penicillin era. Arch Intern Med (Chicago) 118 190, 1966
22. Gelfman R, Levine SA The incidence of acute and subacute bacterial endocarditis in congenital heart disease. Amer J Med Sci 204: 324, 1942.
23. Barker PS: A clinical study of subacute bacterial infection confined to the right side of the heart or the pulmonary artery. Amer Heart J 37: 1054, 1949.
24 Bashour FA, Winchell CP: Right-sided bacterial endocarditis. Amer J Med Sci 240: 411, 1960.
25 Roberts WC. Valvular heart disease. A look at 1000 necropsied patients (In preparation)
26. Roberts WC, Braunwald E, Morrow AG: Acute severe mitral regurgitation secondary to ruptured chordae tendineae. Clinical, hemodynamic, and pathologic considerations. Circulation 33: 58, 1966.
27. Olesen KH, Fabricius J: Pulmonic valvular regurgitation during twenty-seven years after gonorrheal endocarditis Report of a case with catheterization data Amer Heart J 52: 791, 1956.
28 Levin HS, Runco V, Wooley CF, Ryan JM. Pulmonic regurgitation following staphylococcal endocarditis. An intracardiac phonocardiographic study Circulation 30: 411, 1964
29 Garcia R, Taber RE: Bacterial endocarditis of the pulmonic valve Association with atrial septal defect of the ostium secundum type Amer J Cardiol 18: 275, 1966
30. Laniado S, Frater RWM, Jordan A, Kafka EC, Kadish AS, Zelefsky M. Endocarditis of the pulmonic valve simulating cardiac tumor. Chest 59: 464, 1971.
31. Arbulu A, Thoms NW, Chiscano A, Wilson RF. Total tricuspid valvulectomy without replacement in the treatment of Pseudomonas endocarditis Surg Forum 22: 162, 1971.
32 Barger AC, Roe BB, Richardson GS· Relation of valvular lesions and of exercise to auricular pressure, work tolerance, and to development of chronic, congestive failure. in dogs. Amer J Physiol 169· 384, 1952

Left-Sided Valvular Active Infective Endocarditis

A Study of Forty-Five Necropsy Patients

NEIL A. BUCHBINDER, M.D.
WILLIAM C. ROBERTS, M.D.
Bethesda, Maryland

Clinical and anatomic features are described in forty-five necropsy patients with left-sided valvular active infective endocarditis. Vegetations in 53 per cent of the patients involved previously anatomically normal valves, and 76 per cent of all patients had previously functionally normal valves. Predisposing factors allowing entrance of virulent or unusual organisms or alterations of host defense mechanisms appear to account for the frequency of infective endocarditis on normal valves. Valvular dysfunction resulting from infective endocarditis occurred in at least 59 per cent and possibly as high as 74 per cent of the forty-five patients causing congestive heart failure in all. Myocardial lesions were present in 87 per cent of the thirty-eight patients in whom multiple histologic sections were examined, but in none did heart failure appear to result from these lesions. Papillary muscle necrosis was present in 58 per cent, but in none did it appear to cause mitral regurgitation. Congestive heart failure could not be attributed in any patient to myocardial lesions. Pericarditis occurred in eight patients (20 per cent), and in each a site of direct extension of the inflammation into the pericardium was apparent. Ring abscesses occurred in twelve of thirty-one patients with aortic valve vegetations and in none of twenty-six with mitral valve vegetations. Ring abscesses indicate severe destruction of valvular cusps and severe valvular dysfunction.

Infective endocarditis before the advent of antibiotics was virtually always a fatal disease and consequently received particular attention from many pathologists. With the introduction of antibiotics and therefore definitive therapy for the first time, the pathologic features of infective endocarditis became less important, and attention was focused on proper diagnosis and choice of antibiotic(s). It became increasingly evident, however, that antibiotic therapy often was not curative. During recent years cardiac valve replacement or rarely cuspal repair has afforded another form of therapy for infective endocarditis, and now surgery is being increasingly used in treatment of both active and healed infective endocarditis. Relatively few morphologic studies on infective endocarditis have appeared since the introduction of antibiotics or open cardiac surgery, thus a review of the autopsy data on patients with this entity primarily from the anatomic viewpoint seemed appropriate.

From the Section of Pathology, National Heart and Lung Institute, National Institutes of Health, Bethesda, Maryland 20014. Requests for reprints should be addressed to Dr. William C. Roberts, Bldg 10A, Room 3E-30, Section of Pathology, National Heart and Lung Institute, National Institutes of Health,
Manuscript received November 4, 1971; revised January 18, 1972

Summarized here are clinicopathologic observations in forty-five patients with left-sided infective endocarditis who died between 1955 and 1971

PATIENTS STUDIED AND METHODS

Clinical and necropsy records of all patients were reviewed: twenty-three patients were studied clinically and at necropsy at the Clinical Center of the National Institutes of Health; the remaining twenty-two were studied clinically elsewhere, and their hearts were submitted to the Section of Pathology, National Heart and Lung Institute, for examination Patients with endocarditis after cardiac valve replacement [1–3] and patients with vegetations occurring exclusively on mural endocardium were excluded [4] Three of the forty-five patients had histories of successful therapy for previous episodes of infective endocarditis The heart of every patient was studied originally by one of us (W C.R.) and forty were reexamined by both of us At reexamination, additional histologic sections were cut in thirty-eight patients, and old histologic sections of heart were reviewed in forty-two patients At least four hematoxylin and eosin stained histologic sections of heart were examined in every patient including at least one special stain for bacteria (Brown and Brenn) or fungi (methenamine silver)

The forty-five patients ranged in age from seventeen to seventy years (average thirty-nine years) (Figure 1), thirty-two were men, and thirteen were women One patient was less than twenty years of age and two were more than sixty-five years of age.

RESULTS

The sites of the cardiac vegetations are shown in Table I. Of 180 cardiac valves present in the forty-five patients, fifty-seven (32 per cent) contained vegetations: the aortic valve was involved alone or in combination with other valves in thirty-one (69 per cent) and the mitral valve in twenty-six (58 per cent)

The status of the infected valve before infective endocarditis is shown in Table II. Of forty-five patients with vegetations on cardiac valves, twenty-four (53 per cent) had anatomically normal valves before infective endocarditis and twenty-one (47 per cent) had anatomically abnormal valves. The abnormality was rheumatic in ten, congenital in eight (bicuspid aortic valves in six) and of uncertain etiology in three. Of the twenty-one anatomically abnormal valves, ten functioned normally before the onset of infective endocarditis as judged by the absence of signs or symptoms of cardiac dysfunction before the onset of infective endocarditis, and by necropsy evaluation of the involved valve Thus, infective endocarditis occurred on functionally abnormal cardiac valves in only eleven (24 per cent) of the forty-five patients: seven valves were stenotic with or without an element of incompetency and four were purely incompetent. Of the seven patients with stenotic valves, operative commissurotomies (mitral in three, aortic in one) were performed just before the appearance of infective endocarditis in four of them; the fifth patient had systemic crytococcosis and at necropsy fungal vegetations were present on both mitral

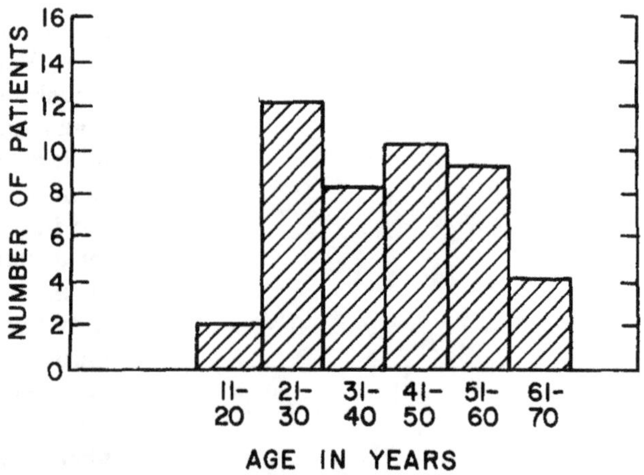

Figure 1. *Age distribution of the forty-five patients with active valvular infective endocarditis*

TABLE I **Valves Involved in Left-Sided Infective Endocarditis (45 Necropsy Patients)**

Sites of Vegetations	Patients No.	Patients %
Aortic valve	19	42
Mitral valve	14	31
Aortic and mitral valves	12	27
Totals	45	100

TABLE II **Status of Left-Sided Cardiac Valve Before Onset of Infective Endocarditis (45 Necropsy Patients)**

Status		Patients No.	Patients %
Valve anatomically normal		24	53
Valve anatomically abnormal		21	47
Functionally normal	10		
Functionally abnormal	11		
Aortic stenosis* (AS) 3			
Pure aortic regurgitation . . . 3			
Mitral stenosis* (MS) 3			
Pure mitral regurgitation . . . 1			
AS + MS 1			

* With or without associated valvular regurgitation.

TABLE III **Organism Causing Left-Sided Infective Endocarditis (IE) and Status of Valve Before Infection (45 Necropsy Patients)**

Causative Organism		No. Patients	Status of Valve Before IE: Anatomically Normal	Anatomically Abnormal: Functionally Normal	Anatomically Abnormal: Functionally Abnormal
Bacterium					
Staphylococcus aureus	31	10	5	3	2*
Staphylococcus epidermidis		2	1		1
Alpha Streptococcus		4	1	1	2
Beta Streptococcus		2		2	
Streptococcus faecalis		3	1	2	
Diplococcus pneumonia		4	4		
L forms corynebacterium and Streptobacillus moniliformis		1	1		
Gram positive coccus†		5	3		2*
Fungus					
Candida species	7	5	2		3‡
Cryptococcus neoformans		1			1
Histoplasma capsulatum		1	1		
Unknown		7	5	1	1
Totals		45	24	9	12

* One developed infective endocarditis after cardiac surgery.
† Organisms identified only on histologic sections of vegetations.
‡ Each developed infective endocarditis after cardiac surgery.

and aortic valves, each of which had been stenotic previously [5,6]; the remaining two patients had infective endocarditis superimposed on stenotic, heavily calcified aortic valves. One of the latter had a congenitally unicommissural valve [7], and the other, a seventy year old man, had degenerative type of aortic stenosis on a three-cuspid valve [8]. Of the four purely incompetent valves, none of which was calcified, before the occurrence of infective endocarditis, two aortic valves were congenitally bicuspid; the third was rheumatically deformed and three-cuspid; the one scarred mitral valve was rheumatic in origin.

The organisms causing infective endocarditis and the relationship of the causative organisms to the underlying status of the valves are summarized in Table III. Of the thirty-one with infective endocarditis caused by bacteria, twelve (39 per cent), and possibly as many as seventeen (55 per cent), were due to Staphylococcus species and only four (13 per cent) to alpha hemolytic Streptococcus. Blood cultures, performed in thirty-six patients, were positive in twenty-nine (81 per cent) and negative in seven (19 per cent). No organisms were cultured from blood or observed on histologic examination of vegetations in three patients, but each had been treated with antibiotics and each otherwise had typical clinical and necropsy findings of infective endocarditis. The valves were normal in five of ten patients with infective endocarditis caused by Staph. aureus and in all four with infective endocarditis caused by Diplococcus pneumoniae. In contrast, three of the four patients with infective endocarditis caused by alpha hemolytic Streptococcus had anatomically abnormal valves before the appearance of infective endocarditis. In forty-three patients the infection was primary in the heart; in the other two the cardiac infection was secondary to infection primary in other organs of tissues, and fungi were the cause in both of them.

Predisposing factors (Table IV) were found in thirty patients (67 per cent). Heroin addiction, alcoholism, malignancy and cardiac surgery accounted for more than 75 per cent of the predisposing factors. A predisposing factor was found in six of twelve patients with infective endocarditis caused by either Staph. aureus or Staph. epidermidis, in four of seven caused by fungi and in all four caused by Pneumococcus. All four patients with pneumococcal endocarditis were alcoholics. Of six heroin addicts the aortic valve alone was involved in four patients, the mitral valve alone in one and both the aortic and mitral valves in one; the causative organism was Staph. aureus in two patients, Staph. epidermidis in one, gram-positive coccus in one, Candida species in one and unknown in one. Three of the four patients with infective endocarditis due to alpha hemolytic Streptococcus had infection on aortic valves which previously had been anatomically abnormal: one had been made incompetent by jet lesions from discrete subaortic stenosis [9], the second had an incompetent rheumatically-deformed three-cuspid aortic valve and the third had an incompetent congenitally bicuspid aortic valve.

The functional status of the cardiac valves after infection is summarized in Table V. Valvular dysfunction occurred in thirty-three patients, twenty-six of whom had dysfunction in whole or in part from infective endocarditis. Further dysfunction from superimposed infective endocarditis in the other seven patients with already abnormally functioning valves due to underlying disease could not be clearly demonstrated. All thirty-three patients with valvular dysfunction had congestive cardiac failure. Of the twelve patients without valvular dysfunction only two had congestive cardiac failure and each of them had coronary heart disease. The principal causes of death in the forty-five patients are summarized in Table VI. Although congestive cardiac failure occurred in thirty-five patients, it appeared to be the principal cause of death in only twenty-one; in the other fourteen, it was a contributing factor. The type valve damage resulting from infective endocarditis and the mechanism of the resulting valve dysfunction are summarized in Table VII. Infective endocarditis caused thirty valves to function abnormally in twenty-six patients: twenty-eight valves were made incompetent, and two valves appeared to have been made stenotic by large vegetations. One of the latter was an aortic valve infected by Candida parapsilosis [10], the other was a mitral valve infected by beta hemolytic Streptococcus (group B) [10].

The physical signs are summarized in Table VIII Six patients presented with acute meningitis and one with cerebrovascular accident. Of forty-one patients with electrocardiograms, thirty-three had sinus rhythm, seven had atrial fibrillation, and one had atrial flutter. Three patients had P-R intervals of more than 0.20 second; one other had second degree atrioventricular block. In the latter patient the inflammatory process extended into the area of the atrioventricular bundle. The clinical diagnosis of active infective endocarditis was established before death in twenty-four patients, strongly suspected in twelve and never considered in nine. Embolic episodes were diagnosed clinically in nineteen patients. The duration of illness (onset of symptoms to death) was known in thirty-two patients: it was less than six weeks in ten (31 per cent) and more than six weeks in twenty-two (69 per cent). Antibiotics were given to forty-one of the forty-five patients although the diagnosis of infective endocarditis had been suspected clinically in only thirty-six: thirty patients received the proper dosage of the proper antibiotic recommended for active infective endocarditis but not necessarily for a sufficient duration, five received a questionably appropriate antibiotic, and six definitely received an improper antibiotic.

Necropsy Findings. Various necropsy findings are illustrated in Figures 2 through 15. Colonies of organisms were found in thirty-five (87 per cent) of forty patients in whom histologic sections of vegetations were available. Organisms were observed histologically in twenty-two of twenty-five patients with positive blood cultures and in four of seven patients with negative blood cultures. The types and frequencies of acute myocardial lesions (Fig-

TABLE IV Predisposing Factors in Left-Sided Infective Endocarditis (IE) and Status of Valve Before Infection

Factor	No. Patients	Status of Valve Before IE: Normal	Abnormal
None	15	7	8
Malignancy*	7	7	0
Heroin addiction	6	3	3
Alcoholism	5	4	1
Cardiac operation	5	0	5
Dental procedure	2	1	1
Genitourinary procedure	2	1	1
Skin infection	1	0	1
Intravenous catheter	1	1	0
Septic abortion	1	0	1
Totals	45	24	21

* Six patients received chemotherapy.

TABLE V Valve Function in Left-Sided Infective Endocarditis (IE) (45 Necropsy Patients)

Valve Function		Patients No.	%
Valve dysfunction		33	74
From IE	22 (50%)		
From IE worsening underlying valve dysfunction	4 (9%)		
From underlying valve dysfunction alone	7 (15%)		
No valve dysfunction		12	26
Totals		45	100

ures 4–6, 10, 14 and 15) are summarized in Table IX and the gross anatomic cardiac findings in Table X. Acute myocardial lesions were observed in thirty-three of thirty-eight (87 per cent) patients in whom histologic sections of walls of each cardiac chamber and of both left ventricular papillary muscles were examined. Foci of myocardial necrosis were found in twenty-three patients (61 per cent) but limited to papillary muscle in eighteen. The papillary muscles in twenty-two patients (58 per cent) were focally (eleven patients) or diffusely (eleven patients) necrotic. Papillary muscle necrosis (Figure 13) occurred in ten (62 per cent) of sixteen patients with infective endocarditis in-

TABLE VI **Principal Cause of Death in Left-Sided Infective Endocarditis (45 Necropsy Patients)**

Type		Patients No.	Patients %
Cardiovascular		24	53
Congestive heart failure . . .	21		
Arrhythmia	1		
Cardiac tamponade	1		
Pulmonary embolus	1		
Central nervous system		9	20
Embolus	6		
Meningitis	3		
Generalized infection		3	7
Acute pneumonia		1	2
Unknown		8	18
Totals		45	100

TABLE VII **Valve Dysfunction Resulting from Left-Sided Infective Endocarditis (30 Valves)**

Dysfunction	Valve (no.) Aortic	Valve (no.) Mitral
Pure regurgitation	19	9
Cuspal perforation	14	3
Cuspal destruction	5	0
Ruptured chordae tendineae	0	6
Stenosis	1	1

TABLE VIII **Physical Signs in Left-Sided Infective Endocarditis (45 Necropsy Patients)**

Signs	% of Patients*
Fever (>100°F)	95
Precordial murmur	91
Dermal petechiae	38
Splenomegaly	33
Retinal lesions	5
Janeway lesions	5
Subungual hemorrhages	2
Clubbing	2
Osler's nodes	2

* Percentages based only on cases in which clinical information was sufficient to allow evaluation regarding presence or absence of the particular physical sign.

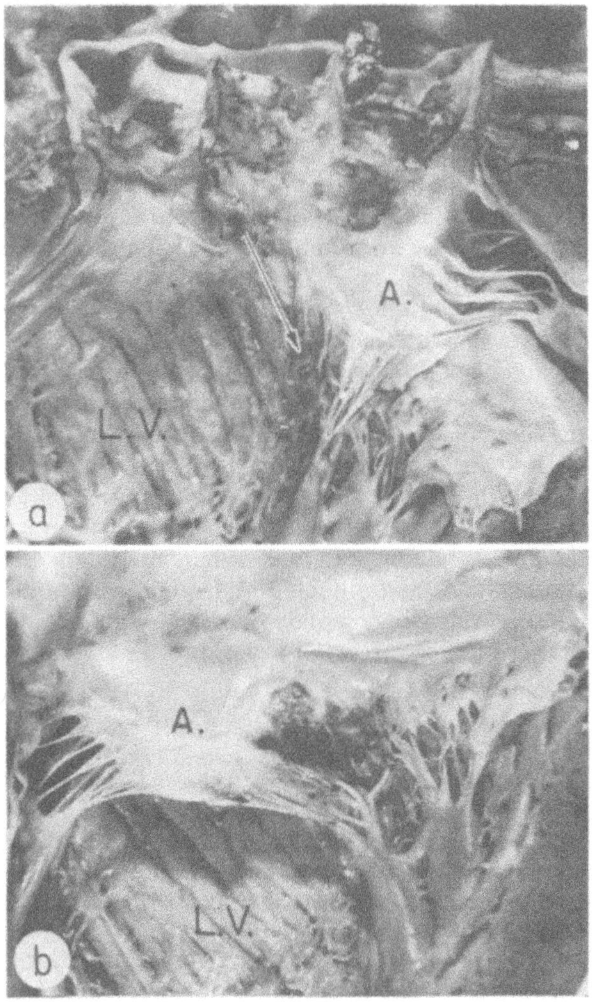

Figure 2. *Strep. faecalis endocarditis involving both aortic and mitral valves in a sixty-one year old man (DCGH No. 71A-120). Symptoms and signs of infective endocarditis appeared three weeks after catheterization of his urinary bladder. Both aortic and mitral valves were probably normal before they became sites of infection.* ***a,*** *opened left ventricle (L.V.) and aortic valve. The vegetations have partially destroyed each cusp causing severe aortic regurgitation. Vegetation on the left ventricular outflow endocardium and mitral leaflet and chordae tendineae almost certainly resulted from retrograde spread of the aortic vegetations by the aortic regurgitant stream* ***(arrow).*** *A. = anterior mitral leaflet.* ***b,*** *opened mitral valve showing vegetations at the posteromedial commissure. A number of chordae tendineae are ruptured.*

volving only the aortic valve and in five (42 per cent) of twelve patients with infective endocarditis limited to the mitral valve. Papillary muscle necrosis was present in twenty (67 per cent) of thirty patients with valvular dysfunction and in one (12 per cent) of eight patients without valvular dysfunction ($p < 0.02$). Three patients with papillary muscle necrosis had coronary heart disease; one had more than 50 per cent luminal narrowing of the three major extramural coronary arteries by atherosclerosis as well as by an embolus to one extramural coronary artery; two patients had coronary arterial emboli to intramural coronary arteries located in a papillary muscle in one patient and in left ventricular free wall in the other. Nine patients without papillary muscle necrosis had coronary arterial disease: one due to atherosclerosis, eight due to emboli. The latter involved extramural coronary arteries in two and intramural vessels in six. Myocardial inflammation was observed histologically in twenty-three patients, nine of whom had abscesses. Myocardial inflammation was extensive in only one patient who had an eosinophilic myocarditis possibly due to a drug reaction. Interstitial myocardial fibrosis, observed in twenty-two of thirty-nine patients, was patchy and mild or minimal in all. One other patient had a healed transmural myocardial infarct. With the exception of papillary muscle necrosis, the presence or absence of other myocardial lesions (necrosis of ventricular free walls, inflammation, or fibrosis) did not correlate with the presence or absence of congestive heart failure.

Aortic valve cusps were perforated (fifteen patients) or otherwise partially destroyed (four patients) (Figures 2–6 and 12) in nineteen (65 per cent) of thirty-one patients with aortic valve vegetations, and all nineteen had aortic regurgitation and congestive heart failure. Mitral valve leaflets were perforated in three (12 per cent) of twenty-six patients with mitral vegetations. Ruptured chordae tendineae (Figure 2) were found in nine (35 per cent) of twenty-six patients with mitral valve vegetations.

Valve ring abscesses (Figures 3–6) were found in twelve patients, and each had aortic valve vegetations. The infective endocarditis in these patients was caused by D. pneumoniae in three, Staph. aureus in two, Staph. epidermidis in one, beta Streptococcus in one, Strep. faecalis in one, gram-positive coccus in two and was unknown in two. In only two patients were organisms seen in histologic sections of the ring abscesses. Of twenty patients with aortic regurgitation resulting from infective endocarditis, eleven had ring abscesses. Of twelve patients with aortic valve ring abscesses, eleven had severe regurgitation, and one had a previously stenotic valve. Two patients

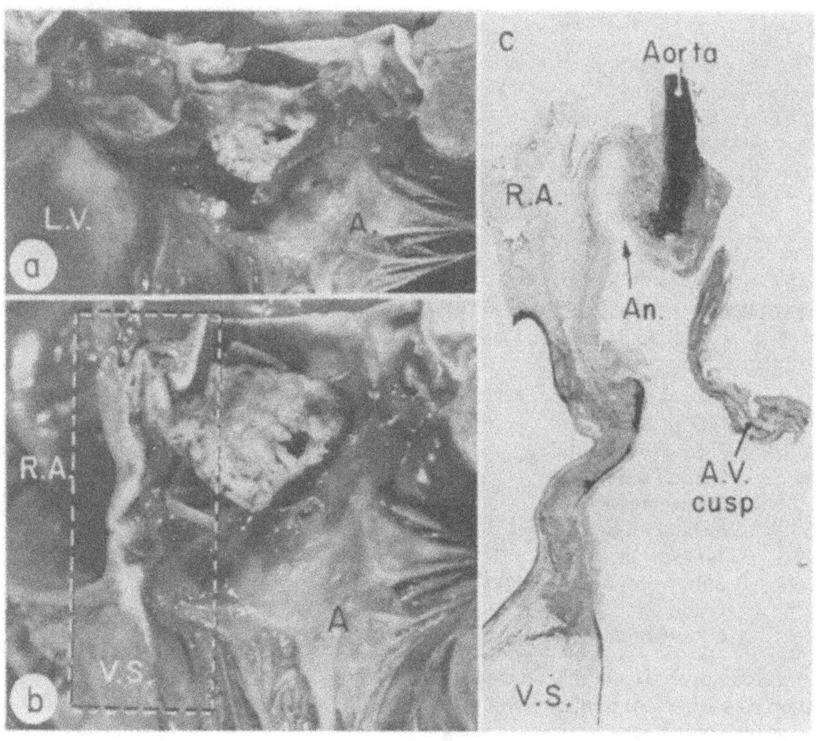

Figure 3. *Staph. epidermidis endocarditis in a twenty-two year old heroin addict (A69-313). The infection was on a congenitally bicuspid aortic valve which, although mildly incompetent before becoming infected, produced no symptoms.* ***a,*** *opened bicuspid aortic valve. L.V. = left ventricle; A. = anterior mitral leaflet.* ***b,*** *longitudinal section showing a huge perforation in one cusp and a subcuspal aneurysm, resulting from partial healing of a "ring" abscess. R.A. = right atrium; V.S. = ventricular septum. A photomicrograph of the area in brackets is shown in* ***c.*** *An. = aneurysm; A.V. = aortic valve. Elastic van Gieson stain; original magnification × 2, reduced by 19 per cent. A pericardial friction rub developed during hospitalization. Progressive aortic regurgitation and heart failure caused death twenty-one days after initiation of antibiotic therapy.*

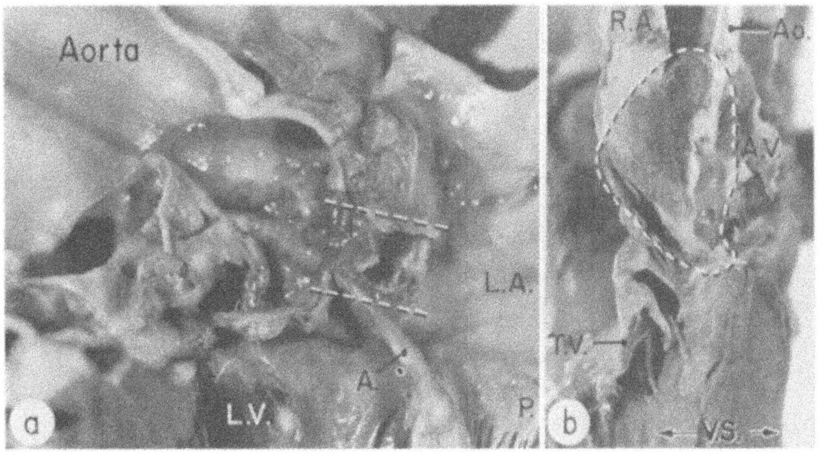

Figure 4. *Aortico-left atrial fistula caused by pneumococcal endocarditis in a fifty-four year old man with alcoholism (SH No. A71-28). After a one month history of cough and weakness he was hospitalized with overt signs of acute pneumonia, acute meningitis and congestive heart failure; he died within twenty-four hours. His blood pressure was 120/0 mm Hg.* ***a,*** *longitudinal section through aorta, aortic valve, anterior mitral leaflet (A.), left ventricle (L.V.) and left atrium (L.A.). The fistula, outlined by the dashed lines, presumably resulted from rupture of a "ring" abscess. The aortic valve is virtually destroyed by the infection. It was normal before the infection appeared. P. = posterior mitral leaflet.* ***b,*** *longitudinal section through aorta (Ao.), aortic valve (A.V.), ventricular septum (V.S.) and right atrial wall (R.A.). The infective process has extended into the right atrial and right ventricular walls. The area of the "ring" abscess is enclosed by the dashed lines. T.V. = septal tricuspid leaflet.*

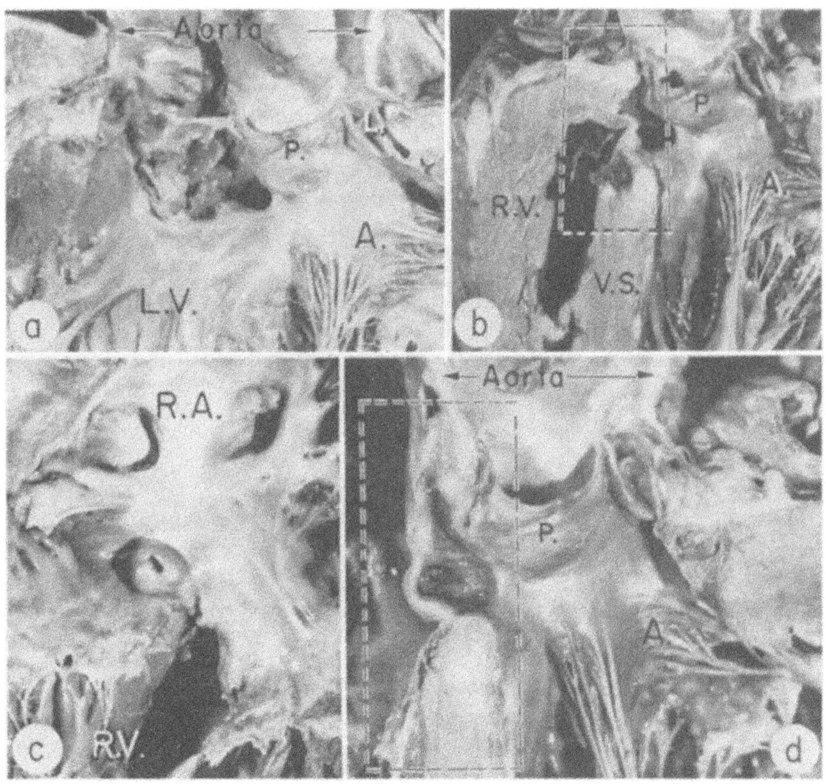

Figure 5. *Staph. epidermidis endocarditis in a seventeen year old boy with an aneurysm of the membranous ventricular septum (A69-42), possibly congenital in origin. Fever and exertional dyspnea developed four weeks before death. At hospitalization, ten days before death, systolic and diastolic precordial basal murmurs were heard. Despite antibiotic therapy, aortic regurgitation progressed, and he died of intractable heart failure.* ***a,*** *opened aortic valve and left ventricular (L.V.) outflow tract. The right cusp is virtually destroyed by the infective process. P. = posterior or noncoronary cusp; L. = left cusp; A. = anterior mitral leaflet.* ***b,*** *longitudinal section through right (R.V.) and left ventricles and ventricular septum (V.S.). An abscess is present in the most cephalad portion of the V.S. A photomicrograph of the area in brackets is shown in Figure 6a.* ***c,*** *opened right atrium (R.A.), tricuspid valve and right ventricle (R.V.) showing extension of the aneurysm of the membranous V.S. into the right atrium. A perforation is present in the aneurysm.* ***d,*** *longitudinal section through aorta and ventricular septum showing protrusion of aneurysm into the right atrium. A photomicrograph of the area in brackets is shown in Figure 6b.*

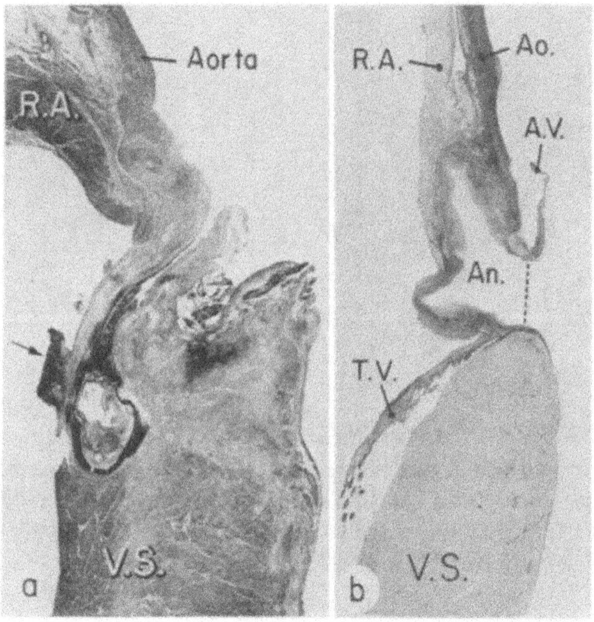

Figure 6. *Photomicrographs of longitudinal sections of ventricular septum (V.S.) at two levels in the patient described in Figure 5.* ***a,*** *section showing extension of the infective process through the entire thickness of the muscular V.S. A small vegetation (arrow) is apparent on the endocardium of the right side of the heart. R.A. = right atrium.* ***b,*** *section includes aneurysm (An.) of membranous portion of V.S. The dashed line represents the normal site of the membranous V.S. T.V. = tricuspid valve leaflet; A.V. = aortic valve cusp; Ao. = aorta. Phosphotungstic acid-hematoxylin stains; original magnification each × 2.9, reduced by 19 per cent.*

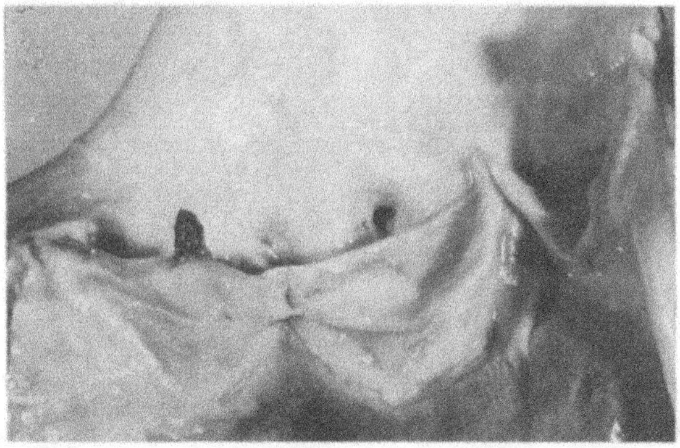

Figure 7. *Small vegetation on one aortic valve cusp in a fifty-three year old man with carcinoma of the prostate (A56-119). Endocarditis was not primary but occurred as part of a generalized staphylococcal septicemia. Organisms were present in this vegetation on histologic examination. Small vegetations like this one cause no cardiac dysfunction.*

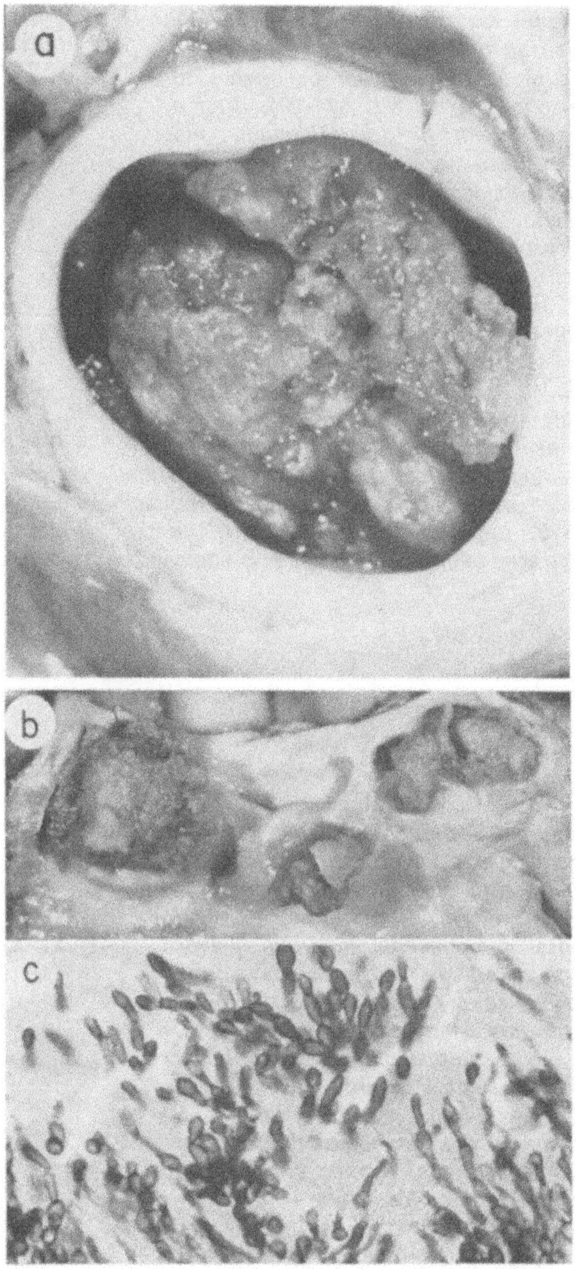

Figure 8. *C. parapsilosis endocarditis involving aortic valve of a twenty-six year old male heroin addict (A60-36). This patient, who was described elsewhere [56], lived for eight months after initial symptoms and signs of infective endocarditis appeared. He had an embolus to the left anterior descending coronary artery with a huge transmural acute myocardial infarct two months before death.* ***a,*** *aortic valve viewed from above. The large vegetations appear to obstruct the valve orifice.* ***b,*** *opened valve showing vegetations on each cusp.* ***c,*** *photomicrograph of vegetation showing pseudomycelia of C. parapsilosis. Methenamine silver stain; original magnification × 775, reduced by 9 per cent.*

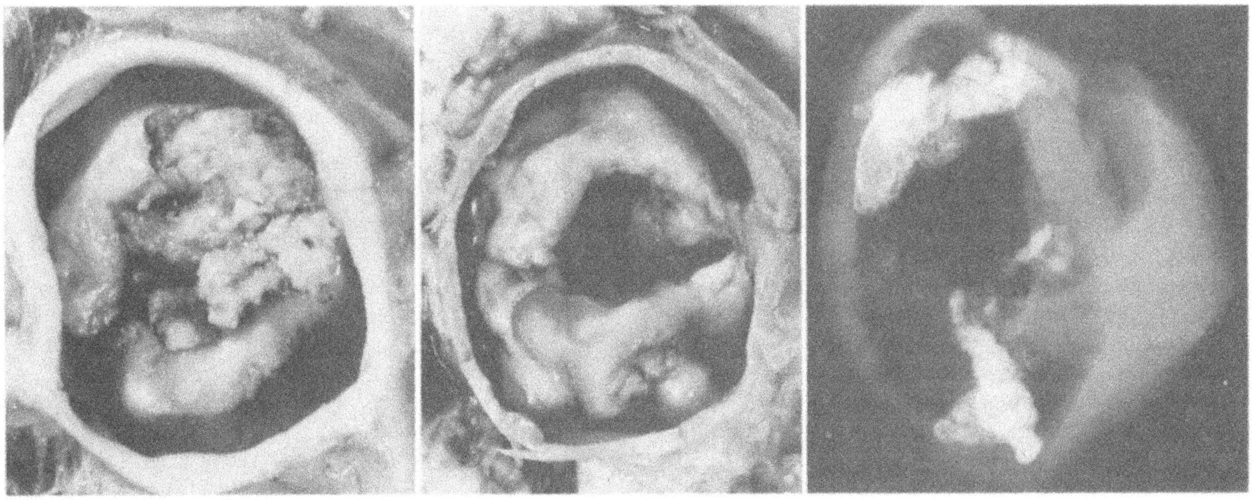

Figure 9. *Infective endocarditis on a calcified congenitally unicommissural aortic valve in a thirty-five year old male heroin addict (A70-181). Although a precordial murmur was present at age eighteen years he never had symptoms of cardiac dysfunction before endocarditis occurred. Ten weeks before death his left arm swelled after using a nonsterile needle for intravenous heroin injections. Seven weeks before death he noted painful red spots on his palms and soles. When hospitalized, six weeks before death, he had dermal and conjunctival petechiae, Roth's spots, Janeway lesions, a grade 5/6 systolic precordial murmur in the aortic area, a grade 2/6 diastolic blow of aortic regurgitation and a grade 3/6 apical systolic murmur; he was semistuporous. Electrocardiogram showed left ventricular hypertrophy. Numerous blood cultures were negative. Death resulted from congestive heart failure which developed after admission.* ***a,*** *aortic valve from above showing vegetations.* ***b,*** *aortic valve after removal of vegetations showing the densely fibrotic cusp with only one commissure (located at 3 o'clock).* ***c,*** *roentgenogram of aortic valve showing calcific deposits.*

with ring abscesses also had fistulas (Figures 4 and 5).

Mycotic aneurysm (Figure 12) of the proximal ascending aorta occurred in twelve patients, two of whom also had a mycotic aneurysm of the anterior mitral leaflet.

Acute pericarditis occurred in fourteen patients: in six of them it resulted from operation. Thus, eight (20 per cent) of the thirty-nine nonoperated patients had acute pericarditis. In none of the eight were organisms demonstrable in histologic sections of epicardium. All eight had fibrinofibrous pericarditis. One patient with a 1,200 ml serosanguineous pericardial effusion died of cardiac tamponade. The pericarditis in these eight patients resulted from extension of the inflammatory process into pericardium from ring abscesses (seven patients) or from a septic embolus to an extramural coronary artery (one patient).

Coronary arterial emboli (Figure 15) were seen in twelve patients: in three the embolus occluded an extramural coronary artery with resultant acute transmural myocardial infarct in two; in the other nine emboli were found on histologic examination only and in intramural coronary arteries.

Gross infarcts in various body organs occurred in twenty-nine (65 per cent) of the forty-five patients (Table XI), and, in addition, five patients had emboli to systemic arteries without infarcts. Multiple organs contained infarcts in twenty patients. Only nineteen of the thirty patients with organ infarcts were suspected clinically of having emboli.

Splenomegaly (weight more than 300 gm) was present in 52 per cent of the patients.

Histologic sections of kidney were reexamined in thirty-seven patients. Abnormalities were observed in twenty-nine patients (78 per cent); five had clinically significant renal disease. Acute pyelonephritis or interstitial inflammation was the most common renal lesion observed.

COMMENTS

Active infective endocarditis occurring on previously normal valves has been considered unusual. Of 1,056 necropsy patients with infective endocarditis summarized from several studies [11–22] in Table XII, 26 per cent had previously normal valves. In the present study of forty-five patients, 53 per cent had anatomically normal valves before the infection, and almost half of the remaining 47 per cent with anatomically abnormal valves had functionally normal valves. Thus, 76 per cent of our forty-five patients had functionally normal

Figure 10. *Pneumococcal endocarditis on the mitral valve of a forty-three year old man with alcoholism (DCGH No. 71A-70). Two weeks before death he noted nausea, vomiting and diarrhea, and six days before death he was hospitalized for acute pneumonia and acute meningitis. He never had signs of cardiac dysfunction and died of gastrointestinal hemorrhage.* ***a,*** *opened left ventricle showing small amount of vegetative material on the ventricular surface of the anterior mitral leaflet.* ***b,*** *atrial aspect of anterior mitral leaflet showing one vegetation. The valve cusps otherwise are normal.* ***c,*** *longitudinal section through the apical portion of the left ventricular wall showing an area of transmural necrosis.* ***d,*** *photomicrograph of area in* ***c*** *showing extensive myocardial necrosis. An extramural coronary artery* ***(arrow)*** *is occluded by vegetative material. Hematoxylin and eosin stain; original magnification × 2.5, reduced by 21 per cent.*

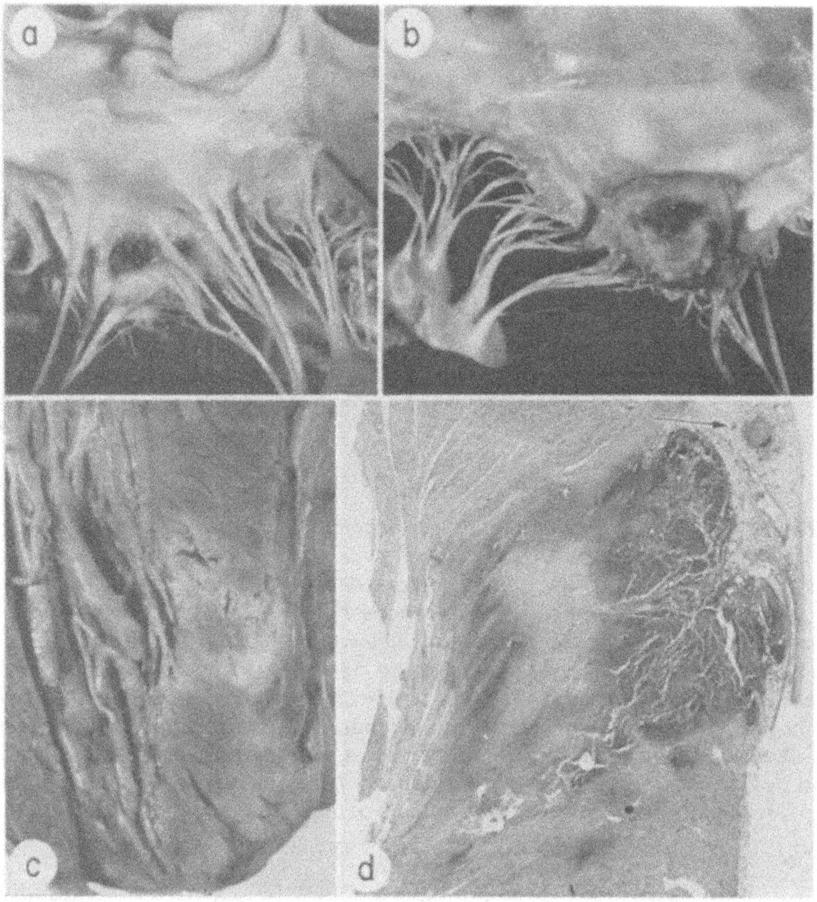

Figure 11. *C. parapsilosis endocarditis on a previously normal mitral valve of a sixty-eight year old man with chronic lung disease and coronary heart disease (A60-126). Five months before death he had fever, and forty-five days later he was hospitalized. A grade 2/6 apical systolic murmur was present. Despite amphotericin B therapy, blood cultures remained positive, and he died of congestive heart failure. A large embolus to the left common iliac artery occurred during hospitalization.* ***a,*** *mitral valve viewed from left atrium showing huge vegetations on both leaflets.* ***b,*** *opened left heart showing large vegetations on both mitral leaflets.* ***c,*** *photomicrograph of portion of vegetation showing spores and pseudomycelia of Candida species. Methenamine silver stain; original magnification × 500, reduced by 25 per cent.*

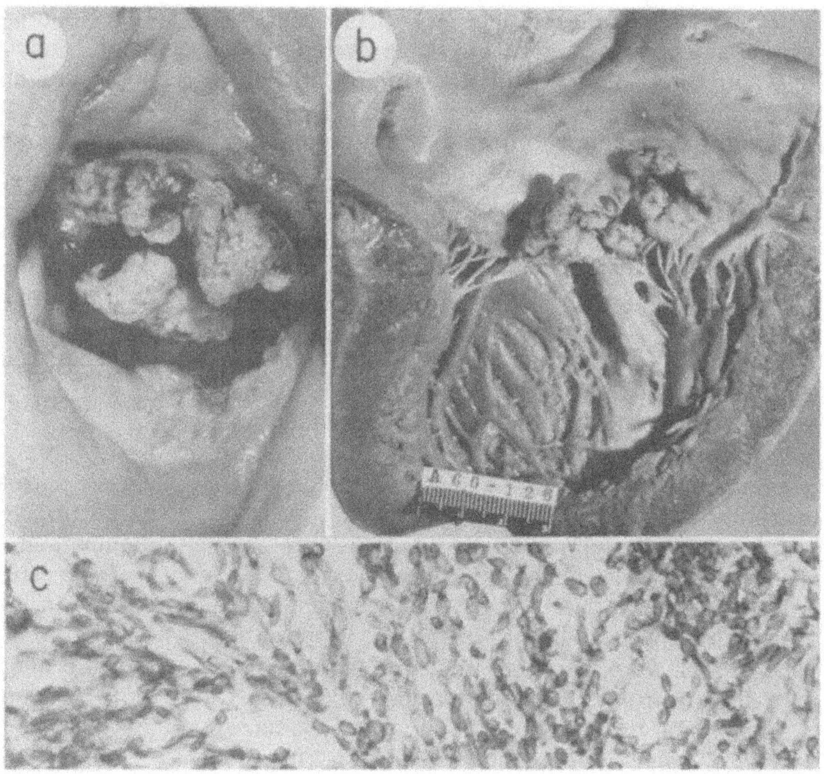

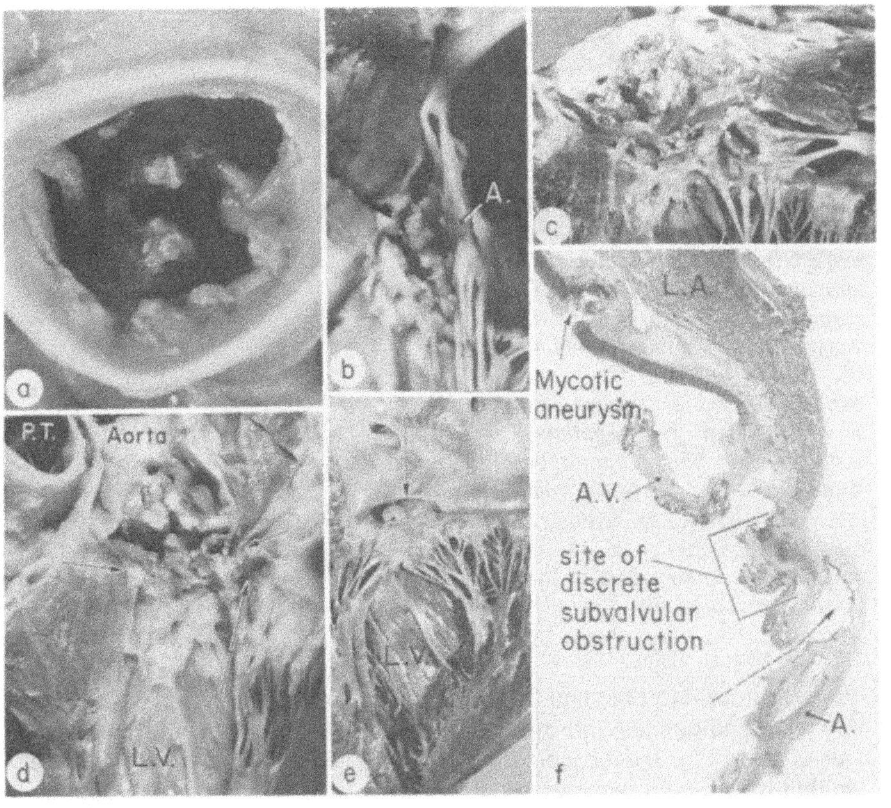

Figure 12. *Alpha hemolytic streptococcus endocarditis complicating congenitally discrete subaortic stenosis in a twenty-eight year old man (A64-20). The infection, which appeared about nine months before death, produced severe valvular aortic regurgitation. This patient was described previously [9].* ***a,*** *aortic valve as viewed from above.* ***b,*** *left ventricular outflow tract viewed from below showing vegetative material on the subvalvular "membrane" adjacent to the anterior mitral leaflet (A).* ***c,*** *opened left ventricular outflow tract showing vegetations on each aortic cusp and on the subvalvular "membrane" and ventricular surface of anterior mitral leaflet.* ***d,*** *longitudinal section showing the left ventricular outflow tract. The area of subaortic stenosis is well seen (between the solid arrows), and a mycotic aneurysm (dashed arrow) is seen in the anterior mitral leaflet. The mitral aneurysm is in the high pressure portion of the left ventricle (L.V.), i.e., below the discrete subvalvular obstruction. P.T. = pulmonary trunk.* ***e,*** *opened mitral valve showing atrial aspect of the mycotic aneurysm (dashed arrow) on the anterior leaflet.* ***f,*** *photomicrograph of section through aorta, left atrium (L.A.), aortic valve (A.V.) cusp, subvalvular "membrane," and anterior mitral leaflet (A.). A mycotic aneurysm is present in the ascending aorta as well as in the anterior mitral leaflet (dashed arrow). Vegetations are present on the aortic valve cusp and on the subvalvular membrane. Hematoxylin and eosin stain; original magnification × 3.2, reduced by 39 per cent.*

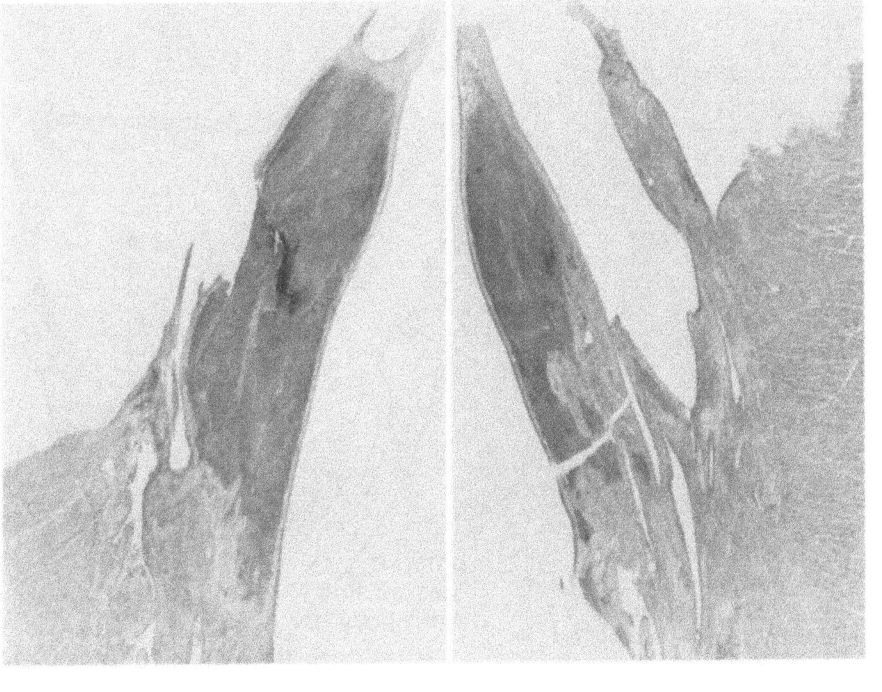

Figure 13. *Photomicrographs of both left ventricular papillary muscles of the patient described in Figure 3. Extensive necrosis is present in each papillary muscle while the left ventricular free wall is normal. Hematoxylin and eosin stain; original magnification × 4, reduced by 16 per cent.*

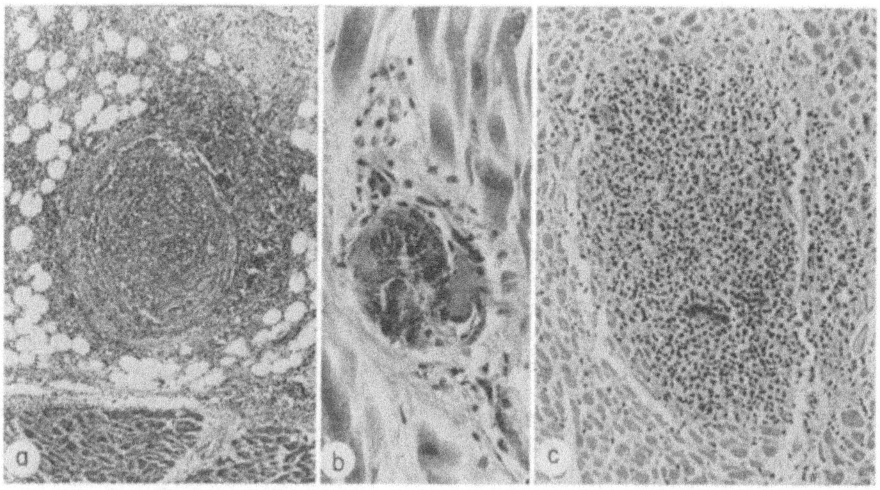

Figure 14. *Photomicrographs of acute inflammatory lesions in the heart in active infective endocarditis.* ***a,*** *extramural coronary artery occluded by vegetative material with resultant extension of the acute inflammation through the vessel wall and into epicardium and myocardium. Hematoxylin and eosin stain; original magnification × 80, reduced by 39 per cent.* ***b,*** *intramural coronary artery occluded by vegetative material containing numerous organisms. This thirty-six year old man (A65-8) had mycosis fungoides and generalized staphylococcal septicemia. Hematoxylin and eosin stain; original magnification × 400, reduced by 39 per cent.* ***c,*** *myocardial abscess with organisms in same patient described in* ***a.*** *Patient died of overwhelming pneumonia and renal failure without signs of cardiac dysfunction. Hematoxylin and eosin stain; original magnification × 220, reduced by 39 per cent.*

valves before the onset of infective endocarditis. When an anatomically normal cardiac valve is the site of infection, the organism is usually a highly virulent one (Staph. species, Pneumococcus) or a very unusual one (fungus, for example). When an anatomically abnormal valve is the site of infection, the organism tends to be a less virulent one (alpha hemolytic Streptococcus, for example). Thayer [12] noted infective endocarditis on previously normal valves in 63 per cent of seventy patients with pneumococcal or staphylococcal endocarditis but in only 20 per cent of patients with infective endocarditis caused by alpha hemolytic Streptococcus. Finland and Barnes [23] found clinically normal valves in 185 (68 per cent) of 271 episodes of infective endocarditis caused by an organism other than alpha hemolytic Streptococcus or Staph. epidermidis.

Infective endocarditis involving previously anatomically normal valves would appear to have a higher mortality than infective endocarditis involving previously anatomically and/or functionally abnormal valves [24]. In a study by Rabinovich et al. [25] ten (83 per cent) of twelve patients with

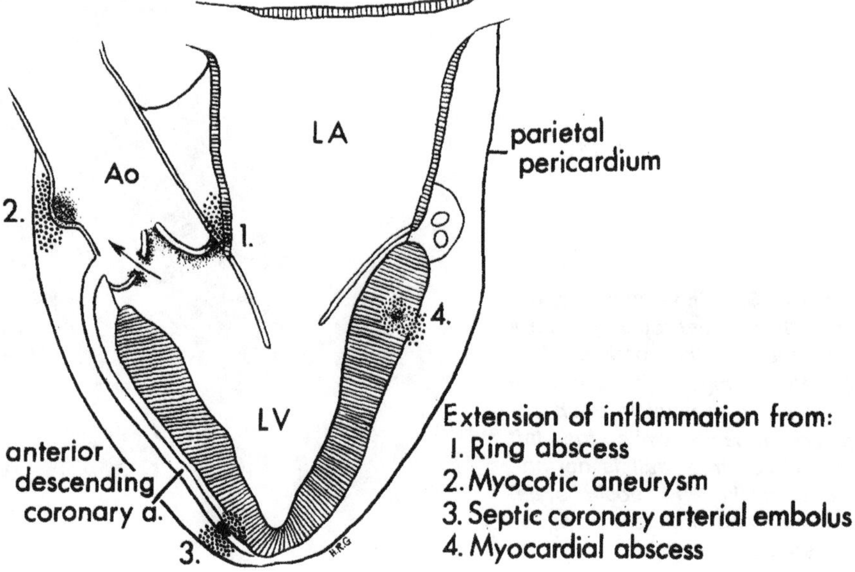

Figure 15. *Schematic portrayal of the pathogenesis of pericarditis in infective endocarditis. Ao = aorta; LV = left ventricle; LA = left atrium.*

infective endocarditis on normal valves died, whereas sixty-one (48 per cent) of 129 patients with infective endocarditis on previously abnormal valves died.

Predisposing factors were apparent in seventeen (71 per cent) of our twenty-four patients with infective endocarditis on previously normal valves and in thirteen (62 per cent) of twenty-one patients with infective endocarditis on previously abnormal valves. Of the thirty patients with predisposing factors eighteen were alcoholics, heroin addicts or had a malignancy, and fourteen (78 per cent) had previously anatomically normal valves before the onset of infective endocarditis. The presence of these various predisposing factors increases the likelihood that infective endocarditis will occur on previously normal valves, that it will be caused by an unusual or virulent organism and that it will carry a high mortality.

Myocardial lesions are frequent in patients with active infective endocarditis [11,12,16,17,21, 26–36] (Table XIII). Clawson [27], Buch-

TABLE IX Acute Myocardial Lesions in Left-Sided Infective Endocarditis (33* of 38† Patients = 87%)

Myocardial Lesion		Patients No.	Patients %
Necrosis‡		23	61
Papillary muscle only	18		
Papillary muscle + LV free wall	4		
Left ventricular free wall only	1		
Myocytolysis		21	55
Inflammation		23	61
Interstitial and perivascular (nonsuppurating myocarditis)	14		
Abscesses	2		
Both	7		

* Eleven patients with one or more of the three myocardial lesions listed had coronary arterial emboli and one other patient had severe coronary atherosclerosis.
† Includes only those subjects in whom sections of both left ventricular papillary muscles as well as left ventricular free wall or septum were available for examination.
‡ Unassociated with myocardial abscesses.

TABLE X Cardiac Findings in Left-Sided Infective Endocarditis (45 Necropsy Patients)

Lesion		Patients No.	Patients %
Perforated or partially destroyed cusp*		22	49
Aortic	19		
Mitral	3		
Mycotic aneurysm		12	27
Ascending aorta	12		
Anterior mitral leaflet	2†		
Ring abscess		12	27
Ruptured chordae tendineae		9	20
Mitral	9		
Pericarditis‡		8	20

* One patient each had a perforated aortic and mitral valve cusp as a result of a previous episode of IE.
† Each patient also had mycotic aneurysms of the ascending aorta.
‡ Six patients with operatively-induced pericarditis were excluded.

TABLE XI Gross Embolic Infarcts* in Left-Sided Infective Endocarditis (29 Patients = 65% of Total of 45)

Site	Patients No.	Patients %
Kidney	19	42
Spleen	17	38
Brain	15	33
Liver	3	7
Heart	2	4
Lung	1	2
Pancreas	1	2

* Total infarcts = fifty-eight of possible 203 organs of twenty-nine patients. In addition, five patients had emboli to systemic arteries without infarction.

TABLE XII Necropsy Incidence of Infective Endocarditis on Normal Valves

Source	Patients Total No.	With Normal Valves No.	With Normal Valves %
Clawson [11] 1924	132	47	36
Thayer [12,13] 1926, 1931	306*	92	30
Seabury [14] 1947	58	10	17
Traut et al. [15] 1949	94†	18	19
Cates, Christie [16] 1951	86	0	0
Perry et al. [17] 1952	52	19*	37
Morgan, Bland [18] 1959	56	8	14
Kalman et al. [19] 1962	80	34*	42
Wilson [20] 1963	103	16	16
Guze, Pearce [21] 1963	64	17	27
Lerner, Weinstein [22] 1966	25	8	32
Totals	1,056‡	269	26
Present series	45	24	53

* Refers to absence of congenital or rheumatic heart disease.
† Only patients more than sixty years old were included.
‡ At least 116 of these 1,056 patients had vegetations on right-sided cardiac valves [11,13,15–17,20,21]. Thus, if they could be excluded the number with normal valves would probably be about 20 per cent rather than 26 per cent.

binder and Saphir [29], Saphir [28] and Perry et al. [17] each observed myocardial lesions in 88 to 100 per cent of 187 patients studied by them at necropsy. Acute myocardial lesions were observed in thirty-three (87 per cent) of our thirty-eight necropsy patients in whom numerous histologic sections of myocardium were examined. The significance of the myocardial lesions observed in patients with infective endocarditis has been debated. Clawson [27] and Correll et al. [34] considered the lesions to be a major cause of congestive heart failure in patients with active infective endocarditis. de Navasquez [30] and Perry et al. [17], however, believed that congestive heart failure in patients with infective endocarditis was rarely the result of myocardial lesions. In none of our patients could we attribute congestive cardiac failure to the acute myocardial lesions. With the exception of two patients with severe coronary heart disease, congestive cardiac failure occurred in our patients only when valvular dysfunction was also present.

The location in the left ventricular wall of acute myocardial lesions in patients with active infective endocarditis has, to our knowledge, not been commented on previously. Although it has been described in infective endocarditis as the result of coronary arterial emboli [37,38], papillary muscle necrosis has not been commented on previously in patients with infective endocarditis in whom coronary narrowing was not present. Foci of necrosis were observed in left ventricular papillary muscles in twenty-two of our thirty-eight patients with active infective endocarditis, and in eleven they were diffusely necrotic. Only three of the twenty-two patients had coronary arterial narrowing: by emboli to intramural coronary arteries in two and by severe (more than 50 per cent luminal narrowing) atherosclerosis in one. The significant ($p < 0.02$) correlation between papillary muscle necrosis and valve dysfunction resulting in congestive heart failure suggests that the necrosis results from poor arterial perfusion associated with the heart failure since the papillary muscles are the last to be supplied by arterial blood [39]. Despite papillary muscle necrosis, no patient had mitral regurgitation in the absence of destruction of mitral leaflets or ruptured chordae tendineae. No patient with papillary muscle necrosis, however, had necrosis in the free wall beneath the papillary muscles.

Valvular dysfunction is the leading cause of congestive cardiac failure in patients with infective endocarditis. Of our forty-five patients with infec-

TABLE XIII Myocardial Lesions in Active Infective Endocarditis (IE)

Source	No. Necropsy Patients*	% Necrosis	% Fibrosis	Inflammation: % Nonsuppurating	Inflammation: % Suppurative	% Coronary Emboli	Total % With Lesions
Blumer [26] 1923	150	3	...	7	2	...	20†
Clawson [11] 1924	103	...	...	24	...	...	...
Thayer‡ [12] 1926	92	...	...	53§ 42#	23	...	...
Clawson [27] 1928	60	...	64	>74	22	...	88
Saphir [28] 1935	35	83¶	43	32	27‖	51	100
Buchbinder, Saphir [29] 1939	40	68	58	48	35‖	50	98
de Navasquez [30] 1939	20	...	...	95	...	80**	...
Middleton, Burke [31] 1939	49	14	47	10	4	...	...
Flaxman [32] 1943	252	...	...	...	3	...	...
Hildebrand, Priest [33] 1947	10	...	...	100	10	...	...
Correll et al. [34] 1951	44	...	...	80	...	...	...
Cates, Christie [16] 1951	442	...	...	..	...	4	...
Perry et al. [17] 1952	52	90‖	40	>51	>8	...	98
Pankey [35] 1961	60	...	...	...	...	8	...
Pankey [36] 1962	48	...	...	22	35	10	...
Guze, Pearce [21] 1963	64	...	...	74	...	...	...

* A few had IE involving right-sided cardiac valves but the exact number is uncertain.
† Includes 12 patients with "cloudy swelling."
‡ Includes patients with staphylococcal, pneumococcal, and streptococcal IE.
§ Acute inflammatory cells.
\# Chronic inflammatory cells.
¶ Abscess used synonymously with focal necrosis.
‖ Refers to miliary infarcts.
** Refers to inflammation in areas with vessels; does not specify actual presence of emboli.

TABLE XIV Necropsy Evidence of Pericarditis

Source	Patients No.	With Pericarditis No.	With Pericarditis %
Blumer [26] 1923	150	16	11
Clawson [11] 1924	132	24	21
Thayer [12] 1926	166*	16	10
Thayer [40] 1931–32	186	7	4
Middleton, Burke [31] 1939	49	12	24
Beck [41] 1942	43	8	16
Traut et al. [15] 1949	94	13	14
Pankey [35] 1961	60	9	15
Pankey [36] 1962	48	13	27
Robinson, Ruedy [42] 1962	267	37	14
Guze, Pearce [21] 1963	50	9	18
Totals	1,245	164	14
Present series	39†	8†	20

* Patients with pneumococcal, streptococcal and staphylococcal endocarditis only.

† Excludes six patients with operatively-induced pericarditis.

tive endocarditis, thirty-five had congestive cardiac failure, and thirty-three of them had severe valvular dysfunction. The remaining two had severe coronary heart disease. Although it is well appreciated that destruction of valvular cusps and chordae tendineae causes regurgitation, it is less well appreciated that vegetations may be large enough to actually obstruct a valve orifice. Valvular stenosis from large vegetations appears to have occurred in two of our patients [10].

The frequency of pericarditis in infective endocarditis is presented in Table XIV [11,12,15,21, 26,31,35,36,40–42]. Middleton and Burke [31] reported pericardial rubs in 6 per cent of eighty-eight patients with active infective endocarditis. Even when recognized, pericarditis usually has been attributed to factors other than infective endocarditis, such as uremia [43], active rheumatic carditis [11] or myocardial infarction [44]. Pericarditis has been described in association with myocardial abscesses in the area of valve rings [41,45–47] and in association with mycotic aneurysms [41,48,49]. A site of extension of inflammation into the pericardium was found in each of our eight patients with pericarditis. The mechanisms of pericarditis resulting from infective endocarditis are shown in Figure 15.

Sheldon and Golden [50] called attention to the occurrence of ring abscesses in acute bacterial endocarditis. Infective endocarditis in their twelve patients was caused by Staph. aureus and D. pneumoniae. They did not find abscesses in eleven patients with subacute bacterial endocarditis. Ring abscesses were found in twelve of our forty-five patients. They occurred in patients with clinical courses longer than six weeks and in whom the causative organism was Strep. faecalis and Staph. epidermidis as well as Staph. aureus and D. pneumoniae. Aortic valve ring abscesses occurred in twelve of our thirty-one patients with aortic vegetations, eleven had severe aortic regurgitation and one had previous aortic stenosis. Several investigators have commented on the problem of valve replacement when the infection has extended into the "annulus." Wallace et al. [51] considered ring abscesses to probably preclude successful valve replacement. Stason et al. [52] postulated that annular involvement may contribute to postoperative paraprosthetic leaks. Several workers [53–55] have noted good operative results in the presence of ring abscesses.

REFERENCES

1 Cohn LH, Roberts WC, Rockoff SD, Morrow AG: Bacterial endocarditis following aortic valve replacement. Clinical and pathologic correlations. Circulation 33: 209, 1966.

2. Archard HO, Roberts WC· Bacterial endocarditis after dental procedures in patients with aortic valve prostheses. J Amer Dent Ass 72: 648, 1966.

3 Roberts WC, Morrow AG: Bacterial endocarditis involving prosthetic mitral valves. Clinical and pathologic observations. Arch Path (Chicago) 82: 164, 1966.

4. Buchbinder NA, Roberts WC: Active infective endocarditis confined to mural endocardium. A study of 6 necropsy patients. Arch Path (Chicago) (in press).

5 Lombardo TA, Rabson AS, Dodge HT· Mycotic endocarditis Amer J Med 22. 664, 1957.

6. Merchant RK, Louria DB, Geisler PH, Edgcomb JH, Utz JP. Fungal endocarditis. review of the literature and report of three cases. Ann Intern Med 48. 242, 1958.

7 Falcone MW, Roberts WC, Morrow AG, Perloff JG: Congenital aortic stenosis resulting from a unicommissural valve: clinical and anatomic features in 21 adult patients Circulation 44: 272, 1971

8. Roberts WC, Perloff JK, Constantino T: Severe valvular aortic stenosis in patients over 65 years of age A clinicopathologic study. Amer J Cardiol 27: 499, 1971.

9. Morrow AG, Fort L III, Roberts WC, Braunwald E: Discrete subaortic stenosis complicated by aortic valvular regurgitation Clinical, hemodynamic, and pathologic studies and results of operative treatment. Circulation 31· 163, 1965.

10. Roberts WC, Ewy GA, Glancy DL, Marcus FI· Valvular stenosis produced by active infective endocarditis. Circulation 36: 449, 1967.

11. Clawson BJ· An analysis of two hundred and twenty cases of endocarditis with special reference to the subacute bacterial type. Arch Intern Med (Chicago) 33: 157, 1924.

12. Thayer WS Studies on bacterial (infective) endocarditis. Johns Hopkins Hosp Rep 22. 1, 1926.
13. Thayer WS: Bacterial or infective endocarditis Edinburgh Med J 38. 237, 1931.
14. Seaburg JH. Subacute bacterial endocarditis: experiences during the past decade Arch Intern Med (Chicago) 79. 1, 1947.
15. Traut EF, Carter JB, Gumbiner SH, Hench RN. Bacterial endocarditis in the elderly. Geriatrics 4· 205, 1949
16. Cates JE, Christie RV. Subacute bacterial endocarditis A review of 442 patients treated in 14 centers appointed by the Penicillin Trials Committee of the Medical Research Council. Quart J Med 20. 93, 1951.
17 Perry EL, Fleming RG, Edwards JE. Myocardial lesions in bacterial endocarditis Ann Intern Med 36 126, 1952
18. Morgan WL, Bland EF: Bacterial endocarditis in the antibiotic era. Circulation 19 753, 1959.
19. Kalman C, Thomison JB, Shapiro JL Bacterial endocarditis. autopsy experience over a thirty year period. Southern Med J 55: 1208, 1962
20 Wilson LM: Pathology of fatal bacterial endocarditis before and since the introduction of antibiotics. Ann Intern Med 58: 84, 1963.
21 Guze LB, Pearce ML. Hospital-acquired bacterial endocarditis Arch Intern Med (Chicago) 112: 102, 1963.
22 Lerner PI, Weinstein L: Infective endocarditis in the antibiotic era. New Eng J Med 274. 199;259;388, 1966.
23. Finland M, Barnes MW Changing etiology of bacterial endocarditis in the antibacterial era Ann Intern Med 72: 341, 1970
24 Kerr A Jr· Subacute Bacterial Endocarditis, Springfield, Ill., Charles C Thomas, 1955, p 225.
25. Rabinovich S, Evans J, Smith IM, January LE: A long term view of bacterial endocarditis. Ann Intern Med 63. 185, 1965
26. Blumer G Subacute bacterial endocarditis. Medicine 2 105, 1923.
27 Clawson BJ: Myocarditis. Amer Heart J 4: 1, 1928.
28. Saphir O Myocardial lesions in subacute bacterial endocarditis Amer J Path 11· 143, 1935.
29. Buchbinder WC, Saphir O: Heart failure in subacute bacterial endocarditis. Arch Intern Med (Chicago) 64 336, 1939.
30. de Navasquez S· The incidence and pathogenesis of myocardial lesions in subacute bacterial endocarditis J Path 49. 33, 1939
31 Middleton WS, Burke M: Streptococcus viridans endocarditis lenta Amer J Med Sci 198: 301, 1939
32 Flaxman N. Myocardial abscess. JAMA 122: 804, 1943.
33. Hildebrand E, Priest W. Cardiac lesions in subacute bacterial endocarditis treated with penicillin Amer J Clin Path 17· 345, 1947.
34. Correll HL, Lubitz JM, Lindert MCF: Bacterial endocarditis: clinicopathologic studies of untreated, treated and cured patients. Ann Intern Med 35: 45, 1951.
35 Pankey GA· Subacute bacterial endocarditis at the University of Minnesota Hospital, 1939 through 1959 Ann Intern Med 55· 550, 1961
36. Pankey GA: Acute bacterial endocarditis at the University of Minnesota Hospital, 1939 through 1959 Amer Heart J 64. 583, 1962.
37 Case records of the Massachusetts General Hospital. Weekly clinicopathological exercises New Eng J Med 284 1084, 1971
38 Edwards JE Mitral insufficiency resulting from "overshooting" of leaflets Circulation 43 606, 1971
39 Estes EH, Dalton FM, Entman ML, Dixon HB III, Hackel DB The anatomy and blood supply of the papillary muscles of the left ventricle Amer Heart J 71, 356, 1966.
40 Tahyer WS Observations on rheumatic pericarditis and infective endocarditis. Ann Intern Med 5: 247, 1931–32
41. Beck D: Pericarditis and subacute bacterial endocarditis J Mount Sinai Hosp NY 8: 364, 1942
42 Robinson MJ, Ruedy J Sequelae of bacterial endocarditis. Amer J Med 32: 922, 1962.
43 Friedberg CK Diseases of the Heart, Philadelphia, W. B. Saunders, 1966, p 1384
44 Libman E Subacute bacterial endocarditis Brit Med J 2· 301, 1920
45. Gross L, Kugel MA: Topographic anatomy and histology of the valves of the human heart Amer J Path 7 445, 1931
46 Ryon DS, Pastor BH, Myerson RM. Abscess of the myocardium Amer J Med Sci 251: 698, 1966.
47 Berger HR, Kossmann CE: Solitary myocardial abscess in subacute bacterial endocarditis. Ann Intern Med 35 1125, 1951.
48. Pirani CL· Erosive (mycotic) aneurysm of the heart with rupture Arch Path (Chicago) 36· 579, 1943.
49 Bristow JD, Parker BM, Hang WA: Hemopericardium following rupture of a bacterial aortic sinus aneurysm Amer J Cardiol 6: 355, 1960.
50 Sheldon WH, Golden A: Abscesses of the valve rings of the heart, a frequent but not well recognized complication of acute bacterial endocarditis. Circulation 4: 1, 1951.
51. Wallace AG, Young WG Jr, Osterhout S Treatment of acute bacterial endocarditis by valve excision and replacement. Circulation 31: 450, 1965.
52. Stason WB, DeSanctis RW, Weinberg AN, Austen WG: Cardiac surgery in bacterial endocarditis. J Thorac Cardiovasc Surg 54: 491, 1967
53. Krutschmer KP, Lawrence GH. Valve replacement in patients with bacterial endocarditis. Amer J Surg 118 273, 1969
54 Symbas PN, Parr JA. Early surgical treatment for acute pneumococcal aortic valvulitis with aortic insufficiency, acquired ventricular septal defect, and aortico-right ventricular shunt. Ann Surg 167 580, 1968
55 Hurley EJ, Eldridge FL, Hultgren HN. Emergency replacement of valves in endocarditis. Amer Heart J 73 798, 1967.
56 Andriole VT, Kravetz M, Roberts WC, Utz JP Candida endocarditis. Clinical and pathologic studies. Amer J Med 32 251, 1962.

Alcoholism

An Important but Unemphasized Factor Predisposing to Infective Endocarditis

Neil A. Buchbinder, MD, William C. Roberts, MD, Bethesda, Md

We studied the clinical and anatomic features in 14 habitual alcoholics who had infective endocarditis. Alcoholism is frequently associated with fatal infective endocarditis. When infective endocarditis develops in alcoholics, the causative organism is usually *Diplococcus pneumoniae* (10 of 14 patients). The endocarditis, however, is usually not the most prominent clinical feature of their illness. Acute pneumonia (11 patients) and acute meningitis (nine patients) overshadows the endocarditis. Often, alcoholism is part of the tetrad of pneumococcal endocarditis, pneumonitis, meningitis, and chronic alcoholism.

It is now widely appreciated that narcotic addicts are highly prone to the development of infective endocarditis. The organism usually responsible for the infective endocarditis is *Staphylococcus*, and the vegetations may be located on either the right or left side of the heart. A far more common type of addiction, however, is to alcohol, and heretofore virtually no association has been demonstrated between alcoholism and infective endocarditis. This report describes chronic alcoholism and infective endocarditis in 14 patients and calls attention to the frequent but unemphasized syndrome of pneumococcal endocarditis, meningitis, and pneumonitis in habitual alcoholics (Fig 1).

Received for publication Aug 7, 1972; accepted Feb 12, 1973.

From the Section of Pathology, National Heart and Lung Institute, National Institutes of Health, Bethesda, Md.

Reprint requests to Section of Pathology, National Heart and Lung Institute, Bethesda, MD 20014 (Dr. Roberts).

Patients Studied

Certain clinical and necropsy observations in the 14 patients are summarized in the Table. According to the testimony of their families, all 14 patients were habitual alcoholics and were unemployed because of their addiction. Their ages ranged from 36 to 65 years (average, 53); 12 were men, two were women; 13 were black and one was an Eskimo. Nine patients had clinical evidence of acute meningitis, and 11 had evidence of acute pneumonia. Thus, 12 of the 14 patients had either acute meningitis or acute pneumonitis, or both. Patient 12 had pneumococcal meningitis as well as acute pneumococcal arthritis of one knee. Patient 6 had only diarrhea and fever, and he later developed cardiac tamponade. In only one patient (No. 5) was cardiac dysfunction the most prominent clinical feature, and he had severe aortic regurgitation. Nine patients, however, had precordial murmurs on admission. Infective endocarditis was suspected clinically in only four patients on admission. Blood cultures or spinal fluid cultures, or both, were positive in all patients: *Diplococcus pneumoniae* in ten patients, *Streptococcus faecalis* in two, *Staphylococcus aureus* in one, and *Escherichia coli* in one. Each patient received antibiotics to which the causative organism was susceptible. In addition to the one patient who had valve dysfunction (aortic regurgitation) on admission, nine others developed valvular incompetence with evidence of congestive cardiac failure during hospitalization. In only five patients, however, could death be attributed directly to congestive cardiac failure; one of them had cardiac tamponade secondary to rupture of an aortic valve "ring" abscess into the pericardium. Death in the remaining nine patients resulted from meningitis or pneumonia, or both.

At necropsy, vegetations were located only on left-sided cardiac valves in nine patients, on both left and right-sided valves in four, and only on right-sided cardiac valves in one. In 13 patients, portions of the valve leaflets not containing vegetative material were normal, and in patient 1, these portions were mildly thickened. Thus, in 13 patients, the valves appear to have been both anatomically and functionally normal before the

Clinical and Necropsy Data in 14 Patients With Chronic Alcoholism and Active Infective Endocarditis

Patient/ Age/Race/ Sex	Duration of Fatal Acute Illness, Days	Acute Pneu-monia	Acute Menin-gitis	Infective Endo-carditis Diagnosed Clinically	Organism Causing Infective Endocarditis	Precor-dial Mur-mur	CHF	Cause of Death
Left-Sided Endocarditis								
1/63/B/M	5	+	0	0	*Strep faecalis*	+	+	Pneumonia
2/44/E/M	2	+	+	0	*D pneumoniae*	+	+	Meningitis
3/56/B/M	14	+	0	0	*D pneumoniae*	0	+	Pneumonia
4/43/B/M	14	+	+	0	*D pneumoniae*	0	0	Pneumonia meningit
5/61/B/M	120	0	0	+	*Strep faecalis*	+	+	CHF
6/51/B/F	45	0	0	0	*E coli*	0	+	Tamponade
7/36/B/F	42	+	+	+	*D pneumoniae*	+	+	CHF
8/54/B/M	30	+	+	0	*D pneumoniae*	0	+	CHF
9/45/B/M	7	+	+	0	*D pneumoniae*	0	+	Pneumonia meningit
Left- and Right-Sided Endocarditis								
10/52/B/M	45	0	+	0	*D pneumoniae*	+	0	Meningitis
11/55/B/M	4	+	0	0	*Staph aureus*	+	0	Pneumonia
12/55/B/M	21	+	+	+	*D pneumoniae*	+	+	CHF
13/58/B/M	2	+	+	0	*D pneumoniae*	+	+	Pneumonia meningit
Right-Sided Endocarditis								
14/65/B/M	90	+	+	+	*D pneumoniae*	+	+	Pneumonia meningit

* AV indicates aortic valve; B, Black; CHF, congestive heart failure; E, Eskimo; F, female; M, male; MV, mitral valve; PV, pulmonic valve; TV, tricuspid valve.

Fig 1.—The tetrad.

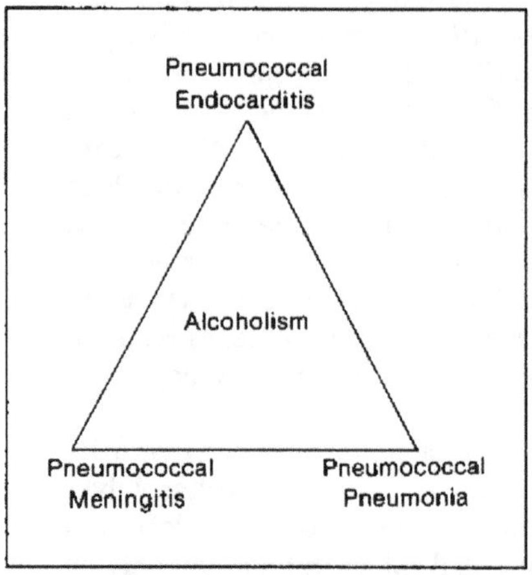

Fig 2.—Patient 3 (Table). Pneumococcal endocarditis in a 56-year-old man who had acute pneumonia. Left, Opened aortic valve showing endocarditis of noncoronary cusp, which is perforated. Right, Opened right atrium, tricuspid valve, and right ventricle. Discoloration above tricuspid valve caused by extension of aortic ring abscess into right atrial wall.

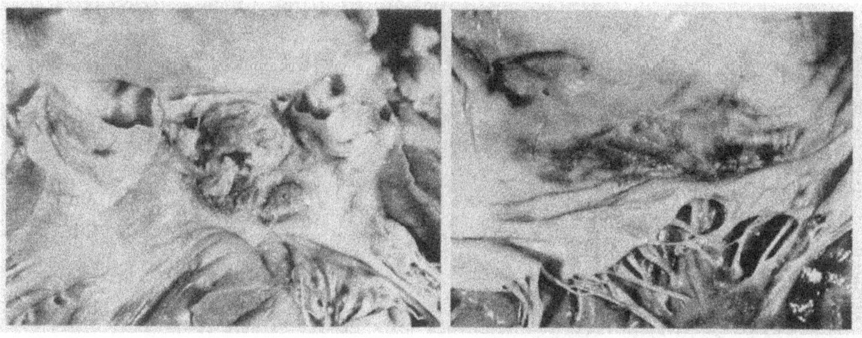

onset of infective endocarditis. Of the 56 cardiac valves present in the 14 patients, 23 contained one or more vegetations; the aortic valve was involved in 11 patients; mitral, in 7; tricuspid, in 4; and pulmonic, in 1. Only one valve contained vegetations in six patients, and in eight patients, two or more valves contained vegetations. Of the 23 valves containing vegetations, 12 were partially destroyed and made incompetent by the infective process. Nine of 11 patients with aortic valvular vegetations had perforated or destroyed cusps, and eight of them also had ring abscesses. In patient 6, the abscess burrowed through to the pericardial space, causing fatal cardiac tamponade. In another patient, a left ventricular-right atrial fistula was produced by an aortic ring abscess burrowing through the ventricular septum. Extension of an aortic valve ring abscess into the cephalad portion of the muscular ventricular septum in another patient led to complete heart block. One of seven

Locaton of Valve Vegetations				Val-vular Regur-gitation	Perfo-ration AV Cusp	Valve Ring Ab-scess
V	MV	PV	TV			
+	+	0	0	+	+	+
+	0	0	0	+	+	0
+	0	0	0	+	+	+
0	+	0	0	0	0	0
+	+	0	0	+	+	0
+	0	0	0	+	+	+
+	0	0	0	+	+	+
+	+	0	0	+	+	+
+	+	0	0	+	+	+
+	0	0	+	0	0	0
[illegible]	+	+	0	0	0	0
+	0	0	+	+	+	+
+	+	0	+	+	+	+
0	0	0	+	+	0	0

patients with mitral vegetations and one of four with tricuspid valve vegetations had ruptured chordae tendineae. Certain anatomic cardiac findings in several patients are illustrated in Fig 2 to 5. None of the 14 patients had hepatic cirrhosis.

Comment

This study calls attention to the association of chronic alcoholism and fatal active infective endocarditis. In addition, it points out the association of pneumonitis and meningitis with the endocarditis, which usually is due to *D pneumoniae*. Although observed in 1% to 14% of reported patients with infective endocarditis,[1-4] alcoholism has not been emphasized as a common underlying disorder. The 14 patients included herein represent 24% of 59 patients with fatal active infective endocarditis who were studied by us.[5,6]

Little information is available on the type of organism causing infective endocarditis in habitual alcoholics. Of ten alcoholic patients studied by Pearce and Guze,[4] infective endocarditis was caused by *D pneumoniae* in three, *Strep species* in two, *Staph aureus* in one, and a Gram-negative rod in four. Of our 14 patients, *D pneumoniae* was the causative organism in ten. Furthermore, among our 50 patients with fatal active infective endocarditis, the pneumococcus was never responsible for causing this disease in the nonalcoholics. Although none of the immunodeficiencies[7-10] of alcoholics are known to account for a specific susceptiblity to pneumococcal infections, the frequency with which *D pneumoniae* is the causative organism suggests that such a specific susceptibility to pneumococcal infections may exist.

Although observed more than 100 years ago,[11] the association of endocarditis, pneumonitis, and meningitis remains an underemphasized observation. In the presence of extracardiac infection, endocarditis may be overlooked. Despite extensive valve destruction, extracardiac infections, ie, pneumonia or meningitis, or both,

Fig 3.—Patient 6. *E coli* endocarditis in a 51-year-old woman hospitalized because of fever and persistent diarrhea. Left, Longitudinal section through left atrium (LA), left ventricle (LV), aorta, ventricular septum (VS), and right ventricle (RV). Ring abscesses are enclosed by dots. Center, Longitudinal section through aortic root, aortic valve, and LV. Ring abscess has extended through left ventricular wall (arrows). Right, section through aorta, AV, coronary artery (Cor Art), LA, and anterior mitral leaflet (A). Aorta and LA are separated by a large ring abscess (enclosed by dots).

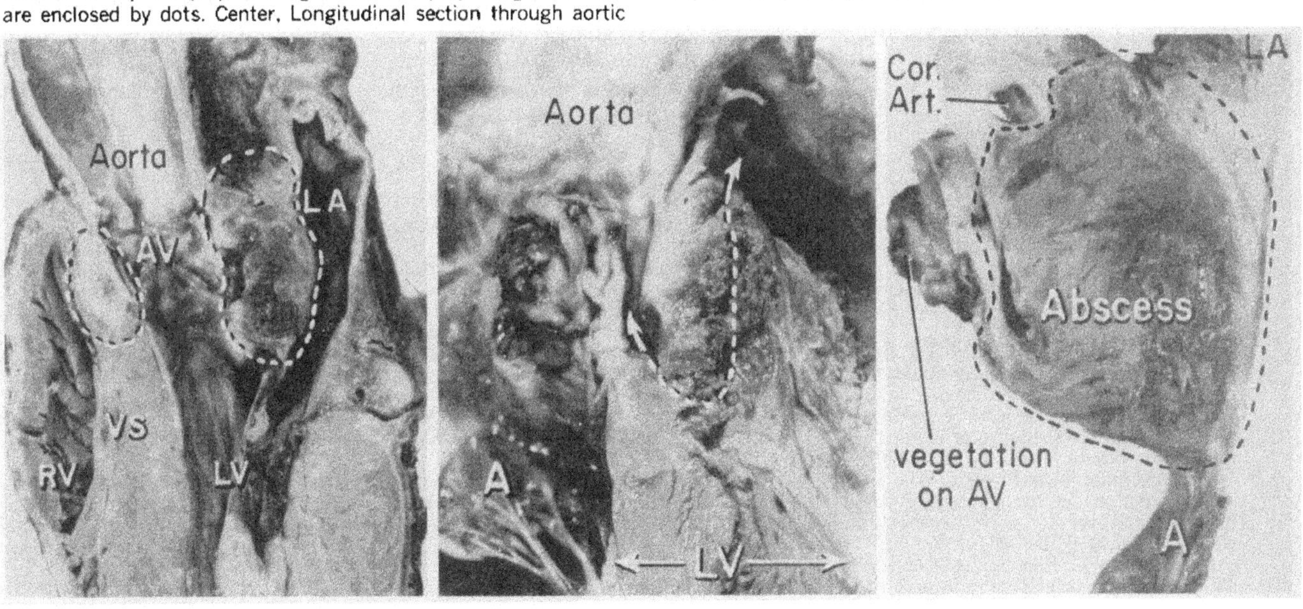

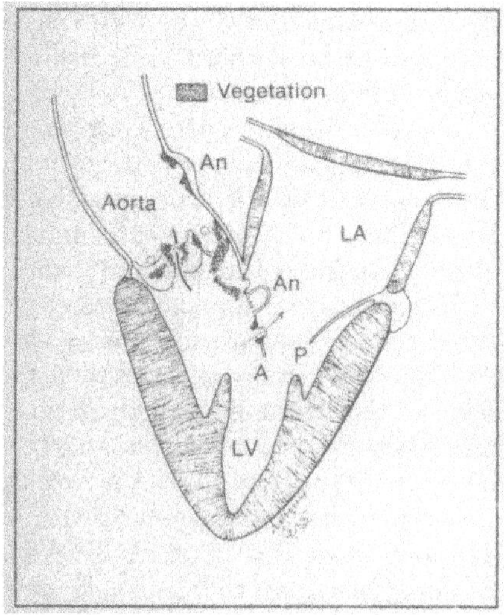

Fig 4.—Patient 1. Diagrammatic representation of pneumococcal endocarditis involving aortic and mitral valves of a 63-year-old man, who had a five-day illness characterized by disorientation and lethargy. Vegetative material also had extended to anterior mitral leaflet (A) and aorta causing an infective aneurysm (An) of each. LV indicates left ventricle; LA, left atrium; P, posterior mitral leaflet.

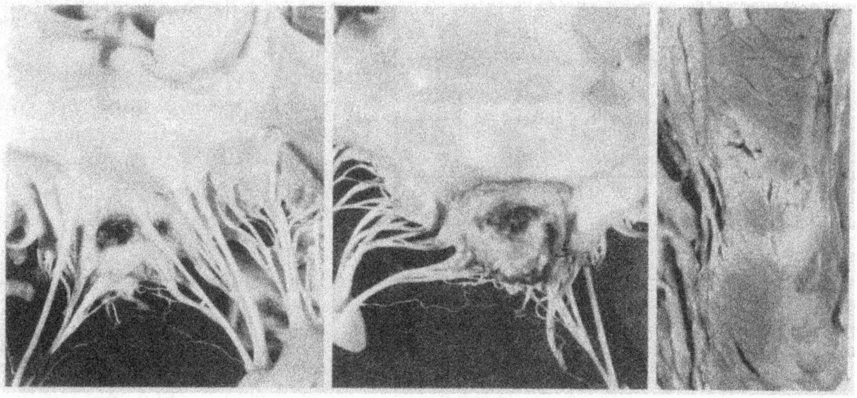

Fig 5.—Patient 4. Pneumococcal endocarditis of mitral valve of a 43-year-old man with acute pneumonitis and meningitis. Left, Ventricular aspect of anterior mitral leaflet, showing a small vegetation. Center, Atrial aspect of anterior mitral leaflet. Right, Longitudinal section through left-ventricular free wall showing transmural necrosis resulting from occlusion of an extramural coronary artery by a septic embolus.

were the major cause of death in 9 of 12 patients in whom they were present. Pneumonitis may be associated with infective endocarditis in patients without alcoholism. The heroin addict with infective endocarditis, for example, often has pneumonia, but in him the infective endocarditis is usually the primary infection, and the pneumonia is secondary to septic emboli from right-sided vegetations.[6] In contrast, in most patients with alcoholism and infective endocarditis, the pneumonitis appears to be the primary infection and infective endocarditis probably develops from bacteremia caused by the pneumonia. Among 51 patients with pneumococcal infective endocarditis who were analyzed from several series,[4,12-15] 32 had pneumonitis and 34 had meningitis. At least 16 of the 51 patients, and probably as many as 26, had both pneumonitis and meningitis. Meningitis was present in nine of our ten patients with pneumonitis and meningitis; it was present in nine of our ten patients with pneumococcal endocarditis, and in three with infective endocarditis caused by organisms other than *D pneumoniae*. Pneumonia was present in nine of our ten patients with pneumococcal endocarditis, and in three with infective endocarditis caused by organisms other than *D pneumoniae*. The pneumonia in one of the latter three patients was probably due to septic pulmonary emboli from tricuspid valve vegetations. The frequency of pneumonitis and meningitis in alcoholic patients with infective endocarditis appears to be more related to the frequency with which *D pneumoniae* is the causative organism rather than to the alcoholism itself.

References

1. Lerner PI, Weinstein L: Infective endocarditis in the antibiotic era. *N Engl J Med* 274:199-206, 1966.
2. Vogler WR, Dorney ER: Bacterial endocarditis in the normal heart. *Bull Emory Univ Clinic* 1:21-31, 1961.
3. Uwaydah MM, Weinberg AN: Bacterial endocarditis—a changing pattern. *N Engl J Med* 273:1231-1235, 1965.
4. Pearce ML, Guze LB: Some factors affecting prognosis in bacterial endocarditis. *Ann Intern Med* 55:270-282, 1961.
5. Buchbinder NA, Roberts WC: Left-sided valvular active infective endocarditis: A study of forty-five necropsy patients. *Am J Med* 53:20-35, 1972.
6. Roberts WC, Buchbinder NA: Right-sided valvular infective endocarditis: A clinico pathologic study of twelve necropsy patients. *Am J Med* 53:7-19, 1972.
7. McFarland W, Libre EP: Abnormal leukocyte response in alcoholism. *Ann Intern Med* 59:865-877, 1963.
8. DeMeo AN, Andersen BR: Defective chemotaxis associated with a serum inhibitor in cirrhotic patients. *N Engl J Med* 286:735-740, 1972.
9. Straus B, et al: Delayed hypersensitivity in alcoholic cirrhosis. *Am J Dig Dis* 16:509-516, 1971.
10. Wilson ID, et al: Selective immunoglobulin: A deficiency in two patients with alcoholic cirrhosis. *Gastroenterology* 54:253-259, 1968.
11. Hesch L: Pathologisch-anatomische Mittkeilungen aus dem Gratzer all gemeinen Krankenhause: IV. Zur Casuistik und Aetiologie der Endocarditis. *Oesterreichische Z Praktische Heilk* 8:238-242, 1862.
12. Sheldon WH, Golden A: Abscesses of the valve rings of the heart: A frequent but not well recognized complication of acute bacterial endocarditis. *Circulation* 4:1-12, 1951.
13. Preble HB: Pneumococcus endocarditis. *Am J Med Sci* 128:782-797, 1904.
14. Ruesegger JM: Pneumococcic endocarditis. *Arch Intern Med* 62:388-400, 1938.
15. Straus AL, Hamburger M: Pneumococcal endocarditis in the penicillin era. *Arch Intern Med* 118:190-198, 1966.

Valve Ring Abscess in Active Infective Endocarditis

Frequency, Location, and Clues to Clinical Diagnosis from the Study of 95 Necropsy Patients

ERNEST N. ARNETT, M.D., AND WILLIAM C. ROBERTS, M.D.

SUMMARY Analysis of 95 necropsy patients with active infective endocarditis (AIE) involving 128 native cardiac valves (aortic = 59, mitral = 48, tricuspid = 20, and pulmonic = 1) disclosed 27 patients with ring abscesses involving 30 valves: the aortic valve ring was infected in 24 patients and only an atrioventricular valve ring (mitral in two, and tricuspid in one) in three patients. Comparison of the following parameters showed no significant differences between the 27 patients with and the 68 patients without ring abscess: age, sex, antibiotic treatment or length of treatment, status of the cardiac valve(s) before infection, and the kind of infecting organism. Comparison of the following parameters, however, showed significant ($P < 0.05$) differences between the 27 patients with and the 68 patients without valve ring abscess: 1) infection of the aortic valve; 2) occurrence of valvular regurgitation of recent origin; 3) presence of pericarditis; 4) presence of high degree of atrioventricular block; and 5) short duration of symptoms leading to severe debility or death. These five features, therefore, serve as clinical clues to the presence of valve ring abscess in patients with AIE.

IN RECENT YEARS it has become well established that certain patients with active infective endocarditis (AIE) require cardiac valve replacement before completion of adequate antibiotic therapy.[1-6] The most frequent indication for early valve replacement is congestive heart failure from valvular destruction. A major determinant of outcome in patients undergoing cardiac valve replacement during AIE is the presence or absence of a valve ring abscess. If limited to the valve leaflets or chordae, the infective process usually can be totally excised and the valve prosthesis consequently can be inserted into a sterile field. If valve ring abscess is present, however, the infection may persist behind the site of attachment of the prosthesis, or significant paravalvular leak may follow valve replacement. Although several reports[7-12] have described the problems of cardiac valve replacement in patients with AIE, few have described the frequency of, or location of, valve ring abscess in patients with AIE. The present study analyzes the frequency and location of ring abscesses in a large group of necropsy patients with AIE, and determines whether certain clinical features in these patients might be clues to diagnosis of valve ring abscess during life.

Patients Studied, Methods, and Results

The hearts and clinical and necropsy records of all necropsy patients with AIE accessioned in the Section of Pathology, National Heart and Lung Institute, were reexamined. The anulus of each valve containing a vegetation was sectioned at approximately right angles to search specifically for the presence of a ring abscess. A total of 135 patients were analyzed: 95 had AIE involving natural (unoperated) cardiac valves (observations in 57 of them have been reported elsewhere);[13-14] 22 had infection at sites of attachment of prosthetic cardiac valves (prosthetic endocarditis) (unpublished observations); six had AIE associated with intracardiac or great vessel shunts; four had AIE after cardiac valve commissurotomy or anuloplasty operations; and eight had AIE involving only mural endocardium.[15] The present analysis concerns only the 95 patients with AIE involving native (unoperated) cardiac valves. Certain clinical and morphologic features in them are summarized in table 1.

Of the 95 patients with AIE analyzed, 11 had vegetations limited to the right-sided cardiac valves, ten had vegetations involving both right and left-sided cardiac valves, and 74 had vegetations limited to one or both left-sided cardiac valves. Among the 95 patients, 128 valves were infected: aortic in 59 patients; mitral in 48; tricuspid in 20; and pulmonic in one. Valve ring abscess occurred in 27 (28%) of the 95 patients: 24 patients had one valve ring infected, and three patients had abscesses involving two valve rings. Among the 27 patients with ring abscess, the aortic valve ring was infected in 24 (figs. 1-5): isolated in 21; combined with tricuspid valve ring abscess in two, and with mitral in one. The remaining three patients had ring abscess involving only the mitral (two patients) (fig. 6) or tricuspid valve (one patient).

The parameters analyzed in the 95 patients with AIE are shown in table 1. No significant differences were observed among patients with and without ring abscess regarding *age, sex, presence or absence of antibiotic therapy* or *length of therapy, status of the cardiac valve before it became the site of AIE,* i.e., whether or not it was previously functionally normal or abnormal, and *type of infecting bacterium.* Significant ($P < 0.05$) differences were observed, however, among patients with and without ring abscess regarding *duration of symptoms resulting from AIE, presence of valvular regurgitation resulting from valvular destruction by vegetations, evidence of pericarditis,* and *high degrees,* either second or third degree, *of atrioventricular block* (table 1).

Clinical evidence of AIE was present for less than six weeks in 19 (70%) of the 27 patients with and in 31 (46%) of the 68 patients without ring abscess associated with AIE ($P < 0.05$). Valvular regurgitation secondary to the AIE was present in 100% of the 27 patients with ring abscess, and in just over half (54%) of the 68 patients without ring abscess associated with AIE ($P < 0.05$).

Pericarditis was present at necropsy in 14 (52%) of the 27 patients with and in four (6%) of the 68 patients without ring abscess ($P < 0.05$). Of the 18 patients with pericarditis at necropsy, 14 (78%) had a ring abscess and four (22%) did not

From the Section of Pathology, National Heart and Lung Institute, National Institutes of Health, Bethesda, Maryland.

Dr. Arnett's present address is Department of Medicine, The Johns Hopkins Hospital, Baltimore, Maryland.

Address for reprints: William C. Roberts, M.D., Bldg. 10A, Room 3E30, National Institutes of Health, Bethesda, Maryland 20014.

Received January 19, 1976; revision accepted February 19, 1976.

Table 1. *Clinical and Morphologic Observations in 95 Nonoperated Necrospy Patients (Pts) with Active Infective Endocarditis (AIE): Relation to Ring Abscess*

Location of vegetations*	Aortic‡ (59 pts) Ring abscess		Mitral‡ (48 pts) Ring abscess		Tricuspid‡ (20 pts) Ring abscess		Totals§ (95 pts) Ring abscess	
	Present	Absent	Present	Absent	Present	Absent	Present	Absent
Number patients†	24(41)	35(59)	3(6)	45(94)	3(15)	17(85)	27(28)	68(72)
Age(yrs):Range[avg]	17–83[44]	20–77[51]	29–77[60]	15–70[44]	35–55[48]	20–66[45]	17–83[46]	20–70[45]
Sex — M:F	20(40): 4(44)	30(60): 5(56)	3(9):0	30(91): 14(100)	2(15): 1(14)	11(85): 6(86)	21(31): 6(21)	46(69): 22(79)
Duration (days) AIE*	2–150[39]	2–390[109]	14–28[21]	2–420[94]	4–21[13]	2–390[80]	2–150[37]	2–420[99]
< 6 weeks	16(59)	11(41)	3(12)	22(88)	3(30)	7(70)	19(38)	31(62)
> 6 weeks	8(25)	24(75)	0	22(100)	0	10(100)	8(18)	37(82)
Antibiotics								
None	3(38)	5(62)	0	3(100)	1(25)	3(75)	3(25)	9(75)
< 10 days	8(44)	10(56)	2(10)	19(90)	1(20)	4(80)	9(29)	22(71)
> 10 days	13(39)	20(61)	1(4)	22(96)	1(9)	10(91)	15(29)	37(71)
Valve leak (from AIE)*	24(57)	18(43)	3(11)	24(89)	3(43)	4(57)	27(42)	37(58)
Pericarditis*	14(82)	3(18)	1(17)	5(83)	1(33)	2(67)	14(78)	4(22)
Previously normal valve	16(44)	20(56)	2(5)	35(95)	3(15)	17(85)	17(27)	46(73)
Heart block (2° or 3°)*	4(80)	1(20)	1(100)	0	0	0	5(83)	1(17)
Infecting organism								
Staphylococcus	5(36)	9(64)	2(14)	12(86)	1(10)	9(90)	8(24)	26(76)
Pneumonococcus	7(70)	3(30)	0	6(100)	2(40)	3(60)	7(54)	6(46)
Non-alpha streptococci	6(60)	4(40)	0	10(100)	0	0	6(46)	7(54)
Alpha streptococcus	2(20)	8(80)	1(17)	5(83)	0	1(100)	3(30)	7(70)
Other bacterium	2(40)	3(60)	0	2(100)	0	0	1(17)	5(83)
Fungus	1(33)	2(67)	0	3(100)	0	2(100)	1(17)	5(83)
Negative blood cultures	0	4(100)	0	5(100)	0	2(100)	0	7(100)
Absent blood cultures	1	2	0	2(100)	0	0	1(17)	5(83)

All numbers in parentheses represent percentages. All numbers in brackets represent averages.

*$P < 0.05$ comparing values for patients with to values for patients without ring abscess.

†Among the 95 patients, 128 cardiac valves contained vegetations: 67 patients had AIE involving only one valve, and 28 patients had AIE involving more than one valve.

‡The figures in these vertical columns refer to numbers of patients with vegetations on that particular valve. Thus, patients with vegetations on more than one valve are listed in more than one column.

§These vertical columns apply only to the total number of patients, i.e., 95, and not to the number of valves containing vegetations, i.e., 128. Therefore, the numbers in these 2 columns are not sums of the columns to their left.

($P < 0.05$). A pericardial friction rub had been heard during life in eight of the 18 patients with pericarditis at necropsy. The pericarditis in the 18 patients resulted from extension of a valve ring abscess through the cardiac wall into epicardium in 13 patients; from transmural acute myocardial infarction in two patients; from extension of a myocardial abscess into epicardium in one patient; and from uncertain cause(s) in the remaining two patients.

High degrees of atrioventricular block (complete heart block in five and Mobitz type II block in one patient) occurred in five (19%) of the 27 patients with and in one (1%) of the 68 patients without ring abscess associated with AIE ($P < 0.05$). Of the six patients with high degrees of heart block, five (83%) had a ring abscess and one did not ($P < 0.05$). The block in the latter patient resulted from severe narrowing of the lumens of the major extramural

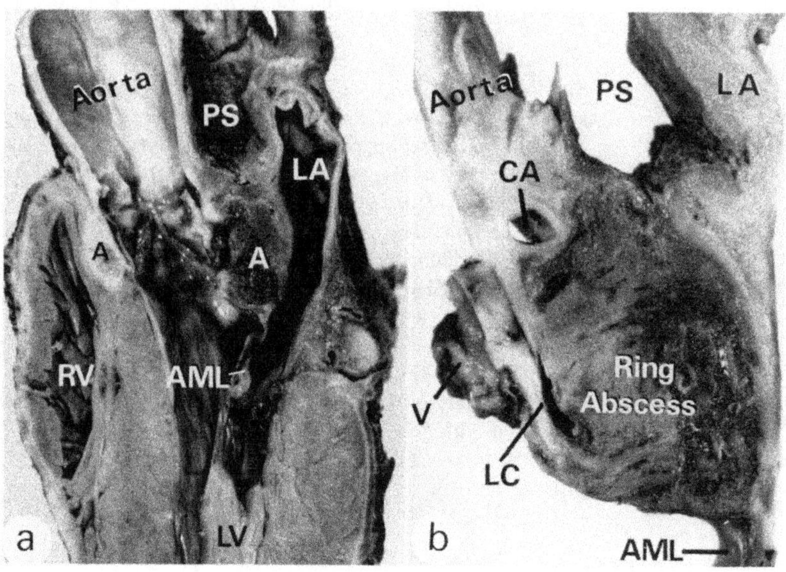

Figure 1. *Hemorrhagic pericarditis from rupture of an aortic valve ring abscess in a 51-year-old woman (72A-22) with* Escherichia coli *endocarditis. She presented with acute pericardial tamponade and infective endocarditis was never suspected clinically.* a) *Longitudinal section showing the ring abscess (A) in the angle between the aortic valve, left atrial (LA) wall and anterior mitral leaflet (AML). RV = right ventricle; LV = left ventricle: PS = pericardial space.* b) *Close-up of the ring abscess behind the left coronary (LC) cusp. CA = coronary artery; V = vegetation.*

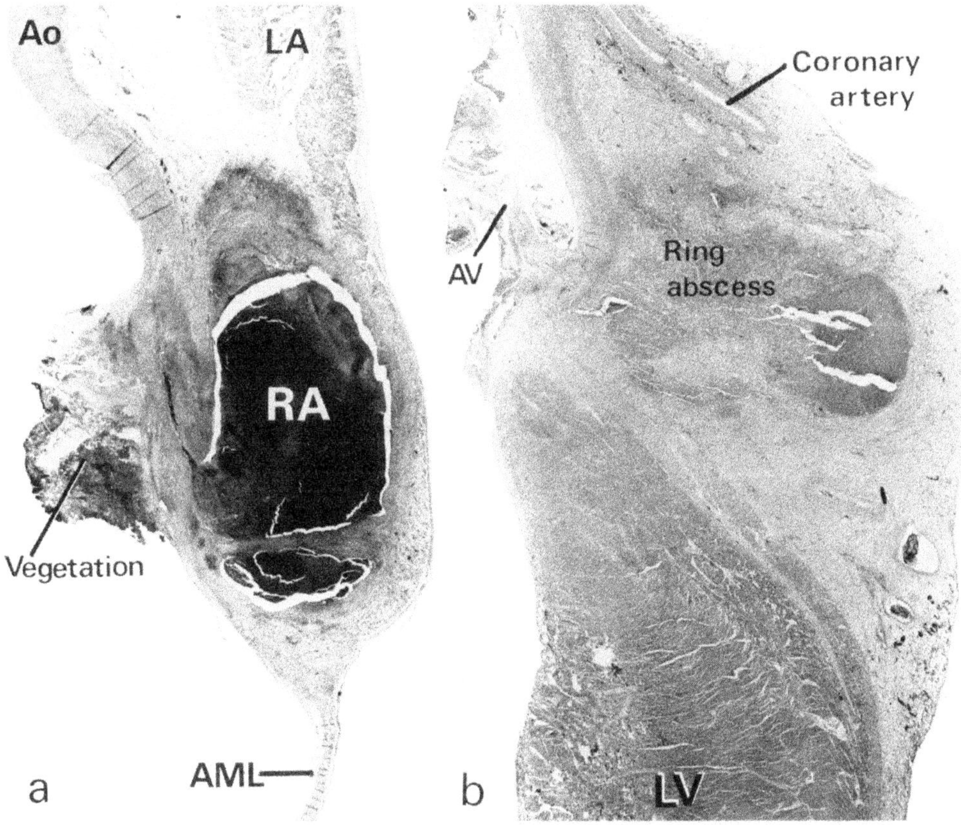

FIGURE 2. *Aortic valve ring abscess in two patients.* a) *This 29-year-old male heroin addict (A67-108) had had symptoms of congestive cardiac failure for only two weeks before death. He arrived at the hospital one day before death and his blood pressure was 135/0 mm Hg and a loud decrescendo aortic diastolic murmur was present. The causative organism was not identified in life, but large colonies of Gram-positive organisms were present in histologic sections of the aortic valve. Histologic section through aorta (Ao), infected aortic valve, anterior mitral leaflet (AML), and left atrial (LA) wall showing the ring abscess (RA). Hematoxylin and eosin stain × 3.* b) *Aortic valve infective endocarditis in a 25-year-old woman (A68-46). She presented with fever and palpitations and a "scratchy" precordial sound was heard. Thyrotoxicosis was suspected clinically; infective endocarditis was never suspected. This histologic section shows a ring abscess in the subepicardial adipose tissue of the left atrioventricular sulcus. AV = aortic valve cusp; LV = left ventricle. Hematoxylin and eosin stain × 4.*

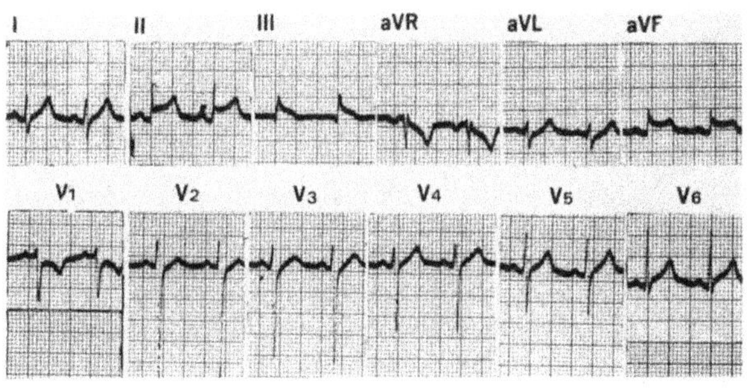

FIGURE 3. *Infective endocarditis in a 40-year-old man (A56-95) with previous mild aortic regurgitation from a congenitally bicuspid aortic valve. Chills, fever and symptoms of congestive cardiac failure began one week after a dental procedure. Examination disclosed dermal petechiae, subungual hemorrhages, Osler's nodes and a loud murmur of aortic regurgitation. Blood cultures were positive for* beta hemolytic streptococcus. *One week after hospitalization he complained of chest pain and* electrocardiogram showed ST-T changes of acute pericarditis. *Despite antibiotics, signs of left ventricular failure increased and he died 35 days after the onset of symptoms of infection.*

coronary arteries from atherosclerosis. The heart block in the other five patients resulted from destruction of the atrioventricular bundle by extension of the ring abscess into the most cephalad portion of the muscular ventricular septum. One patient had complete right bundle branch block from spread of an aortic valve ring abscess through the membranous ventricular septum and destruction of the right side of the most cephalad portion of the muscular ventricular septum (fig. 6). No patient had complete left bundle branch block.

No significant differences were observed among patients with and without ring abscess when comparing specific organisms. Ring abscess occurred in a third of the patients (21 of 61) with AIE due to a so-called virulent bacterium (staphylococcus, pneumococcus, non-alpha streptococcus) and also in a third of the patients (3 of 10) with AIE due to a so-called non-virulent bacterium *(alpha streptococcus)*. Among our 95 patients, however, AIE resulted from *alpha streptococcus* in only ten patients, and therefore, the AIE in nearly all of the remaining 85 patients probably resulted from infection by so-called virulent organisms.

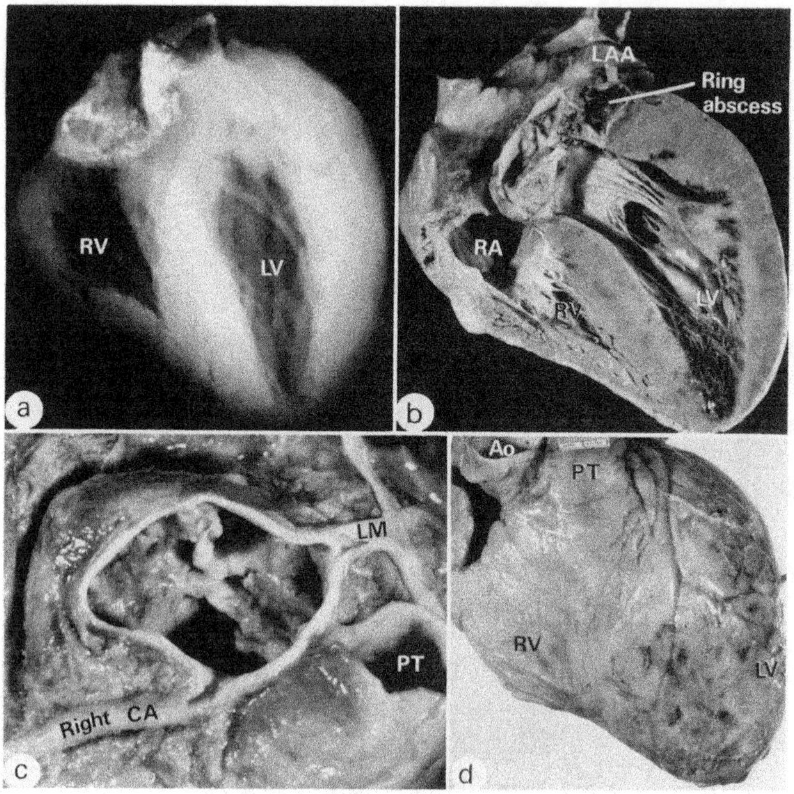

FIGURE 4. *The heart in a 54-year-old man (A75-55) with infective endocarditis involving a calcified, stenotic, congenitally bicuspid aortic valve. Fever and syncope occurred several weeks after tooth extraction and blood cultures yielded* alpha streptococcus. *Despite antibiotic therapy, signs of left ventricular failure increased, and he died 23 days after the onset of symptoms of infection.* a) *Postmortem roentgenogram of the heart showing a large amount of calcium in the aortic valve. RV = right ventricle; LV = left ventricle. b) Longitudinal section through the aortic valve showing a large ring abscess. The abscess has burrowed to the epicardial surface and is contained only by a thin layer of fibrous tissue. Multiple small vegetations are present on the mitral valve chordae, but no chordae are ruptured. The distal third of the anterolateral papillary muscle is necrotic. RA = right atrium; LAA = left atrial appendage.* c) *Aortic valve viewed from above. The orifice of the valve is markedly stenotic. The ring abscess lies beneath the left main (LM) coronary artery (CA). PT = pulmonary trunk.* d) *Exterior of the heart showing focal fibrinous pericarditis. The pericarditis resulted from extension of the ring abscess into the pericardial space. Ao = aorta.*

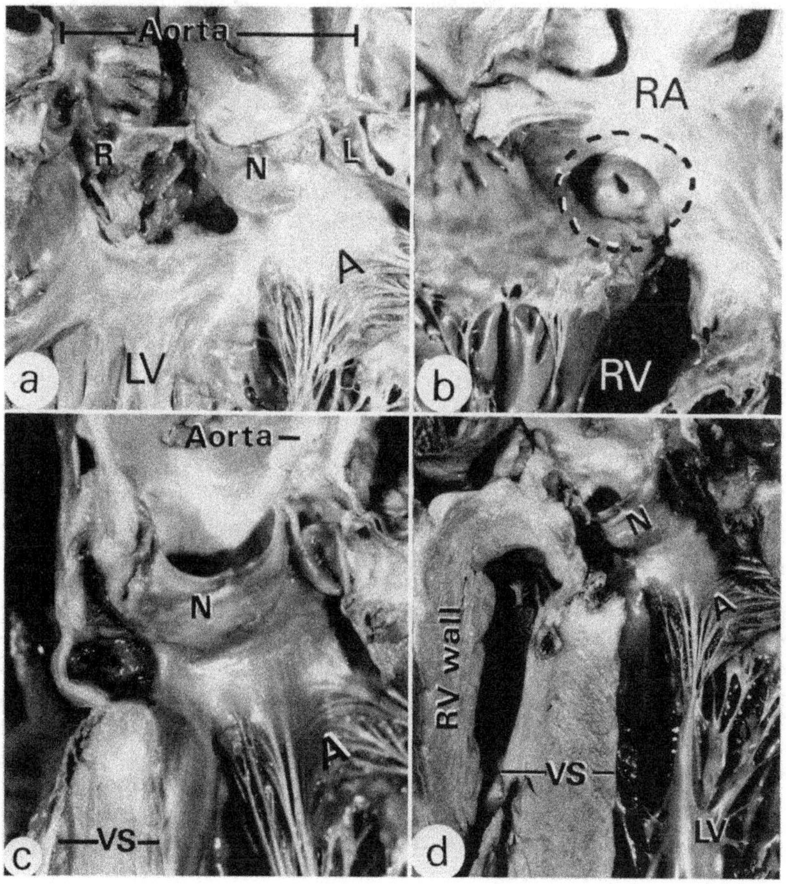

FIGURE 5. Staphylococcus epidermidis *aortic valve endocarditis in a 17-year-old boy (A69-4). Massive aortic regurgitation and right bundle branch block developed during the infection and he died 28 days after the onset of symptoms of infection.* a) *Opened aortic valve and left ventricle. The right (R) coronary cusp is destroyed by the infection and a ring abscess is present behind this cusp. N and L = non and left coronary cusps; A = anterior mitral leaflet; LV = left ventricle.* b) *Opened right atrium (RA), tricuspid valve and right ventricle (RV) showing a bulging membranous ventricular septum (dashed circle) with a perforation in its center.* c) *Longitudinal section through the aneurysm in the ventricular septum (VS).* d) *Longitudinal section anterior to* c *showing a ring abscess in the muscular portion of the ventricular septum.*

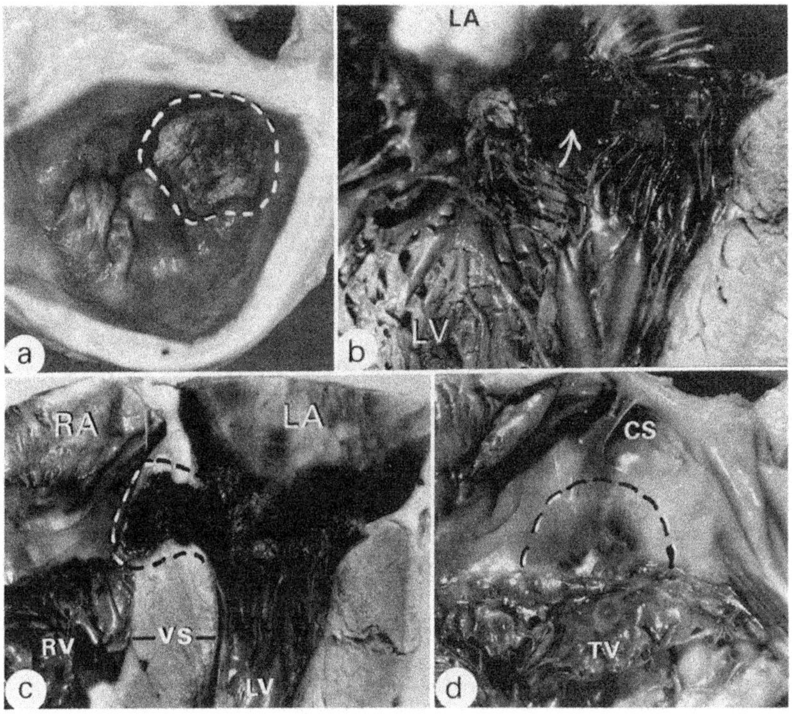

FIGURE 6. *Ring abscess in a 66-year-old diabetic man with mitral valve active infective endocarditis.* Staphylococcus aureus *septicemia appeared during hospitalization for treatment of an infected foot. Complete heart block developed and he died soon thereafter. At necropsy, vegetations were present on the mitral valve in the area of the posteromedial commissure. The infection had extended through the mitral anulus and burrowed deeply into the atrial and ventricular septa.* a) *Mitral valve viewed from the left atrium. Vegetations are indicated by the dashed line.* b) *Opened left atrium (LA), mitral valve, and left ventricle (LV). The location of the ring abscess is indicated by the arrow.* c) *Longitudinal cut of the heart. The ring abscess (dashed line) has burrowed deeply into the atrial septum and the cephalad portion of the ventricular septum (VS).* d) *Opened right atrium, tricuspid valve (TV), and right ventricle. The abscess is visible in the right atrial wall between the base of the tricuspid valve (TV) and the ostium of the coronary sinus (CS).*

Comments

The present study of 95 necropsy patients with active infective endocarditis (AIE) resulted in the following firm observations: 1) that ring abscess is common at necropsy in patients in AIE, occurring in nearly one-third of them; 2) that ring abscess is common among necropsy patients with AIE involving the aortic valve but is quite uncommon in patients with AIE isolated to any of the other three cardiac valves; 3) that there are five clinical clues which suggest the presence of a valve ring abscess during life. These include a) AIE involving the aortic valve; b) presence of valvular regurgitation of recent origin; c) evidence of pericarditis; d) evidence of high degrees of atrioventricular block, and e) a short duration of symptoms caused by AIE resulting in severe debility.

Although it occurred in nearly a third of our 95 necropsy patients, ring abscess was common only among the patients with AIE involving the aortic valve. Of 59 patients with vegetations on the aortic valve, ring abscess occurred in 24 (41%), whereas among 36 patients with AIE without aortic valve vegetations, ring abscess occurred in only three (6%). Of the six patients with ring abscess involving either the mitral or tricuspid valves, three also had aortic valve ring abscess. One of the three patients with isolated mitral ring abscess had the infection superimposed on a heavily calcified mitral anulus.[16, 17] Thus, of the clues suggesting the presence of a ring abscess, infection of the aortic valve, rather than any of the other three valves, is nearly a prerequisite.

Valvular regurgitation is always present in patients with valve ring abscess. All of our 27 patients with ring abscess had signs of valvular regurgitation resulting from AIE, i.e., of recent onset, whereas signs of valvular regurgitation were present in only 54% of the 68 patients with AIE without ring abscess. Classical signs of aortic regurgitation, however, may be absent in patients with acute aortic regurgitation, and this observation should be borne in mind regarding any patient suspected of having AIE.[18-20]

The most common cause of pericarditis in patients with AIE is extension of the valvular ring abscess into epicardium. Thus, the occurrence of a pericardial friction rub or pericardial effusion during the course of AIE is highly suggestive of ring abscess. As early as 1856, Rokitansky[21] recognized that ring abscess may be associated with pericarditis and myocarditis, and that it may cause a cardiac aneurysm which may rupture into a cardiac chamber or pericardial space. Ponfick[22] in 1873 again noted the association of AIE with pericarditis, and Osler[23] in 1885 noted the tendency of valve ring abscess to burrow into adjacent structures. Of 43 consecutive necropsy patients with AIE studied by Beck,[24] eight (16%) had pericarditis and five of them had an aortic valve ring abscess with perforation into the pericardial space. McColl[25] reported a patient with pericarditis due to mycotic aneurysm resulting from AIE, and concluded from a review of previously reported cases that perforation of a ring abscess was the most frequent cause of pericarditis in patients with AIE. A similar observation was made by Buchbinder and Roberts.[13] Among 38 patients with aortic valve AIE reported by Utley and Mills,[26] 15 had ring abscess and five of them had pericarditis. Evidence of pericardial disease was evident at necropsy in 18 of our 95 necropsy patients with AIE and 14 of them had a ring abscess. In 13 of the 14 patients the pericarditis was the result of extension of the inflammatory process from the ring abscess into epicardium. Although only half of our patients with evidence of pericardial disease at necropsy were noted to have a pericardial friction rub during life, this sign clearly was not sought in most of the other patients.

Either complete heart block or a high degree of second degree heart block appearing suddenly in a patient with AIE is highly suggestive of the presence of a ring abscess, which has extended into the area of the atrioventricular node or bundle.[27-31] Of our six patients with either complete heart block (five patients) or Mobitz type II atrioventricular block, five had a valve ring abscess. In addition, the appearance of complete right or left bundle branch block during AIE is also highly suggestive of the presence of a ring abscess with extension into the most cephalad portion of the muscular ventricular septum. Although only one of our patients developed complete right bundle branch block and none developed complete left bundle branch block, the latter has been reported in AIE by Roberts and Somerville.[27]

In this study, the duration of symptoms attributable to AIE was significantly shorter among patients with ring abscess than among patients without ring abscess. Symptoms of AIE were present for less than six weeks in 70% of the 27 patients with and in 46% of the 68 patients without ring abscess. Utley and Mills[26] also found a significantly shorter duration of symptoms leading to death or severe debility among patients with ring abscess, than among patients without ring abscess. The explanation for this shorter symptomatic period is uncertain. The difference could not be attributed to the type of infecting bacterium, or to the presence of a previously normal or abnormal valve. Furthermore, this shorter duration of symptomatic illness could not be attributed to the presence or absence of, or length of, antibiotic administration: 43 patients received either no antibiotics or antibiotics for less than ten days, and 12 (28%) of them had ring abscess; 52 patients received antibiotics for longer than ten days and 15 (29%) of them had a ring abscess.

A study of ring abscess during AIE by Sheldon and Golden in 1951[32] emphasized that this complication resulted when the infecting process was due to a highly virulent organism, like pneumococcus and staphylococcus. The infecting organism in each of their 12 patients with ring abscess was caused by one or the other of these two organisms, whereas among their 11 patients with *alpha streptococcus* endocarditis, none had a ring abscess. Likewise, among 38 patients with aortic valve endocarditis reported by Utley and Mills,[26] anular involvement was less common when the infection was due to *alpha streptococcus* than when it was due to *Staphylococcus aureus* or non-*alpha streptococci.* Among our 95 necropsy patients with AIE, the infecting organism, when known, also was usually a highly virulent one. When, however, the patients were grouped according to the presence or absence of ring abscess, no significant differences between types of causative organisms were observed.

References

1. Wallace AG, Young WG, Osterhout S: Treatment of acute bacterial endocarditis by valve excision and replacement. Circulation **31:** 450, 1965
2. Wilson LC, Wilcox BR, Sugg WL, Peters RM: Valvular regurgitation in acute infective endocarditis: early replacement. Arch Surg **101:** 756, 1970
3. Okies JE, Bradshaw MW, Williams TW Jr: Valve replacement in bacterial endocarditis. Chest **63:** 898, 1973
4. Griffin FM Jr, Jones G, Cobbs CC: Aortic insufficiency in bacterial endocarditis. Ann Intern Med **76:** 23, 1972
5. Manhas DR, Mohri H, Hessel EA 2d, Merendino KA: Experience with surgical management of primary infective endocarditis: a collected review of 139 patients. Am Heart J **84:** 738, 1972
6. Black S, O'Rourke RA, Karliner JS: Role of surgery in the treatment of primary infective endocarditis. Am J Med **56:** 357, 1974
7. Stason WB, DeSanctis RW, Weinberg AN, Austen WG: Cardiac surgery in bacterial endocarditis. Circulation **38:** 514, 1968
8. Manhas DR, Hessel EA, Winterscheid LC, Dillard DH, Merendino KA: Open heart surgery in infective endocarditis. Circulation **41:** 841, 1970
9. Hatcher CR Jr, Symbas PN, Logan WD Jr, Mansour KA, Abbott OA: Surgical management of complications of bacterial endocarditis. Ann Surg **173:** 1045, 1971
10. Buckley MJ, Mundth ED, Daggett WM, Austen WG: Surgical management of the complications of sepsis involving the aortic valve, aortic root, and ascending aorta. Ann Thorac Surg **12:** 391, 1971
11. Crosby IK, Carrell R, Reed WA: Operative management of valvular complications of bacterial endocarditis. J Thorac Cardiovasc Surg **64:** 235, 1972
12. Danielson GK, Titus JL, DuShane JW: Successful treatment of aortic valve endocarditis and aortic root abscesses by insertion of prosthetic valve in ascending aorta and placement of bypass grafts to coronary arteries. J Thorac Cardiovasc Surg **67:** 443, 1974
13. Roberts WC, Buchbinder NA: Right-sided valvular infective endocarditis. A clinicopathologic study of twelve necropsy patients. Am J Med **53:** 7, 1972
14. Buchbinder NA, Roberts WC: Left-sided valvular active infective endocarditis. A study of forty-five necropsy patients. Am J Med **53:** 20, 1972
15. Buchbinder NA, Roberts WC: Active infective endocarditis confined to mural endocardium. Arch Pathol **93:** 435, 1972
16. Burnside JW, DeSanctis RW: Bacterial endocarditis on calcification of the mitral annulus fibrosus. Ann Intern Med **76:** 615, 1972
17. Case records of the Massachusetts General Hospital. Weekly clinicopathological exercises. Case 5-1975. N Engl J Med **292:** 255, 1975
18. Wigle ED, Labrosse CJ: Sudden, severe aortic insufficiency. Circulation **32:** 708, 1965
19. Wise JR Jr, Oakley CM, Goodwin JF: Acute aortic regurgitation in patients with infective endocarditis. The distinctive clinical features and the role of premature mitral valve closure. J Maine Med Assoc **63:** 273, 1972
20. Mann T, McLaurin L, Grossman W, Craige E: Assessing the hemodynamic severity of acute aortic regurgitation due to infective endocarditis. N Engl J Med **293:** 108, 1975
21. Rokitansky C: Lehrbuch der Pathologischen Anatomie. Wein, Wilhelm Braumüller, 1856, Vol II
22. Ponfick: Ueber embolische aneurysmen, nebst bemerkungen über das acute herzaneurysma (herzgeschwür). Virchow Arch Pathol Anat **58:** 528, 1873
23. Osler W: Malignant endocarditis. Lancet **1:** 415, 459, 505, 1885
24. Beck D: Pericarditis and subacute bacterial endocarditis. J Mt Sinai Hosp **8:** 364, 1941
25. McColl I: Pericarditis due to a mycotic aneurysm in subacute bacterial endocarditis. Report of a case affecting congenitally stenosed quadricuspid aortic valve. Guys Hosp Rep **107:** 34, 1958
26. Utley JR, Mills J: Annular erosion and pericarditis. Complications of endocarditis of the aortic root. J Thorac Cardiovasc Surg **64:** 76, 1972
27. Roberts NK, Somerville J: Pathological significance of electrocardiographic changes in aortic valve endocarditis. Br Heart J **31:** 395, 1969
28. Meshel JC, Wachtel HL, Graham J: Bacterial endocarditis presenting as heart block. Am J Med **48:** 254, 1970
29. Kleid JJ, Kim ES, Brand B, Eckles S, Gordon GM: Heart block complicating acute bacterial endocarditis. Chest **61:** 301, 1972
30. Wang K, Gobel F, Gleason DF, Edwards JE: Complete heart block complicating bacterial endocarditis. Circulation **46:** 939, 1972
31. Katz D, Cooper JA, Frieden J: Bacterial endocarditis presenting as complete heart block with paradoxical (left-to-right) pulmonary emboli. Am Heart J **85:** 108, 1973
32. Sheldon WH, Golden A: Abscesses of the valve rings of the heart, a frequent but not well recognized complication of acute bacterial endocarditis. Circulation **4:** 1, 1951

Prosthetic Valve Endocarditis

Clinicopathologic Analysis of 22 Necropsy Patients With Comparison of Observations in 74 Necropsy Patients With Active Infective Endocarditis Involving Natural Left-Sided Cardiac Valves

ERNEST N. ARNETT, MD
WILLIAM C. ROBERTS, MD, FACC

Bethesda, Maryland

Clinical and morphologic features are described in 22 necropsy patients with endocarditis involving rigid-framed prosthetic valves: aortic in 15 patients and mitral in 7. The interval from valve replacement to onset of symptoms of prosthetic valve endocarditis was less than 2 months in 8 patients and longer than 2 months in 14 patients. The most frequent infecting organism was the Staphylococcus (13 patients). In each of the 22 patients the infection was located behind the site of attachment of the prosthesis to the valve ring, and the infection spread to adjacent structures in 13 patients, 11 of whom had aortic prostheses. Prosthetic detachment causing severe regurgitation occurred in 12 of the 15 patients with an infected aortic valve prosthesis, and in 2 of the 7 with an infected mitral valve prosthesis. Prosthetic obstruction by vegetative material occurred in 5 of 7 patients with prosthetic mitral infection and in only 1 of 15 with prosthetic aortic infection. High degrees of conduction defects developed in seven patients with aortic prosthetic valve endocarditis: complete heart block in five, and complete left bundle branch block in two.

Comparison of observations in the 22 patients with prosthetic valve endocarditis with those in 74 patients with active infective endocarditis involving natural left-sided cardiac valves revealed significant (*P* <0.05) differences in the percent with ring abscess, hemodynamic consequences of the endocarditis (valve stenosis), frequency of Staphylococcus as the causative organism and percent with complete heart block or left bundle branch block. No significant differences were observed between the two groups when comparing age, sex, type of underlying valve disease or frequency of organ infarcts or splenomegaly.

From the Pathology Branch, National Heart and Lung Institute, National Institutes of Health, Bethesda, Md. Manuscript received January 16, 1976; revised manuscript received March 29, 1976, accepted March 31, 1976.
Address for reprints: William C. Roberts, MD, Bldg. 10A, Room 3E-30, National Institutes of Health, Bethesda, Md. 20014.

Among 450 consecutive patients with one or more rigid-framed prosthetic cardiac valves studied by us at necropsy,[1–7] 22 (5 percent) had infection involving a prosthetic valve. These 22 patients represent 17 percent of the 127 patients with active valvular infective endocarditis studied in this laboratory.[8–10] Although many reports are available on patients with fatal active infective endocarditis involving natural cardiac valves, surprisingly little information is available on the morphologic features of endocarditis involving prosthetic cardiac valves. This report consequently focuses on the clinicopathologic features in 22 patients with prosthetic valve endocarditis and compares them with the features we observed in 74 nonsurgical necropsy patients with active infective endocarditis involving natural left-sided cardiac valves.

Patients Studied

Clinical observations: Clinical and morphologic observations in the 22 patients with prosthetic valve

TABLE I

Prosthetic Valve Endocarditis: Type of Prosthesis Infected

	Aortic Valve	Mitral Valve	Totals
Caged ball	9*	6*	15*
Tilting disc	5†	0	5†
Poppet disc	1‡	1§	2
Totals	15	7	22

* Starr-Edwards; † Björk-Shiley; ‡ Hufnagel; § Kay-Shiley.

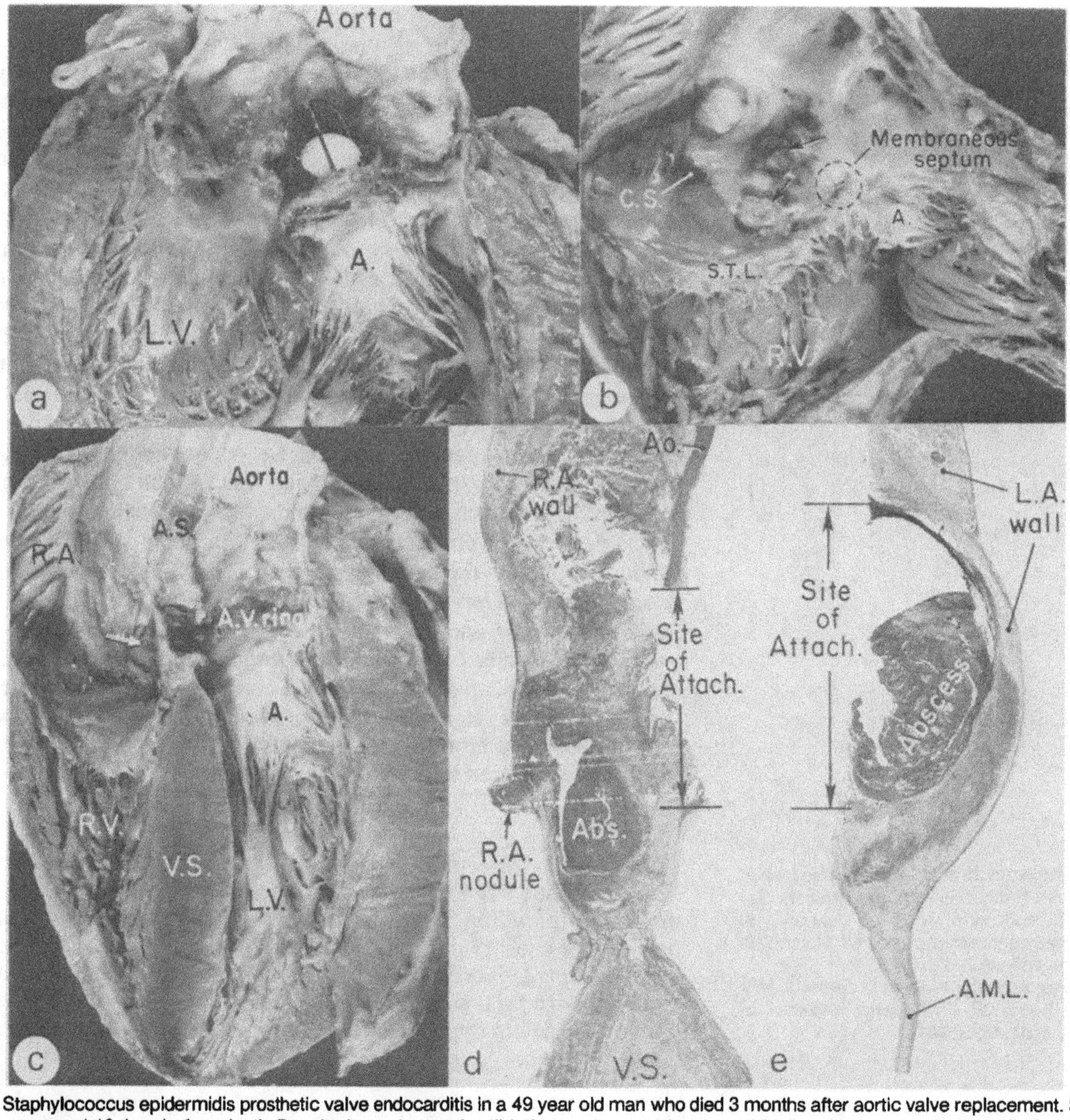

FIGURE 1. Staphylococcus epidermidis prosthetic valve endocarditis in a 49 year old man who died 3 months after aortic valve replacement. Symptoms of infection appeared 16 days before death. Despite large doses of antibiotic agents, complete heart block and severe aortic regurgitation developed. **a,** opened aorta, aortic valve and left ventricle (L.V.) showing a necrotic anulus to which the prosthesis is only partially attached. A. = anterior mitral leaflet. **b,** opened right atrium, tricuspid valve and right ventricle (R.V.) showing vegetative material **(arrows)** that had burrowed through the atrial septum from the necrotic aortic valve ring. C.S. = ostium of coronary sinus; S.T.L. = septal tricuspid leaflet; A. = anterior tricuspid leaflet. **c,** longitudinal section of the heart with the anterior portion removed. The necrotic aortic valve (A.V.) ring is again seen and the penetration of the infective process through the atrial septum (A.S.) is apparent. An **arrow** indicates the vegetation in the right atrium (R.A.). V.S. = ventricular septum. **d** and **e,** histologic sections through the ring abscess. The site of attachment (Attach.) of the prosthesis, which has been removed, is indicated. The infected nodule, an extension of the ring abscess (Abs.), is showing in the right atrium. Ao. = aortic wall; L.A. = left atrium; A.M.L. = anterior mitral leaflet.

TABLE II

Prosthetic Endocarditis: Clinical Observations in 22 Cases

Prosthesis Infected	Patients: no.	Patients: Age Range and Average (yr)	Sex: M	Sex: F	Preop Lesion: Stenosis	Preop Lesion: Pure Regurgitation	Interval From Valve Replacement to Infection: <2 mo	Interval From Valve Replacement to Infection: >2 mo	Duration of Signs and Symptoms of Infection: <60 Days	Duration of Signs and Symptoms of Infection: >60 Days	Patients Receiving Antibiotics >7 Days (no.)	Conduction Disturbance: LBBB	Conduction Disturbance: CHB	Prosthetic Dysfunction: Regurgitation	Prosthetic Dysfunction: Stenosis
Aortic	15	37–69 (54)	13	2	12	3	5	10	10	5	9	2	5	11	1
Mitral	7	37–65 (52)	3	4	7	0	3	4	6	1	2	0	0	0	0
Totals	22	37–69 (53)	16	6	19	3	8	14	16	6	13	2	5	11	1

CHB = complete heart block; LBBB = left bundle branch block; Preop = preoperative.

endocarditis are summarized in Tables I to V, and some of the morphologic features are illustrated in Figures 1 to 11. Certain observations in several of these patients have appeared elsewhere.[1–3,11–13] Patients with active infective endocarditis at the time of valve replacement were excluded. The 22 patients had 27 prosthetic cardiac valves; 17 patients had one prosthetic valve and 5 had two prosthetic valves. Of the 27 prosthetic valves, 22 were infected (Table I): the aortic prosthesis in 15 patients and the mitral in 7. Clinical evidence of infective endocarditis was present less than 2 months after operation in 8 patients (early deaths) (Table II), and from 3 months to 10 years after valve replacement in 14 patients. In 6 of the latter 14 patients clinical evidence of infection did not appear until more than 1 year after valve replacement. The duration of signs and symptoms of infective endocarditis ranged from 14 days to 13 months. In 16 patients, the duration of illness was less than 60 days and, in 6 patients, more than 60 days. Factors predisposing to development of endocarditis were apparent in only 5 of the 14 patients who died late: tooth extraction (2 patients), skin graft infection (1 patient), prolonged use of an intravenous catheter (1 patient) and prolonged use of a transthoracic pacing wire (1 patient). It is presumed that the infection in the eight patients who died early either was incurred at operation or was secondary to a wound infection.

The infecting organisms (cultured from the blood during life in 20 patients) are listed in Table III. Staphylococcus was the responsible organism in 13 patients, and a different organism in each of the other 9. Fungi caused the endocarditis in two patients who had negative blood cultures during life. Evidence of prosthetic dysfunction was present clinically in 12 of the 15 patients with an infected aortic valve prosthesis

TABLE III

Prosthetic Valve Endocarditis: Infecting Organism

Organism	Onset From Valve Replacement: <2 mo	Onset From Valve Replacement: >2 mo	Totals
I. Gram-positive bacterium	6	11	17
Staphylococcus epidermidis	3	7	10
Staphylococcus aureus	2	1	3
Streptococcus pneumoniae	0	1	1
Group-D streptococcus	0	1	1
Diphtheroids	1	0	1
Listeria monocytogenes	0	1	1
II. Gram-negative bacterium	1	2	3
Proteus mirabilis	1	0	1
Klebsiella species	0	1	1
Serratia marcescens	0	1	1
III. Fungus	1	1	2
Candida species	0	1	1
Aspergillus fumigatus	1	0	1
Totals	8	14	22

TABLE IV

Prosthetic Valve Endocarditis: Necropsy Observations in 22 Cases

Prosthesis Infected	Patients (no.)	Ring Abscess	Ring Organisms	Prosthetic Valve Detachment (Regurgitation)	Prosthetic Valve Stenosis
Aortic	15	15	8	12	1
Mitral	7	7	5	2	5
Totals	22	22	13	14	6

TABLE V

Prosthetic Valve Endocarditis: Organ Weights and Infarcts in 22 Cases

Prosthesis Infected	Patients (no.)	Organ Weight (g) (range and average): Spleen	Organ Weight (g) (range and average): Liver	Gross Infarcts (no. of patients): Spleen	Gross Infarcts (no. of patients): Kidney	Gross Infarcts (no. of patients): Brain
Aortic	15	120–1000 (470)	1450–2950 (2140)	7	3	3
Mitral	7	170–920 (370)	1350–2000 (1755)	5	4	4
Totals	22	120–1000 (460)	1350–2950 (2050)	12	7	7

(regurgitation in 11 and stenosis plus regurgitation in 1), but in none of the 7 patients with an infected mitral valve prosthesis. High grade conduction disturbances occurred in 7 patients, all in the group of 15 with an infected aortic prosthesis: left bundle branch block in 2 and complete heart block in 5. Thirteen of the 22 patients received appropriate antibiotic therapy for more than 7 days. Three patients underwent valve replacement for prosthetic endocarditis. The principal causes of death in the 22 patients were congestive heart failure (19 patients), central nervous system embolus (2 patients) and generalized infection (1 patient).

Morphologic observations: Among the 22 patients, 17 had one valve prosthesis and 5 had two valve prostheses. In each of the five latter patients, only the "downstream" prosthesis was infected: the aortic prosthesis in the three patients with mitral and aortic prostheses, and the mitral prosthesis in the two patients with tricuspid and mitral prostheses. Twelve of the 15 infected aortic valve prostheses and 2 of the 7 infected mitral valve prostheses were partially or completely detached. In contrast, 5 of the 7 infected mitral prostheses and only 1 of the 15 infected aortic prostheses were obstructed by vegetative material.

Ring abscesses (Table IV) were present in each of the 22 infected prostheses; in one the abscess was visible only by histologic examination. The ring abscess involved the entire valve anulus in 14 patients and only portions of the anulus in the other 8. In 13 of the 22 patients the infective process spread to adjacent

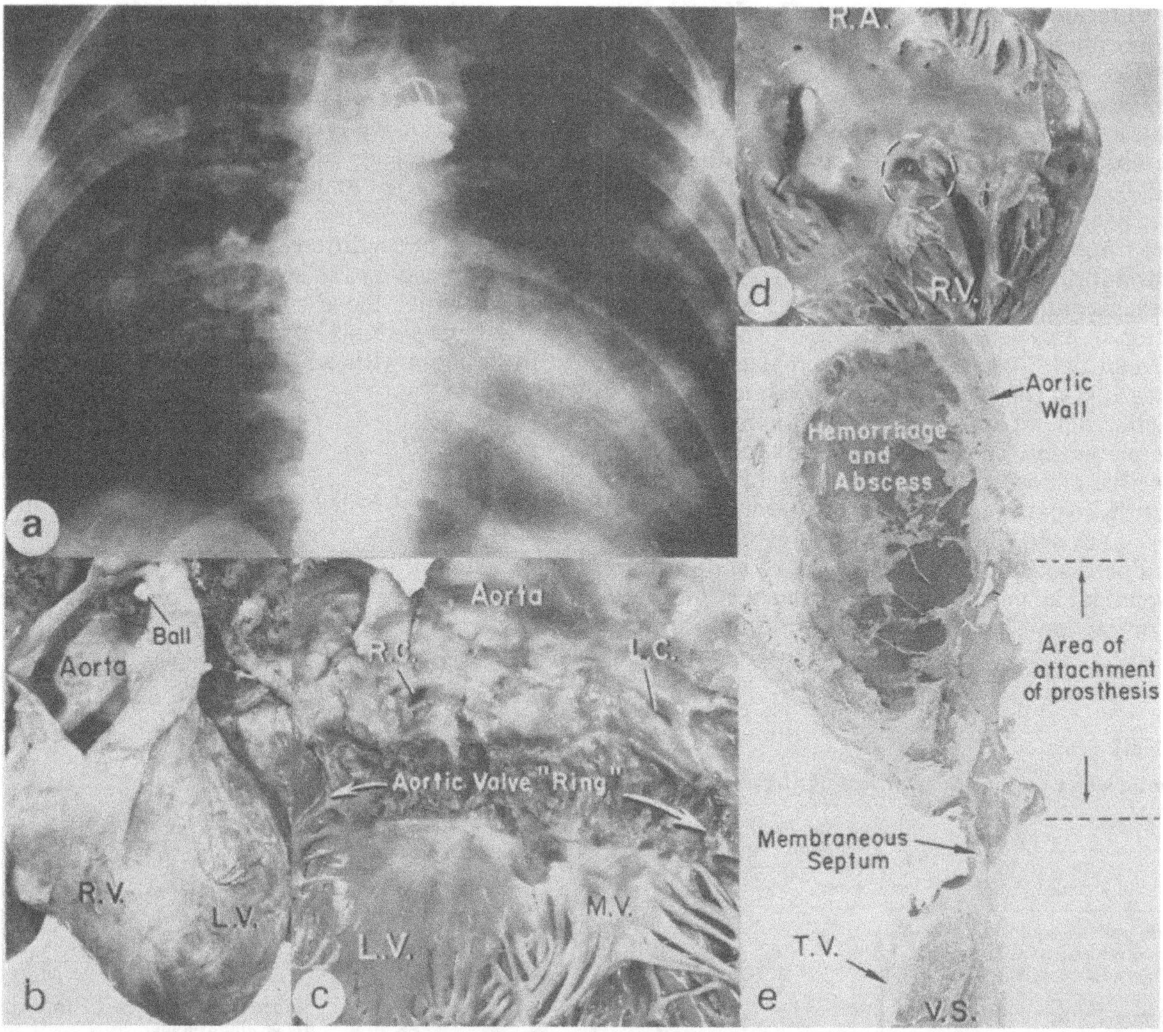

FIGURE 2. Staphylococcus epidermidis prosthetic aortic valve endocarditis in a 48 year old man. He had been well for 11 months after insertion of the Starr-Edwards prosthesis when, 1 month before death and 6 weeks after dental extraction, shaking chills appeared and blood cultures were positive for Staphylococcus epidermidis. Despite intensive antibiotic therapy, signs of aortic regurgitation appeared, and minutes before death he complained of "feeling funny." **a,** chest roentgenogram immediately after death revealed that the prosthesis had dislodged and migrated to the aortic arch. **b,** anterior view of the heart and opened ascending aorta. The detached prosthesis ball is visible, lodged in the transverse aorta. L.V. = left ventricle; R.V. = right ventricle. **c,** opened aorta, aortic valve "ring" and left ventricle showing a totally necrotic aortic anulus. L.C. = ostium of left coronary artery; M.V. = anterior mitral leaflet; R.C. = ostium of right coronary artery. **d,** opened right atrium (R.A.), tricuspid valve and right ventricle showing a ring abscess **(dashed circle)** that had extended from the prosthetic aortic valve anulus. **e,** photomicrograph through the aortic valve "ring" showing a large ring abscess and the necrotic aortic anulus material that extended through the membranous ventricular septum into the right atrium. T.V. = tricuspid valve leaflet; V.S. = ventricular septum. (Hematoxylin-eosin ×2, reduced by 24 percent.)

structures. In 11 of the 15 patients with an infected aortic aortic valve prosthesis the ring abscess burrowed into adjacent structures: through the ascending aorta into the periaortic space (7 patients); through the atrial septum into the right atrium (9 patients) or into the left atrium (2 patients); through the ventricular septum into the right ventricle (8 patients); and into the anterobasal left ventricular wall (2 patients). In two patients with an infected mitral valve prosthesis the ring abscess burrowed through the atrial wall into the pericardial space. Histologic examination of the infected rings disclosed colonies of organisms in 13 of the 22 patients.

Both arterial emboli and gross organ infarcts were common with both prosthetic aortic and prosthetic mitral valve endocarditis (Table V). Grossly visible infarcts were present in the spleen in 12, the kidney in 7 and the brain in 7 of the 22 patients. Two patients had a bowel infarct, one a pancreatic infarct and one a transmural myocardial infarct. In addition, mycotic aneurysms were present in the ascending aorta of three patients: in two patients, aneurysms resulted from jet lesions from the infected prosthesis and, in the third, the cage of the partially detached prosthesis burrowed into the wall of a weakened aorta (after an aortotomy performed weeks earlier) causing a sacular aneurysm.

The spleen ranged in weight from 120 to 1,000 g (average 460) and in 14 of the 22 patients it weighed more than 300 g. The liver ranged in weight from 1,350 to 2,950 g (average 2,050).

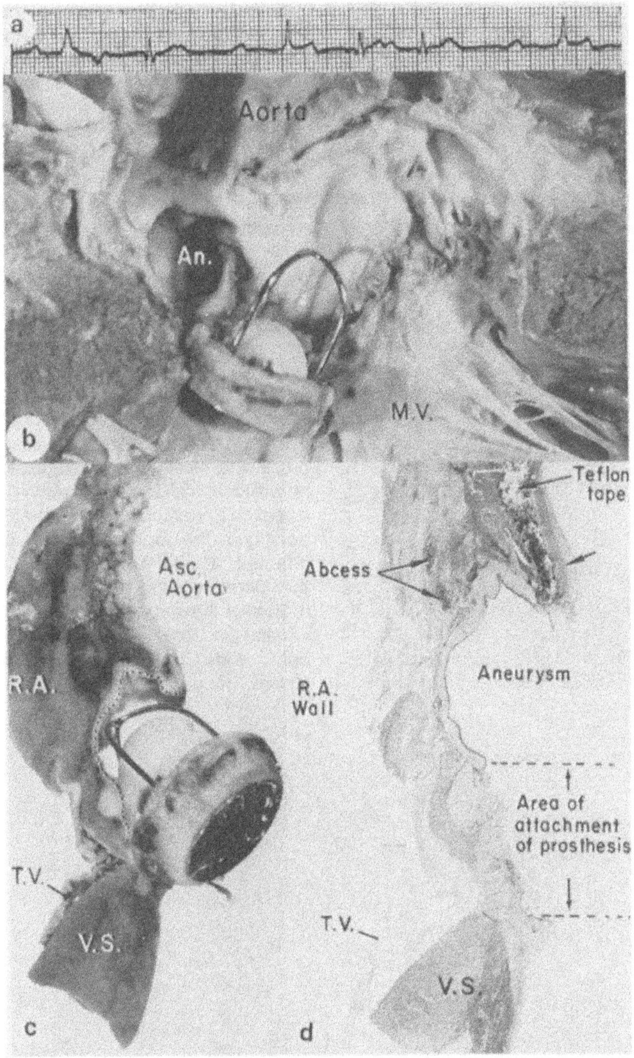

FIGURE 3. Staphylococcus epidermidis prosthetic aortic valve endocarditis in a 55 year old man. The Starr-Edwards prosthesis was used to replace an infected trileaflet Teflon® (Muller) valve 45 days before death. **a,** electrocardiogram revealing complete heart block and signs of massive aortic regurgitation that appeared despite antibiotic therapy. **b,** opened aorta, aortic valve and left ventricle. The aortic valve ring is necrotic, and the prosthesis is almost totally detached. The cage of the prosthesis has burrowed into the wall of the aorta causing a saccular aneurysm (An.). M.V. = mitral valve. **c,** longitudinal section showing the caged ball prosthesis burrowing into the ascending (Asc.) aorta, producing the aneurysm. R.A. = right atrium; T.V. = septal tricuspid valve leaflet; V.S. = ventricular septum. **d,** photomicrograph through the same area after removal of the prosthesis. (Hematoxylin-eosin X2, reduced by 25 percent.)

Comments

Clinical Features

Incidence: Study of our 22 necropsy patients and analysis of more than 150 necropsy cases of prosthetic valve endocarditis reported by others[14–47] allows certain general conclusions regarding this condition. It is a devastating complication of cardiac valve replacement,

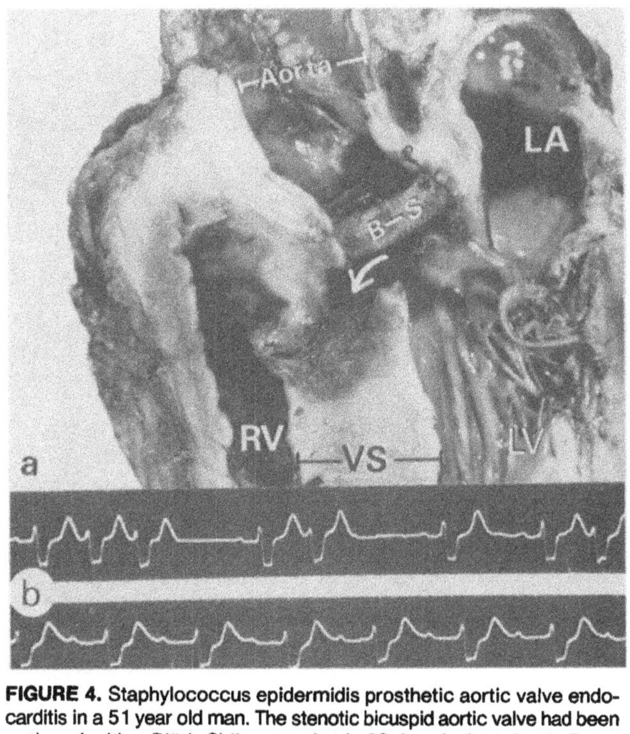

FIGURE 4. Staphylococcus epidermidis prosthetic aortic valve endocarditis in a 51 year old man. The stenotic bicuspid aortic valve had been replaced with a Björk-Shiley prosthesis 83 days before death. Fever was present in the early postoperative period, and shortly before death complete heart block and signs of congestive heart failure appeared. **a,** longitudinal section of the heart with the anterior portion removed. The Björk-Shiley (B-S) prosthesis is partially detached and the ring abscess **(arrow)** has burrowed through the ventricular septum (VS) into the right ventricle (RV). LA = left atrium; LV = left ventricle. **b,** rhythm strip obtained shortly before death revealing complete heart block.

but fortunately it is infrequent. The exact incidence rate is uncertain but it is clearly less than 1 percent annually among patients with prosthetic cardiac valves.[37,39,45,48] Although prospective studies[49,50] have been inconclusive, retrospective studies[16,17,51,52] have shown a reduction in the frequency of early (less than 2 months after valve replacement) endocarditis coincident with the use of prophylactic antibiotic therapy. Late prosthetic valve infection now appears to be more common than early infection,[37,45] presumably because there are now so many persons with prosthetic cardiac valves. Although the mortality rate is high for both groups,

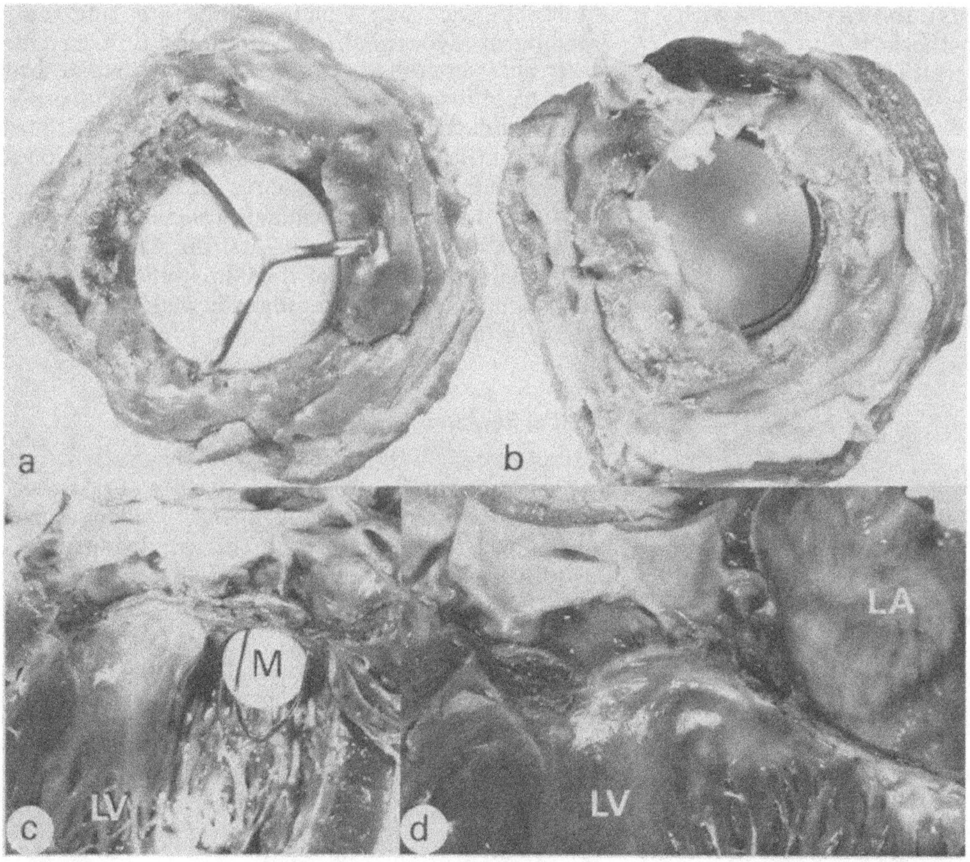

FIGURE 5. Serratia marcescens prosthetic aortic valve endocarditis in a 57 year old man whose infection occurred 4 months after replacement of both aortic and mitral valves. The apparent source of the infection was an intravenous catheter. Left bundle branch block and signs of aortic regurgitation appeared and, despite massive doses of antibiotic agents, he died 3 months after the onset of symptoms of infection. **a,** view of the aortic prosthesis from above. Infected thrombus is present on its anulus. **b,** view of the prosthesis as it appeared from the left ventricle. Some of the infected thrombus became detached during excision of this prosthesis at necropsy. The primary orifice is partially obstructed by the infected material. **c,** opened aortic root, aortic valve and left ventricle (LV) after removal of the aortic prosthesis. Most of the aortic ring is necrotic. In addition, the portion of mitral (M) prosthesis in direct apposition to the aortic anulus also is infected. **d,** view after excision of the mitral prosthesis showing extension of the aortic anular infection into the junctional area between the aortic and mitral anuli. LA = left atrium.

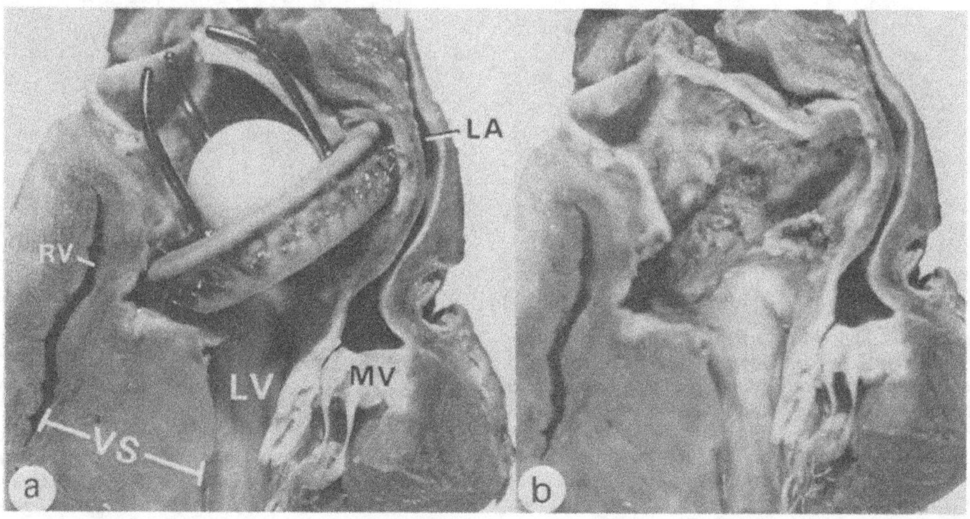

FIGURE 6. Staphylococcus epidermidis endocarditis originally involving a Björk-Shiley aortic valve prosthesis that was excised and replaced with a Magovern prosthesis 28 days before death in a 69 year old man. Fever and signs of aortic regurgitation appeared 7 months after aortic valve replacement with the Björk-Shiley prosthesis. After replacement with the Magovern prosthesis, a murmur of aortic regurgitation reappeared. At necropsy, the sewing ring of the Magovern prosthesis had burrowed deeply into the necrotic anulus, causing the ball of the prosthesis to strike the nonnecrotic portion of the aortic wall, probably producing prosthetic aortic stenosis. **a,** longitudinal section of the heart through the aortic anulus with the Magovern prosthesis in place; **b,** section after removal of the prosthesis. The frame of the prosthesis has burrowed deeply into the necrotic anulus. LA = left atrium; LV = left ventricle; MV = mitral valve; RV = right ventricular cavity; VS = ventricular septum.

early prosthetic valve infection apparently is more often fatal than late infection.[37,39,45,48]

Etiology: Most early infections either are incurred at operation or result from a wound infection.[25,29,37,39,48] Those at operation appear to result from contamination of the cardiopulmonary bypass equipment.[53,54] Staphylococcus is the organism cultured most frequently from cardiopulmonary bypass equipment and it is the most frequent cause of early prosthetic valve endocarditis.[14,16–18,25,30,37,39,44,45] When gram-negative bacteria or fungi cause endocarditis early, they are usually also recovered from the operating room equipment or from a wound infection.[28,39] Late infections usually result from transient bacteremias.[37,39,45,48] Although both staphylococci and streptococci are frequent causes of clinically diagnosed late prosthetic valve endocarditis,[37,39,45] the former have caused most cases of necropsy-proved late endocarditis and the latter relatively few. In none of our 22 necropsy patients was the infection caused by Streptococcus. Staphylococcus was the most common cause of endocarditis in our patients whether the infection occurred early or late.

Blood cultures: Among patients with prosthetic valve endocarditis, blood cultures are almost always positive, except when the infections are caused by certain fungi.[27,28,31,32,37,39,44,45,48] Blood cultures were positive during life in each of our 20 patients with endocarditis caused by bacteria and were negative in each of our 2 patients with fungal endocarditis. Blood cultures were positive in only 3 of 39 patients with endocarditis caused by Aspergillus species in a series reviewed by Kammer and Utz.[55]

Prosthetic valve dysfunction: Signs of prosthetic valve dysfunction are usually present when the aortic prosthesis is infected and usually absent when the mitral prosthesis is infected. Clinical signs of aortic regurgitation were present in 11 of our 15 patients with an infected aortic valve prosthesis. In three of the four

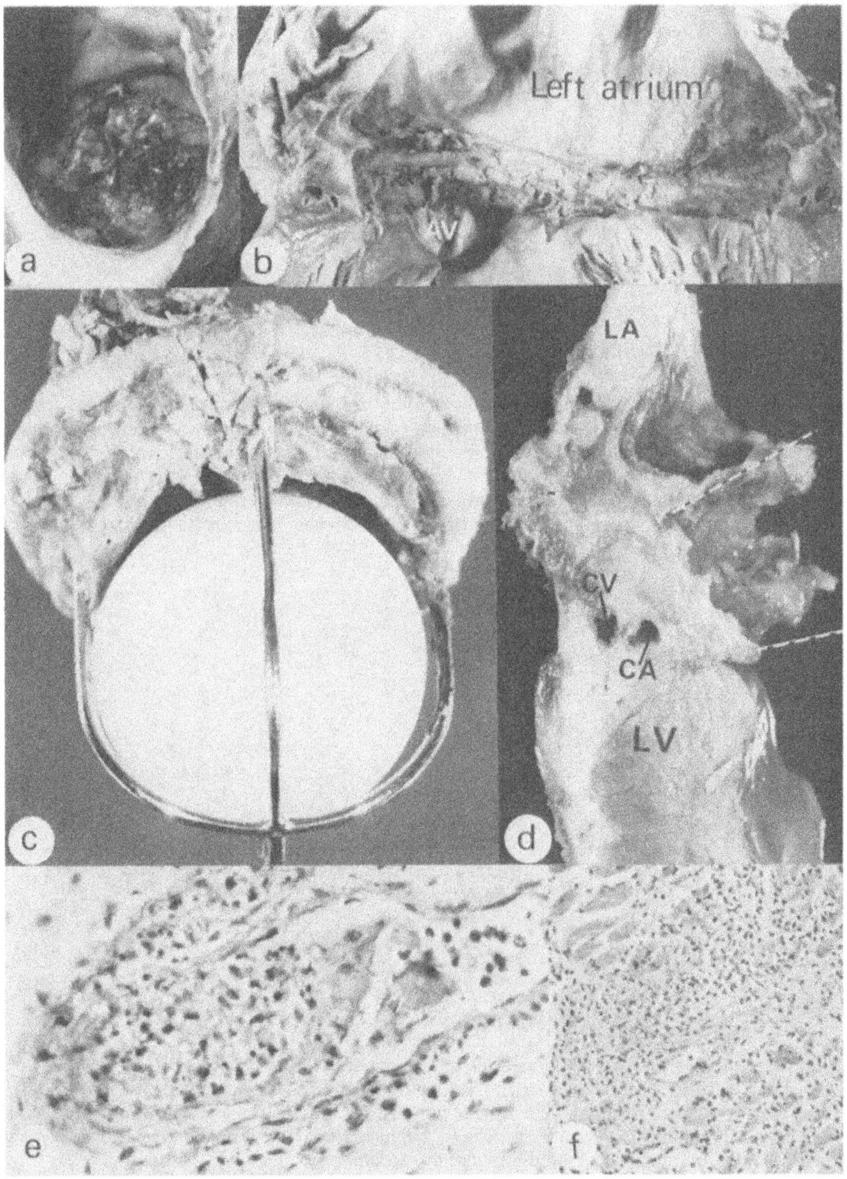

FIGURE 7. Staphylococcus aureus prosthetic mitral valve endocarditis in a 47 year old man who had the onset of symptoms of infective endocarditis 4 months after valve replacement. He had done well during the first 3 months after operation, but symptoms of infection developed after grafting of a cutaneous ulcer. Signs of prosthetic dysfunction were never detected clinically. **a,** prosthetic mitral valve orifice obstructed by vegetative material, as viewed from the left atrium. **b,** opened left atrium, mitral anulus and left ventricle after removal of the mitral prosthesis. The entire anulus is necrotic. AV = aortic valve. **c,** mitral valve prosthesis showing infected thrombus at its base. **d,** longitudinal section through the left atrium (LA), mitral anulus and left ventricle (LV). The former site of attachment of the prosthesis is designated by the **dashed lines.** The infective process burrowed through the wall of the heart and caused pericarditis. CA = coronary artery; CV = coronary vein in the right atrioventricular sulcus. **e** and **f,** hematoxylin-eosin-stained histologic sections of the left ventricle remote from the infected mitral anulus. **e,** infected embolus in an intramural coronary artery. **f,** microscopic-sized myocardial abscess. (×400 [**e**] and ×160 [**f**], reduced by 24 percent.)

patients without clinical signs of aortic regurgitation, the prosthesis was not detached at necropsy. Among patients with acute aortic regurgitation, however, classic signs of aortic regurgitation may be absent.[56–59] Signs of aortic regurgitation were not detected in three of nine necropsy patients with prosthetic aortic valve endocarditis described by Madison et al.,[44] but all three had prosthetic detachment at necropsy.

In contrast, patients with infection involving the mitral valve prosthesis usually have no clinical signs of prosthetic mitral valve dysfunction. Clinical signs of such dysfunction were not detected in any of our seven patients with prosthetic mitral valve endocarditis although the prosthesis was significantly obstructed by vegetative material in five of the seven and partially detached from the anulus in two.[12] McAllister et al.[43] reported on two patients with virtual total obstruction of the mitral prosthesis.

Morphologic Features

Valve ring abscess: The most consistent morphologic feature of prosthetic valve infection in our 22 patients was infection behind the site of attachment of the valve prosthesis, resulting in valve ring abscess. Ring abscess was present in each of our 22 patients, and in 14 the infection involved the entire circumference of the valve anulus. In several patients, however, only a portion of the circumference of the valve anulus was involved and, in one patient, histologic examination of the anulus disclosed infection that had not been apparent on gross examination. Extension of the ring infection to adjacent cardiac structures was common, especially when the aortic prosthesis was infected. This extension resulted in the frequent occurrence of both intracardiac fistulas and complete heart block or left bundle branch block. Among nine necropsy patients with prosthetic aortic valve endocarditis described by Madison et al.,[44] each had infection at the site of attachment of the prosthesis, and atrioventricular conduction defects developed in 7 (44 percent) of their entire group of 16 patients with prosthetic aortic valve endocarditis. Obviously, it is the occurrence of the infection behind the site of attachment of the prosthesis that makes reoperation so hazardous. Were the infection limited to the interior por-

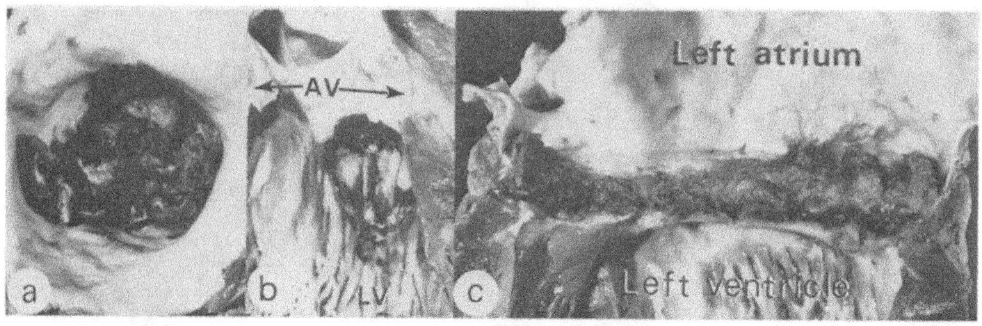

FIGURE 8. Staphylococcus epidermidis prosthetic mitral valve endocarditis in a 46 year old man who died 16 months after mitral valve replacement with a Starr-Edwards prosthesis. Eight months postoperatively, when he was asymptomatic, cardiac catheterization disclosed normal left atrial pressure and cardiac output. Signs of infection appeared 15 months after valve replacement. Despite antibiotic therapy, fatal congestive heart failure developed. **a,** mitral valve prosthesis as viewed from the left atrium. A large infected thrombus virtually occludes the mitral valve orifice. **b,** opened aorta, aortic valve (AV) and left ventricle (LV) showing infected thrombus on the cage of the mitral prosthesis. **c,** opened left atrium and ventricle showing a completely necrotic mitral valve anulus. The prosthesis has been removed.

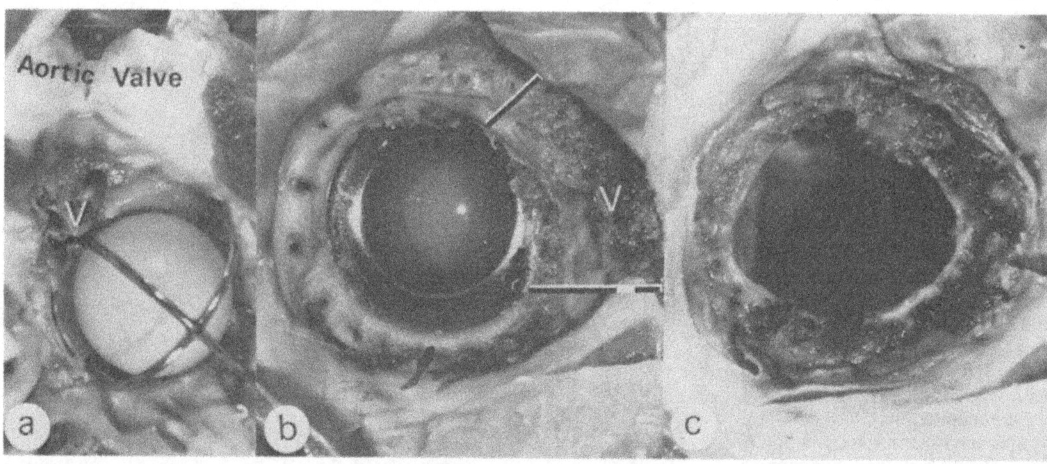

FIGURE 9. Staphylococcus epidermidis prosthetic mitral valve endocarditis in a 59 year old woman. The infection appeared 10 years after replacement of both mitral and tricuspid valves. At necropsy, only the mitral prosthesis was infected. **a,** infected mitral valve prosthesis viewed from the left ventricle. Vegetative material (V) is present on the prosthetic anulus just below the aortic valve. **b,** prosthesis as viewed from the left atrium showing vegetations (V) at the junction of the prosthetic and natural valve anuli. **c,** same view after removal of the prosthesis showing even greater extensiveness of the infection at the site of attachment of the prosthesis.

tion of the prosthesis, excision of the prosthesis should eliminate the infection. Unfortunately, as demonstrated in our patients and in those described by others,[20,35,38,43,44,47] the tissues behind the site of attachment of the prosthesis usually are involved by the infective process.

Treatment

Replacement of infected prosthesis: The occurrence of a grossly necrotic anulus at the time of reoperation for prosthetic valve endocarditis does not necessarily mean that valve replacement will be fruitless. Although it may be grossly necrotic, the anulus may be free of colonies of organisms and cultures of the necrotic anulus may be negative. In 9 of our 22 patients with prosthetic valve endocarditis and ring abscess, no stainable organisms were found in histologic sections from the prosthetic anulus.

One hazard of inserting a prosthesis in a necrotic anulus at the time of valve replacement for prosthetic valve endocarditis is burrowing of the sewing ring of the new prosthesis into the necrotic anulus with resulting impingement on movement of the poppet of the prosthesis by adjacent tissue. This sequence occurred in one of our patients and resulted in prosthetic aortic stenosis from inability of the ball to ascend in the cage (Fig. 6).

Tissue valve endocarditis: Although prosthetic valve endocarditis in patients with rigid-framed prostheses (the kind present in our 22 patients) usually indicates infection behind the site of attachment of the prosthesis, that is, the sewing ring, ring abscess may be less frequent with endocarditis involving tissue valves. Indeed, in animals and in man, the infective process may be limited to the cusps of the tissue valve, as when infective endocarditis involves natural valves.[60,61] Thus, the chance of cure, either by antibiotic therapy or valve replacement, or both, when infective endocarditis is superimposed on a homograft or heterograft (porcine valve, for example) is much better than when endocarditis involves a rigid-framed prosthesis.[61] This, then, is an advantage, although a small one, of the tissue valve (porcine) over the rigid-framed prosthesis.

Diagnosis: Establishment of the diagnosis of prosthetic valve endocarditis, particularly in the early postoperative period at times may be difficult, as pointed out by several investigators.[48,62,63] Diagnosis in the late postoperative period, in contrast, is usually

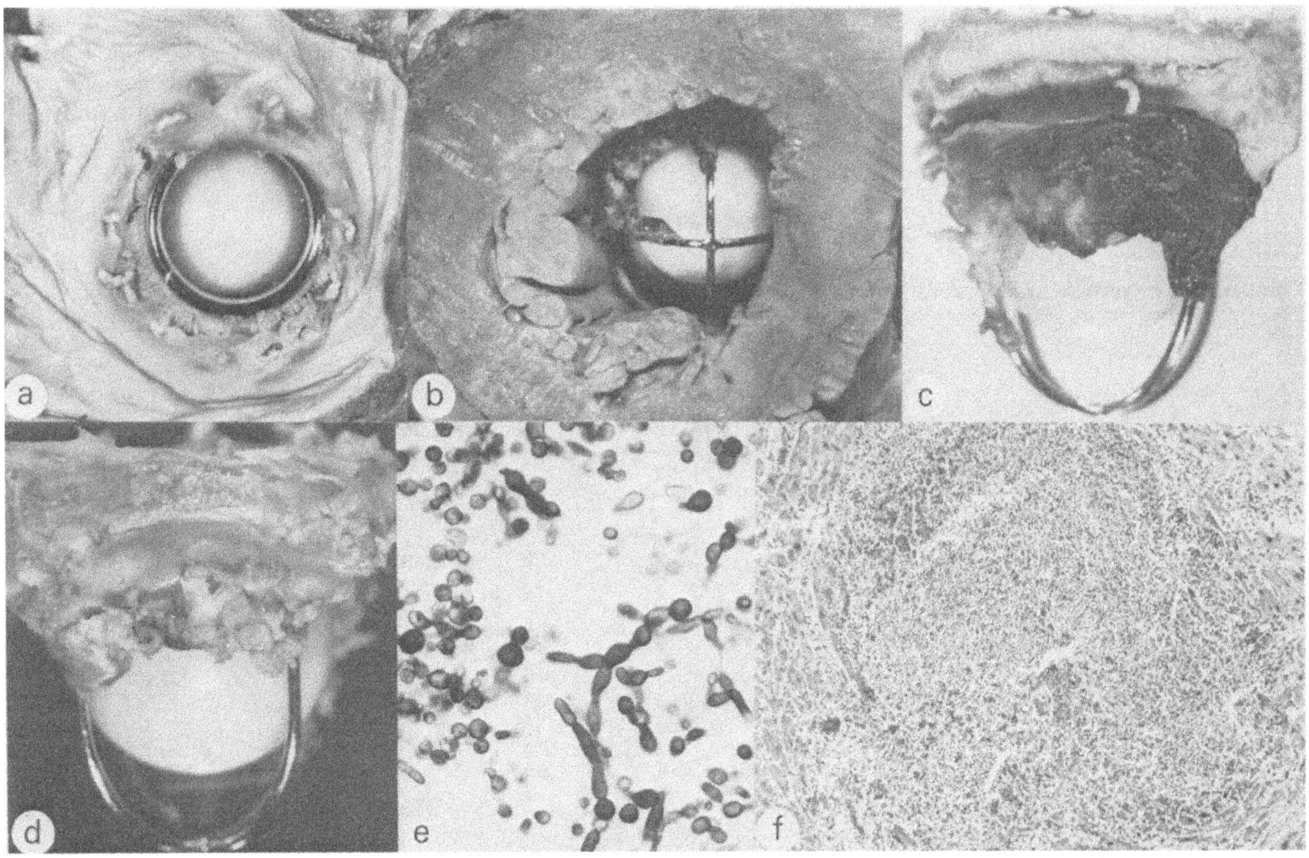

FIGURE 10. Candida species prosthetic mitral valve endocarditis in a 37 year old woman who underwent valve replacement 125 months before death because of mitral stenosis (mean mitral gradient 7 mm Hg) and regurgitation. Her tricuspid valve was replaced with a porcine xenograft because of severe tricuspid regurgitation 66 days before death. Postoperatively, she required prolonged use of a transthoracic pacing wire, which was the apparent source of the infection. She died from central nervous system embolism. Necropsy disclosed infection of the mitral valve prosthesis. **a,** mitral valve prosthesis viewed from the left atrium; **b,** prosthesis viewed from the left ventricle. Large vegetations are present on the base and struts of the prosthesis. **c** and **d,** removed mitral valve prosthesis viewed from two different sides showing large vegetations. **e,** photomicrograph of Candida species in the mitral vegetations. (Methenemine silver stain ×860, reduced by 23 percent.) **f,** photomicrograph of microabscess in the left ventricular myocardium. (Hematoxylin-eosin ×80, reduced by 23 percent.)

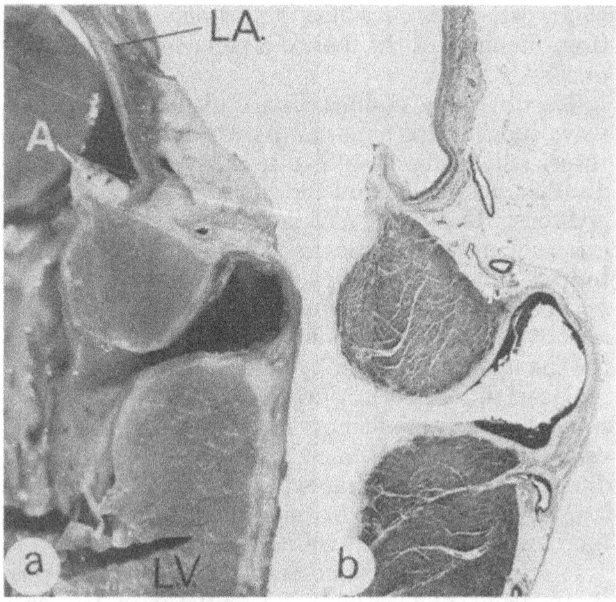

FIGURE 11. Left ventricular aneurysm simulating prosthetic valve endocarditis in a 46 year old woman. She had almost daily fever after mitral valve replacement 4 months before death and one of many blood cultures grew Staphylococcus epidermidis and diphtheroids. The clinical diagnosis was prosthetic valve endocarditis and she was treated with prolonged intravenous antibiotic therapy. She died from central nervous system embolism. At necropsy, an aneurysm was present in the basal portion of the left ventricular free wall. The prosthesis and its anulus were free of signs of infection. **a,** longitudinal cut of the left atrial (LA.) wall, mitral anulus (A) and left ventricular (L.V.) wall through the aneurysm. **b,** histologic section of the aneurysm (Movat stain). Thrombus is present in the aneurysm.

made quite readily.[48,62,63] It is worth emphasizing, however, that the combination of fever and a positive blood culture in a patient with a prosthetic cardiac valve does not always indicate the presence of prosthetic valve infection. We recently studied a patient at necropsy who was diagnosed during life as having prosthetic mitral valve endocarditis on the basis of fever, cerebral episodes consistent with emboli, and one blood culture that grew Staphylococcus epidermidis and diphtheroids. She received antibiotic treatment during most of her 4 month postoperative period and at necropsy no endocarditis was found. A left ventricular aneurysm was present immediately caudal to the mitral anulus and a sterile thrombus was present in the aneurysm (Fig. 11). The latter was the likely source of the cerebral emboli.

Antibiotic agents: There seems to be a general view that prosthetic valve endocarditis can at times be cured by antibiotic drugs. For such cure to be established, however, it is necessary that prosthetic valve endocarditis be confirmed during life, and this unequivocal confirmation can be obtained only by examination of the prosthetic valve and its anulus (site of attachment) at reoperation. In other words, to establish cure of prosthetic valve endocarditis it is necessary to be absolutely positive of the diagnosis. Although this confirmation is usually not obtained, it has now been obtained in enough patients to support the view that prosthetic valve endocarditis can indeed be cured in some patients.[16,17,21,23,24,29,30,37,39,44,45,48,64,65]

TABLE VI

Comparison between Active Infective Endocarditis (IE) Involving Prosthetic Cardiac Valves and Natural Cardiac Valves

	Mitral Valve				Aortic Valve			
	Prosthetic		Natural		Prosthetic		Natural	
	no.	%	no.	%	no.	%	no.	%
Necropsy patients (no.)	7		22		15		52*	
Age (yr) (range and average)	37–65 (52)		15–74 (43)		37–69 (54)		17–83 (45)	
Sex ratio (male:female)	3:4		12:10		13:2		41:11	
Underlying valve disease	7	100	7	32	15	100	26	50
Rheumatic	—	—	6	27	—	—	4	8
Congenital	—	—	0	0	—	—	12	23
Other	—	—	1†	5	—	—	10‡	19
None	—	—	15	68	—	—	26	50
Previous episode IE	1	14	0	0	1	7	3	6
Infecting organism								
Staphylococcus §	4	57	7	32	9	60	13	25
Alpha streptococcus	0	0	0	0	0	0	9	17
Pneumococcus	0	0	2	9	1	7	6	12
Valve regurgitation (from IE)	2	29	14	64	12	80	36	69
Valve stenosis (from IE) §	5	71	1	5	1	7	1	2
Valve-ring abscess §	7	100	1	5	15	100	21	40
Complete heart block §	0	0	1	5	5	33	4	8
Left bundle branch block §	0	0	0	0	2	13	0	0
Organ infarcts	5	71	17	77	9	60	31/47	66
Spleen >300 g	2/6	33	3	20	12	80	19/38	50

* Eighteen of the 52 also had infection of the mitral valve, but in at least 13 of them the mitral valve infection appeared to be secondary to the aortic valve infection.
† Floppy mitral valve.
‡ Degenerative (5 patients); previous infective endocarditis that healed (3 patients) and uncertain origin (2 patients).
§ $P < 0.05$.

Comparison With Endocarditis Involving Natural Valves

Comparison of observations in our 22 patients with prosthetic valve endocarditis with our observations in 74 nonsurgically treated necropsy patients with active infective endocarditis involving natural left-sided cardiac valves disclosed certain clear differences between the two groups (Table VI): (1) Ring abscess was always present in patients with prosthetic valve endocarditis regardless of the site of the prosthesis, but was present in only 30 percent of the comparison group and then, with rare exception, only when the aortic valve was infected. (2) The hemodynamic consequences were different. Prosthetic valve endocarditis caused valve obstruction nearly as often as valve regurgitation, whereas valve stenosis from active infective endocarditis involving natural cardiac valves was extremely rare.[10,66] (3) Spread of ring abscess was more extensive in patients with prosthetic valve endocarditis than in patients with natural valve endocarditis, and consequently the frequency of high grade conduction defects was much greater in the former patients. (4) The infecting organism in fatal prosthetic valve endocarditis was most commonly the Staphylococcus. Alpha streptococcus, which remains a common cause of fatal active infective endocarditis in patients with natural cardiac valves, is a rare cause of fatal prosthetic valve endocarditis.

Valve ring abscess: Among patients with infective endocarditis involving native cardiac valves, ring abscess when present almost always (95 percent of cases) involves the aortic valve.[67] Among our necropsy patients with active infective endocarditis involving a natural aortic valve, 40 percent had a valve ring abscess, whereas only 5 percent of patients with endocarditis involving a natural mitral valve had a ring abscess. In contrast, each of our 22 patients with prosthetic valve endocarditis had a ring abscess. Thus, valve ring abscess is the usual morphologic feature of prosthetic valve endocarditis, regardless of the valve infected.

Ring abscesses in patients with infection involving prosthetic valves are generally more extensive than those in patients with active infective endocarditis involving natural cardiac valves. This appears to be a consequence of the rigid nature of the prosthetic frame. Once the prosthesis is loosened by the infection, the rocking-rigid frame promotes spread of the infection. The greater turbulence across the aortic valve prosthesis probably accounts for the generally more extensive nature of ring abscess with prosthetic aortic than with prosthetic mitral endocarditis. A consequence of this extension is the greater frequency of complete heart block and left bundle branch block in patients with prosthetic aortic valve endocarditis (32 percent) than in patients with natural aortic valve endocarditis (8 percent).

Infecting organism: *Staphylococcus* (either aureus or epidermidis) is the most common cause of prosthetic valve endocarditis (59 percent). Many different organisms cause the remainder of the infections. Although alpha streptococcus was the responsible organism in 17 percent of our 74 patients with natural aortic valve infection, this bacterium was not the causative organism in any of our 22 patients with prosthetic valve endocarditis.

Valve dysfunction: The hemodynamic consequences of prosthetic valve endocarditis vary with the site of the infected prosthesis. Valve regurgitation developed in 12 of the 15 patients (80 percent) with prosthetic aortic valve endocarditis and in 2 of the 7 patients (28 percent) with prosthetic mitral valve infection. In contrast, valve obstruction developed from the infection in 5 of the 7 patients (71 percent) with prosthetic mitral valve endocarditis, and in 1 of the 15 patients (7 percent) with prosthetic aortic valve endocarditis. Among patients with natural left-sided valve infection, 65 percent (64 percent of those with mitral valve disease and 69 percent of those with aortic valve disease) had valve regurgitation from active infective endocarditis, and relatively few (3 percent) had valve obstruction from the endocarditis.[10] Thus, aortic prosthetic valve endocarditis almost alv ıys causes valve regurgitation and mitral prosthetic valve endocarditis most often causes valve obstruction.

Splenomegaly (greater than 300 g) is common both in patients with prosthetic valve endocarditis (64 percent) and in patients with native left-sided valve endocarditis (37 percent). The frequency of infarcts in other body organs is similar in both groups (64 and 70 percent, respectively).

References

1. **Roberts WC, Morrow AG:** Anatomic studies of hearts containing caged-ball prosthetic valves. John Hopkins Med J 121:271–295, 1967
2. **Roberts WC, Morrow AG:** Causes of death and other anatomic observations after cardiac valve replacement. Adv Cardiol 7: 226–247, 1972
3. **Roberts WC, Bulkley BH, Morrow AG:** Pathologic anatomy of cardiac valve replacement: a study of 224 necropsy patients. Prog Cardiovasc Dis 15:539–587, 1973
4. **Fishbein MC, Roberts WC, Golden A, et al:** Cardiac pathology after aortic valve replacement using Hufnagel trileaflet prostheses: a study of 20 necropsy patients. Am Heart J 89:443–448, 1975
5. **Roberts WC, Fishbein MC, Golden A:** Cardiac pathology after valve replacement by disc prosthesis. A study of 61 necropsy patients. Am J Cardiol 35:740–760, 1975
6. **Fishbein MC, Roberts WC:** Late postoperative anatomic observations after insertion of Hufnagel caged-ball prosthesis in descending thoracic aorta. Chest 68:6–11, 1975
7. **Roberts WC, Hammer WJ:** Cardiac pathology after valve replacement with a tilting disc prosthesis (Björk-Shiley type): a study of 46 necropsy patients and 49 Björk-Shiley prostheses. Am J Cardiol 37:1024–1033, 1976
8. **Roberts WC, Buchbinder NA:** Right-sided valvular infective endocarditis. A clinicopathologic study of twelve necropsy patients. Am J Med 53:7–19, 1972
9. **Buchbinder NA, Roberts WC:** Left-sided valvular active infective endocarditis. A study of forty-five necropsy patients. Am J Med 53:20–35, 1972
10. **Arnett EN, Roberts WC:** Pathology of active infective endocarditis. A clinicopathologic study of 137 necropsy patients. Current

Problems in Cardiology, in press.
11. **Cohn LH, Roberts WC, Rockoff SD, et al:** Bacterial endocarditis following aortic valve replacement. Clinical and pathological correlations. Circulation 33:209–217, 1966
12. **Roberts WC, Morrow AG:** Bacterial endocarditis involving prosthetic mitral valves. Clinical and pathologic observations. Arch Pathol 82:164–169, 1966
13. **Arnett EN, Roberts WC:** Prosthetic valve endocarditis. A study of 18 patients at necropsy (abstr). Am J Cardiol 35:120, 1975
14. **Björk VO:** Aortic valve replacement. Thorax 19:369–378, 1964
15. **Newman WH, Cordell AR:** Aspergillus endocarditis after open-heart surgery. Report of a case and review of literature. J Thorac Cardiovasc Surg 48:652–660, 1964
16. **Amoury RA, Bowman FO Jr, Malm JR:** Endocarditis associated with intracardiac prostheses. Diagnosis, management and prophylaxis. J Thorac Cardiovasc Surg 51:36–48, 1966
17. **Stein PD, Harken DE, Dexter L:** The nature and prevention of prosthetic valve endocarditis. Am Heart J 71;393–407, 1966
18. **Fraser RS, Rossall RE, Dvorkin J:** Bacterial endocarditis occurring after open heart surgery. Can Med Assoc J 96:1551–1558, 1967
19. **Leffert RC, Hackett RL:** Aspergillus aortitis following replacement of aortic valve. J Thorac Cardiovasc Surg 53:866–874, 1967
20. **McConnell EM, Roberts C:** Pathological findings in three cases of fungal endocarditis complicating open-heart surgery. J Clin Pathol 20:555–560, 1967
21. **Geraci JE, Forth RJ, Ellis FH:** Postoperative prosthetic valve endocarditis due to *Corynebacterium xerosis.* Mayo Clin Proc 42: 736–743, 1967
22. **Cheng TO, Kinhal V, Tice DA:** Fatal thrombosis of the Starr-Edwards mitral valve prosthesis associated with bacterial endocarditis. Diagnostic significance of a disappearing prosthetic click. Chest 57:151–155, 1970
23. **Hairston P, Lee WH Jr:** Management of infective prosthetic heart valves. Ann Thorac Surg 9:229–237, 1970
24. **Killen DA, Collins HA, Koenig MG, et al:** Prosthetic cardiac valves and bacterial endocarditis. Ann Thorac Surg 9:238–246, 1970
25. **Shafer RB, Hall WH:** Bacterial endocarditis following open heart surgery. Am J Cardiol 25:602–607, 1970
26. **Sutton GC, Wright JEC:** Major detachment of aortic prosthetic valves. Br Heart J 32:337–343, 1970
27. **Chaudhuri MR:** Fungal endocarditis after valve replacements. J Thorac Cardiovasc Surg 60:207–214, 1970
28. **Gage AA, Dean DC, Schimert G, et al:** Aspergillus infection after cardiac surgery. Arch Surg 101:384–387, 1970
29. **Block PC, DeSanctis RW, Weinberg AN, et al:** Prosthetic valve endocarditis. J Thorac Cardiovasc Surg 60:540–548, 1970
30. **Okies JE, Viroslav J, Williams TW Jr:** Endocarditis after cardiac valvular replacement. Chest 59:198–202, 1971
31. **Ostermiller WE Jr, Dye WS, Weinberg M:** Fungal endocarditis following cardiovascular surgery. J Thorac Cardiovasc Surg 61: 670–675, 1971
32. **Lawrence T, Shockman AT, Macvaugh H 3rd:** Aspergillus infection of prosthetic aortic valves. Chest 60:406–414, 1971
33. **Robinson MJ, Greenberg JJ, Korn M, et al:** infective endocarditis at autopsy: 1965–1969. Am J Med 52:492–498, 1972
34. **Levin S, Balagtas R, Susmano A, et al:** Meningococcus endocarditis at the site of Starr-Edwards mitral prosthesis. Arch Intern Med 129:963–966, 1972
35. **Joassin A, Edward JE:** Late causes of death after mitral valve replacement. J Thorac Cardiovasc Surg 65:255–263, 1973
36. **Vlachakis ND, Gazes PC, Hairston P:** Nocardial endocarditis following mitral valve replacement. Chest 63:276–278, 1973
37. **Slaughter L, Morris JE, Starr A:** Prosthetic valvular endocarditis. A 12-year review. Circulation 47:1319–1326, 1973
38. Case records of the Massachusetts General Hospital. Weekly clinicopathological exercises. Case 24, 1973. N Engl J Med 288:1290–1296, 1973
39. **Dismukes WE, Karchmer AW, Buckley MJ, et al:** Prosthetic valve endocarditis. Analysis of 38 cases. Circulation 48:365–377, 1973
40. **Jackson G, Saunders K:** Prosthetic valve diphtheroid endocarditis treated with sodium fusidate and erythromycin. Br Heart J 35: 931–936, 1973
41. **Harris JA, Cobbs CG:** Serratia endocarditis in patients with a Starr-Edwards valve: report of a case of bacteriologic cure with antimicrobial therapy. South Med J 66:1117–1120, 1973
42. **Hall WJ 3rd:** Penicillium endocarditis following open heart surgery and prosthetic valve insertion. Am Heart J 87:501–506, 1974
43. **McAllister RG, Samet J, Mazzoleni A, et al:** Endocarditis on prosthetic mitral valves. Fatal obstruction to left ventricular inflow. Chest 66:682–686, 1974
44. **Madison J, Wang K, Gobel FL, et al:** Prosthetic aortic valvular endocarditis. Circulation 51:940–949, 1975
45. **Wilson WR, Jaumin PM, Danielson GK, et al:** Prosthetic valve endocarditis. Ann Intern Med 82:751–756, 1975
46. **Rubenstein E, Noriega ER, Simberkoff MS, et al:** Fungal endocarditis: analysis of 24 cases and review of the literature. Medicine 54:331–344, 1975
47. **Robboy SJ, Kaiser J:** Pathogenesis of fungal infection on heart valve prostheses. Human Pathol 6:711–715, 1975
48. **Kloster FE:** Diagnosis and management of complications of prosthetic heart valves. Am J Cardiol 35:872–885, 1975
49. **Conte JE, Cohen SN, Roe BB, et al:** Antibiotic prophylaxis and cardiac surgery. A prospective double-blind comparison of single-dose versus multiple-dose regimens. Ann Intern Med 76: 943–949, 1972
50. **Goodman JS, Schaffner W, Collins HA, et al:** Infection after cardiovascular surgery: clinical study including examination of antimicrobial prophylaxis. N Engl J Med 287:117–123, 1968
51. **Nelson RM, Jenson CB, Peterson CA, et al:** Effective use of prophylactic antibiotics in open-heart surgery. Arch Surg 90:731–735, 1965
52. **Herr R, Starr A, McCord CW, et al:** Special problems following valve replacement. Embolus, leak, infection, red cell damage. Ann Thorac Surg 1:403–415, 1965
53. **Ankeney JL, Parker RF:** Staphylococcal endocarditis following open heart surgery related to positive intraoperative blood cultures. In, Prosthetic Heart Valves (Brewer LA III, ed). Springfield, Ill, Charles C Thomas, 1969, p 719–730
54. **Blakemore WS, McGarrity GJ, Thurer RJ, et al:** Infection by airborne bacteria with cardiopulmonary bypass. Surgery 70: 830–838, 1971
55. **Kammer RB, Utz JP:** Aspergillus species endocarditis. The new face of a not so rare disease. Am J Med 56:506–521, 1974
56. **Wigle ED, Labrosse CJ:** Sudden, severe aortic insufficiency. Circulation 32:708–720, 1965
57. **Wise JR, Bentall HH, Cleland WP, et al:** Urgent aortic-valve replacement for acute aortic regurgitation due to infective endocarditis. Lancet 2:115–121, 1971
58. **Wise JR Jr, Oakley CM, Goodwin JF:** Acute aortic regurgitation in patients with infective endocarditis. The distinctive clinical features and the role of premature mitral valve closure. J Maine Med Assoc 63:273–278, 1972
59. **Mann T, McLaurin L, Grossman W, et al:** Assessing the hemodynamic severity of acute aortic regurgitation due to infective endocarditis. N Engl J Med 293:108–113, 1975
60. **Yarbrough JW, Roberts WC, Reis RL:** Structural alterations in tissue cardiac valves implanted in patients and in calves. J Thorac Cardiovasc Surg 65:364–375, 1973
61. **Clarkson PM, Barratt-Boyes BG:** Bacterial endocarditis following homograft replacement of the aortic valve. Circulation 42:987–991, 1970
62. **Sande MA, Johnson WD Jr, Hook EW, et al:** Sustained bacteremia in patients with prosthetic cardiac valves. N Engl J Med 286: 1067–1070, 1972
63. **Weinstein L:** Infected prosthetic valves: a diagnostic and therapeutic dilemma. N Engl J Med 286:1108–1109, 1972
64. **Watanakunakorn C, Hamburger M:** Staphylococcus epidermidis endocarditis complicating a Starr-Edwards prosthesis. A therapeutic dilemma. Arch Intern Med 126:1014–1018, 1970
65. **Walker SR, Shumway NE, Merigan TC:** Management of infected cardiac valve prostheses. JAMA 208:531–533, 1969
66. **Roberts WC, Ewy GA, Glancy DL, et al:** Valvular stenosis produced by active infective endocarditis. Circulation 36:449–451, 1967
67. **Arnett EN, Roberts WC:** Valve ring abscess in active infective endocarditis. Frequency, location, and clues to clinical diagnosis from the study of 95 necropsy patients. Circulation 54:140–145, 1976

ACTIVE INFECTIVE ENDOCARDITIS: A CLINICOPATHOLOGIC ANALYSIS OF 137 NECROPSY PATIENTS

ERNEST N. ARNETT
WILLIAM C. ROBERTS

Ernest N. Arnett

is Assistant Chief of Service and Instructor in Medicine in the Department of Medicine of Johns Hopkins Hospital. Doctor Arnett graduated from the University of Cincinnati College of Medicine in 1972 and completed an internship and assistant residency in medicine at the Johns Hopkins Hospital. Prior to his current position he was a staff associate in the Pathology Section of the National Heart and Lung Institute. Doctor Arnett's principal research interests are in the clinical and morphologic aspects of infective endocarditis, coronary heart disease and pulmonary hypertension.

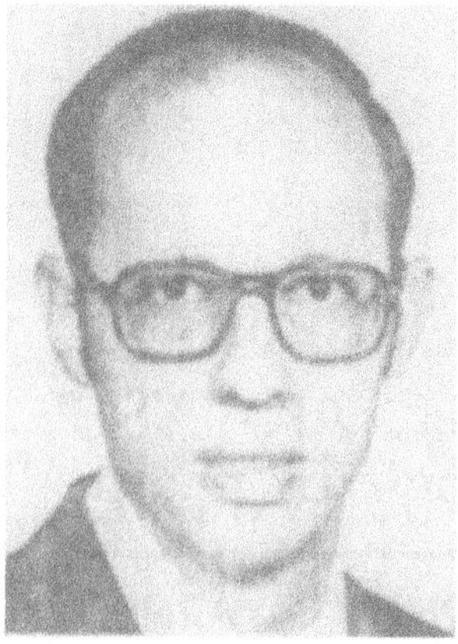

William C. Roberts

is Chief, Pathology Branch, National Heart, Lung and Blood Institute and Clinical Professor of Medicine and Pathology, Georgetown University. Doctor Roberts received his M.D. degree from Emory University School of Medicine in 1958 and served an internship in medicine at Boston City Hospital. From 1959 to 1962 he was a resident in anatomic pathology in the Laboratory of Pathology, National Cancer Institute. Subsequently he took a residency in medicine at the Johns Hopkins Hospital, Baltimore, returning to Bethesda to spend a year on the heart surgery ward and in the cardiac catheterization laboratory at NHLBI. Doctor Roberts has written more than 250 publications that deal primarily with structural alterations produced by various cardiovascular diseases and he is on the editorial boards of five medical journals.

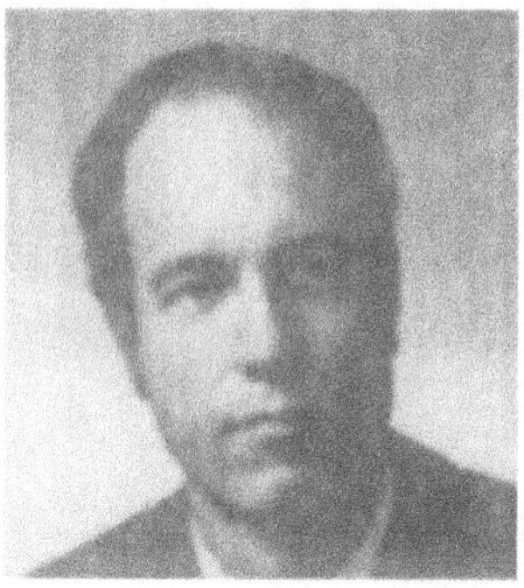

INFECTIVE ENDOCARDITIS (IE) in the preantibiotic era virtually always was fatal and consequently its morphologic aspects received particular attention. With the introduction of antibiotics, the morphologic features of IE became less emphasized and attention focused more on proper diagnosis and choice of antibiotics. During recent years, cardiac valve replacement or repair has afforded another form of therapy for both active and

TABLE 1.—CLASSIFICATION OF 137 PATIENTS WITH ACTIVE INFECTIVE ENDOCARDITIS (IE)

GROUP	PATIENTS No.	%
I. *IE involving right sided valves*	23	(17)
A. Isolated = 13		
B. Combined with left-sided IE = 10		
II. *IE limited to left-sided valve(s)*	74	(54)
A. Aortic valve (AV) = 34		
B. Mitral valve (MV) = 22		
C. AV + MV = 18		
III. *IE involving prosthetic valves*	22	(16)
A. Aortic valve = 15		
B. Mitral valve = 7		
IV. *IE after valvulotomy or valvuloplasty*	4	(3)
A. Aortic valve = 1		
B. Mitral valve = 3		
V. *IE complicating congenital cardiac disease with a shunt*	6	(4)
VI. *IE limited to mural endocardium*	8	(6)
TOTAL	137	(100)

healed IE. Thus, the morphologic features of IE once again have become important.

For information derived from the study of large numbers of necropsy patients with IE to be clinically useful, separation of the patients by site(s) of vegetations appears appropriate (Tables 1 and 2). Patients with IE involving right-sided cardiac valves, for example, usually have different clinical and morphologic features than patients with IE involving left-sided cardiac valves. Similarly, patients with IE involving prosthetic cardiac valves usually have different clinical and morphologic features than patients with IE involving natural cardiac valves. Therefore, patients with IE involving right-sided cardiac valves, those with IE limited to one or both left-sided valves and patients with prosthetic valve IE are presented separately (Table 3). In addition, patients with IE complicating congenital cardiac disease with shunt(s), those with IE after open heart surgery and those with vegetations limited to mural endocardium present special problems and, therefore, each of these three groups is discussed separately.

ACTIVE INFECTIVE ENDOCARDITIS INVOLVING RIGHT-SIDED CARDIAC VALVES WITH OR WITHOUT INVOLVEMENT OF LEFT-SIDED CARDIAC VALVES

Twenty-three (17%) of our 137 necropsy patients had vegetations on right-sided cardiac valves: in 13 patients, vegetations were limited to the tricuspid valve; in the other 10 patients, vegetations involved one right-sided (tricuspid in 9; pulmonic in

TABLE 2.—SITES OF VEGETATIONS IN ACTIVE VALVULAR INFECTIVE ENDOCARDITIS
(129 Necropsy Patients)

	GROUP I	GROUP II	GROUP III	GROUP IV	GROUP V	
Location of Vegetations	Right-Sided (with or without Left)	Left Only	Prosthetic	PO Valvulotomy	In Congenital Cardiac Disease with Shunt	Totals
1. Aortic valve (AV) only	—	34	15	1	2*	52
2. Mitral valve (MV) only	—	22	7	3	0	32
3. MV + AV	0	18	0	0	1†	19
4. Tricuspid valve (TV) only	13	—	0	0	0	13
5. TV + MV + AV	5	0	0	0	1	6
6. TV + MV	2	0	0	0	0	2
7. TV + AV	2	0	0	0	0	2
8. Pulmonic valve (PV) only	0	—	0	0	2	2
9. PV + MV	1	0	0	0	0	1
10. PV + AV	0	0	0	0	0	0
11. TV + PV	0	0	0	0	0	0
	23	74	22	4	6	129

*Truncus valve in 1 patient with persistent truncus arteriosus.
†Mitral valve + truncus valve.

1) and one or both left-sided cardiac valves. Clinical and morphologic observations in the 23 patients are shown in Table 3, and certain morphologic features of the IE in them are illustrated in Figures 1–7.

None of the 23 patients had a history of previous cardiac dis-

TABLE 3. - ACTIVE INFECTIVE ENDOCARDITIS: CLINICAL AND NECROPSY OBSERVATIONS

	GROUP I		GROUP II	GROUP III	
	Right-Sided IE Isolated	Right and Left	Left-Sided IE	Prosthetic IE	Totals
1. Number of patients	13 (11)	10 (8)	74 (62)	22 (18)	119 (100)
2. Ages (Years): Range [avg]	22–77 [47]	1–66 [45]	15–83 [45]	37–69 [53]	1–83 [47]
3. Males: Females	6:7	9:1	53:21	16:6	84:35
4. Predisposing factors					
a. None	0	0	21 (28)	9 (41)	30 (25)
b. Opiate addiction	5 (38)	1 (10)	10 (14)	0	16 (13)
c. Alcoholism	3 (28)	6 (60)	17 (23)	0	26 (22)
d. Neoplasm and chemotherapy	3 (23)	1 (10)	7 (9)	0	11 (9)
e. Miscellaneous	2 (15)	2 (20)	19 (26)	13 (59)	36 (30)
5. Other infection					
a. Acute pneumonia	12 (92)	8 (80)	14 (19)	2 (9)	36 (30)
b. Acute meningitis	3 (23)	4 (40)	10 (14)	2 (9)	19 (16)
6. Underlying heart disease					
a. Rheumatic	0	0	10 (14)	0	10 (8)
b. Congenital	0	0	12 (16)	0	12 (10)
c. Degenerative	0	0	5 (7)	0	5 (4)
d. Floppy	0	0	2 (2)	0	2 (2)
e. Previous IE (healed)	0	0	3 (4)	0	3 (3)
f. Other	0	0	2 (3)	22 (100)	24 (20)
7. Status of valve before IE					
a. Anatomic status					
1) Normal	13 (100)	10 (100)	41 (55)	0	64 (54)
2) Abnormal	0	0	33 (45)	22 (100)	55 (46)
b. Functional status					
1) Normal	13 (100)	10 (100)	45 (61)	0	68 (57)
2) Abnormal	0	0	29 (39)	22 (100)	51 (43)
a) Purely incompetent	0	0	10 (14)	–	10 (8)
b) Stenotic	0	0	19 (26)		19 (16)
8. Valve function after IE					
a. Normal	6 (46)	3 (30)	11 (15)	3 (14)	23 (19)
b. Abnormal	7 (54)	7 (70)	63 (85)	19 (86)	96 (81)
9. Valve dysfunction from IE					
a. Pure regurgitation	5 (38)	7 (70)	53 (72)	13 (59)	78 (66)
b. Stenosis	2 (15)	0	2 (3)	6 (27)	10 (8)
10. Infecting organism					
a. Bacterium					
1) Staphylococcus	8 (62)	3 (30)	20 (27)	13 (59)	44 (37)
2) Streptococcus	0	1 (10)	22 (30)	1 (5)	24 (20)
3) Pneumococcus	2 (15)	4 (40)	8 (11)	1 (5)	15 (33)
4) Other	1 (8)	0	4 (5)	3 (14)	8 (7)
b. Fungus	1 (8)	1 (10)	4 (5)	2 (9)	8 (7)
c. Unknown or negative	1 (8)	1 (10)	16 (22)	0	18 (15)
11. Ring abscess	2 (15)	2 (20)	24 (32)	22 (100)	50 (42)
12. Acute pericarditis	1 (8)	2 (20)	16 (22)	9 (41)	28 (24)
13. Acute myocarditis	8 (62)	7 (70)	[illegible] (62)	22 (100)	78 (70)
14. Embolism (gross organ infarcts)					
a. Systemic					
1) Heart	0	2 (20)	5 (7)	1 (5)	8 (7)
2) Spleen	0	2 (20)	33 (45)	12 (55)	47 (39)
3) Kidney	0	1 (40)	31 (42)	7 (32)	42 (35)
4) Brain	0	2 (20)	27 (36)	7 (32)	36 (30)
5) Lung	11 (87)	8 (80)	3 (4)	0	22 (18)
6) Other	0	0	10 (14)	3 (14)	13 (11)
b. Pulmonary	11 (87)	8 (80)	3 (4)	0	22 (18)
15. Splenomegaly (> 300 gm)	6 (46)	3 (30)	21 (28)	14 (67)	44 (37)
16. Principal cause of death					
a. Cardiovascular	1 (8)	5 (50)	45 (61)	19 (86)	70 (59)
1) CHF	1 (8)	5 (50)	40 (54)	19 (86)	65 (55)
2) Other	0	0	5 (7)	0	5 (4)
b. CNS	2 (15)	2 (20)	17 (23)	2 (9)	23 (19)
1) Embolism	0	0	12 (16)	2 (9)	14 (12)
2) Meningitis	2 (15)	2 (20)	5 (7)	0	9 (8)
c. Pneumonia	2 (15)	0	1 (1)	0	3 (2)
d. Generalized infection	3 (23)	0	7 (9)	1 (5)	11 (9)
e. Other	4 (31)	3 (30)	4 (5)	0	11 (9)
17. Heart weight (gm) Range [avg]	220–540 [365]	220–500 [360]	200–900 [485]	400–880 [610]	200–900 [490]
18. Location of primary infection					
a. Heart	10 (77)	8 (80)	73 (99)	22 (100)	13 (95)
b. Other	3 (23)	2 (20)	1 (1)	0	6 (5)

*All numbers in ( ) represent percentages and all numbers in [ ] represent averages.

ease. Factors associated with an increased risk of developing IE, however, were present in each: habitual alcoholism (9 patients), opiate addiction (6 patients), malignant neoplasm (4 patients), infected intravenous catheters (2 patients), extensive body burns (1 patient) and hereditary immune deficiency disease (a 1-year-old boy).

Signs and/or symptoms of IE were present from 2 to 390 days (avg 67). Fever (temperature > 100°F) was present in all 23 patients. Precordial murmurs were present in 15 patients, but in 7 of them the murmurs resulted from left-sided valve dysfunction (aortic regurgitation in 5 and mitral regurgitation in 2). Thus, of the 23 patients with vegetations on right-sided cardiac valves, only 8 had murmurs suggestive of right-sided IE. Similarly, although signs of congestive heart failure were present in 13 patients, only 6 of the 16 patients without left-sided valve dysfunction had signs of congestive heart failure. Seven of the 23 patients

Fig. 1.—Tricuspid valve endocarditis due to *Staphylococcus aureus* and *Enterobacter cloacae* in a 26-year-old male heroin addict (A75–84). He was hospitalized 4½ months before death with fever (104° F), malaise, dyspnea, proteinuria (up to 14 gm per 24 hr), multiple pulmonary infiltrates and a grade 3/6 holosystolic murmur that increased with inspiration. Following 6 weeks of intravenous antibiotic therapy, he was discharged but returned to the hospital 43 days later, just hours before death, with severe dyspnea and massive edema. **a,** tricuspid valve viewed from right atrium. **b,** posterior portion and **c,** anterior portion of a longitudinal cut through right atrium *(RA)*, tricuspid valve and right ventricle *(RV)*. A huge vegetation virtually fills the tricuspid valve orifice. A hemorrhagic abscess is present in the cephalad portion of the ventricular septum *(VS)*. **d,** microscopic-sized abscess in left ventricular myocardium (hematoxylin and eosin stain; ×450).

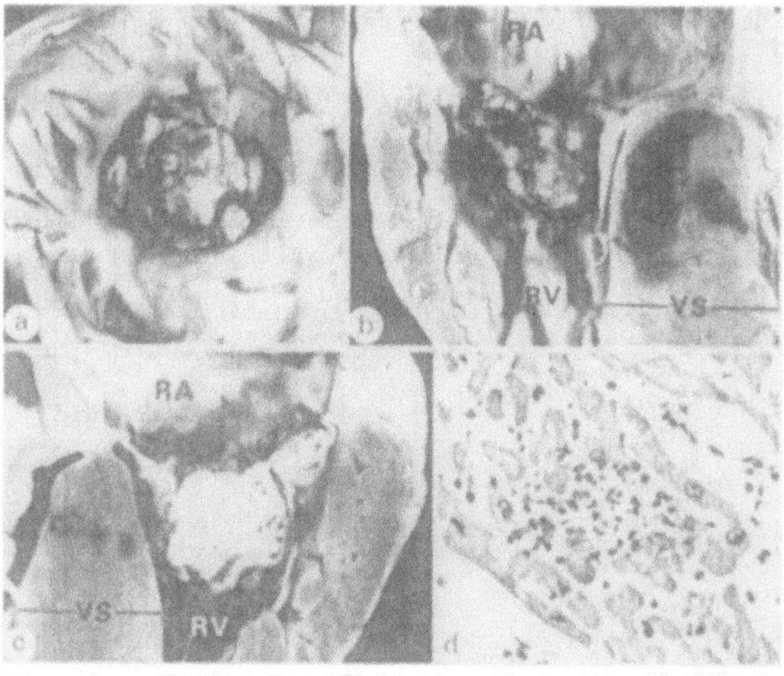

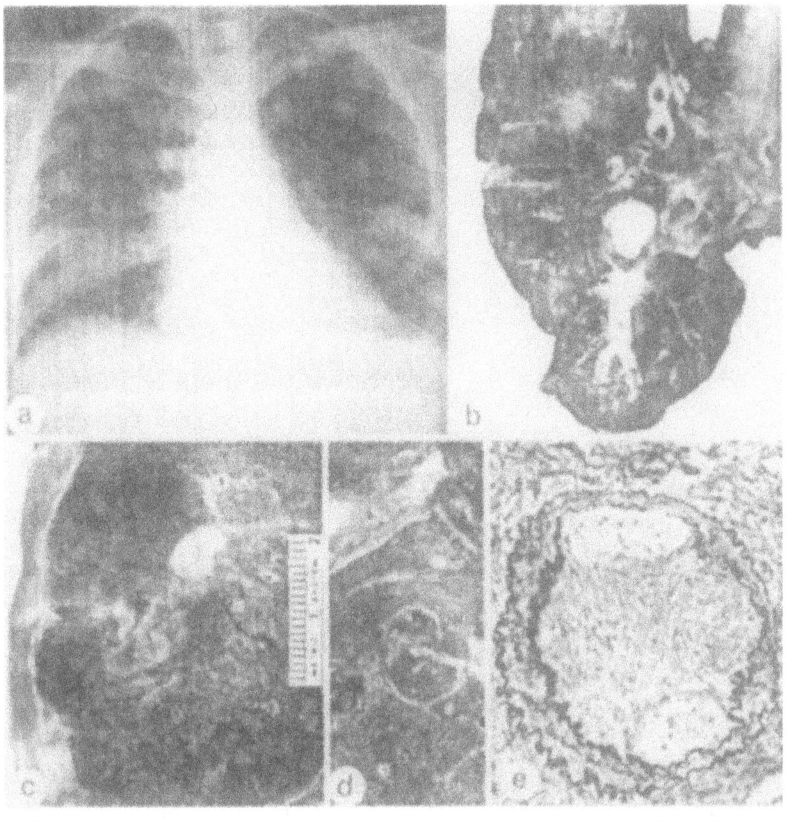

Fig. 2.—Same patient as Figure 1. **a,** chest roentgenogram at time of initial hospitalization. Multiple infiltrates are present in both lungs. **b,** longitudinal cut through the right lung. The lumen of a large pulmonary artery is totally obstructed by a septic embolus. **c** and **d,** close-up of lung showing multiple small infarcts and abscesses. **e,** small muscular pulmonary artery with occluded but partially recanalized lumen (elastic van Gieson stain; ×80).

presented with acute meningitis, and 20 had acute pneumonia. Five had palpable spleens.

► ANTONIO C. DE LEON, JR.: The significant frequency of absence of a diagnostic murmur with right-sided (tricuspid) endocarditis is dramatically pointed out by these data. Severe tricuspid regurgitation resulting in "ventricularization" of right atrial pressure may not result in an audible murmur or, more frequently, result in a short, early systolic (rather than the typical holosystolic) murmur and thus is mistaken for an innocent systolic murmur. Careful auscultation with respiration usually will demonstrate an inspiratory increase in the murmur or bring out a murmur that otherwise is inaudible. Careful observation of the jugular venous pulse (and/or presence of systolic hepatic expansion) usually will enable the recognition of severe tricuspid regurgitation in the absence of any audible murmur.

► W. PROCTOR HARVEY: Just to elaborate on Doctor de Leon's comments: Personally observed have been patients with tricuspid valve insufficien-

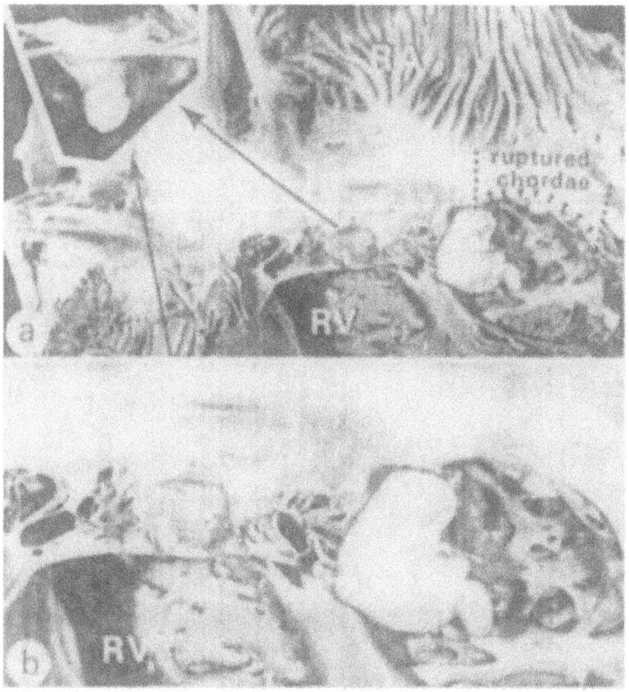

Fig. 3.—*Diplococcus pneumoniae* tricuspid valve endocarditis in a 56-year-old female chronic alcoholic (A76–3) who had been treated for pneumococcal meningitis 3 months earlier. She was brought to the hospital 3 days before death because of mental confusion. She was febrile, dehydrated and had a murmur of tricuspid regurgitation. Chest roentgenogram revealed multiple pulmonary infiltrates and blood cultures were positive. **a,** opened right atrium *(RA)*, tricuspid valve and right ventricle *(RV)*. Two vegetations are present. The inset shows the vegetation as it would appear from the right atrium. **b,** close-up of the tricuspid valve. The ruptured chordae are apparent.

cy and *no* systolic murmur was detected—until one listened specifically along the lower left sternal border searching for a murmur coincident with inspiration but not heard with expiration. This murmur could be termed "silent" had not the physician paid close attention to respiration affecting a murmur. Sometimes the first clue as to the presence of tricuspid insufficiency has been the detection of a significant "c-v" wave of the jugular venous pulse. In addition, a more prominent "a" wave may occur with acute tricuspid valve endocarditis; on auscultation, an atrial sound (S_4) may also be heard along the lower left sternal border that increases in intensity with inspiration. I suspect that there will be fewer silent tricuspid valve lesions if we pay more attention to these simple points.

Blood cultures were positive in 21 and negative in 2 of the 23 patients. *Staphylococcus aureus* was the most frequent infecting organism (11 patients) and caused the infection in 8 of the 13 patients with isolated right-sided vegetations. *Staphylococcus aureus* caused the infection in each of the 6 opiate addicts.

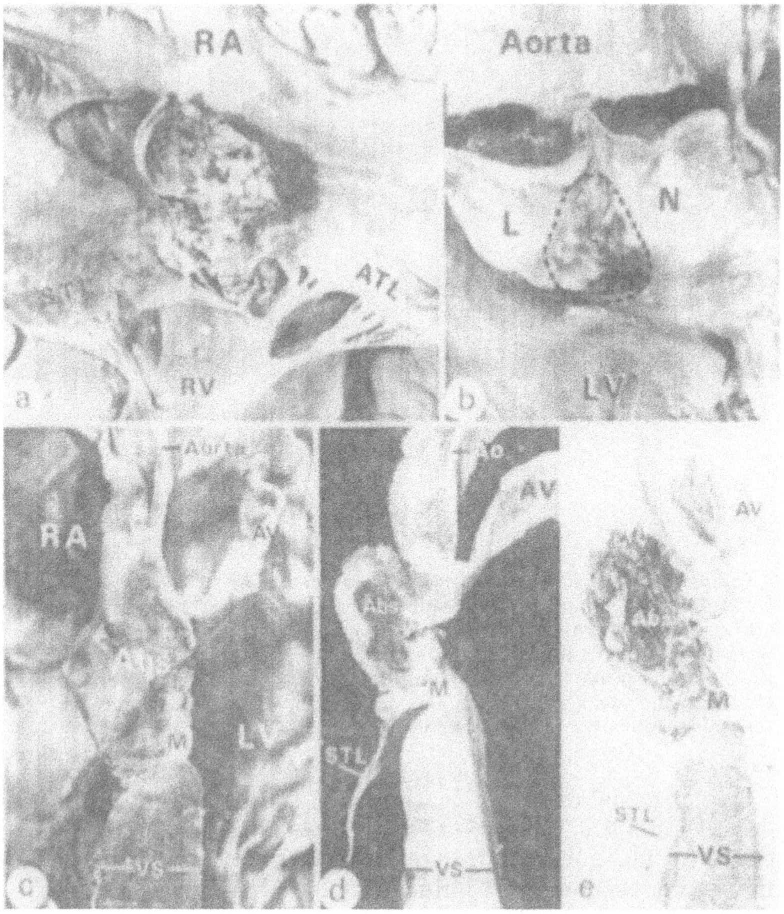

Fig. 4.—*Staphylococcus aureus* tricuspid valve endocarditis with ring abscess in a 77-year-old male chronic alcoholic (A76–1). He was hospitalized 3 weeks before death for open reduction of a fractured femur. Postoperatively, he developed fever and positive blood cultures. Despite intravenous antibiotic therapy, he died several days later. **a,** opened right atrium *(RA)*, tricuspid valve and right ventricle *(RV)*. A large vegetation is present on the septal tricuspid leaflet *(STL)*. *ATL* = anterior tricuspid valve leaflet. **b,** opened aortic valve. The infection has burrowed through the membranous ventricular septum *(circle)* and is visible between the left *(L)* and noncoronary *(N)* aortic valve cusps. *LV* = left ventricle. **c** and **d,** longitudinal cuts through the atrial septum, aortic valve cusp, septal tricuspid leaflet *(STL)*, membranous *(M)* and muscular ventricular septum *(VS)*. The vegetation has extended cephalad from the base of the septal tricuspid leaflet, producing a large abscess *(Abs)* in the membranous *(M)* ventricular septum. **e,** histologic section of **d.** The dark stained material is composed of fibrin, leukocytes and colonies of gram-positive cocci (Movat stain; ×2).

Diplococcus pneumoniae was the second most frequent infecting organism (6 patients) and caused the infection in 6 of the 9 chronic alcoholics. Fungi caused the infection in 2 patients; 1 was receiving cytotoxic drugs for acute leukemia and the other had an hereditary immune deficiency disease.

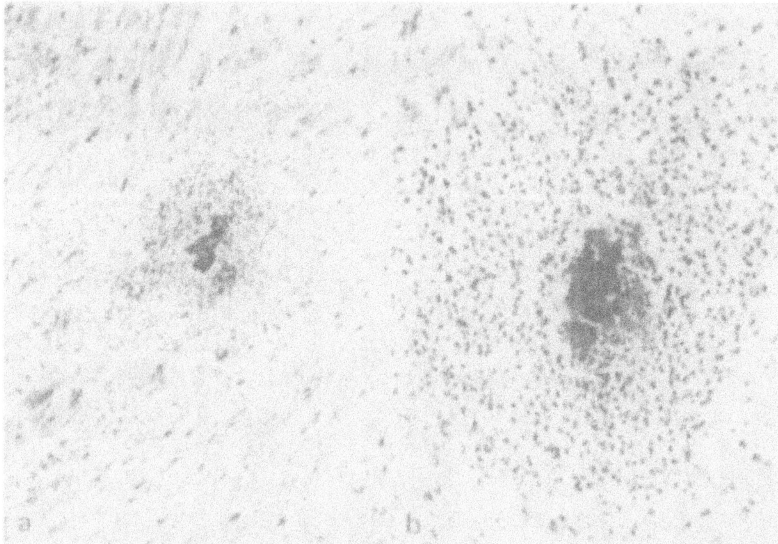

Fig. 5.—Myocardial abscesses in a 66-year-old woman (A74–177) with *Staphyloccus aureus* tricuspid valve endocarditis. She died of hepatoma and the septicemia appeared during the last few weeks of life. At necropsy, vegetations were present on the tricuspid valve and multiple small abscesses, as seen here, were present in the myocardium, both right and left, and also in several other organs (hematoxylin and eosin stains: **a,** ×140; **b,** ×350). The dark areas represent collections of gram-positive cocci.

The principal causes of death among the 13 patients with isolated right-sided vegetations were: generalized infection (3 patients), acute pneumonia (2 patients), acute meningitis (2 patients), congestive heart failure (1 patient), renal failure (1 patient) and causes unrelated to IE (4 patients) (malignant neoplasm in 3 and extensive body burns in 1). Among the 10 patients with vegetations on both right- and left-sided cardiac valves, 5 died of congestive heart failure, 2 from acute meningitis and 3 from causes unrelated to IE. IE was diagnosed during life in 16 patients (70%); of the 7 in whom IE was not diagnosed during life, 6 died from causes unrelated to IE.

Necropsy findings.—In 18 of the 23 patients, infection was primary in the heart; in the other 5 patients, the heart was one of many organs involved by a generalized infection. In each of the 23 patients, the cardiac valves appeared to have been normal, both functionally and anatomically, before the onset of IE.

Vegetations were present on the tricuspid valve in 22 of the 23 patients, including each of the 13 patients with isolated right-sided IE (Figs. 1–5). Vegetations were present on the tricuspid valve in 9 of the 10 patients with IE involving both right- and left-sided cardiac valves (Figs. 6 and 7), and in 8 of them the IE appeared to have initially involved the tricuspid valve. In 1

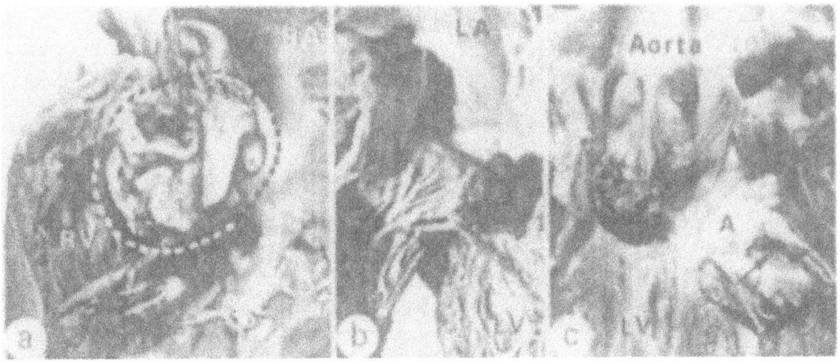

Fig. 6.—*Diplococcus pneumoniae* endocarditis involving the right- and left-sided cardiac valves in a 55-year-old male chronic alcoholic (A74–108). Although symptoms of acute pneumonia had appeared 2 weeks earlier, he was not hospitalized until 1 day before death, when signs of extensive pneumonia and meningitis were obvious. Cultures of both blood and spinal fluid were positive. **a,** opened right atrium *(RA),* tricuspid valve and right ventricle *(RV)* showing a large vegetation *(circle)* on the valve. **b,** opened left atrium *(LA),* mitral valve and left ventricle *(LV).* A large vegetation is present on the anterior leaflet. **c,** opened aorta, aortic valve and left ventricle *(LV).* A vegetation is present on the right aortic valve cusp. In addition, a perforation *(arrow)* is present in the anterior mitral leaflet *(A).*

patient, vegetations were present on the pulmonic and mitral valves. Among the 10 patients with IE involving both right- and left-sided cardiac valves, 8 had vegetations on the mitral valve and 7 on the aortic valve.

IE appeared to have caused tricuspid regurgitation in 8 of the 22 patients with tricuspid valve vegetations. Each of these 8 patients had tears or defects in the tricuspid valve leaflets and ruptured chordae tendineae. IE caused aortic regurgitation in 6 of the 7 patients with aortic valve vegetations and mitral regurgitation in 2 of the 8 patients with mitral vegetations. Large vegetations appeared to obstruct the tricuspid valve orifice in 2 patients (Fig. 1).

Valve ring abscesses were present in 4 of the 22 patients with tricuspid valve vegetations: 2 of them had isolated tricuspid valve IE; the other 2 also had aortic valve vegetations and aortic ring abscess. In 2 patients, the tricuspid ring abscess burrowed into the membranous ventricular septum (Fig. 4) and in another patient the ring abscess burrowed through the right atrial wall into the pericardial sac.

Acute myocardial lesions were present in 13 of the 23 patients, including 6 of the 13 patients with isolated right-sided vegetations (Fig. 5). Each of these 13 patients had microscopic-sized foci of interstitial and perivascular inflammation, and 10 of them also had microscopic-sized myocardial abscesses. Septic emboli were present in the lumina of intramural coronary arteries in 7 patients, 6 of whom had vegetations on left-sided cardiac valves.

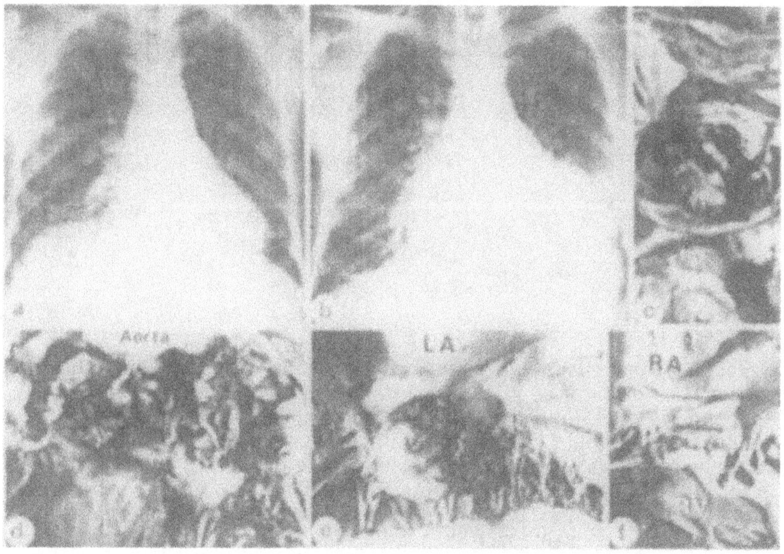

Fig. 7.—Alpha streptococcus endocarditis involving right- and left-sided cardiac valves in a 43-year-old man (A72-226). Hematuria and edema appeared 2 years before death and a renal biopsy showed resolving glomerulonephritis. Ten months later, a murmur of aortic regurgitation and signs of congestive cardiac failure appeared, but blood cultures were negative. Six months before death, fever and myalgias appeared, the serum complement was low and a test for rheumatoid factor was positive. Fever persisted and signs of congestive cardiac failure increased, but blood cultures continued to be negative throughout life. **a,** chest roentgenogram 2 years before death and **b,** 1 month before death. **c,** aortic valve as viewed from above. **d,** opened aorta, aortic valve and left ventricle *(LV)*. Vegetations are present on all three aortic valve cusps and each has been severely damaged by the infection. Postmortem culture of one aortic valve vegetation was positive for alpha streptococcus. Vegetative material also is present on the anterior mitral leaflet. **e,** opened left atrium *(LA)*, mitral valve and left ventricle. A large vegetation is present on the anterior mitral leaflet. **f,** opened right atrium *(RA)*, tricuspid valve and right ventricle *(RV)*. A vegetation is present on the anterior tricuspid leaflet.

Septic infarcts were present in the lungs in 19 of the 23 patients. In contrast, infarcts were present in other organs in only 4 patients, all of whom had vegetations on left-sided cardiac valves.

Splenomegaly (> 300 gm) was present in 9 of the 19 patients in whom the spleen weight was known, excluding 2 patients with hematologic malignancy. In 6 of the 13 patients with isolated right-sided vegetations, the spleen weighed more than 300 gm.

Comments on Right-Sided Infective Endocarditis

Certain features of right-sided IE are evident from our data and from review of previous reports on this subject. (1) It is considerably less frequent than left-sided IE. (2) The clinical presentation usually is that of acute pneumonia, not heart disease, and precordial murmurs often are absent. (3) Predisposing factors nearly always are present, the most frequent being opiate addiction, habitual alcoholism and malignant neoplasm. (4) It usually is caused by a highly virulent organism. *Staphylococcus aureus* or *Diplococcus pneumoniae* are causative in about 75% of the patients. (5) The involved right-sided valve nearly always is both anatomically and functionally normal before the onset of IE. (6) The tricuspid valve is involved in 95% of the patients and the pulmonic valve in only 5%. (7) About half the patients also have infection of left-sided cardiac valves.

As early as 1856, Rokitansky[1] wrote that the frequency of right-sided IE was rare compared to the frequency of left-sided IE. In 1885, Osler[2] reported vegetations on right-sided cardiac valves in 34 of more than 200 patients with IE, and in only 9 of them were vegetations limited to right-sided cardiac valves. In the early 1900s, Preble,[3] Clawson[4] and Thayer[5] found vegetations on right-sided cardiac valves in from 5% to 10% of necropsy patients with IE and in 1942 Goldburgh and associates[6] found right-sided vegetations in 53 (8%) of 646 necropsy patients with IE. Following the introduction of penicillin in 1943, however, Wilson[7] found a statistically significant increase in the incidence of right-sided IE. Right-sided vegetations were present in 17% of our 137 necropsy patients with active IE and in 23% of our patients with infection of natural cardiac valves, excluding 6 patients with congenital shunt lesions.

Two major reasons have been advanced as the explanation for the lower incidence of right-sided compared to left-sided IE. The first is that pressures in the right side of the heart are lower and there appears to be a direct relationship between the pressure on a valve and the frequency with which that valve becomes infected. Allen[8] and, later, Lepeschkin[9] showed that the frequency of right-sided compared to left-sided valve vegetations was numerically very near the ratio of right-to-left ventricular systolic pressure. The second explanation for the lower incidence of right-sided IE is the lower incidence of other diseases affecting the right-sided valves compared to the left-sided ones.[10] Deformed valves are particularly prone to be sites of vegetations and the tricuspid and pulmonic valves are less frequently deformed than their left-sided counterparts.[11, 12]

Patients with right-sided IE usually present with acute pneumonia rather than with symptoms of cardiac disease.[6, 13] Of our 23 patients with vegetations on right-sided cardiac valves, 20 had pulmonary infiltrates on chest roentgenogram and septic pulmonary infarcts were present in the lung at necropsy in 19 of them. Only 8 (35%) of the 23 patients had murmurs from right-sided valvular dysfunction. In each of these 8 patients, IE had caused destruction of the tricuspid valve leaflets and rupture of chordae tendineae. Although the infection was caused by highly virulent organisms in 14 of the other 15 patients, none had extensive damage to the valve apparatus. The lower pressures in the right side of the heart probably also account for the lower frequency of severe leaflet destruction in right-sided compared to left-sided IE.[11]

Right-sided IE usually is caused by highly virulent bacteria, and circumstances associated with an increased risk of developing IE almost always are present.[15-17] Opiate addiction, a well-recognized predisposing factor to infection on either side of the heart,[18-23] was present in 6 (26%) of our patients with right-sided vegetations. *Staphylococcus aureus*, the most frequent cause of IE among opiate addicts,[19-21, 24-29] caused the infection in each. *S. aureus* was the causative organism in 15 of 16 patients with heroin-associated tricuspid valve endocarditis reviewed by Louria and associates.[20] Of 62 opiate addicts with fatal IE reviewed by Sapira,[21] *S. aureus* was the causative organism in 9 of 13 patients (69%) with isolated right-sided vegetations. In 1958, Bain and associates[16] reported 23 necropsy patients with right-sided IE observed at the Mayo Clinic between 1910 and 1955; staphylococcus was the causative organism in 11 of their 19 patients in whom the organism was identified. Among 104 patients with staphylococcal endocarditis reviewed by Dowling and associates,[30] 25% had vegetations on right-sided cardiac valves.

Nine of our 23 patients (39%) with right-sided IE were habitual alcoholics, and *Diplococcus pneumoniae* caused the infection in each.[31] Seven of these 9 patients presented with acute pneumococcal meningitis and in 4 it was fatal. In 1904, Preble[3] reviewed 141 cases of pneumococcal endocarditis and found vegetations on right-sided cardiac valves in 18% of them. He calculated that the pneumococcus infected the tricuspid valve 20 times more often than all other organisms combined. Among 646 necropsy patients with IE studied at the Philadelphia General Hospital, Goldburgh and associates[6] found vegetations on right-sided cardiac valves in 53 (8%); in 62 patients, the infection was caused by pneumococcus and in 9 (15%) of them vegetations were limited to the tricuspid valve. Straus and Hamburger[32] reported 15 patients seen at the Cincinnati General Hospital with pneumococcal endocarditis, 3 (20%) of whom had involvement of the tricuspid valve. Thirteen (87%) of their 15 patients also had pneumococcal meningitis. Of the 141 patients reported by Preble,[3] 60% also had pneumococcal meningitis.

Patients with right-sided IE almost always have vegetations on the tricuspid valve,[6, 7, 9, 16, 17, 19-25] and the involved valve, with rare exception, is anatomically and functionally normal before the onset of IE.[15-17, 19-29] In 22 (96%) of our 23 patients, vegetations were present on the tricuspid valve and on the pulmonic valve in only 1. In each of the 23 patients, the involved valve(s), as well as the uninvolved valves, were normal before the onset of IE. Of 54 patients with active bacterial endocarditis (82% caused by *Staphylococcus aureus*) reported by Pankey,[33] 34 (67%) had no underlying cardiac disease and in 29% the tricuspid valve was involved. Rheumatic tricuspid valve disease is uncommon and, when present, the mitral valve always is stenotic, and often the aortic valve is involved also.[11, 12] IE rarely involves hearts with deformed right- and left-sided valves; when it does, it almost always attacks one or both left-sided valves and spares the right-sided valves. Infection of congenitally malformed, particularly stenotic, pulmonic valves, although described,[34-37] is rare.

Patients with infection on right-sided cardiac valves frequently also have vegetations on left-sided cardiac valves.[2-6, 15-17, 38] Ten (43%) of our 23 patients with right-sided vegetations also had left-sided valvular infection, and among these patients signs of left-sided valvular infection predominated. Seven had signs of left-sided valvular dysfunction and left ventricular failure and 4 had systemic emboli with gross infarcts in other organs.

Splenomegaly is as common in patients with isolated right-sided vegetations as it is in patients with left-sided vegetations. Splenomegaly (> 300 gm) was present at necropsy in 9 of our 23 patients in whom the spleen weight was known, including 6 of the 13 patients with isolated right-sided vegetations. Infection appears to be a more important cause of splenomegaly than congestive failure. In 1922, Arnett[39] analyzed the frequency of splenomegaly among 286 necropsy patients dying from IE, from nonendocardial streptococcal infections or from congestive heart failure due to causes other than IE. He found that although splenomegaly was quite frequent among the patients with IE, it was more frequent among patients with nonendocardial streptococcal infections than among patients with congestive heart failure from causes other than IE.

INFECTIVE ENDOCARDITIS LIMITED TO ONE OR BOTH LEFT-SIDED CARDIAC VALVES

Seventy-four (54%) of our 137 necropsy patients had vegetations limited to one or both left-sided cardiac valves: 22 had vegetations only on the mitral valve and 52 had vegetations on the aortic valve, alone (34 patients) or in combination with the mitral valve (18 patients). Clinical and necropsy observations in these 74 patients are summarized in Tables 3–5, and certain morphologic features in them are illustrated in Figures 8–25.

Underlying valvular disease was present in 33 (45%) and 5 had associated coronary heart disease. Signs and symptoms of IE were present from 2 to 420 days (avg 86). Fever (> 100° F) was the most frequent sign, present in 69 patients (93%). Precordial murmurs were present in 65 patients (88%): new murmurs in 42, changed murmurs in 2 and murmurs unchanged from those present before infection in 21. Nine patients had no

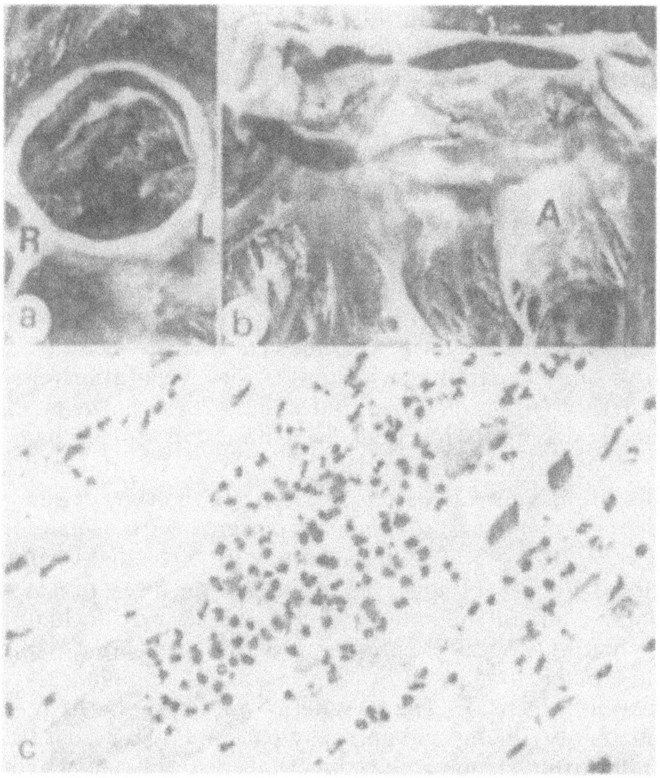

Fig. 8.—*Staphylococcus aureus* endocarditis involving a congenitally bicuspid aortic valve in a 55-year-old woman (A66–62). She had never had symptoms of heart disease when chills, fever and mental confusion appeared 4½ months before death. Blood cultures were positive for *S. aureus*, and penicillin, 40 million units per day intravenously for 4 weeks followed by 24 million units per day intramuscularly for 2 weeks was given. A grade 4/6 early diastolic blowing murmur appeared, and the diastolic blood pressure fell to 20 mm Hg. Six days after penicillin was stopped, she had a shaking chill and blood cultures again were positive for *S. aureus*. Over the next 3 months, she was treated with various combinations of penicillin, methicillin, cephalothin and vancomycin but each time antibiotics were withdrawn, blood cultures again grew *S. aureus*. Signs of congestive cardiac failure increased progressively, the diastolic pressure rose to 60 mm Hg and the aortic regurgitation became almost inaudible several days before death. **a,** bicuspid aortic valve viewed from above. Both the right *(R)* and left *(L)* coronaries arise from the anterior sinus. **b,** opened aortic valve and left ventricle. Discrete perforations are present in both aortic valve cusps. *A* = anterior mitral leaflet. **c,** histologic section showing microabscess in left ventricular wall (hematoxylin and eosin stain; ×400).

precordial murmurs. Dermal petechiae were present in 47% and palpable spleens in 33%. Other clinical signs of IE were less frequent. Major central nervous system complications occurred in 30 patients: 20 had embolic strokes and 10 had acute meningitis. Acute pneumonia was present in 13 patients. High-degree conduction defects occurred in 6 patients with aortic valve vegetations: complete heart block in 4, Mobitz II atrioventricular

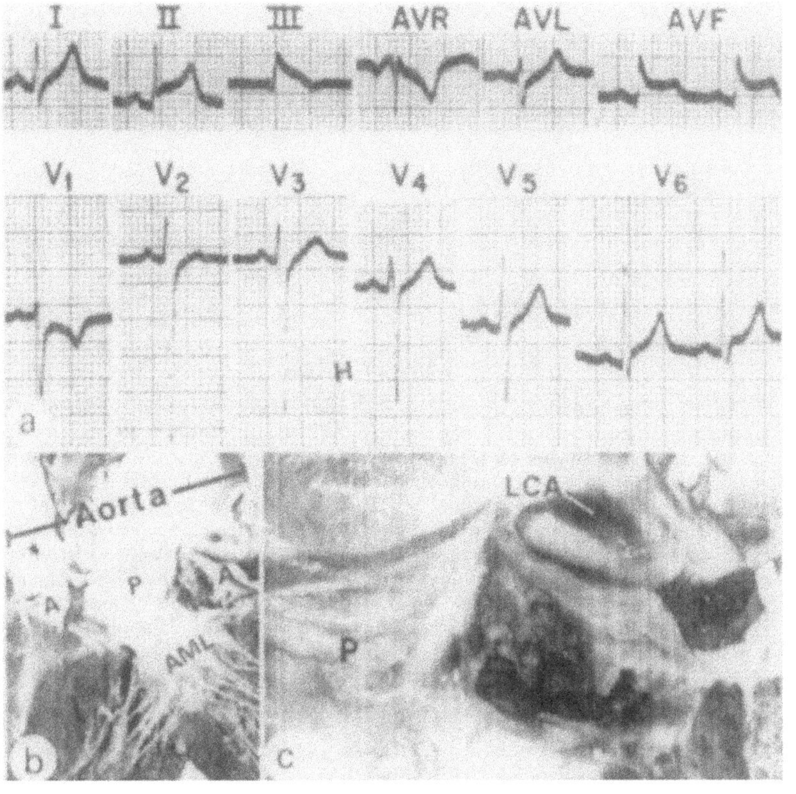

Fig. 9.—Beta hemolytic streptococcus endocarditis in a 40-year-old man (A56–95) with previous mild aortic regurgitation from a congenitally bicuspid aortic valve. Chills, fever and symptoms of congestive cardiac failure began 1 week after a dental procedure. Examination disclosed dermal petechiae, sublingual hemorrhages, Osler's nodes and a loud murmur of aortic regurgitation. Blood cultures were positive. One week after hospitalization, he complained of chest pain and electrocardiogram **(a)** showed ST–T changes of acute pericarditis. Despite antibiotics, signs of left ventricular failure increased and he died 35 days after the onset of symptoms of infection. **b,** opened aortic valve and left ventricle showing a destroyed anterior *(A)* coronary cusp and a large ring abscess at the base of the anterior mitral leaflet *(AML)*. *P* = posterior aortic valve cusp. **c,** close-up of the aortic valve cusp. *LCA* = left coronary arterial ostium. A fibrino-hemorrhagic exudate was present on the epicardium.

block in 1 and complete right bundle-branch block in 1. One patient with isolated mitral valve vegetations had complete heart block.

► ANTONIO C. DE LEON, JR.: The 9 patients with left-sided cardiac valve involvement without any precordial murmur are of special interest. Although acute severe mitral regurgitation may result in a less than holosystolic murmur, it is less likely to result in total absence of a murmur. Acute severe aortic regurgitation, however, can result in markedly elevated left ventricular diastolic pressure and is the more likely cause of cases where no precordial murmurs are noted.

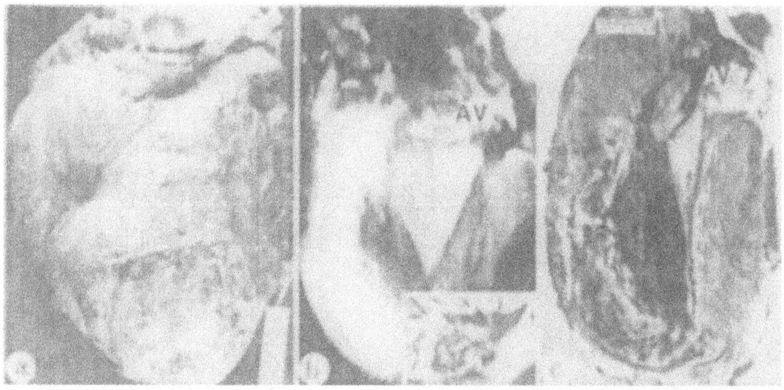

Fig. 10.—*Staphylococcus aureus* endocarditis involving a calcified stenotic 3-cusped aortic valve in a 67-year-old man (A72 - 281). Although asymptomatic, he was known to have had a grade 2/6 aortic systolic ejection murmur for 3 years. Chills and fever appeared 6 weeks before death and blood cultures were positive. Three days later, he sustained an acute anterolateral myocardial infarction followed by the development of a pericardial friction rub. He died suddenly 4 weeks later. **a,** anterior view of the heart. Diffuse fibrinous pericarditis is present. **b,** postmortem roentgenogram of the heart showing heavy calcific deposits in the aortic valve *(AV)*. Inset, vegetation on one aortic valve cusp. **c,** longitudinal cut through the aortic valve *(AV)* and left ventricle showing a huge transmural myocardial infarct with superimposed mural thrombus

► W. PROCTOR HARVEY: The significant incidence (39%) of patients with right-sided infective endocarditis due to *Diplococcus pneumoniae*, especially in chronic alcoholics, is an important reminder to us to be on the alert for this possibility in the alcoholic.

In addition, as documented by the authors in the next paragraph, the alcoholic and the dope addict were the most susceptible to *left*-sided endocarditis involving one or both previously *normal* valves.

Concerning symptoms and signs: fever and a murmur were the most common findings. When these are present, the possibility of infectious endocarditis should be carefully tracked down. Of importance also is to record temperatures rectally. All too often a fever is overlooked or thought unimportant because oral temperatures not properly taken miss this clinical finding. An older observation as a sign of infective endocarditis is a "changing" murmur. This is not, in my experience, one of the frequent signs that we can "hang our hats on," as most patients have not shown this. This is also evident by the authors' correlation of the pathologic material with the clinical findings.

Circumstances associated with an increased risk of developing IE were present in 53 patients (72%), including 34 (83%) of the 41 patients with previously normal cardiac valves. Habitual alcoholism (17 patients = 23%) and opiate addiction (10 patients = 14%) were the two most frequent predisposing factors. Other important predisposing factors were malignant neoplasm (7 patients), dental procedures (5 patients), genitourinary procedures (5 patients) and skin infections (5 patients).

The infecting organisms (Table 4) were identified in 58 pa-

TABLE 4.–ACTIVE INFECTIVE ENDOCARDITIS (IE) INVOLVING ONLY LEFT-SIDED CARDIAC VALVES: CAUSATIVE ORGANISMS AND STATUS OF VALVES BEFORE IE

CAUSATIVE ORGANISM	NO. PTS.	STATUS OF VALVE BEFORE IE Anatomically Normal	Anatomically Abnormal
I. Bacterium	54	29	25
Staphylococcus aureus	17	11	6
Staphylococcus epidermidis	3	1	2
Alpha streptococcus	9	2	7
Beta streptococcus	4	1	3
Streptococcus faecalis	8	6	2
Streptococcus bovis	1	0	1
Diplococcus pneumoniae	8	5	3
Escherichia coli	1	1	0
Diphtheroids	1	1	0
Peptostreptococcus	1	0	1
Serratia marcescens	1	1	0
II. Fungus	4	3	1
Candida paropsilosis	2	2	0
Cryptococcus neoformans	1	0	1
Histoplasma capsulatum	1	1	0
III. Unknown	16*	9	7
TOTAL	74	41	33†

*No blood cultures = 7; negative blood cultures = 7; information unavailable = 2.
†Functionally abnormal also in 29 of the 33.

tients, 57 of whom had positive blood cultures during life. Among these 58 patients, bacteria caused the IE in 54. *Staphylococcus aureus* was the most frequent infecting organism (17 patients = 23%) and more often infected a previously normal valve (11 patients) than a previously abnormal valve (6 patients). *Diplococcus pneumoniae* or *Streptococcus faecalis* caused IE in 16 patients, 11 of whom previously had had normal valves. In contrast, among 9 patients with alpha streptococcus endocarditis, only 2 previously had had normal valves. IE was caused by a gram-negative bacterium in 2 patients and by a variety of other gram-positive bacteria in 10 patients. Fungi caused the IE in 4 patients, but in 3 of them the heart was only one of many organs involved by a generalized fungal infection. Seven patients (9%) had negative blood cultures and 9 patients never had blood cultures. Forty-five patients (61%) died from cardiovascular effects of the IE: congestive heart failure in 40 patients, each of whom had signs of severe valvular dysfunction; arrhythmia in 2 patients; coronary arterial embolism, cardiac tamponade and pulmonary embolism in 1 patient each. Seventeen patients (23%) died from central nervous system complications of IE: embolism in 12 and acute meningitis in 5. Seven patients died from generalized infection and 5 from miscellaneous causes unrelated to IE.

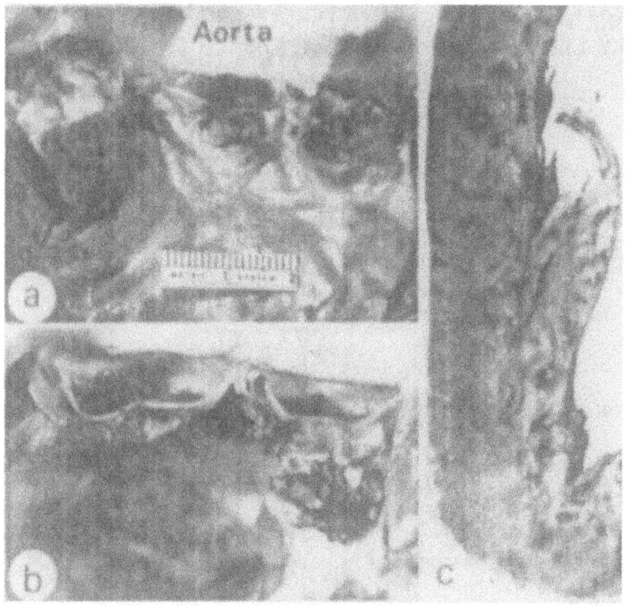

Fig. 11.—*Staphylococcus aureus* aortic valve endocarditis in a 31-year-old male heroin addict (A72 169) Chills and fever appeared 8 days before death and he was hospitalized 4 days later with signs of acute meningitis. Cultures of blood and spinal fluid were positive for *S. aureus* but no precordial murmur was heard and endocarditis was never suspected. **a,** opened aorta, aortic valve and left ventricle. Vegetations are present on all 3 cusps of the previously normal aortic valve. **b,** opened aortic valve viewed from above. The cusps are not destroyed by the vegetations. **c,** section of left ventricular wall including papillary muscle. The papillary muscle is focally necrotic and multiple small abscesses are present in the myocardium.

Necropsy findings.—Among the 74 patients, 92 cardiac valves were infected: the aortic only in 34, the mitral only in 22 and the aortic and mitral in 18. In at least 13 of the last 18 patients, however, the mitral infection appeared to be secondary to the aortic infection. Among the other 5 patients with infection of both aortic and mitral valves, 2 had rheumatic disease of both valves, 1 had degenerative disease of the aortic valve and heavy calcific deposits in the mitral anulus and 1 previously had had normal valves; the remaining patient had a floppy mitral valve, and only in this patient was it certain that the infection appeared initially on the mitral valve. For this reason, patients with vegetations on both left-sided valves are considered together with patients having vegetations limited to the aortic valve.

Among the 52 patients with aortic valve IE (Figs. 8–19), 26 (50%) had anatomically normal and 26 (50%) had anatomically abnormal aortic valves before the onset of IE. Of the latter 26 patients, 23 had functionally abnormal aortic valves (stenosis = 16 and pure regurgitation = 7) before the onset of IE. The most common cause of the underlying aortic valvular disease was

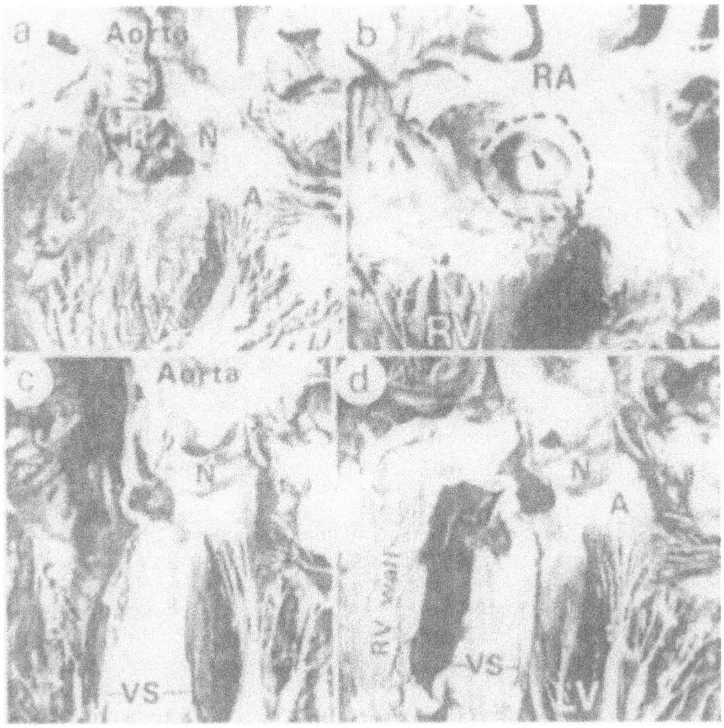

Fig. 12. – *Staphylococcus epidermidis* aortic valve endocarditis in a 17-year-old boy (A69–42). Massive aortic regurgitation and right bundle-branch block developed during the infection and he died 28 days after the onset of symptoms. **a,** opened aortic valve and left ventricle. The right *(R)* coronary cusp is destroyed by the infection and a ring abscess is present behind this cusp. *N* and *L* = non- and left coronary cusps; *A* = anterior mitral leaflet; *LV* = left ventricle. **b,** opened right atrium *(RA)*, tricuspid valve and right ventricle *(RV)* showing a bulging membranous ventricular septum *(circle)* with a perforation in its center. **c,** longitudinal section through the aneurysm in the ventricular septum *(VS)*. **d,** longitudinal section anterior to **c** showing a ring abscess in the muscular portion of the ventricular septum.

congenital malformation: bicuspid valve in 9 patients, unicommissural valve in 1 and discrete subaortic stenosis in 2. Degenerative aortic valve disease was the second most frequent cause of the underlying valve disease (5 patients) and was present in 4 of our 5 patients older than 65 years of age. Four patients had rheumatic disease of the aortic valve (each also had rheumatic mitral disease) and 2 had aortic valve disease of uncertain etiology. Three patients had aortic valve deformity from a previous episode of IE and in each of them the valve appeared to have been normal before the first episode of IE.

The IE caused severe leaflet damage in 37 (71%) of the 52 patients with aortic valve vegetations: 21 had discrete perforations of one or more aortic valve cusps and 16 had destruction of aortic valvular tissue without discrete perforations. The IE caused

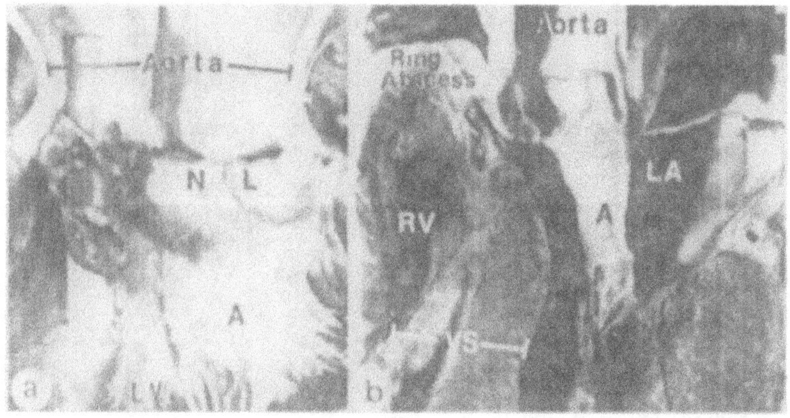

Fig. 13.—*Diplococcus pneumoniae* aortic valve endocarditis in a 36-year-old alcoholic woman (A72-106). She presented to the hospital with signs of acute meningitis and positive blood cultures. With penicillin therapy, the signs of meningitis cleared. A murmur of aortic regurgitation appeared, however, and it was followed by signs of left ventricular failure. She died 42 days after the onset of symptoms of infection. **a,** opened aortic valve showing perforation of the right coronary cusp. *N* and *L* = non- and left coronary cusps; *A* = anterior mitral leaflet; *LV* = left ventricle. **b,** longitudinal section showing a ring abscess behind the right aortic valve cusp. *A* = anterior mitral leaflet; *RV* = right ventricle; *LA* = left atrium; *VS* = ventricular septum

aortic regurgitation in 36 of these patients and aortic stenosis in 1. In the other 15 patients, the aortic valve vegetations caused no functional damage to the cusps. At necropsy, the aortic valve appeared to have been functionally abnormal in 45 of the 52 patients: from IE alone in 22, from IE plus underlying valve defor-

Fig. 14.—*Candida paropsilosis* endocarditis involving the aortic valve of a 26-year-old male heroin addict (A60-36). This patient lived for 8 months after initial symptoms and signs of infective endocarditis appeared. He had an embolus to the left anterior descending coronary artery with a huge transmural acute myocardial infarct 2 months before death. **a,** aortic valve viewed from above. The large vegetations appear to obstruct the valve orifice. **b,** opened valve showing vegetations on each cusp. **c,** photomicrograph of vegetation showing pseudomycelia of *C. paropsilosis* (methenamine silver stain; ×775).

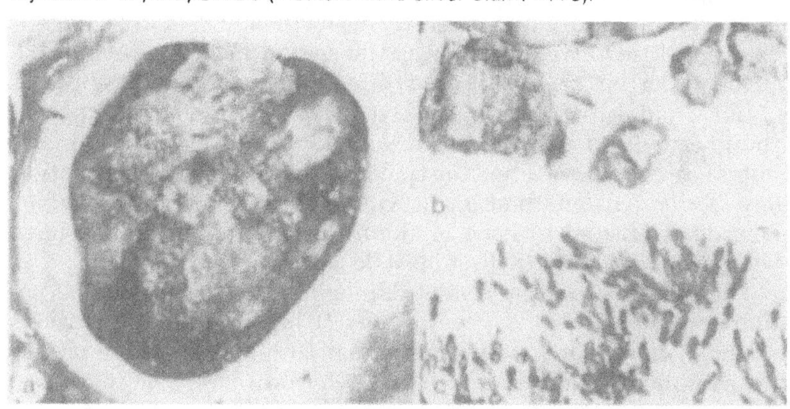

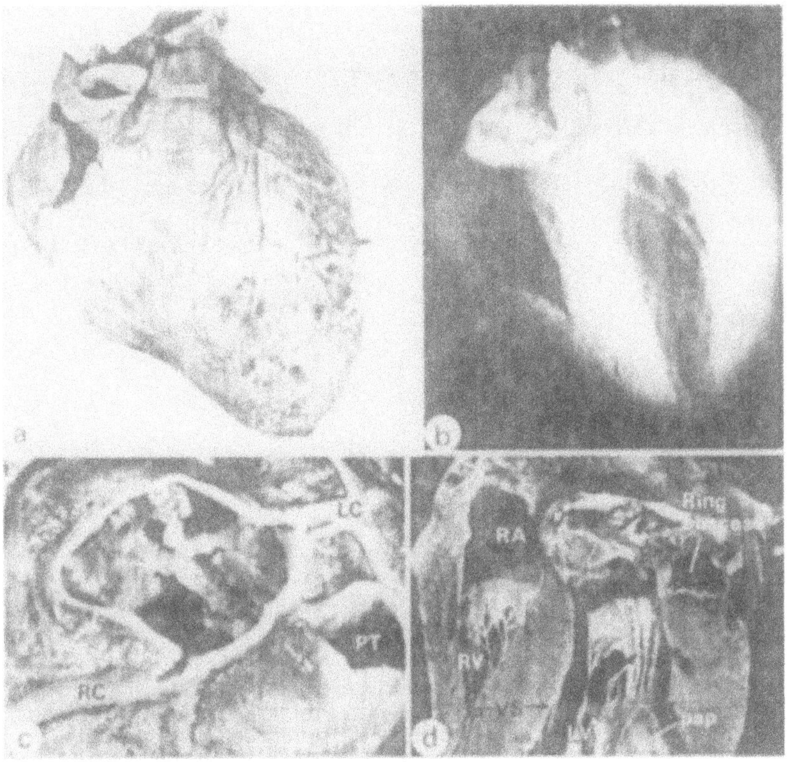

Fig. 15.—Alpha streptococcus endocarditis involving a calcified, stenotic, congenitally bicuspid aortic valve in a 54-year-old man (A75–55). Fever and syncope occurred several weeks after tooth extraction, and blood cultures were positive. Despite antibiotic therapy, signs of left ventricular failure increased, and he died 23 days after the onset of symptoms of infection. **a,** anterior view of the heart showing focal fibrinous pericarditis. **b,** postmortem roentgenogram of the heart. A large amount of calcium is present in the aortic valve. **c,** bicuspid aortic valve viewed from above. *RC* = right coronary artery; *LC* = left coronary artery; *PT* = pulmonary trunk. **d,** longitudinal section through the aortic valve, right atrium *(RA),* tricuspid valve *(TV),* right ventricle *(RV),* ventricular septum *(VS)* and left ventricle *(LV).* A large ring abscess is present. Vegetations are also present on several mitral valve chordae tendineae *(arrow).* The tip of the papillary muscle *(pap)* is necrotic. The pericarditis probably resulted from rupture of the right abscess into the pericardial space.

mity in 18 and from underlying valve deformity alone in 5. Seven patients appeared to have had normal valve function despite the presence of vegetations.

Valve ring abscess was present in 22 (42%) of the 52 patients with aortic valve vegetations. The IE had caused severe leaflet destruction in each of these 22 patients and interruption of major conduction tissue in 5 of them. In 11 of the 22 patients, the aortic ring abscess had ruptured into the pericardial space, causing pericarditis.

Of the 52 patients with aortic valve vegetations, 18 also had vegetations on the mitral valve (Figs. 15–19): in 13 of them, the

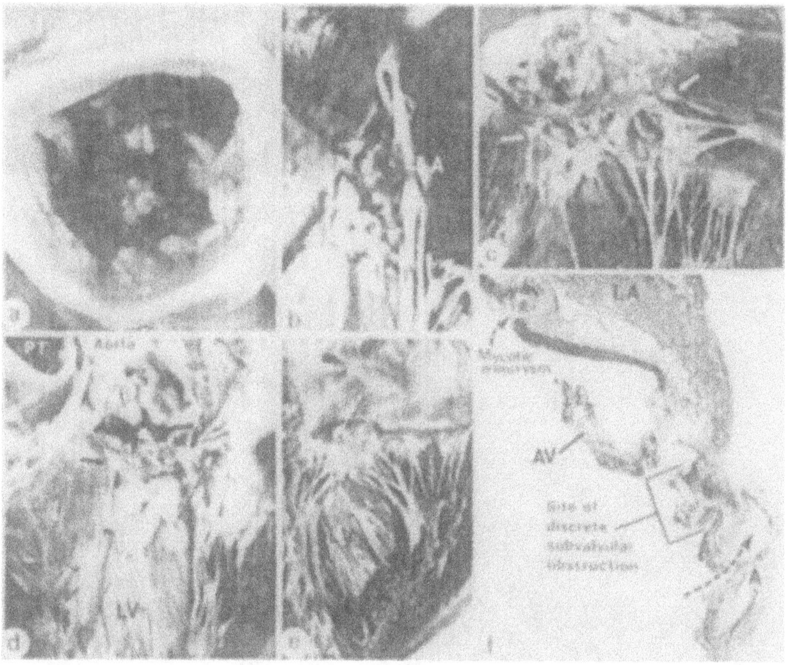

Fig. 16.—Alpha hemolytic streptococcus endocarditis complicating congenital discrete subaortic stenosis in a 28-year-old man (A64–20). The infection, which appeared about 9 months before death, produced severe valvular aortic regurgitation. **a,** aortic valve as viewed from above. **b,** left ventricular outflow tract viewed from below, showing vegetative material on the subvalvular "membrane" adjacent to the anterior mitral leaflet *(A)*. **c,** opened left ventricular outflow tract showing vegetations on each aortic cusp and on the subvalvular "membrane" *(between the solid arrows)* and ventricular surface of anterior mitral leaflet. **d,** longitudinal section showing the left ventricular outflow tract. The area of subaortic stenosis is well seen *(between the solid arrows)* and a mycotic aneurysm *(dashed arrow)* is seen in the anterior mitral leaflet. The mitral aneurysm is in the high pressure portion of the left ventricle *(LV)*, i.e., below the discrete subvalvular obstruction. *PT* = pulmonary trunk. **e,** opened mitral valve showing the atrial aspect of the mycotic aneurysm *(dashed arrow)* on the anterior leaflet. **f,** photomicrograph of section through the aorta, left atrium *(LA)*, aortic valve *(AV)* cusp, subvalvular "membrane" and anterior mitral leaflet *(A)*. A mycotic aneurysm is present in the ascending aorta as well as in the anterior mitral leaflet *(dashed arrows)*. Vegetations are present on the aortic valve cusp and on the subvalvular membrane (hematoxylin and eosin stain; ×3.2).

mitral vegetations caused significant damage to the mitral apparatus and in the other 5 insignificant damage. Of the 13 with significant mitral damage from vegetations, 6 had ruptured chordae tendineae, 3 had defects in the margins of the mitral leaflets (associated with ruptured chordae in 2) and 4 had infected aneurysms of the anterior mitral leaflet. The IE appeared to have caused mitral regurgitation in 9 patients, 6 of whom also had aortic regurgitation.

Twenty-two patients had vegetations confined to the mitral valve (Figs. 20–25). In 15 of them, the mitral valve leaflets ap-

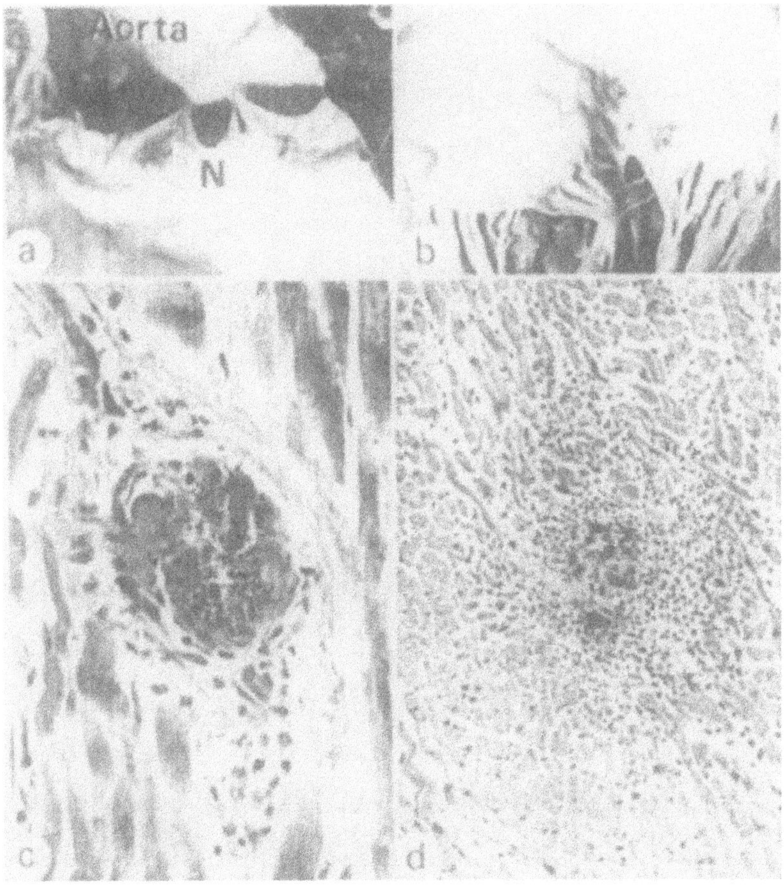

Fig. 17.—*Staphylococcus aureus* endocarditis in a 36-year-old man (A65–8) with mycosis fungoides. Pneumonia, septicemia and renal failure occurred in the terminal phase of his chronic illness, but signs of cardiac dysfunction were never present. **a**, opened aorta and aortic valve. The noncoronary *(N)* cusp is much smaller than the other two cusps, each of which contains vegetations. **b**, opened left atrium, mitral valve and left ventricle. Small vegetations are present at the posteromedial commissure, but there is no valvular destruction. **c**, hematoxylin and eosin stained histologic section of left ventricular myocardium (×400) showing a septic embolus in the lumen of an intramural coronary artery. **d**, hematoxylin and eosin stained section of myocardium (×160) showing a microscopic-sized abscess. The dark material in both **c** and **d** represents colonies of organisms.

peared to have been anatomically normal and in 7 anatomically abnormal before the onset of IE; of the latter, 6 had functioned abnormally (stenosis in 3 and pure regurgitation in 3). One patient with anatomically normal mitral leaflets and chordae had mitral regurgitation from an old myocardial infarct. Of the 7 patients with previously abnormal valves, 6 had rheumatic disease and 1 had a floppy valve.

Fifteen of the 22 patients with isolated mitral valve vegeta-

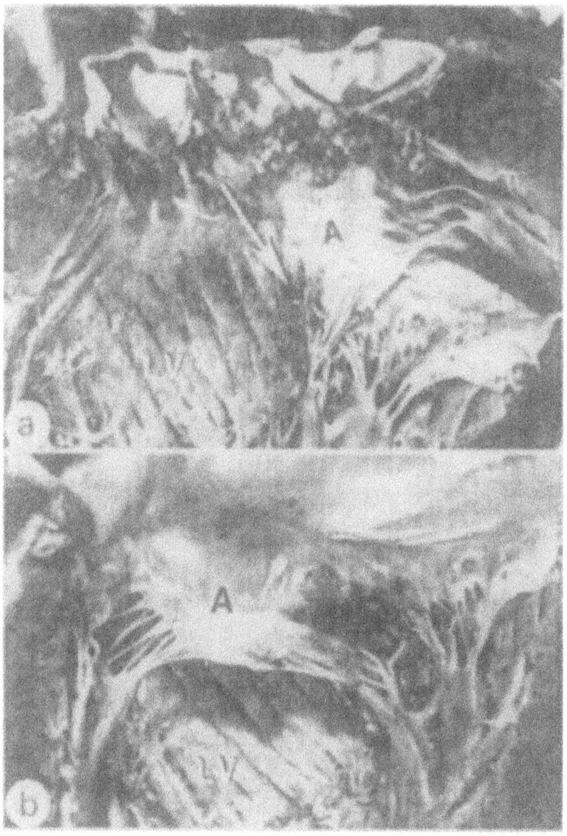

Fig. 18.—*Streptococcus faecalis* endocarditis involving both aortic and mitral valves in a 61-year-old man (A71–120). Symptoms and signs of endocarditis appeared 3 weeks after catheterization of his urinary bladder. Both aortic and mitral valves probably were normal before they became sites of infection. **a,** opened left ventricle *(LV)* and aortic valve. The vegetations have partially destroyed each cusp, causing severe aortic regurgitation. Vegetation on the left ventricular outflow endocardium and mitral leaflet and chordae tendineae almost certainly resulted from retrograde spread of the aortic vegetations by the aortic regurgitant stream *(arrow)*. *A* = anterior mitral leaflet. **b,** opened mitral valve showing vegetations at the posteromedial commissure. A number of chordae tendineae are ruptured

tions had valve dysfunction from the IE. Fourteen developed mitral regurgitation: from leaflet destruction alone in 6, from leaflet destruction and ruptured chordae tendineae in 6 and from ruptured chordae alone in 1. A large vegetation on the anterior leaflet prevented mitral valve closure in another patient. In 1 patient, a huge vegetation obstructed the mitral orifice and also prevented its closure. At necropsy, the mitral valve appeared to have functioned abnormally in 18 patients: from IE alone in 11, from IE plus underlying valve deformity in 4 and from underlying valve deformity alone in 3.

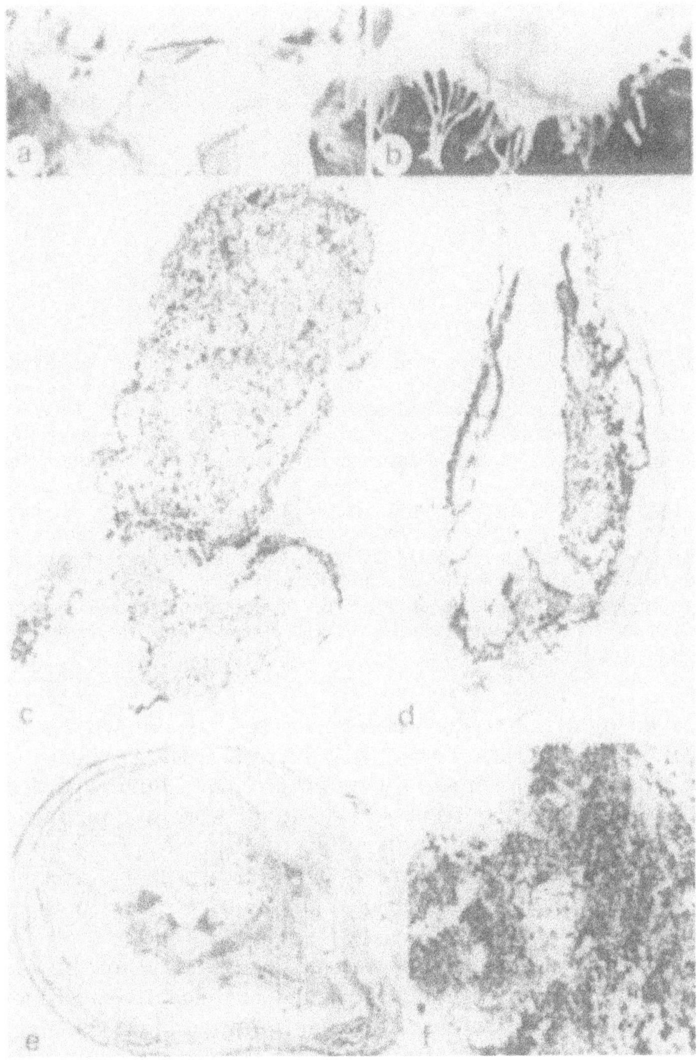

Fig. 19.—Group D streptococcus endocarditis of both aortic and mitral valve in a 56-year-old paraplegic man (A74–63). Chronic urinary tract infection had been present for 1 year before death, and blood cultures intermittently had been positive for Group D streptococcus. One day before death, he was hospitalized because of fever and the sudden appearance of left hemiparesis. Blood cultures again were positive for Group D streptococcus. **a,** opened aortic valve. Small vegetations are present on each of the aortic valve cusps. **b,** opened mitral valve. Vegetations are present along the margin of the anterior leaflet and several chordae tendineae are ruptured. **c,** photomicrograph of aortic valve vegetation. **d,** photomicrograph of ruptured mitral chorda tendineae. The dark staining material represents colonies of gram-positive bacteria. **e,** middle cerebral artery, the lumen of which is occluded by a septic embolus. **f,** histologic section of the embolus shown in **e**. Numerous gram-positive cocci are present. (Brown and Brenn stain [**c, d, f**]; Movat stain [**e**]: ×32 [**c**], ×20 [**d**], ×22 [**e**], ×330 [**f**].)

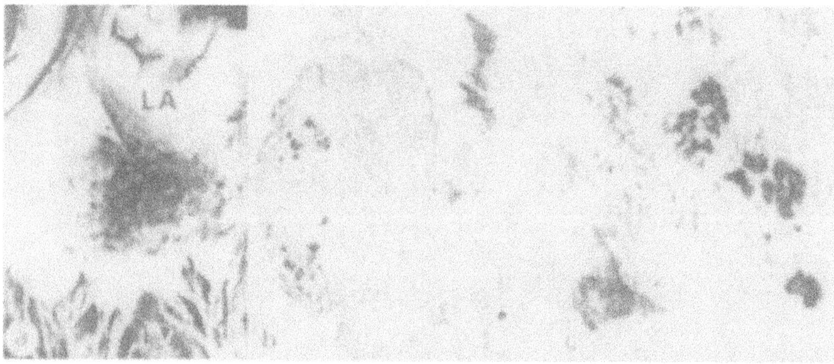

Fig. 20.—*Staphylococcus aureus* mitral valve endocarditis in a 22-year-old drug addict (A75–65). He had acute rheumatic fever at age 13 and murmurs of aortic and mitral regurgitation had been present for several years. He was hospitalized because of fever (105°F), headache, vomiting and mental confusion. Blood cultures were positive and intravenous antibiotics were started. Several days later, he became obtunded and lumbar puncture yielded bloody spinal fluid. He died shortly after the lumbar puncture, and necropsy revealed a large intracerebral hemorrhage. **a,** opened left atrium *(LA)*, mitral valve and left ventricle *(LV)*. The mitral valve leaflets are diffusely thickened and vegetations are present on the posterior leaflet and on left atrial mural endocardium. **b** and **c,** histologic sections of the vegetation. The dark staining material represents gram-positive cocci. (Hematoxylin and eosin stain [**b**] and Brown and Brenn stain [**c**]: ×54 [**b**] and ×350 [**c**].)

Valve ring abscess was present in only 1 patient with isolated mitral valve vegetation (Fig. 24). In this patient, vegetations, located at the posteromedial commissure, had burrowed deeply into the lowermost portion of the atrial septum and into the cephalad portion of the ventricular septum and destroyed the atrioventricular bundle. Another patient with mitral and aortic valve vegetations had an abscess involving a heavily calcified mitral anulus.

Pericarditis was present at necropsy in 16 (22%) of the 74 patients with IE involving only left-sided cardiac valves. Fifteen of the 16 patients had aortic valve vegetations and only 1 had isolated mitral valve vegetations. Among the 16 patients, pericarditis resulted from rupture of an aortic valve ring abscess in 11, from transmural acute myocardial infarction in 2, from rupture of a myocardial abscess into the pericardial space in 1 and from uncertain cause(s) in the remaining 2 patients.

Acute myocardial lesions were present in 56 (85%) of the 66 patients in whom adequate histologic sections were available for examination (Table 5). Myocardial necrosis unassociated with abscess was present in 42 patients (64%). In 26 of them, necrosis was limited to one or both left ventricular papillary muscles; in 14 it involved the left ventricular free wall as well as one or both left ventricular papillary muscles and in 2 patients it was limited to the left ventricular free wall. Myocardial inflammation was present in 41 patients (62%). Twenty-one patients had

TABLE 5. - ACTIVE INFECTIVE ENDOCARDITIS INVOLVING ONLY LEFT-SIDED CARDIAC VALVES: ACUTE MYOCARDIAL LESIONS 56* OF 66† PATIENTS = 85%

MYOCARDIAL LESION		PATIENTS No.	%
I. Necrosis‡		42	(64)
A. Papillary muscle only	26		
B. Papillary muscle + LV free wall	14		
C. Left ventricular free wall only	2		
II. Inflammation		41	(62)
A. Interstitial and perivascular (nonsuppurating myocarditis)	21		
B. Abscesses	7		
C. Both	13		

*Twenty patients with one or more of the myocardial lesions had coronary arterial emboli and 5 other patients had severe coronary atherosclerosis.
†Includes only patients in whom sections of both left ventricular papillary muscles as well as left ventricular free wall and septum were available for examination.
‡Unassociated with myocardial abscesses.

only foci of nonsuppurating interstitial and perivascular inflammation (Bracht-Wächter bodies), 7 patients had only myocardial abscesses and 13 had foci of both suppurating and nonsuppurating myocardial inflammation.

Emboli were present in the lumina of coronary arteries in 23 patients: in intramural coronary arteries only in 16 patients, in both intramural and extramural coronary arteries in 6 patients and in only an extramural coronary artery in 1 patient.

Grossly visible infarcts were present in the viscera of 46 patients (62%). The three most frequently infarcted organs were spleen (33 patients), kidney (31 patients) and brain (27 patients). In addition, 7 patients had hepatic infarcts, 5 had myocardial infarcts, 3 had pulmonary infarcts and 1 each had infarcts in adrenal gland, pancreas and small intestine.

The spleen ranged in weight from 80 to 1000 gm (avg 310); it weighed more than 300 gm in 22 (37%) of the 60 patients in whom the weight was known.

Comments on Left-Sided Infective Endocarditis

Many morphologic observations concerning IE were made in patients dying in the preantibiotic era, when IE was a uniformly fatal disease. Since the introduction of antibiotic therapy, however, a number of important changes have occurred.[7, 40-51] (1) The frequency of rheumatic heart disease as an underlying condition has declined[7, 42, 44-47, 50, 51] and, consequently, the etiologies of the underlying valve disease in patients with IE has changed. (2) The frequency of IE in patients with normal cardiac valves has

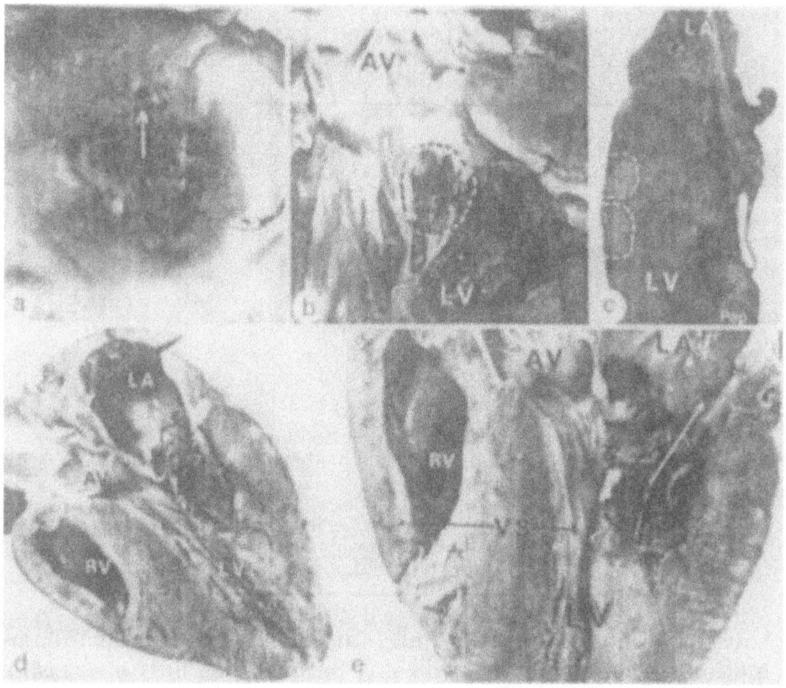

Fig. 21.—*Streptococcus faecalis* mitral valve endocarditis in a 36-year-old male heroin addict (A75–159). Five months before death, he presented with fever and a precordial murmur, and blood cultures were positive. He was treated with antibiotics intravenously, but 4 months later symptoms of congestive heart failure appeared, and blood cultures again were positive for *S. faecalis*. An echocardiogram showed mitral valve vegetations and ruptured chordae tendineae. Despite a second course of intravenous antibiotics, he died from progressive congestive heart failure. **a**, mitral valve viewed from the left atrium. Vegetations are present both on the valve and on the left atrial endocardium *(arrow)*. **b**, opened aortic valve *(AV)* and left ventricle *(LV)*. A perforation *(circle)* is present in the anterior mitral leaflet. **c**, longitudinal cut including portions of left atrial wall *(LA)*, posterior mitral leaflet and left ventricular free wall. A portion of the leaflet curls toward the left atrium. The tip of the papillary muscle *(Pap)* is necrotic and abscesses *(dashed lines)* are present in the left ventricular wall. **d**, longitudinal cut of the heart. There is extensive destruction of the mitral valve. and a portion of the leaflets as well as several ruptured chordae are prolapsed into the left atrium *(LA)*. The papillary muscle is partially necrotic, and multiple abscesses are present in the left ventricular wall. The left atrial cavity is of normal size and the right ventricular *(RV)* wall is thick, suggesting the presence of pulmonary hypertension. **e**, close-up of the mitral valve showing the ruptured chordae and the left atrial mural (jet) vegetations *(arrow)*.

increased.[7, 44, 45, 47, 50, 51] (3) The frequency and mortality of alpha hemolytic streptococcus endocarditis have declined[7, 41, 43, 45, 49, 51] and the frequency of staphylococcal endocarditis has increased.[43, 45, 51] (4) The frequency of aortic valve infection has increased[46, 50] and that of mitral valve infection has decreased.[7, 46] (5) Congestive heart failure has replaced infection as the leading cause of death among patients with IE.[42, 45, 47, 49, 51, 52]

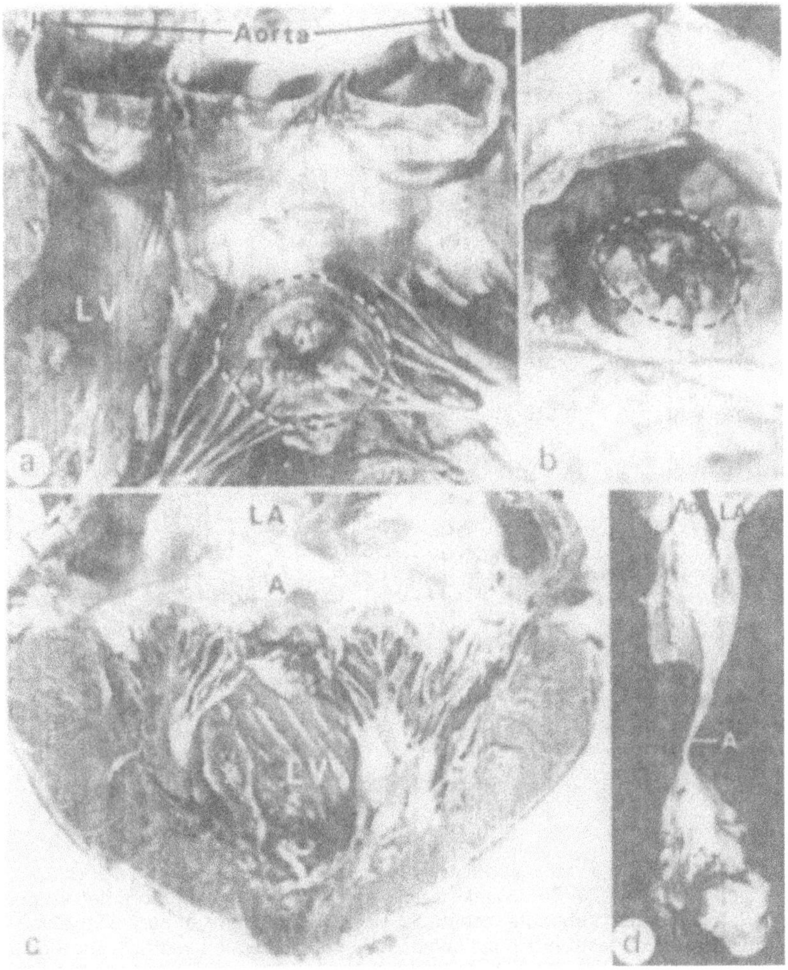

Fig. 22.—*Serratia marcescens* mitral valve endocarditis in a 59-year-old male chronic alcoholic (A75–123). He was hospitalized 16 days before death because of fever and leg pain of sudden onset. Examination disclosed an apical systolic murmur, and an echocardiogram revealed a density between the anterior and posterior mitral valve leaflets. Clinical and roentgenographic signs of acute pneumonia appeared shortly after admission and sputum cultures were positive for *S. marcescens*. Blood cultures were negative until the time of death, but postmortem cultures of the mitral valve vegetation grew *S. marcescens*. **a,** opened aorta, aortic valve and left ventricle *(LV)*. A large perforation *(circle)* is present in the anterior mitral leaflet. **b,** mitral valve with vegetation *(circle)* viewed from the left atrium. **c,** opened left atrium *(LA)*, mitral valve and left ventricle *(LV)*. The large vegetation on the anterior mitral leaflet *(A)* is apparent. **d,** longitudinal section through aorta *(Ao)*, left atrial wall *(LA)*, left coronary cusp *(L)* of aortic valve and anterior mitral leaflet *(A)*, showing the large mitral valve vegetation.

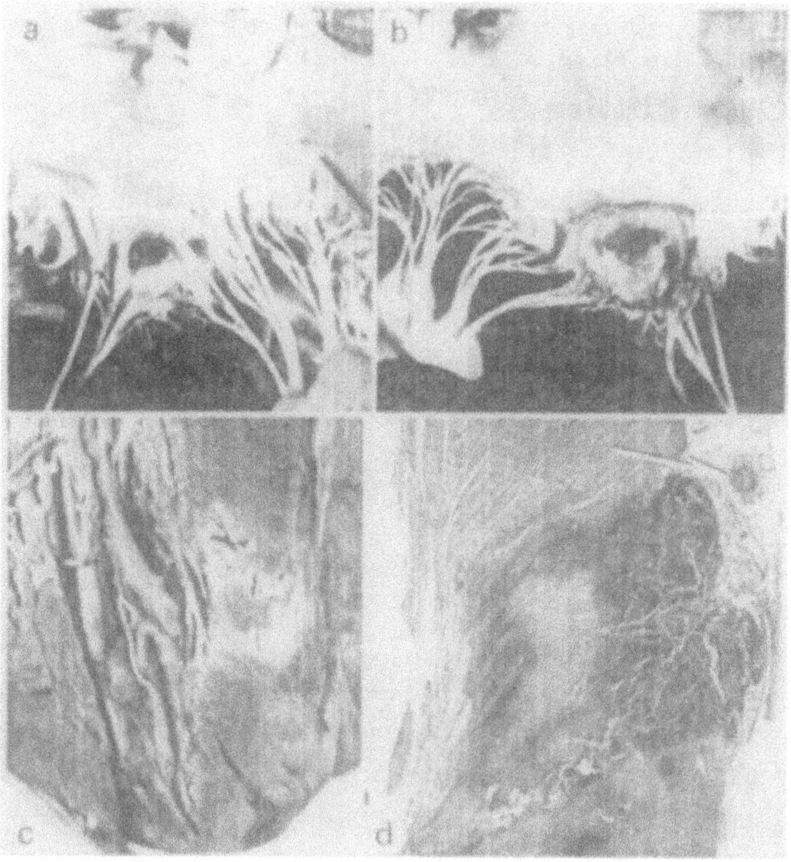

Fig. 23. – Pneumococcal mitral valve endocarditis in a 43-year-old male chronic alcoholic (A71 – 70). Two weeks before death, he was hospitalized because of acute pneumonia and acute meningitis. He never had signs of cardiac dysfunction and died of gastrointestinal hemorrhage. **a,** opened left ventricle showing a small amount of vegetative material on the ventricular surface of the anterior mitral leaflet. **b,** atrial aspect of the anterior mitral leaflet showing a single large vegetation. The valve cusps otherwise are normal. **c,** longitudinal section showing transmural necrosis of the left ventricular wall. **d,** photomicrograph of area in **c** showing extensive myocardial necrosis. An extramural coronary artery *(arrow)* is occluded by vegetative material (hematoxylin and eosin stain; ×2.5).

To emphasize the change in the types of underlying valve disease observed today compared to earlier periods, among our 74 patients, including 22 with isolated mitral valve vegetations, only 10 (13%) had rheumatic valvular disease. Twelve (23%) of the 52 patients with aortic valve vegetations had congenital malformation (bicuspid valves in 9). Only in recent years has it been recognized that isolated aortic valve disease rarely is caused by rheumatic fever.[10, 53-56] Consequently, it is likely that many infected, scarred aortic valves in earlier reports were congenital rather than rheumatic in origin. Of our 5 patients older than 65 years with aortic valve vegetations, 4 had degenerative

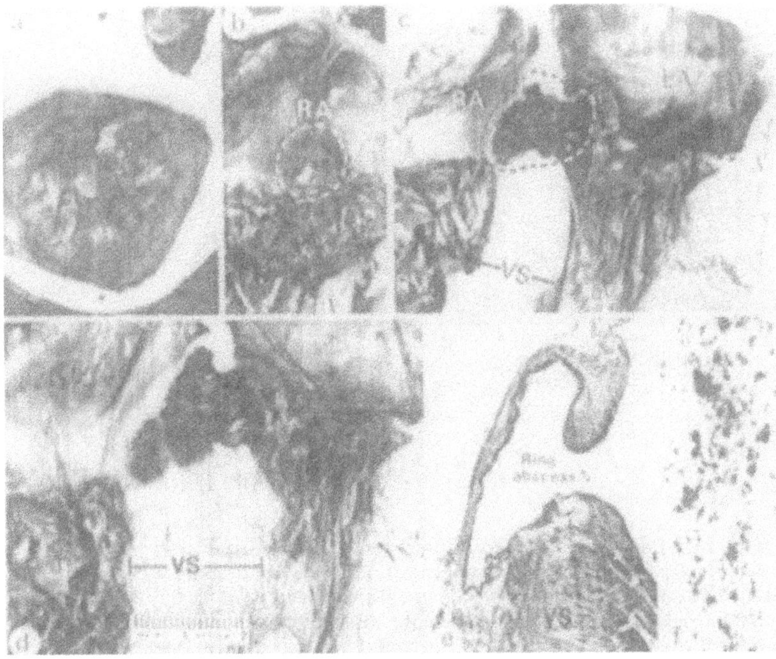

Fig. 24.—*Staphylococcus aureus* mitral valve endocarditis with ring abscess in a 66-year-old diabetic man (A48226). During hospitalization for treatment of an infected foot, fever developed and blood cultures were positive. Complete heart block and a murmur of mitral regurgitation appeared, and he died soon thereafter. **a,** mitral valve viewed from the left atrium. Vegetations are present in the region of the posteromedial commissure. **b,** opened right atrium *(RA),* tricuspid valve and right ventricle *(RV).* Abscess is visible in the membranous septum *(circle).* **c,** longitudinal section through the four cardiac chambers and both atrioventricular valves. The mitral ring abscess *(circle)* has burrowed deeply into the atrial and ventricular septa. *RA* = right atrium; *RV* = right ventricle; *LA* = left atrium; *LV* = left ventricle; *VS* = ventricular septum. **d,** longitudinal section posterior to **c** showing the abscess in the ventricular septum. **e,** histologic section of the ring abscess (Movat stain; ×4). **f,** histologic section showing gram-positive cocci in the ring abscess (Brown and Brenn stain; ×880).

aortic valve disease and 1 previously had had normal valves. Among 94 necropsy patients older than 45 years with IE reported in 1949 by Traut and associates,[57] 46 had isolated aortic valve vegetations and 5 (11%) had underlying degenerative aortic valve disease. Among 42 patients older than 60 years with morphologically proved (41 necropsy, 1 surgical) IE reported by Thell and associates[58] in 1975, 6 (14%) had degenerative aortic valve disease. Three (4%) of our 74 patients had valvular damage from a previous episode of successfully treated IE involving a normal valve. Thus, although patients with multiple episodes of IE usually have congenital heart disease,[59] as emphasized by Austrian[60] in 1957, the advent of antibiotic therapy resulted in a new type of valvular heart disease. Floppy mitral valve, which increases the risk of developing IE,[61-63] was present in 2 of our

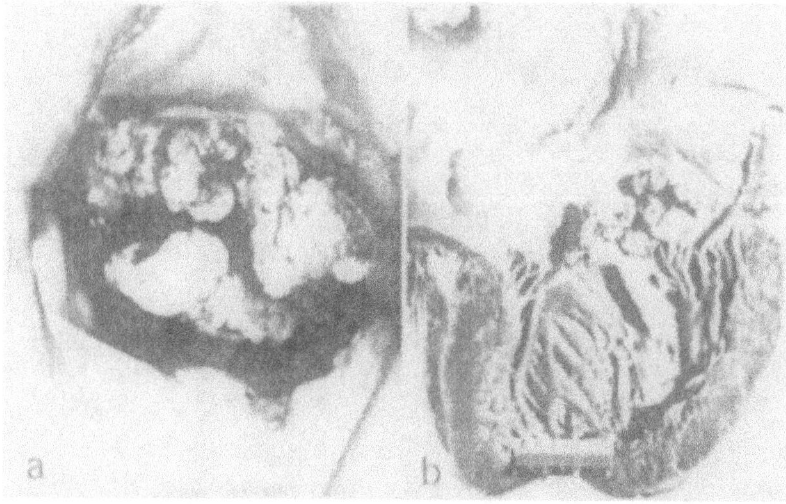

Fig. 25.—*Candida paropsilosis* endocarditis on a previously normal mitral valve of a 68-year-old man with chronic lung disease and coronary heart disease (A60–126). Five months before death, he had fever and 45 days later he was hospitalized. A grade 2/6 apical systolic murmur was present. Despite amphotericin B therapy, blood cultures remained positive, and he died of congestive heart failure. A large embolus to the left common iliac artery occurred during hospitalization. **a,** mitral valve viewed from the left atrium showing large vegetations on both leaflets. **b,** opened left ventricle showing large vegetations on both leaflets.

patients. In contrast, among 399 necropsy patients with IE summarized from several studies[1, 38, 64-66] in the preantibiotic era, 258 (65%) had underlying rheumatic valvular disease. Among 424 patients with IE studied clinically by Christian[67] and by Kelson and White,[68] 381 (90%) had underlying rheumatic valvular disease. The declining frequency of rheumatic heart disease,[69-73] the lowered frequency of IE in patients with rheumatic valvular disease[12] and the increasing age of patients with IE[7, 44, 45, 51] appear to account for these changes.

IE occurring on previously normal valves has been considered unusual. Of 1056 necropsy patients with IE summarized from several studies,[4, 5, 7, 41, 45, 57, 66, 74-77] 26% previously had had normal valves. Among our 74 patients with active left-sided valvular endocarditis, however, 41 (55%) had anatomically normal valves before the onset of IE and 4 of the 33 with anatomically abnormal valves had functionally normal valves before the onset of IE. Thus, 67% of our 74 patients had functionally normal valves before the onset of IE. Morgan and Bland,[41] Wilson,[7] Uwaydah and Weinberg,[44] Lerner and Weinstein[45] and others[47, 50, 51] have noted an increasing number of patients with IE involving previously functionally normal valves. In addition, the mortality from IE now is considerably higher among patients with previously normal valves than among patients with previously abnormal valves.[78] In a study by Rabinovich and associates,[43] the IE was fatal in 10 of 12 patients with IE involving previously normal valves whereas it was fatal in 61 (48%) of 129 patients with IE involving previously abnormal valves. Fifty-one (94%) of 54 patients with active bacterial endocarditis reported by Pankey[33] died, and 63% of them previously had had normal cardiac valves.

► ANTONIO C. DE LEON, JR.: The lower incidence of abnormal valves noted in these cases of necropsy-proved infective endocarditis should not be interpreted to mean that they now are less prone to endocarditis. The total number of individuals with previously normal valves is small compared to the total number of individuals with previously abnormal valves. Furthermore, as the authors emphasize, infective endocarditis involving previously normal valves has a significantly greater mortality than infective endocarditis involving previously abnormal valves. Thus, patients with endocarditis (preponderantly those with previously abnormal valves) who are treated successfully are not included in the above data. Antibiotic prophylaxis against infective endocarditis in patients with abnormal valves continues to be an important and necessary part of management of the patient.

► W. PROCTOR HARVEY: Patients having had no murmur or history of heart disease are less likely to have infective endocarditis considered in differential diagnosis, as compared with the patient with known valvular or congenital heart disease. For this reason, earlier diagnosis and treatment in those with documented heart disease may result; this may be one of the possible explanations of the higher mortality associated with previously normal valves. It is obvious, however, that we should be more alert as to the diagnosis of infective endocarditis in patients without a previous history of heart disease.

When an anatomically normal valve is the site of infection, the causative organism usually is a highly virulent one.[5, 7, 17, 33, 45, 47, 51] Thayer[5] noted IE on previously normal valves in 63% of 70 patients with staphylococcal or pneumococcal endocarditis but in only 20% of patients with IE caused by alpha hemolytic streptococcus. Finland and Barnes[79] found functionally normal valves in 185 (68%) of 271 episodes of IE caused by organisms other than alpha hemolytic streptococcus or *Staphylococcus epidermidis*. In 22 (54%) of our 41 patients with previously normal valves, the infection was caused by *Staphylococcus aureus* in 11 patients, *Diplococcus pneumoniae* in 5 and by *Streptococcus faecalis* in 6. Alpha hemolytic streptococcus was the most frequent causative organism among our patients with abnormal valves, but accounted for only 7 (21%) of the infections in these 33 patients. Highly virulent bacteria generally cause a more acute illness, and mortality is higher both among patients with infection caused by highly virulent bacteria[30, 32, 33, 41, 80] and among patients with shorter duration of symptoms before diagnosis.[43, 81]

Among necropsy patients with IE occurring after the introduction of antibiotic therapy, the frequency of aortic valve infection has increased and the frequency of mitral valve infection has decreased.[7, 46, 50] Of our 74 patients, 52 (70%) had infection of the aortic valve and 36 (49%) had infection of the mitral valve. Of the latter 36 patients, however, 18 also had aortic valve infection, and in at least 13 (72%) of them, the mitral infection appeared to be secondary to the aortic valve IE.[82-85] In a study of 656 patients with IE seen at the Columbia-Presbyterian Medical Center between 1938 and 1967, Cherubin and Neu[18] found a progressive increase in aortic valve involvement over the three decades and a decline in mitral valve infection. Of 28 necropsy patients with IE dying in 1969 in Kampala, Uganda, 15 (54%) had isolated aortic valve vegetations.[50]

Congestive heart failure has replaced infection as the leading cause of death among patients with IE, and damage to the aortic valve is the most common cause of the failure in patients with IE.[42, 45, 47, 49, 51, 52] Of our 74 patients, 45 (61%), including 33 with aortic valve vegetations, died from congestive heart failure, and in each of them the IE had caused severe valve destruction. In a study by Robinson and Ruedy,[42] congestive heart failure was the cause of death in only 6% of patients with IE in the preantibiotic era but caused death in 61% of those with fatal IE after the introduction of antibiotic therapy. The increased frequency of congestive heart failure resulted from the increased frequency of valve destruction by the vegetation: 16% of patients with fatal IE in the preantibiotic era and 45% in the antibiotic era had cuspal perforations. In nearly all patients in both eras, the perforations involved the aortic valve. Among 33 patients with IE studied by Cohen and Freedman,[52] damage to the aortic valve was the most common cause of death. Of 14 patients with acute aortic regurgitation from IE reported by Fowler and associates,[86] 10 developed severe congestive heart failure within 4 months of the onset of IE, and 9 of them died.

► ANTONIO C. DE LEON, JR.: The severe congestive heart failure that can occur with acute severe aortic regurgitation at times precludes completion of antibiotic therapy before considering surgical intervention. Early surgical intervention to correct the hemodynamic deficit appears to be a significant factor in trying to reduce the high mortality seen in this group of patients.

► W. PROCTOR HARVEY: It now is well appreciated that when heart failure with significant aortic insufficiency rapidly develops following acute infective endocarditis, surgery should be promptly considered for definitive treatment. In the past, undue delay in proceeding with operation occurred too often. One reason for postponing aortic valve replacement was the impression that active myocarditis was associated in a number of patients with endocarditis and that more time should be allowed for healing of the myocarditis as well as trying to achieve more control of cardiac decompensation by medical means. However, we, as others, have learned the necessity for early operation.

The hemodynamic consequence of IE almost always is regurgitation. IE caused aortic regurgitation in 36 (69%) of our 52 patients with aortic valve vegetations and mitral regurgitation in 14 (64%) of our 22 patients with isolated mitral vegetations. It also caused mitral regurgitation in 9 of the 52 patients with aortic valve vegetations. Massive vegetations caused valvular stenosis in 1 patient with IE involving the aortic valve and in 1 patient with IE involving the mitral valve.[87]

Valve ring abscess is frequent in patients with IE involving the aortic valve and rare in patients with IE of the mitral valve.[88] Valve ring abscess was present in 24 (32%) of our 74 patients: in 22 (92%), the ring abscess involved the aortic valve and in only 2 (8%) the mitral valve. One of the latter 2 patients had isolated mitral valve infection with ring abscess; the other had aortic valve vegetations and infection of a heavily calcified mitral valve anulus.[89-91] Each of the 24 patients with valve ring abscess had valvular regurgitation from IE.

Pericarditis and atrioventricular block in patients with IE almost always result from ring abscess and, thus, usually are a complication of aortic valve infection.[88] Pericarditis was present in 16 (22%) of our 74 patients and, in 15 of them, vegetations were present on the aortic valve. In 11 of the 16 patients, the pericarditis resulted from rupture of an aortic valve ring abscess into the pericardial space. In 1856, Rokitansky[1] recognized that ring abscess may be associated with pericarditis and myocarditis, and that it may cause a cardiac aneurysm that may rupture into a cardiac chamber or pericardial space. In 1873, Ponfick[92] again noted the association of IE with pericarditis, and in 1885 Osler[2] noted the tendency of valve ring abscess to burrow into adjacent structures. Of 43 consecutive necropsy patients with IE studied by Beck,[93] 8 (16%) had pericarditis and 5 of them had an aortic valve ring abscess with perforation into the pericardial space. McColl[94] reported a patient with pericarditis due to mycotic aneurysm from IE, and concluded from a review of previously reported cases that perforation of an aortic valve ring abscess was the most frequent cause of pericarditis in patients with IE. A similar observation was made by Buchbinder and Roberts.[47] Among 38 patients with aortic valve IE reported by Utley and Mills,[81] 15 had ring abscess and 5 of them had pericarditis. Thus, the occurrence of a pericardial friction rub or pericardial effusion during the course of IE is highly suggestive of ring abscess.

Either complete heart block or a high degree of heart block appearing suddenly in a patient with IE is highly suggestive of the presence of a ring abscess, which has extended into the area of the atrioventricular node or bundle.[88, 95-99] Of our 6 patients with either complete (5 patients) or Mobitz type II atrioventricular block, 5 had a ring abscess, aortic valve in 4 of them. In addition, the appearance of complete right or left bundle-branch block during IE is also highly suggestive of the presence of a ring abscess with extension into the most cephalad portion of the muscular ventricular septum. Although only 1 of our patients developed complete right bundle-branch block and none developed complete left bundle-branch block, the latter has been reported in aortic valve endocarditis by Roberts and Somerville.[95]

Acute myocardial lesions are frequent in patients with IE. Clawson,[4] Buchbinder and Saphir,[100] Saphir[101] and Perry and associates[75] observed myocardial lesions in 88–100% of 187 patients with IE studied by them at necropsy. Acute myocardial lesions were observed in 56 (85%) of our 66 patients in whom numerous histologic sections of myocardium were examined. The significance of myocardial lesions in patients with IE has been debated. Clawson[4] and Correll and associates[102] considered the lesions to be a major cause of congestive heart failure in patients with active IE. de Navasquez[103] and Perry and associates,[75] however, believed that congestive heart failure in patients with IE rarely was the result of myocardial lesions. In none of our patients could we attribute congestive cardiac failure to the acute myocardial lesions.

Papillary muscle necrosis is common in patients with fatal IE with or without associated coronary arterial narrowing.[47] Foci of necrosis was observed in the left ventricular papillary muscles in 39 (59%) of our 66 patients in whom sections of both left ventricular papillary muscles were examined. Only 13 of the 39 patients had significant coronary arterial narrowing: by emboli to intramural coronary arteries in 5, by emboli to both intramural and extramural coronary arteries in 5[104] and by severe (> 75% luminal narrowing) atherosclerosis in 3, 1 of whom also had coronary arterial emboli. The significant correlation ($p < 0.02$) between papillary muscle necrosis and valve dysfunction resulting in congestive heart failure[47] suggests that the necrosis results from poor arterial perfusion associated with the congestive heart failure because the papillary muscles are the last portion of myocardium to be supplied by arterial blood.[105] Despite papillary muscle necrosis, no patient had mitral regurgitation in the absence of destruction of mitral leaflets or ruptured chordae tendineae.

INFECTIVE ENDOCARDITIS INVOLVING PROSTHETIC CARDIAC VALVES

Among approximately 450 patients with one or more rigid-framed substitute cardiac valves studied by us at necropsy,[106-112] 22 (5%) had infection involving a prosthetic valve. These 22 patients represent 17% of the 129 patients with active valvular IE studied by us.[17, 47, 113-115]

Clinical and morphologic observations in the 22 patients with

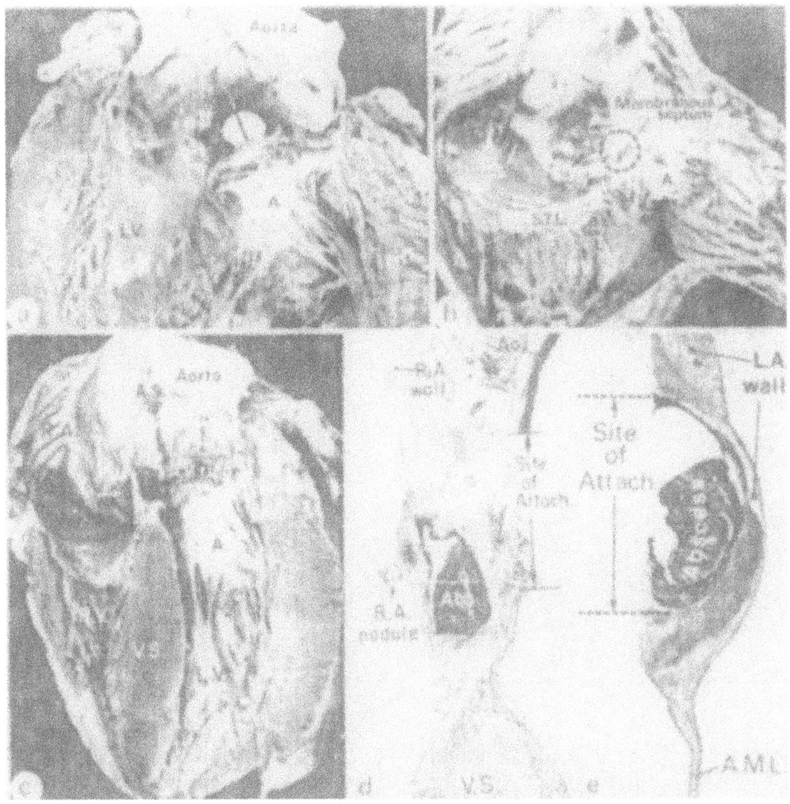

Fig. 26.—*Staphylococcus epidermidis* prosthetic valve endocarditis in a 49-year-old man (A67–22) who died 3 months after aortic replacement. Symptoms of infection appeared 16 days before death. Despite large doses of antibiotics, complete heart block and wide-open aortic regurgitation developed. **a,** opened aorta, aortic valve and left ventricle *(L.V.)* showing a necrotic anulus to which the prosthesis is only partially attached. *A.* = anterior mitral leaflet. **b,** opened right atrium, tricuspid valve and right ventricle *(R.V.)* showing vegetative material *(arrows)* that had burrowed through the atrial septum from the necrotic aortic valve ring. *C.S.* = ostium of coronary sinus; *S.T.L.* = septal tricuspid leaflet; *A.* = anterior tricuspid leaflet. **c,** longitudinal section of the heart with the anterior portion removed. The necrotic aortic valve *(A.V.)* ring again is seen and the penetration of the infective process through the atrial septum *(A.S.)* is apparent. An arrow again designates the vegetation in the right atrium *(R.A.)*. *V.S.* = ventricular septum. **d** and **e,** histologic sections through the ring abscess. The site of attachment of the prosthesis, which has been removed, is indicated. The infected nodule, an extension of the ring abscess *(Abs.)*, is showing in the right atrium *(R.A.)*. *Ao.* = aortic wall; *L.A.* = left atrium. *A.M.L.* = anterior mitral leaflet.

prosthetic valve endocarditis (PVE) are summarized in Table 3 and certain morphologic features in them are illustrated in Figures 26–37. Patients with active IE at the time of valve replacement were excluded. Among the 22 patients, 27 cardiac valves had been replaced: 17 patients had one prosthetic valve and 5 had two prosthetic valves. Of the 27 prosthetic valves, 22 were infected: aortic in 15 patients and mitral in 7 patients. Clinical

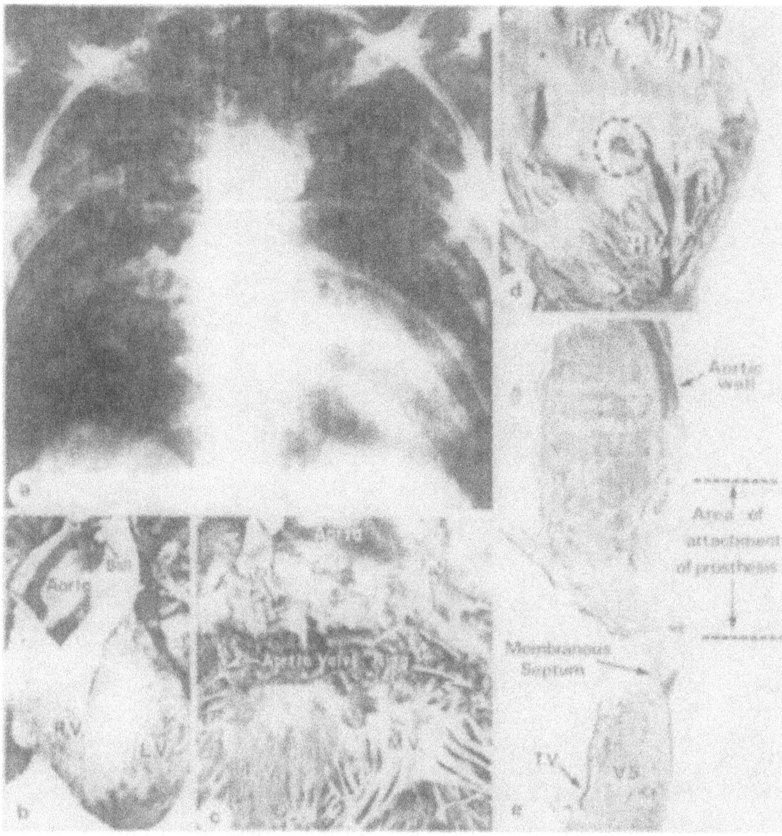

Fig. 27.—*Staphylococcus epidermidis* prosthetic aortic valve endocarditis in a 48-year-old man (A64-189). He had been well for 11 months following insertion of the Starr-Edwards prosthesis when, 1 month before death and 6 weeks after dental extraction, shaking chills appeared and blood cultures were positive for *Staphylococcus epidermidis*. Despite intensive antibiotic therapy, signs of aortic regurgitation appeared, and minutes before death he complained of "feeling funny." **a,** chest roentgenogram immediately post mortem revealed that the prosthesis had dislodged and migrated to the aortic arch. **b,** anterior view of the heart and opened ascending aorta. The detached prosthesis ball is visible lodged in the transverse aorta. *L.V.* = left ventricle; *R.V.* = right ventricle. **c,** opened aorta, aortic valve "ring" and left ventricle showing a totally necrotic aortic anulus. *M.V.* = anterior mitral leaflet; *R.C.* = ostium of right coronary artery, *L.C.* = ostium of left coronary artery. **d,** opened right atrium *(R.A.)*, tricuspid valve and right ventricle *(R.V.)* showing a ring abscess *(circle)* that had extended from the aortic prosthetic anulus. **e,** photomicrograph through the aortic valve "ring" showing a large ring abscess and the necrotic aortic anulus material, which extended through the membranous ventricular septum into the right atrium. Hematoxylin and eosin stain; original magnification ×2. *T.V.* = tricuspid valve leaflet; *V.S.* = ventricular septum.

evidence of IE was present within 2 months after operation in 8 patients (early deaths) and from 3 months to 10 years after valve replacement in 14 patients. In 6 of the latter 14 patients, clinical evidence of infection did not appear until more than 1 year after valve replacement. The length of signs and symptoms

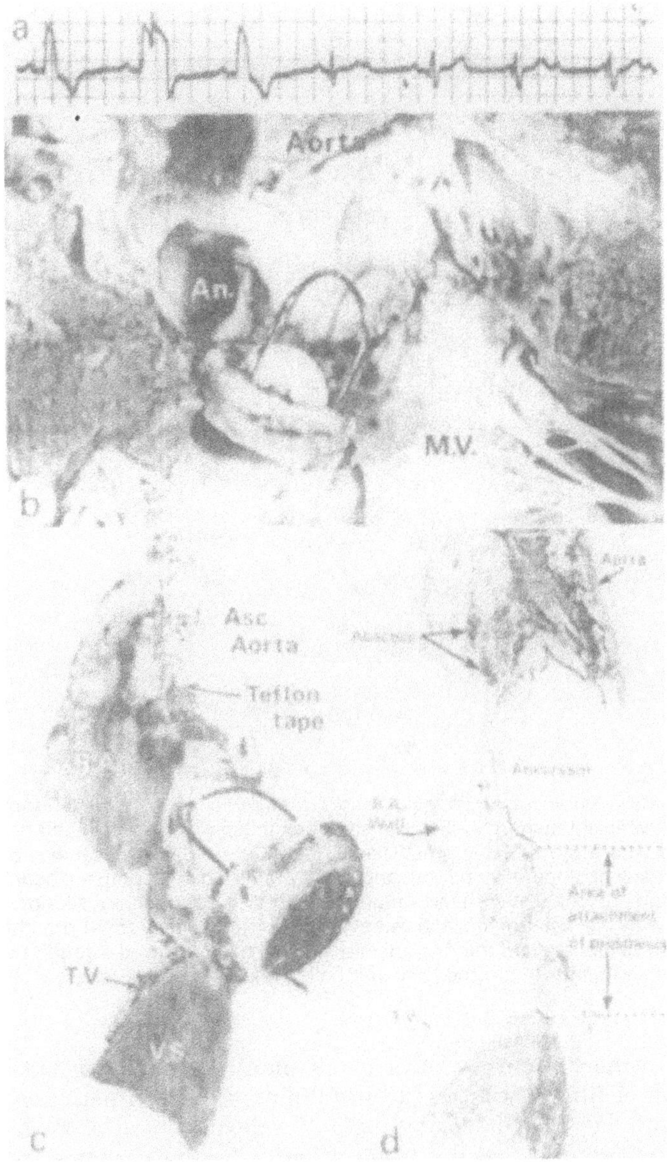

Fig. 28.—*Staphylococcus epidermidis* prosthetic aortic valve endocarditis in a 55-year-old man (A63–176). The Starr-Edwards prosthesis was used to replace an infected trileaflet Teflon (Müller) valve 45 days before death. **a,** complete heart block and signs of massive aortic regurgitation appeared despite antibiotic therapy. **b,** opened aorta, aortic valve and left ventricle. The aortic valve ring is necrotic and the prosthesis is almost totally detached. The cage of the prosthesis has burrowed into the wall of the aorta, causing a saccular aneurysm *(An.)*. *M.V.* = mitral valve. **c,** longitudinal section showing the caged-ball prosthesis burrowing into the ascending *(Asc.)* aorta, producing the aneurysm. *R.A.* = right atrium; *T.V.* = septal tricuspid valve leaflet. *V.S.* = ventricular septum. **d,** photomicrograph through the same area after the prosthesis has been removed (hematoxylin and eosin stain; original magnification ×2).

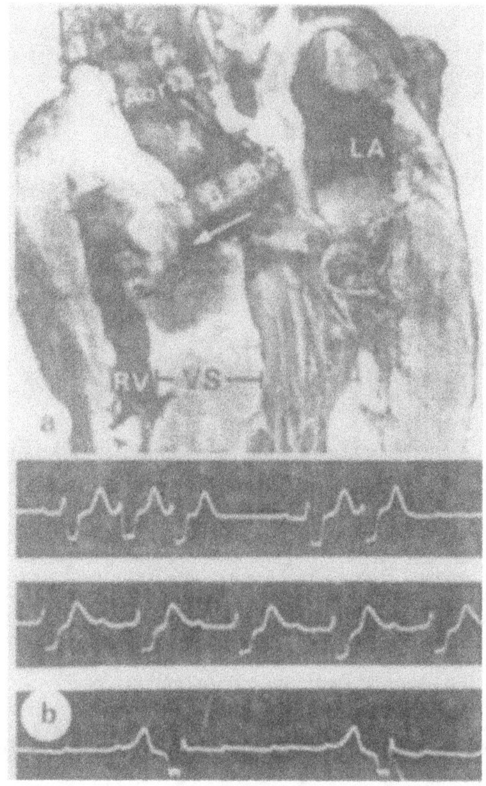

Fig. 29.—*Staphylococcus epidermidis* prosthetic aortic valve endocarditis in a 51-year-old man (A74–51). His stenotic bicuspid aortic valve had been replaced with a Björk-Shiley prosthesis 83 days before death. Fever was present in the early postoperative period, and shortly before death complete heart block and signs of congestive heart failure appeared. **a,** longitudinal section of the heart with the anterior portion removed. The Björk-Shiley *(B-S)* prosthesis is partially detached, and the ring abscess *(arrow)* has burrowed through the ventricular septum *(VS)* into the right ventricle *(RV)*. *LA* = left atrium.

of IE ranged from 14 days to 13 months. In 16 patients, the length of illness was less than 60 days and in 6 patients more than 60 days. Predisposing factors to development of PVE were apparent in only 5 of the 14 late deaths: tooth extraction in 2 patients, skin-graft infection in 1, prolonged use of an intravenous catheter in 1 and prolonged use of a transthoracic pacing wire in 1. It is presumed that the infection in the 8 early deaths either was incurred at operation or was secondary to a wound infection.

Of the infecting organisms (cultured from the blood during life in 20 patients), the staphylococcus was responsible in 13 patients and a different organism in each of the other 9 patients. Fungi caused the PVE in 2 patients, and in each of them blood cultures during life were negative. Evidence of prosthetic dys-

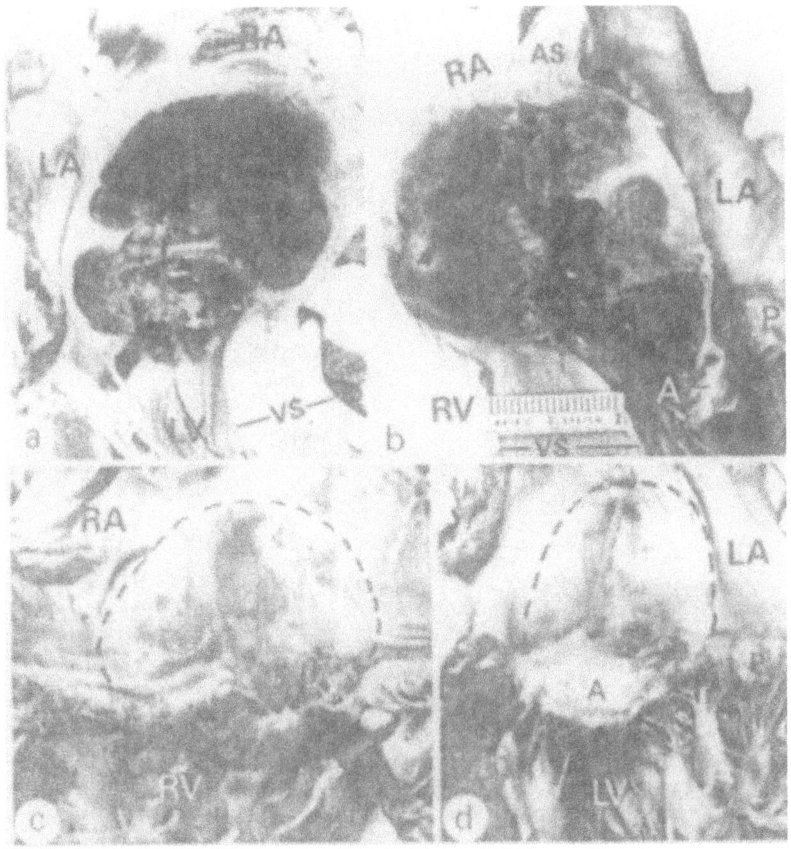

Fig. 30.—*Diplococcus pneumoniae* aortic prosthetic endocarditis in a 40-year-old man (A74–82). The preoperative hemodynamic lesion was aortic regurgitation, which was caused by a previous episode of pneumococcal endocarditis. Evidence of infection was apparent clinically 10 months after valve replacement with a Björk-Shiley prosthesis. When he was brought to the hospital shortly before death, complete heart block and signs of prosthetic valve obstruction were present. **a,** infected hematoma about the aortic prosthesis. This is a view of the anterior half of the heart from the posterior position. The disk of the prosthesis is totally immobilized by the infected thrombus. *LA* = left atrium; *LV* = left ventricle; *RA* = right atrium; *VS* = ventricular septum. **b** is a view of the posterior half of the heart. The prosthesis is not present here. *AS* = atrial septum; *A* = anterior mitral leaflet; *P* = posterior mitral leaflet. **c,** opened right atrium *(RA),* tricuspid valve and right ventricle *(RV)* showing extension of the infected thrombus *(half circle)* into the right atrium. **d,** opened left atrium *(LA),* mitral valve and left ventricle *(LV)* showing the infected thrombus extending into the left atrium.

function was present clinically in 12 of the 15 patients with infected aortic prostheses (regurgitation in 11 and stenosis in 1) but in none of the 7 patients with infected mitral prostheses. High-grade conduction disturbances occurred in 7 patients, all of whom had infected aortic valve prostheses: left bundle-branch block in 2 and complete heart block in 5. Thirteen of the 22 pa-

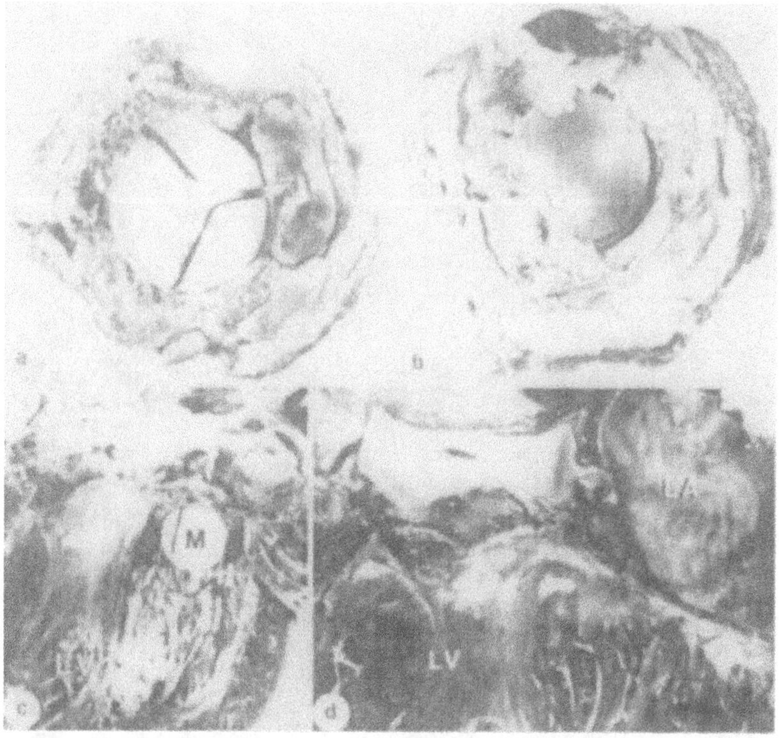

Fig. 31.—*Serratia marcescens* prosthetic aortic valve endocarditis in a 57-year-old man (A68–33) who became infected 4 months after replacement of both aortic and mitral valves. The apparent source of the infection was an intravenous catheter. Left bundle-branch block and signs of aortic regurgitation appeared and, despite massive doses of antibiotics, he died 3 months after onset of symptoms of infection. **a,** view of aortic prosthesis from above. Infected thrombus is present on its anulus. **b,** view of prosthesis as it appeared from the left ventricle. Some of the infected thrombus became detached during excision of this prosthesis at necropsy. The primary orifice is partially obstructed by the infected material. **c,** opened aortic root, aortic valve and left ventricle *(LV)* after removal of the aortic prosthesis. Most of the aortic ring is necrotic. In addition, the portion of mitral *(M)* prosthesis in direct apposition to the aortic anulus also is infected. **d,** view after excision of the mitral prosthesis showing extension of the aortic anular infection into the junctional area between aortic and mitral anuli. *LA* = left atrium; *LV* = left ventricle.

tients received appropriate antibiotic therapy for longer than 7 days. Three patients underwent valve replacement for PVE. The principal causes of death in the 22 patients were congestive heart failure (19 patients), central nervous system emboli (2 patients) and generalized infection (1 patient).

Among the 22 patients, 27 valves were replaced: 1 valve in 17 patients and 2 valves in 5 patients. In each of the 5 patients with 2 prosthetic valves, only the "downstream" valve was infected: the aortic valve in the 3 patients with mitral and aortic prostheses and the mitral in the 2 patients with tricuspid and

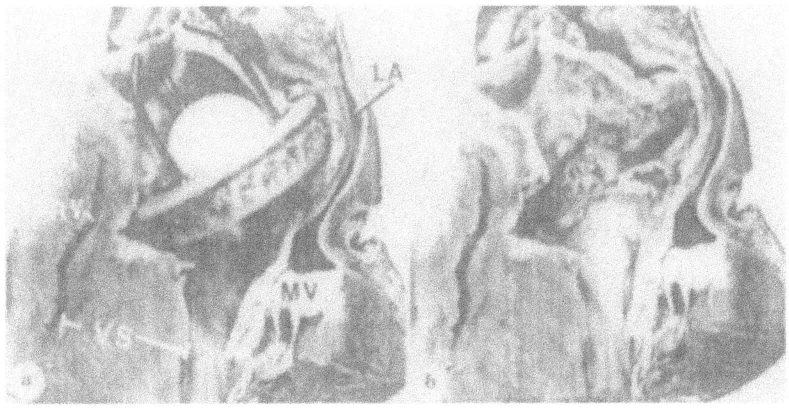

Fig. 32.—*Staphylococcus epidermidis* endocarditis originally involving a Björk-Shiley aortic valve prosthesis, which was excised and replaced with a Magovern prosthesis 28 days before death in a 69-year-old man (A75-200). Fever and signs of aortic regurgitation appeared 7 months following aortic valve replacement with the Björk-Shiley prosthesis. After replacement with the Magovern prosthesis, a murmur of aortic regurgitation reappeared. At necropsy, the sewing ring of the Magovern prosthesis had burrowed deeply into the necrotic anulus and caused the ball of the prosthesis to strike the non-necrotic portion of the aortic wall, probably producing prosthetic aortic stenosis. **a**, longitudinal section of the heart through the aortic anulus with the Magovern prosthesis in place, and **b** after removal of the prosthesis. The frame of the prosthesis has burrowed deeply into the necrotic anulus. *VS* = ventricular septum; *RV* = right ventricular cavity; *MV* = mitral valve; *LA* = left atrium.

mitral prostheses. Twelve of the 15 infected aortic prostheses and 2 of the 7 infected mitral prostheses were either partially or completely detached. In contrast, 5 of the 7 infected mitral prostheses and only 1 of the 15 infected aortic prostheses were obstructed by vegetative material.

Ring abscesses were present with each of the 22 infected prostheses, but, in 1, the abscess was visible only by histologic examination. The ring abscess involved the entire valve anulus in 14 patients and only portions of the anulus in the other 8 patients. In 13 of the 22 patients, the infective process spread to adjacent structures. In 11 of the 15 patients with infected aortic prostheses, the ring abscess burrowed into adjacent structures: through the ascending aorta into the periaortic space (7 patients); through the atrial septum into the right atrium (9 patients) or into the left atrium (2 patients); through the ventricular septum into the right ventricle (8 patients); and into the anterobasal left ventricular wall (2 patients). In 2 patients with infected mitral prostheses, the ring abscess burrowed through

Fig. 33.—*Staphylococcus aureus* prosthetic mitral valve endocarditis in a 47-year-old man (A65-186) who had the onset of symptoms of infective endocarditis 4 months after valve replacement. He had done well during the first 3 months following operation but developed symptoms of infection following

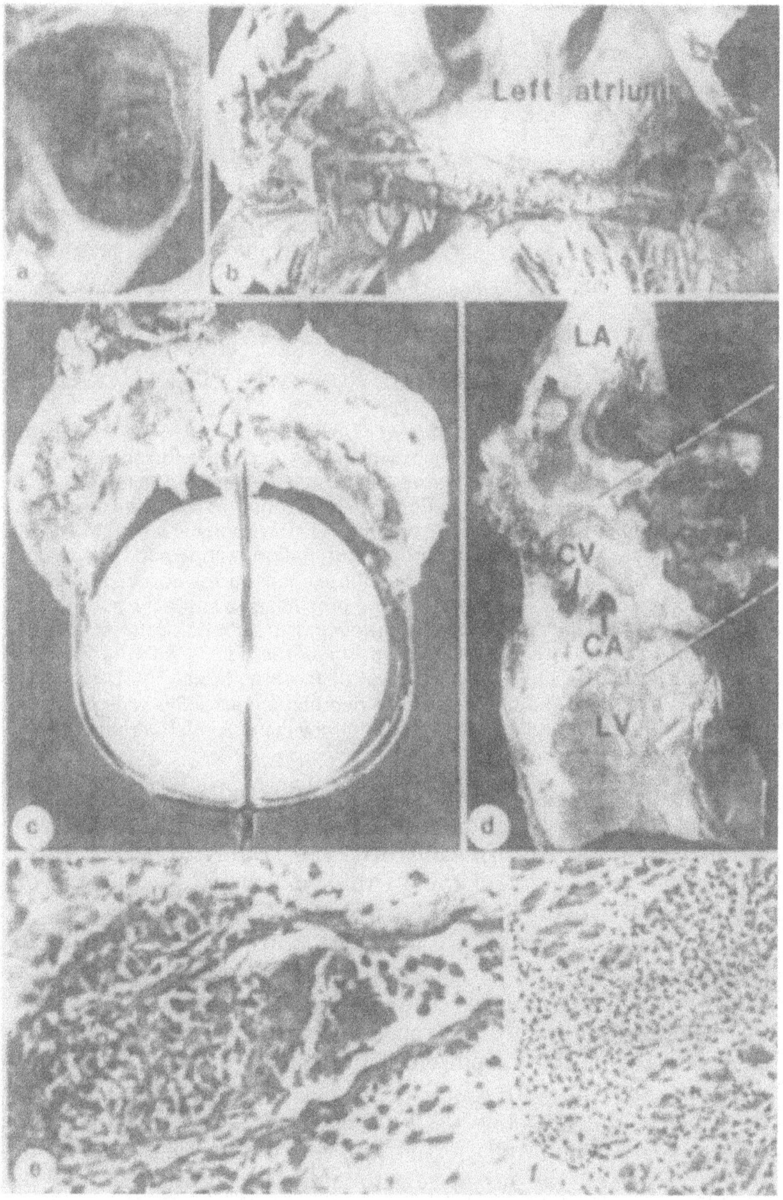

grafting of a cutaneous ulcer. Signs of prosthetic dysfunction were never detected clinically. **a,** prosthetic mitral orifice obstructed by vegetative material, as viewed from the left atrium. **b,** opened left atrium, mitral anulus and left ventricle after removal of the mitral prosthesis. The entire anulus is necrotic. *AV* = aortic valve. **c,** mitral prosthesis showing infected thrombus at its base. **d,** longitudinal section through left atrium *(LA)*, mitral anulus and left ventricle *(LV)*. The former site of attachment of the prosthesis is designated by the dashed lines. The infective process burrowed through the wall of the heart and caused pericarditis. *CA* = coronary artery; *CV* = coronary vein in the right atrioventricular sulcus.

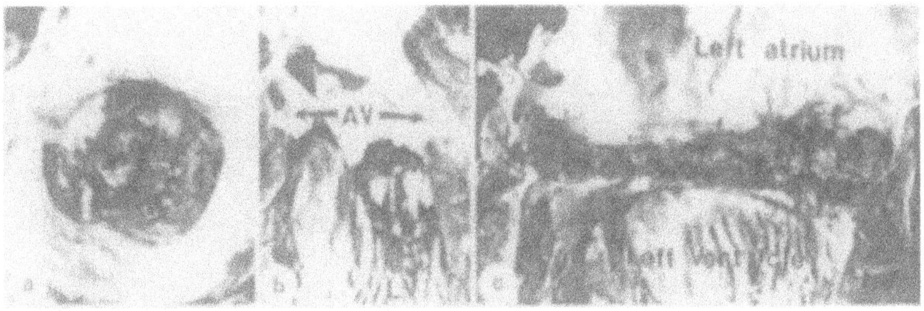

Fig. 34.—*Staphylococcus epidermidis* prosthetic mitral valve endocarditis in a 46-year-old man (A65-221) who died 16 months after mitral replacement with a Starr-Edwards prosthesis. Eight months postoperatively, when he was asymptomatic, cardiac catheterization disclosed normal left atrial pressure and cardiac output. Signs of infection appeared 15 months after valve replacement. Despite antibiotics, he developed fatal congestive heart failure. **a,** mitral prosthesis as viewed from the left atrium. A large infected thrombus virtually occludes the mitral orifice. **b,** opened aorta, aortic valve *(AV)* and left ventricle *(LV)* showing infected thrombus on the cage of the mitral prosthesis. **c,** opened left atrium and ventricle showing a completely necrotic mitral anulus. The prosthesis has been removed.

the atrial wall into the pericardial space. Histologic examination of the infected rings disclosed colonies of organisms in 13 of the 22 patients.

Both arterial emboli and gross organ infarcts were common with both aortic and mitral PVE. Of the 22 patients, grossly visible infarcts were present in the spleen in 12, kidney in 7 and brain in 7. Two patients had bowel infarcts, 1 had a pancreatic infarct and 1 a transmural myocardial infarct. In addition, mycotic aneurysms were present in the ascending aorta of 3 patients: in 2 patients, aneurysms resulted from jet lesions from

Fig. 35.—*Staphylococcus epidermidis* prosthetic mitral valve endocarditis in a 59-year-old woman (A74-196). The infection appeared 10 years after replacement of both mitral and tricuspid valves. At necropsy, only the mitral prosthesis was infected. **a,** infected mitral prosthesis viewed from the left ventricle. Vegetative material *(V)* is present on the prosthetic anulus just below the aortic valve. **b,** mitral prosthesis as viewed from the left atrium showing vegetations *(V)* at the junction of the prosthetic and natural valve anuli. **c,** same view after removal of the prosthesis, showing even greater extensiveness of the infection at the site of attachment of the prosthesis.

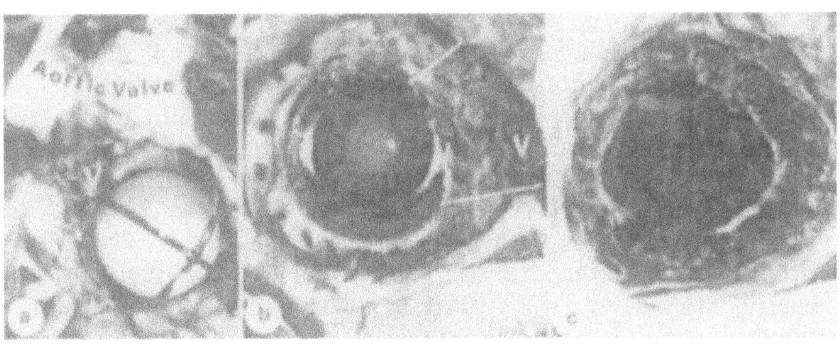

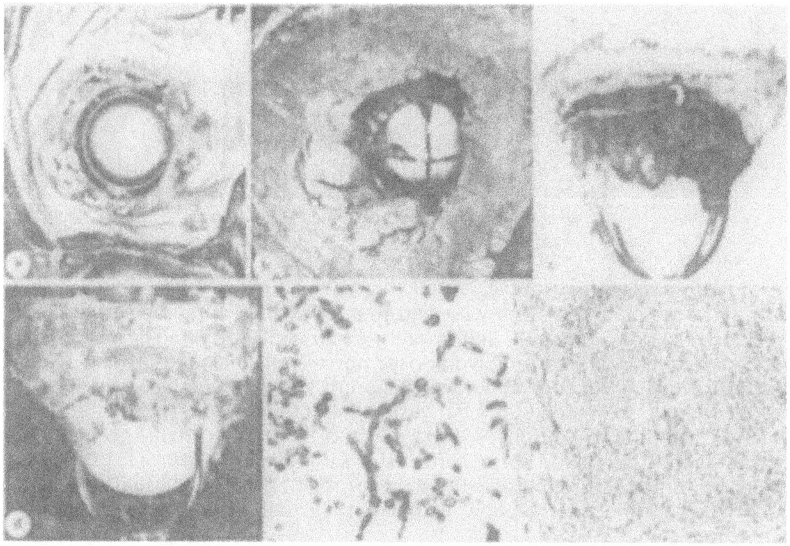

Fig. 36. – Candida species prosthetic mitral valve endocarditis in a 37-year-old woman (A75-242) who had undergone valve replacement 125 months before death because of mitral stenosis (mean mitral gradient 7 mm Hg) and regurgitation. Her tricuspid valve was replaced with a porcine xenograft because of severe tricuspid regurgitation 66 days before death. Postoperatively, she required prolonged use of a transthoracic pacing wire, which was the apparent source of the infection. She died from central nervous system embolism. Necropsy disclosed infection of the mitral prosthesis. **a,** mitral prosthesis viewed from the left atrium and, **b,** from the left ventricle. Large vegetations are present on the base and struts of the prosthesis. **c** and **d,** removed mitral valve prosthesis from two different sides showing large vegetations. **e,** photomicrograph of Candida species in the mitral vegetations (methenamine silver stain; original magnification ×860). **f,** photomicrograph of microabscess in left ventricular myocardium (hematoxylin and eosin stain; original magnification ×80).

the infected prosthesis and, in the third, the cage of the partially detached prosthesis burrowed into the wall of a weakened aorta (from an aortotomy – weeks earlier), causing a saccular aneurysm. In 14 of the 22 patients, the spleen weighed more than 300 gm.

Comments on Prosthetic Valve Endocarditis

Study of our 22 necropsy patients and analysis of more than 150 necropsy patients with prosthetic valve endocarditis (PVE) reported by others[116, 117] allows certain general conclusions regarding this condition. PVE is a devastating complication of cardiac valve replacement but, fortunately, it is infrequent. Its exact frequency is not certain but it clearly is less than 1% per year among patients with prosthetic cardiac valves.[137, 139, 145, 148] Although prospective studies[149, 150] have been inconclusive, retrospective studies[118, 119, 151, 152] have shown a reduction in the frequency of early (< 2 months after valve replacement) PVE coinci-

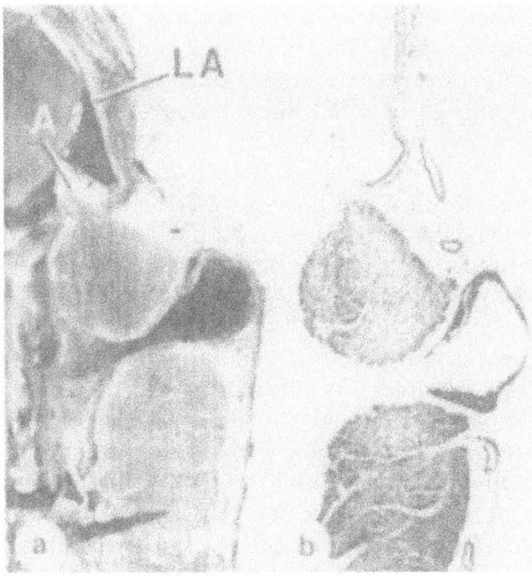

Fig. 37. – Left ventricular aneurysm misdiagnosed as prosthetic valve endocarditis in a 46-year-old woman (A75–17). She had almost daily fever following mitral valve replacement 4 months before death and one of many blood cultures grew *Staphylococcus epidermidis* and diphtheroids. The clinical diagnosis was prosthetic valve endocarditis and she was treated with prolonged intravenous antibiotic therapy. She died from central nervous system embolism. At necropsy, an aneurysm was present in the basal portion of the left ventricular free wall. The prosthesis and its anulus were free from signs of infection. **a,** longitudinal cut of the left atrial *(LA)* wall, mitral anulus *(A)* and left ventricular *(LV)* wall through the aneurysm. **b,** histologic section of the aneurysm (Movat stain). Thrombus is present in the aneurysm.

dent with the use of prophylactic antibiotics. Late infection now appears to be more common than early infection,[137, 145] presumably because there now are so many persons with prosthetic cardiac valves. Although the mortality rate is high for both groups, early infection from PVE apparently is fatal more often than late infection.[137, 139, 145, 148]

Most early infections either are incurred at operation or result from a wound infection.[126, 129, 137, 139, 147] The former most often appears to result from contamination of the cardiopulmonary bypass equipment.[153, 154] Staphylococcus is the most frequent organism cultured from cardiopulmonary bypass equipment and staphylococcus is the most frequent cause of early PVE.[116, 118-120, 126, 130, 137, 139, 144, 145] When gram-negative bacteria or fungi cause PVE early, they usually are also recovered from the operating room equipment or from a wound infection.[128, 139] Late infections usually result from transient bacteremia.[137, 139, 145, 148] Although both staphylococci and streptococci are frequent causes of clinically diagnosed late PVE,[137, 139, 145] the former have caused most cases of necropsy-proved late PVE and the latter relatively few. In none of our 22 necropsy patients with PVE was the infection caused by streptococcus. Staphylococcus was the most common cause of PVE in our patients irrespective of whether the infection occurred early or late.

Among patients with PVE, blood cultures almost always are positive, except when the infections are caused by certain fungi.[127, 128, 131, 132, 137, 139, 144, 145, 146, 148] Blood cultures were positive during life in each of our 20 patients with PVE caused by bacteria and were negative in each of our 2 patients with fungal PVE. Among 39 patients with endocarditis caused by *Aspergillus* species reviewed by Kammer and Utz,[155] blood cultures were positive in only 3.

Signs of prosthetic dysfunction usually are present when the aortic prosthesis is infected and usually absent when the mitral prosthesis is infected. Clinical signs of aortic regurgitation were present in 11 of our 15 patients with prosthetic aortic infection. In the 4 patients without clinical signs of aortic regurgitation, no prosthetic detachment was present at necropsy. Among patients with acute aortic regurgitation, however, classic signs of aortic regurgitation may be absent.[156-159] Signs of aortic regurgitation were not detected in 3 of 9 necropsy patients with aortic PVE reported by Madison and associates,[141] but in each of them prosthetic detachment was present at necropsy.

In contrast, patients with infection involving the mitral prosthesis usually have no clinical signs of mitral prosthetic dysfunction. Clinical signs of mitral prosthetic dysfunction were not detected in any of our 7 patients with mitral PVE; yet, the prosthesis was significantly obstructed by vegetative material in 5 of them and partially detached from the anulus in 2. McAllister and associates[143] reported 2 patients with virtual total obstruction of the mitral prosthesis by infected thrombus.

► Antonio C. de Leon, Jr.: Mitral prosthetic perivalvular leak is another cause of a "silent" regurgitant lesion. Severe regurgitation across a mitral valve prosthesis has been shown to occur without a corresponding audible murmur. The higher incidence of mitral prosthetic obstruction rather than insufficiency resulting from infective endocarditis may also account for the paucity of clinical evidence for prosthetic dysfunction in the 7 patients with a mitral valve prosthesis. Auscultatory findings other than a cardiac murmur can also be helpful in the recognition of mitral valve prosthetic dysfunction. The timing and intensity of the mitral prosthetic closure and opening sound has been shown to be helpful in the assessment of mitral prosthetic valve function.

The most consistent morphologic feature of prosthetic valve infection in our 22 patients was infection behind the site of attachment of the valve prosthesis, resulting in valve ring abscess.[115] Ring abscess was present in each of our 22 patients, and in two thirds of them the infection involved the entire circumference of the valve anulus. In several patients, however, only a portion of the circumference of the valve anulus was involved, and, in 1 patient, histologic examination of the anulus disclosed infection that had not been apparent on gross examination. Extension of the ring infection to adjacent cardiac structures was common, especially with aortic prosthetic infection. This extension resulted in the frequent occurrence of complete heart block or left bundle-branch block and of intracardiac fistulae. Among 9 necropsy patients with aortic PVE reported by Madison and associates,[144] each had infection at the site of attachment of the prosthesis, and among their entire group of 16 patients with aortic PVE, 7 (44%) developed atrioventricular conduction defects. Obviously, it is the occurrence of the infection behind the site of attachment of the prosthesis that makes reoperation so hazardous. Were the infection limited to the interior portion of the prosthesis, excision of the prosthesis should eliminate the infection. Unfortunately, as demonstrated by our patients and by those reported by others,[121, 135, 138, 143, 144, 147] the tissues behind the site of attachment of the prosthesis usually are involved by the infective process.

The occurrence of a grossly necrotic anulus, however, at the time of reoperation for PVE does not mean that valve replacement will be fruitless. Although it may be grossly necrotic, the anulus may be free from colonies of organisms and cultures of the necrotic anulus may be negative. In 9 of our 22 patients with PVE and ring abscess, no stainable organisms were found in histologic sections from the prosthetic anulus.

One hazard of inserting a prosthesis in a necrotic anulus at the time of valve replacement for PVE is burrowing of the sewing ring of the new prosthesis into the necrotic anulus, with resulting impingement on movement of the poppet of the prosthesis by adjacent tissue. This sequence occurred in one of our patients and resulted in prosthetic aortic stenosis from inability of the ball to ascend in the cage (Fig. 31).

Although PVE in patients with rigid-framed prostheses, as were present in our 22 patients, usually indicates the presence of infection behind the site of attachment of the prosthesis, i.e., sewing ring, ring abscess may not be so frequent with endocarditis involving tissue valves. Indeed, both experimentally and in humans, the infective process may be limited to the cusps of the tissue valve, just like the situation with infective endocarditis involving natural valves.[160, 161] Thus, the chance of cure, by either antibiotics or valve replacement or both, when IE is superimposed on a homograft or heterograft (porcine valve, for example) is much better than when IE involves a rigid-framed prosthesis. This, then, is an advantage, although a small one, of the tissue valve (porcine) over the rigid-framed prosthesis.

Establishment of the diagnosis of PVE, particularly in the early postoperative period, at times may be difficult, as pointed out by a number of authors.[148, 162, 163] Diagnosis in the late postoperative period, in contrast, usually is made quite readily.[148, 162, 163]

It is worth emphasizing, however, that the combination of fever and a positive blood culture in a patient with a prosthetic cardiac valve does not always indicate the presence of PVE. Recently, we studied a patient at necropsy who was diagnosed during life as having mitral PVE on the basis of fever, cerebral episodes consistent with emboli and one blood culture that grew *Staphylococcus epidermidis* and diphtheroids. She received antibiotics during most of her 4-month postoperative period, and at necropsy no PVE was found. A left ventricular aneurysm, however, was present immediately caudal to the mitral anulus and a sterile thrombus was present in the aneurysm (Fig. 37). The latter was the likely source of the cerebral emboli.

There is a general view that at times PVE can be cured by antibiotics. For cure of PVE to be established, however, it is necessary that PVE be confirmed during life, and this unequivocal confirmation can be obtained only by examination of the prosthetic valve and its anulus (site of attachment) at reoperation. In other words, to establish cure of PVE it is necessary to be absolutely positive of the diagnosis of PVE. Although usually not obtained, this confirmation now has been obtained in enough patients to support the view that PVE can indeed be cured in some patients.[118, 119, 122, 124, 125, 129, 130, 137, 139, 144, 145, 148, 164, 165]

Comparison of observations in our 22 patients with PVE to those in 74 not operated on necropsy patients with active IE involving natural *left*-sided cardiac valves disclosed certain clear differences (Table 3): (1) Ring abscess always was present in patients with PVE regardless of the site of the prosthesis and, in contrast, it was present in 32% of our 74 patients with active IE involving natural left-sided valves, and then, with rare exception, only when the aortic valve was infected. (2) The hemodynamic consequences were different. Prosthetic valve endocarditis caused valve obstruction nearly as often as valvular regurgitation whereas valvular stenosis from active IE involving natural cardiac valves was extremely rare.[87] (3) Spread of ring abscess was more extensive in patients with PVE than in patients with natural valve IE and, consequently, the frequency of high-grade conduction defects was much greater in patients with PVE. (4) The infecting organism in fatal PVE most commonly was the staphylococcus. Alpha streptococcus, which remains a common cause of fatal active IE in patients with natural cardiac valves, is a rare cause of fatal PVE.

Among patients with IE involving native cardiac valves, ring abscess, when present, almost always (95%) involves the aortic valve. Among our necropsy patients with active IE involving natural aortic valves, 40% had a ring abscess whereas only 5% of patients with IE involving natural mitral valves had a ring abscess. In contrast, each of our 22 patients with PVE had a ring abscess. Thus, valve ring abscess is the usual morphologic feature of PVE, regardless of the valve infected.

Ring abscesses in patients with PVE generally are more extensive than those in patients with IE involving natural cardiac valves. This occurrence appears to be a consequence of the rigid nature of the prosthetic frame. Once the prosthesis is loosened by the infection, the rocking rigid frame promotes spread of the infection. The greater turbulence across the aortic valve prosthesis probably accounts for the generally more extensive nature of ring abscess with aortic PVE than with mitral PVE. A consequence of this extension is the greater frequency of complete heart block and left bundle-branch block in patients with aortic PVE (32%) compared to patients with natural aortic valve endocarditis (8%).

Staphylococcus (either *aureus* or *epidermidis*) is the most common cause of PVE (59%). Many different organisms cause the remainder of the infections. Although alpha streptococcus was the responsible organism in 17% of our 74 patients with IE on natural valves, this bacterium was not the causative organism in any of our 22 patients with PVE.

The hemodynamic consequences of PVE vary with the site of the infected prosthesis. Twelve of the 15 patients (80%) with aortic PVE and 2 of the 7 patients with prosthetic mitral valve infection developed valvular regurgitation from PVE. In contrast, 5 of the 7 patients (71%) with mitral PVE and 1 of the 15 patients (7%) with aortic PVE developed valvular obstruction from the infection. Among patients with natural left-sided valvular IE, 65% (64% of the mitral and 69% of the aortic patients) developed valvular regurgitation from active IE and relatively few (3%) developed valvular obstruction from the IE.[87] Thus, aortic PVE almost always causes valvular regurgitation and mitral PVE most often causes valvular obstruction.

Splenomegaly (> 300 gm) is common both in patients with PVE (64%) and in patients with native left-sided valve IE (37%). Similarly, the frequency of infarcts in other body organs is similar in both PVE (64%) and native valve endocarditis (70%).

INFECTIVE ENDOCARDITIS AFTER VALVE COMMISSUROTOMY OR VALVULOPLASTY

In 4 of our 137 patients, IE followed valve commissurotomy or valvuloplasty operations (Table 6): mitral valve procedures in 3 and aortic valve in 1. Signs of IE appeared in the early (< 2 months) postoperative period in 3 patients and 80 days after operation in the other patient. In each of them, the IE presumably was acquired at operation. Species of Candida caused the IE in 3 and *Staphylococcus aureus* in 1. Two patients died from congestive heart failure and 2 from generalized infection.

The etiology of the underlying valvular deformity was rheumatic in the 3 patients with mitral valve disease and not certain in the 1 patient with isolated aortic valve disease. Among the 3

TABLE 6. – ACTIVE INFECTIVE ENDOCARDITIS (IE) AFTER VALVULOTOMY OR VALVULOPLASTY*: OBSERVATIONS IN 4 NECROPSY PATIENTS

PATIENT	AGE	SEX	HEMODYNAMIC LESION	TYPE OF OBSERVATION	INTERVAL (DAYS) OP-SIGNS IE	CAUSATIVE ORGANISMS	SITE OF VEGETATIONS	CAUSE OF DEATH
1	45	M	MS	Mitral commissurotomy	Early postop	*Candida paropsilosis*	MV	CHF
2	39	F	MS MR	Mitral valvuloplasty	80	*Candida guilliermondi*	MV	CHF
3	48	M	AS	Transaortic valvuloplasty	45	*Candida guilliermondi*	AV	Generalized infection
4	36	F	MS	Mitral commissurotomy	Early postop	*Staphylococcus aureus*	MV	Generalized infection

*Excludes patients with prosthetic cardiac valves.

patients with rheumatic mitral disease, 2 also had aortic valve disease and 1 had mitral, aortic and tricuspid valve disease. In each of the 4 patients, however, the vegetations were limited to the valve on which the operation was performed.

Comments on Infective Endocarditis after Valve Commissurotomy or Valvuloplasty

Although direct trauma to cardiac valves is a means of producing experimental IE,[166, 167] valvular infection after valve operations (excluding replacement) is uncommon.[120, 126, 168, 171] Of 1333 patients who had open heart operations for valvular heart disease reported by Koiwai and Nahas,[168] 11 (1%) developed IE postoperatively. Of 1889 patients undergoing nonreplacement valvular operations reported by Denton and associates,[169] 19 (1%) developed IE postoperatively. Shafer and Hall[126] reported IE in 13 of 2288 patients (0.5%) surviving open heart operations at the University of Minnesota Hospital.

Among patients undergoing open heart operations, the frequency of IE is lower in those in whom no prosthetic materials are used. Yeh and associates[171] reported IE in 18 of 400 patients (4.5%) following open heart operations; 14 of the 18 infections, however, occurred among 242 patients in whom prosthetic materials were used and only 2 among 158 patients in whom no prosthetic materials were used.

When IE follows commissurotomy or valvuloplasty procedures, the valve operated on generally is the site of the infection. In each of our 4 patients, 3 of whom had multivalvular disease, vegetations were limited to the valve operated on. Dalton and associates[172] reported 2 necropsy patients with IE following mitral valvulotomy and, in both, vegetations were limited to the mitral valve.

IE following commissurotomy or valvuloplasy operations usually is acquired at the time of operation. Staphylococcus is the organism most often cultured from cardiopulmonary bypass equipment[153, 154] and it is the most frequent cause of IE in patients surviving open heart operations.[116, 118, 120, 126, 130, 137, 139, 141, 145, 168, 169, 171] Staphylococcus caused the IE in 9 of the 11 patients reported by Koiwai and Nahas[168] and in 14 of the 19 patients reported by Denton and associates[169] with IE following valvular commissurotomy or valvulotomy. Opportunistic fungi, however, may cause IE following these operative procedures.[117, 121, 127, 128, 131] Candida species caused the IE in 3 of our patients and *Staphylococcus aureus* in the remaining patient.

INFECTIVE ENDOCARDITIS COMPLICATING CONGENITAL HEART DISEASE WITH A SHUNT

Six (4%) of our 137 patients with active IE had congenital heart disease with an intracardiac shunt (Table 7). Two had iso-

TABLE 7.—ACTIVE INFECTIVE ENDOCARDITIS (IE) IN CONGENITAL HEART DISEASE WITH SHUNT: OBSERVATIONS IN 6 NECROPSY PATIENTS

PATIENT	AGE	SEX	TYPE OF CONGENITAL HEART DISEASE	CAUSATIVE ORGANISM	SITE OF VEGETATIONS	FUNCTION OF VALVES BEFORE IE	PRINCIPAL CAUSE OF DEATH
1	2	M	T of F	*Staphylococcus aureus*	PV PT	Stenotic	Acute pneumonia
2	5	F	VSD	Alpha streptococcus	AV MV TV RV endocardium	Normal	CHF
3	17	F	TA + PTA	Unknown	MV truncus valve	Normal	CHF
4	18	M	PTA	*Staphylococcus epidermidis*	Truncus valve	Normal	CHF
5	36	M	T of F	*Candida paropsilosis*	PV PT RA and RV endocardium	Stenotic	Generalized infection
6	63	F	VSD	*Staphylococcus aureus*	AV VSD RV endocardium	Normal	Generalized infection

Abbreviations: AV = aortic valve, MV = mitral valve, PT = pulmonary trunk, PTA = persistent truncus arteriosus, RA = right atrium, RV = right ventricle, TA = tricuspid atresia, T of F = tetralogy of Fallot, TV = tricuspid valve, VSD = ventricular septal defect.

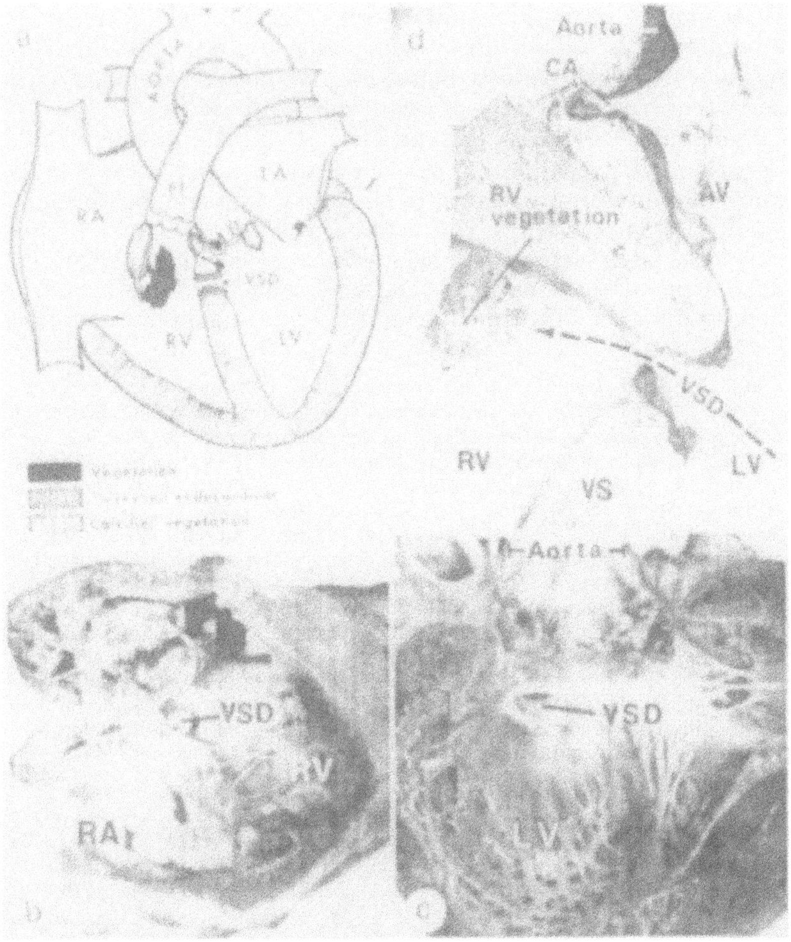

Fig. 38.—Alpha hemolytic streptococcus endocarditis in a 5-year-old girl (A68–260) with congenital ventricular septal defect (VSD). Pneumonia and anemia developed 4 months before death, and 2 months later a grade 2/6 murmur of aortic regurgitation was noted for the first time. Death resulted from a large brain embolus. Vegetation probably formed initially on the jet lesion in the right ventricular outflow tract. Dislodgment of portions of right ventricular vegetation produced septic pulmonary emboli, which presented clinically as "acute pneumonia." The exact mechanism of involvement of the aortic valve by the infective process is not certain. **a,** diagrammatic representation of location of vegetative material. Calcific deposits developed in aortic valve vegetation during the 4-month course. *RA* = right atrium; *RV* = right ventricle; *PT* = pulmonary trunk; *LA* = left atrium; *A* = aneurysm with orifice just below the aortic valve. **b,** view of opened right atrium, tricuspid valve and right ventricle showing the large vegetation *(enclosed by dashed line)* in the right ventricular outflow tract adjacent to the small ventricular septal defect. **c,** view of opened left ventricle, aortic valve and aorta showing partial but extensive destruction of aortic valve cusps by vegetative material. The borders of the ventricular septal defect are free from vegetation. **d,** photomicrograph of section through the ventricular septal defect, including a portion of the aorta, aortic valve *(AV)* cusp and ventricular septum *(VS)*. The endocardium bordering the ventricular septal defect and that in the right ventricular outflow tract is thick. *CA* — coronary artery (elastic van Gieson stain; ×8).

lated small ventricular septal defects (Figs. 38 and 39) (entirely muscular in 1), 2 had tetralogy of Fallot (with a Pott's anastomosis in 1), 1 had persistent truncus arteriosus and 1 had both persistent truncus arteriosus and tricuspid atresia.

Symptoms of IE were present from 21 to 210 days (avg 112). Fever (> 100°) was present in each of the 6 patients. New murmurs appeared in 2 patients; in the other 4, murmurs were unchanged from those present before onset of IE. Two patients developed splinter hemorrhages. Acute pneumonia developed during the IE in 5 patients. Signs of congestive heart failure appeared for the first time during the IE in 4 patients, and in 3

Fig. 39. – *Staphylococcus aureus* endocarditis in a 63-year-old woman (A75-117) with a small congenital membranous ventricular septal defect. She fell at home and was brought to the hospital unconscious. Examination revealed fever (102° F), a systolic precordial murmur and retinal and subungual hemorrhages. Chest roentgenogram showed multiple pulmonary infiltrates. **a,** opened aorta, aortic valve and left ventricle *(LV)*. The right *(R)* coronary cusp is diffusely thickened and a large defect is present at its base. The non- *(N)* and left *(L)* coronary cusps are normal. *A* = anterior mitral leaflet. **b,** longitudinal section through the aorta, right *(R)* coronary cusp, right ventricle *(RV)* and ventricular septum *(VS)*. A small former defect is present in the VS immediately below the right coronary cusp, and an abscess is present in the VS. **c,** longitudinal section anterior to that shown in **b.** The former defect *(VSD)* in the ventricular septum is better seen. The former small ventricular septal defect *(VSD)* is filled with vegetative material. **d,** opened right atrium, tricuspid valve and right ventricle. The right ventricular opening of the ventricular septal defect *(circle)* is filled with vegetative material, and the surrounding endocardium is thickened. *STL* = septal and *ATL* = anterior tricuspid leaflets.

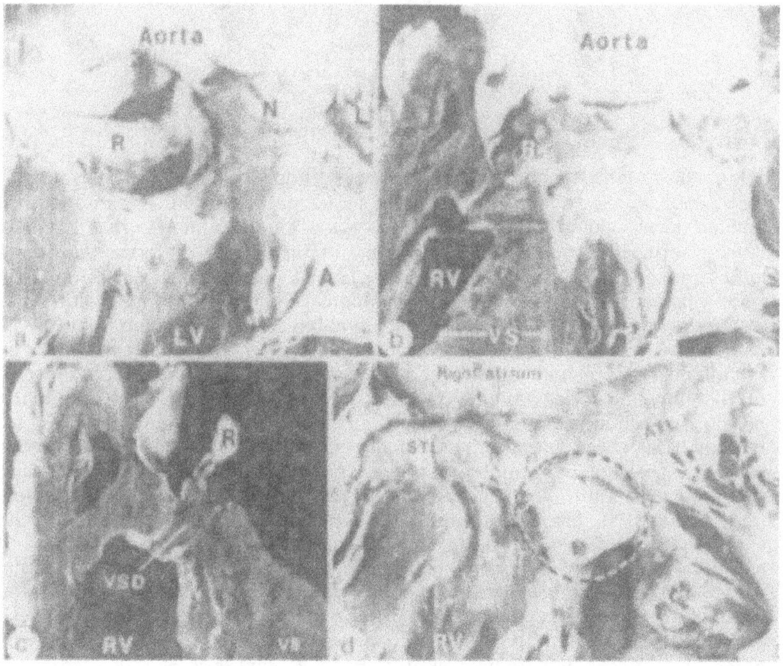

it was fatal. Two patients died from generalized infection and 1 from acute pneumonia. Blood cultures were positive during life in 5 patients and negative in 1. *Staphylococcus* (*aureus* in 2 and *epidermidis* in 1) was the most frequent infecting organism causing the IE in 3 patients. Alpha streptococcus and *Candida paropsilosis* caused the IE in 1 patient each.

► ANTONIO C. DE LEON, JR.: On occasion, in the patient with a ventricular septal defect who develops endocarditis, the involved septal leaflet of the tricuspid valve becomes attached to and effectively closes the VSD. Thus, part of the clinical presentation could include *disappearance* of the cardiac murmur.

At necropsy, vegetations were present in the right side of the heart in 2 patients and in both sides of the heart in 4, including the 2 with persistent truncus arteriosus. In both patients with tetralogy of Fallot, vegetations were present on the pulmonic valve; in 1 of them, vegetations also were present in the pulmonary trunk opposite the Pott's anastomosis and in the right ventricular outflow tract. In each of the 2 patients with isolated ventricular septal defect, vegetations were present in the right ventricle: on the mural endocardium opposite the defect as well as surrounding it in 1 patient and on the ventricular side of the septal tricuspid leaflet in the other. Both patients also had vegetations on left-sided cardiac valves. In 1 (Fig. 38), the IE appeared to have initially involved the tricuspid valve; in the other (Fig. 39), the IE appeared to have initially involved a prolapsing, right coronary aortic valve cusp and then spread via a membranous ventricular septal defect to involve right ventricular mural endocardium. Vegetations were present on the truncus valve in both patients with persistent truncus arteriosus and, in 1 of them, a 17-year-old girl who also had tricuspid atresia, vegetations also were present on the mitral valve. Septic infarcts were present in the lungs of 4 patients.

COMMENTS ON INFECTIVE ENDOCARDITIS COMPLICATING CONGENITAL HEART DISEASE WITH A SHUNT

Patients with congenital heart disease have an increased risk of developing IE. Gelfman and Levine[34] found IE in 35 (7%) of 453 necropsy patients with congenital heart disease, but among their 181 necropsy patients older than 2 years of age, 30 (17%) had IE. In a study of IE in infants and children, Johnson and associates[173] found an absolute increase in the number of hospital admissions for IE in each decade from 1943 to 1972, and this increase appeared to result from a growing population of older patients with congenital heart disease.

Among patients with congenital heart disease, those with small ventricular septal defect, tetralogy of Fallot or patent ductus arteriosus appear to have the greatest risk of developing

IE.[34, 35, 37, 173, 174] Of 164 necropsy patients with ventricular septal defect reported by Gelfman and Levine,[34] 17 (10%) had infective IE, but of the 44 in whom the defect was small, IE occurred in 23%. Two of their 16 patients with tetralogy of Fallot and 4 (3%) of their 134 patients with patent ductus arteriosus had IE. Among patients with congenital heart disease and IE reported by Volger and Dorney,[37] 15 (39%) had ventricular septal defect, 7 (18%) had tetralogy of Fallot and 7 had patent ductus arteriosus. Two of our 6 patients had isolated ventricular septal defect, 2 had tetralogy of Fallot and 2 had persistent truncus arteriosus.

In patients with congenital cardiovascular shunts and IE, the vegetations usually are located on the low-pressure side of the defect, which usually is the site of endocardial trauma.[34, 75] Patients with isolated ventricular septal defect and IE usually have vegetations on right ventricular mural endocardium or tricuspid valve in opposition to this defect.[34, 175] When IE occurs in patients with tetralogy of Fallot who are not operated on, vegetations usually are on the arterial side of the stenotic pulmonic valve.[34] In patients with IE associated with patent ductus arteriosus or tetralogy of Fallot with an operative systemic-pulmonary arterial shunt, the vegetations usually occur on the pulmonary side of the shunt.[34, 175, 176]

Staphylococcus has become a frequent cause of IE among patients with congenital heart disease. Among 141 patients under age 25 years with IE between 1933 and 1972, Johnson and associates[173] found that the frequency with which staphylococcus caused the IE rose from 22% during the first two decades to 33% during the later two decades. Staphylococcus was the most frequent cause (34%) of IE among 38 patients with congenital heart disease reported by Volger and Dorney.[37] In 3 of our 6 patients, the endocarditis was due to staphylococcus.

INFECTIVE ENDOCARDITIS LIMITED TO MURAL ENDOCARDIUM

Eight of our 137 necropsy patients with IE had vegetations limited to mural (nonvalvular) endocardium (Table 8). Six patients had leukemia, 1 had lymphoma and 1 had Waldenström's macroglobulinemia. Each had received cytotoxic drugs. A fungus caused the IE in each: Candida species in 4, Mucor species in 3 and Aspergillus species in 1. None had symptoms or signs of cardiac disease, and endocarditis was not suspected clinically in any of them. Death was attributed to acute pneumonia in 5, to brain abscess in 2 and to hemorrhage in 1.

In all 8 patients, the endocardial vegetations were not primary but resulted from extension of infections originating at other sites. Five patients had vegetations confined to ventricular endocardium: right ventricle in 4 and left ventricular papillary muscle in 1 (Fig. 40). Each of them also had multiple myocardial

TABLE 8.–ACTIVE INFECTIVE ENDOCARDITIS LIMITED TO MURAL ENDOCARDIUM: OBSERVATIONS IN 8 NECROPSY PATIENTS

PATIENT	AGE	SEX	UNDERLYING DISEASE	CAUSATIVE ORGANISM	SITE(S) OF VEGETATIONS	PRINCIPAL CAUSE OF DEATH
1	7	F	AML	*Candida tropicalis*	RV	Acute pneumonia
2	29	M	CML	Candida species	RV	Acute pneumonia
3	65	M	CML	*Candida albicans*	RV	Brain abscess
4	30	F	CML	Candida species	RV	Bleeding
5	15	M	AML	Mucor species	LA	Acute pneumonia
6	27	M	Lymphoma	Aspergillus species	LA	Acute pneumonia
7	33	M	AML	*Mucor pusillus*	SVC, IVC, RA, LA, RPV	Acute pneumonia
8	58	M	Waldenström's macroglobulinemia	Mucor species	LV papillary muscle	Brain abscess

Abbreviations: AML = acute myelogenous leukemia, CML = chronic myelogenous leukemia, RA = right atrium, RV = right ventricle, LA = left atrium, LV = left ventricle, IVC = inferior vena cava, SVC = superior vena cava, RPV = right pulmonary vein.

abscesses from a generalized fungal pyemia and, in each, the vegetations resulted from extension of a myocardial abscess to the endocardium. Two patients had vegetations confined to left atrial endocardium and 1 had vegetations involving left atrial, atrial septal and right atrial endocardium in addition to pulmonary veins. Each of these 3 patients had massive pulmonary mycosis that had extended into the atria via the pulmonary veins.

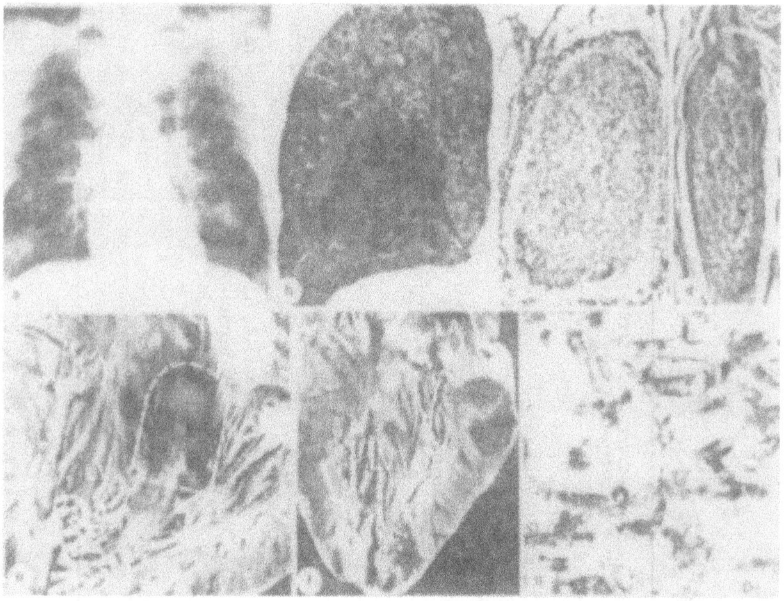

Fig. 40.—Mucor species endocarditis confined to left ventricular mural endocardium in a 58-year-old man (A75–44). Waldenström's macroglobulinemia had been present for $5^{1}/_{2}$ years before death, and he had received various combinations of cytotoxic drugs. Pancytopenia developed and 13 days before death he was hospitalized because of high fever, productive cough and mental confusion. Several days later, a chest roentgenogram **(a)** revealed infiltrates in both lungs. He became progressively more confused and left hemiparesis appeared. Signs or symptoms of cardiac dysfunction were never present. **b,** longitudinal section through the left lung. A large fungal abscess involves the upper and lower lobes. **c,** histologic section of a pulmonary vein (methenamine silver stain; ×108). The lumen is filled with fungal hyphae. **d,** histologic section of an intramural coronary artery in the left ventricular papillary muscle (PAS stain; ×140). The lumen is totally occluded by fungal hyphae. **e,** opened left ventricle *(LV)*. A large fungal vegetation surrounds a portion of the posteromedial papillary muscle. **f,** longitudinal section of heart showing the aortic valve *(AV)*, left atrium *(LA)*, mitral valve *(MV)* and left ventricle *(LV)*. Multiple fungal abscesses are present in the myocardium. **g,** histologic section of a portion of the mural vegetation showing fungal hyphae (methenamine silver stain; ×880).

Comments on Infective Endocarditis Limited to Mural Endocardium

IE confined to mural endocardium is not common in patients without ventricular septal defect. Among 92 necropsy patients with IE reported by Wilson[7] in 1963, none had vegetations limited to mural endocardium. In 1972, Buchbinder and Roberts[177] reported 6 patients with isolated mural endocarditis and found only 14 previously reported patients. Although 6% of our 137 patients with IE had vegetations limited to mural endocardium, many patients studied at necropsy at the Clinical Center of NIH have received cytotoxic drugs for malignant neoplastic disease, and thus the true incidence of IE confined to mural endocardium probably is much lower.

IE confined here to mural endocardium is virtually limited to patients with a debilitating disease, and the mural vegetations rarely represent a site of primary infection. The causative organism usually is a fungus and the mural vegetations most often result from extension of a myocardial abscess to the endocardium.[177] All of our 8 patients had received cytotoxic drugs for leukemia or lymphoma, and a fungus caused terminal infection in each. Five patients with mural vegetations had multiple myocardial abscesses and in each of them the mural vegetations represented extension of myocardial abscesses to the endocardium. Mural vegetations that are not due to extension of myocardial abscesses usually are located in the left atrium and represent extension of pulmonary mycosis via the pulmonary veins.[177]

Isolated mural IE by itself rarely is fatal. None of our 8 patients had symptoms of heart disease and, in each, death was due to a cause other than the endocardial infection. Mural vegetations, however, may embolize[178, 179] and, rarely, may be a primary source of persistent bacteremia.[180]

REFERENCES

1. Rokitansky, C.: *Lehrbuch der Pathologischen Anatomie* (Wien: Wilhelm Braumüller, 1856), Vol.II.
2. Osler, W.: Malignant endocarditis, Lancet 1:415, 459, 505, 1885.
3. Preble, H. B.: Pneumococcus endocarditis, Am. J. Med. Sci. 128:782, 1904.
4. Clawson, B. J.: An analysis of two hundred and twenty cases of endocarditis with special reference to the subacute bacterial type, Arch. Intern. Med. 33:157, 1924.
5. Thayer, W. S.: Bacterial or infective endocarditis. Edinburgh Med. J. 38: 237, 307, 1931.
6. Goldburgh, H. L., Baer, S., and Lieber, M. M.: Acute bacterial endocarditis of the tricuspid valve, Am. J. Med. Sci. 204:319, 1942.
7. Wilson, L. M.: Pathology of fatal bacterial endocarditis before and since the introduction of antibiotics, Ann. Intern. Med. 58:84, 1963.
8. Allen, A. C.: Mechanism of localization of vegetations of bacterial endocarditis, Arch. Pathol. 27:399, 1939.
9. Lepeschkin, E.: On the relation between the site of valvular involvement in endocarditis and the blood pressure resting on the valve, Am. J. Med. Sci. 224:318, 1952.
10. Roberts, W. C., Dangel, J. C., and Bulkley, B. H.: Non-rheumatic valvular cardiac disease: A clinicopathologic survey of 27 different conditions causing valvular dysfunction, Cardiovasc. Clin. 5:333, 1973.
11. Clawson, B. J.: Rheumatic heart disease. An analysis of 796 cases, Am. Heart J. 20:454, 1940.
12. Wallach, J. B., Borgatta, E. F., and Angrist, A. A.: *Rheumatic Heart Disease. Pathology and Clinical Implications – A Summary of Five Hundred and Nine Autopsied Cases* (Springfield, Ill.: Charles C Thomas, Publisher, 1962.
13. Ellis, K., Jaffe, C., Malm, J. R., and Bowman, F. O., Jr.: Infective endocarditis. Roentgenographic considerations, Radiol. Clin. North Am. 11: 415, 1973.
14. Bramwell, B.: On right sided endocarditis, Am. J. Med. Sci. 91:419, 1886.

15. Karotkin, L., and Marcuse, P.: Bacterial endocarditis of the tricuspid valve, South. Med. J. 39:769, 1946.
16. Bain, R. C., Edwards, J. E., Scheifley, C. H., and Geraci, J. E.: Right-sided bacterial endocarditis and endarteritis, Am. J. Med. 24:98, 1958.
17. Roberts, W. C., and Buchbinder, N. A.: Right-sided valvular infective endocarditis. A clinicopathologic study of twelve necropsy patients, Am. J. Med. 53:7, 1972.
18. Luttgens, W. F.: Endocarditis in "main line" opium addicts. Report on eleven cases, Arch. Intern. Med. 83:653, 1949.
19. Hussey, H. H., and Katz, S.: Infections resulting from narcotic addiction. Report of 102 cases, Am. J. Med. 9:186, 1950.
20. Louria, D. B., Hensle, T., and Rose, J.: The major medical complications of heroin addiction, Ann. Intern. Med. 67:1, 1967.
21. Sapira, J. D.: The narcotic addict as a medical patient, Am. J. Med. 45:555, 1968.
22. Reyes, M. P., Palutke, W. A., Wylin, R. F., and Lerner, A. M.: Pseudomonas endocarditis in the Detroit Medical Center 1969–1972, Medicine 52:173, 1973.
23. Mills, J., and Drew, D.: *Serratia marcescens* endocarditis: A regional illness associated with intravenous drug abuse, Ann. Intern. Med. 84:29, 1976.
24. Olsson, R. A., and Romansky, M. J.: Staphylococcal tricuspid endocarditis in heroin addicts, Ann. Intern. Med. 57:755, 1962.
25. Cherubin, C. E., Baden, M., Kavaler, F., Lerner, S., and Cline, W.: Infective endocarditis in narcotic addicts, Ann. Intern. Med. 69:1091, 1968.
26. Ramsey, R. G., Gunnar, R. M., and Tobin, J. R.: Endocarditis in the drug addict, Am. J. Cardiol. 25:608, 1970.
27. Menda, K. B., and Gorbach, S. L.: Favorable experience with bacterial endocarditis in heroin addicts, Ann. Intern. Med. 78:25, 1973.
28. Dreyer, N. P., and Fields, B. N.: Heroin-associated infective endocarditis. A report of 28 cases, Ann. Intern. Med. 78:699, 1973.
29. Banks, R., Fletcher, R., and Ali, N.: Infective endocarditis in heroin addicts, Am. J. Med. 55:444, 1973.
30. Dowling, H. F., Lepper, M., Caldwell, E. R., and Spies, H. W.: Staphylococci endocarditis: An analysis of 25 cases treated with antibiotics together with a review of the recent literature, Medicine 31:155, 1952.
31. Buchbinder, N. A., and Roberts, W. C.: Alcoholism, an important but unemphasized factor predisposing to infective endocarditis, Arch. Intern. Med. 132:689, 1973.
32. Straus, A. L., and Hamburger, M.: Pneumococcal endocarditis in the penicillin era, Arch. Intern. Med. 118:190, 1966.
33. Pankey, G. A.: Acute bacterial endocarditis at the University of Minnesota Hospital, 1939–1959, Am. Heart J. 64:583, 1962.
34. Gelfman, R., and Levine, S. A.: The incidence of acute and subacute bacterial endocarditis in congenital heart disease, Am. J. Med. Sci. 204:324, 1942.
35. Barker, P. S.: A clinical study of subacute bacterial infection confined to the right side of the heart or the pulmonary artery, Am. Heart J. 37:1054, 1949.
36. Bashour, F. A., and Winchell, C. P.: Right-sided bacterial endocarditis, Am. J. Med. Sci. 240:411, 1960.
37. Volger, W. R., and Dorney, E. R.: Bacterial endocarditis in congenital heart disease, Am. Heart J. 64:198, 1962.
38. Horder, T. J.: Infective endocarditis with an analysis of 150 cases and with special reference to the chronic form of the disease, Q. J. Med. 2:289, 1909.
39. Arnett, J. H.: Splenic and hepatic enlargement in endocarditis: A study of two hundred and eighty-six autopsy findings, Am. J. Med. Sci. 163:590, 1922.
40. Angrist, A., and Marquiss, J.: The changing morphologic picture of endocarditis since the advent of chemotherapy and antibiotic agents, Am. J. Pathol. 30:39, 1954.

41. Morgan, W. L., and Bland, E. F.: Bacterial endocarditis in the antibiotic era with special reference to the later complications, Circulation 19:753, 1959.
42. Robinson, M. J., and Ruedy, J: Sequelae of bacterial endocarditis, Am. J. Med. 32:922, 1962.
43. Rabinovich, S., Evans, J., Smith, I. M.., and January, L. E.: A long-term view of bacterial endocarditis: 337 cases 1924 to 1963, Ann. Intern. Med. 63:185, 1965.
44. Uwaydah, M. M., and Weinberg, A. N.,: Bacterial endocarditis – a changing pattern, N. Engl. J. Med. 273:1231, 1965.
45. Lerner, P. I., and Weinstein, L.: Infective endocarditis in the antibiotic era, N. Engl. J. Med. 274:199, 1966.
46. Cherubin, C. E., and Neu, H. C.: Infective endocarditis at the Presbyterian Hospital in New York City from 1938 – 1967, Am. J. Med. 51:83, 1971
47. Buchbinder, N. A., and Roberts, W. C.: Left-sided valvular active infective endocarditis. A study of forty-five necropsy patients, Am. J. Med. 53:20, 1972.
48. Hayward, G. W.: Infective endocarditis: A changing disease – I, Br. Med. J. 2:706, 1973.
49. Hayward, G. W.: Infective endocarditis: A changing disease – II, Br. Med. J. 2:764, 1973.
50. Steiner, I., Patel, A. K., Hutt, M. S. R., and Somers, K.: Pathology of infective endocarditis. A postmortem evaluation, Br. Heart J. 35:159, 1973.
51. Weinstein, L., and Rubin, R. H.: Infective endocarditis – 1973, Prog. Cardiovasc. Dis. 16:239, 1973.
52. Cohen, L., and Freedman, L. R.: Damage to the aortic valve as a cause of death in bacterial endocarditis, Ann. Intern. Med. 55:562, 1961.
53. Roberts, W. C.: The structure of the aortic valve in clinically isolated aortic stenosis. An autopsy study of 162 patients over 15 years of age, Circulation 42:91, 1970.
54. Roberts, W. C.: The congenitally bicuspid aortic valve. A study of 85 autopsy cases, Am. J. Cardiol. 26:72, 1970.
55. Roberts, W. C.: Anatomically isolated aortic valvular disease. The case against its being of rheumatic etiology, Am. J. Med. 49:151, 1970.
56. Roberts, W. C., Perloff, J. R., and Costantino, T.: Severe aortic stenosis in patients over 65 years of age. A clinicopathologic study, Am. J. Cardiol. 27:497, 1971.
57. Traut, E. F., Carter, J. B., Gumbiner, S. H., and Hench, R. N.: Bacterial endocarditis in the elderly. A report of 94 autopsied cases, Geriatrics 4:205, 1949.
58. Thell, R., Martin, F. H., and Edwards, J. E.: Bacterial endocarditis in subjects 60 years of age and older, Circulation 51:174, 1975.
59. Levison, M. E., Kaye, D., Mandell, G. L., and Hook, E. W.: Characteristics of patients with multiple episodes of bacterial endocarditis, JAMA 211:1355, 1970.
60. Austrian, R.: The syndrome of pneumococcal endocarditis, meningitis and rupture of the aortic valve, Arch. Intern. Med. 99:539, 1957.
61. Linhart, J. W., and Taylor, W. J.: The late apical systolic murmur. Clinical, hemodynamic and angiographic observations. Am. J. Cardiol. 18:164, 1966.
62. LeBauer, E. J., Perloff, J. K., and Keliher, T. F.: The isolated systolic click with bacterial endocarditis, Am. Heart J. 73:534, 1967.
63. Case records of the Massachusetts General Hospital. Weekly clinicopathological exercises. Case 30-1974, N. Engl. J. Med. 291:242, 1974.
64. Morrison, H.: A study of the incidence of sub-acute bacterial endocarditis at the Massachusetts General Hospital, Boston Med. Surg. J. 197:46, 1927.
65. Middleton, W. S., and Burke, M.: Streptococcus viridans endocarditis lenta. A clinico-pathologic analysis of the experience in the Wisconsin General Hospital, Am. J. Med. Sci. 198:301, 1939.
66. Seabury, J. H.: Subacute bacterial endocarditis. Experiences during the past decade, Arch. Intern. Med. 79:1, 1947.

67. Christian, H. A.: The determinative background of subacute bacterial endocarditis, Am. J. Med. Sci. 201:34, 1941.
68. Kelson, S. R., and White, P. D.: Notes on 250 cases of subacute bacterial (streptococcal) endocarditis studied and treated between 1927 and 1939, Ann. Intern. Med. 22:40, 1945.
69. Wallace, H. M., and Rich, H.: Changing status of rheumatic fever and rheumatic heart disease in children and youth, Am. J. Dis. Child. 89:7, 1955.
70. Massell, B. F., Fyler, D. C., and Roy, S. B.: The clinical picture of rheumatic fever. Diagnosis, immediate prognosis, course, and therapeutic implications, Am. J. Cardiol. 1:436, 1958.
71. Bland, E. F.: Declining severity of rheumatic fever. A comparative study of the past four decades, N. Engl. J. Med. 262:597, 1960.
72. Massell, B. F., Amezcua, F., and Pelargonio, S.: Evolving picture of rheumatic fever. Data from 40 years at The House of the Good Samaritan, JAMA 188:287, 1964.
73. Stollerman, G. H.: *Rheumatic Fever and Streptococcal Infection* (New York: Grune & Stratton, Inc., 1975), pp. 209–226.
74. Cates, J. E., and Christie, R. V.: Subacute bacterial endocarditis. A review of 442 patients treated in 14 centers appointed by the Penicillin Trials Committee of the Medical Research Council, Q. J. Med. 20:93, 1951.
75. Perry, E. L., Fleming, R. G., and Edwards, J. E.: Myocardial lesions in bacterial endocarditis, Ann. Intern. Med. 36:126, 1952.
76. Kalman, C., Thomison, J. B., and Shapiro, J. L.: Bacterial endocarditis: Autopsy experience over a thirty year period, South. Med. J. 55:1208, 1962.
77. Guze, L. B., and Pearce, M. L.: Hospital-acquired bacterial endocarditis, Arch. Intern. Med. 112:56, 1963.
78. Kerr, A., Jr.: *Subacute Bacterial Endocarditis* (Springfield, Ill.: Charles C Thomas, Publisher, 1955), p. 255.
79. Finland, M., and Barnes, M. W.: Changing etiology of bacterial endocarditis in the antibacterial era. Experiences at Boston City Hospital 1933–1965, Ann. Intern. Med. 72:341, 1970.
80. Watanakunakorn, C., Tan, J. S., and Phair, J. P.: Some salient features of staphylococcus aureus endocarditis, Am. J. Med. 54:473, 1973.
81. Utley, J. R., and Mills, J.: Annular erosion and pericarditis. Complications of endocarditis of the aortic root, J. Thorac. Cardiovasc. Surg. 64:76, 1972.
82. Gonzalez-Lavin, L., Lise, M., and Ross, D.: The importance of the "jet lesion" in bacterial endocarditis involving the left heart. Surgical considerations, J. Thorac. Cardiovasc. Surg. 59:185, 1970.
83. English, T. A., Honey, M., and Cleland, W. P.: Ruptured true aneurysm of mitral valve endocarditis. A complication of aortic valve endocarditis, Br. Heart J. 34:434, 1972.
84. Edwards, J. E.: Mitral insufficiency secondary to aortic valvular bacterial endocarditis, Circulation 46:623, 1972.
85. Weinstein, L., and Schlesinger, J. J.: Pathoanatomic, pathophysiologic and clinical correlations in endocarditis, N. Engl. J. Med. 291:832, 1122, 1974.
86. Fowler, N. O., Hamburger, M. H., and Bove, K. E.: Aortic valve perforation, Am. J. Med. 42:539, 1967.
87. Roberts, W. C., Ewy, G. A., Glancy, D. L., and Marcus, F. I.: Valvular stenosis produced by active infective endocarditis, Circulation 36:449, 1967.
88. Arnett, E. N., and Roberts, W. C.: Valve ring abscess in active infective endocarditis. Frequency, location, and clues to clinical diagnosis from study of 95 necropsy patients, Circulation 54:140, 1976.
89. Burnside, J. W., and DeSanctis, R. W.: Bacterial endocarditis on calcification of the mitral anulus fibrosus, Ann. Intern. Med. 76:615, 1972.
90. Watanakunakorn, C.: Staphylococcus aureus endocarditis on the calcified mitral anulus fibrosus, Am. J. Med. Sci. 266:219, 1973.
91. Case records of the Massachusetts General Hospital. Weekly clinicopathological exercises. Case 5-1975, N. Engl. J. Med. 292:255, 1975.

92. Ponfick, E.: Ueber embolische aneurysmen, nebst bemerkungen über das acute herzaneurysma (herzgeschwür), Virchows Arch. (Pathol. Anat.) 58: 528, 1873.
93. Beck, D.: Pericarditis and subacute bacterial endocarditis, J. Mt. Sinai Hosp. 8:364, 1941.
94. McColl, I.: Pericarditis due to a mycotic aneurysm in subacute bacterial endocarditis. Report of a case affecting congenitally stenosed quadricuspid aortic valve, Guys Hosp. Rep. 107:34, 1958.
95. Roberts, N. K., and Somerville, J.: Pathological significance of electrocardiographic changes in aortic valve endocarditis, Br. Heart J. 31:395, 1969.
96. Meshel, J. C., Wachtel, H. L., and Graham J.: Bacterial endocarditis presenting as heart block, Am. J. Med. 48:254, 1970.
97. Kleid, J. J., Kim, E. S., Brand, B., Eckles, S., and Gordon, G. M.: Heart block complicating acute bacterial endocarditis, Chest 61:301, 1972.
98. Wang, K., Gobel, F., Gleason, D. F., and Edwards, J. E.: Complete heart block complicating bacterial endocarditis, Circulation 46:939, 1972.
99. Katz, D., Cooper, J. A., and Frieden, J.: Bacterial endocarditis presenting as complete heart block with paradoxical (left-to-right) pulmonary emboli, Am. Heart J. 85:108, 1973.
100. Buchbinder, W. C., and Saphir, O.: Heart failure in subacute bacterial endocarditis, Arch. Intern. Med. 64:336, 1939.
101. Saphir, O: Myocardial lesions in subacute bacterial endocarditis, Am. J. Pathol. 11:143, 1935.
102. Correll, H. L., Lubitz, J. M., and Lindert, M. C. F.: Bacterial endocarditis: Clinicopathologic studies of untreated, treated and cured patients, Ann. Intern. Med. 35:45, 1951.
103. de Navasquez, S.: The incidence and pathogenesis of myocardial lesions in subacute bacterial endocarditis, J. Pathol. Bacteriol. 49:33, 1939.
104. Wenger, N. K., and Bauer, S.: Coronary embolism: Review of literature and presentation of 15 cases, Am. J. Med. 25:549, 1958.
105. Estes, E. H., Dalton, F. M., Entman, M. L., Dixon, H. B., III, and Hackel, D. B.: The anatomy and blood supply of the papillary muscles of the left ventricle, Am. Heart J. 71:356, 1966.
106. Roberts, W. C., and Morrow. A. G.: Anatomic studies of hearts containing caged-ball prosthetic valves, Johns Hopkins Med. J. 121:271, 1967.
107. Roberts, W. C., and Morrow, A. G.: Causes of death and other anatomic observations after cardiac valve replacement, Adv. Cardiol. 7:226, 1972
108. Roberts, W. C., Bulkley, B. H., and Morrow, A. G.: Pathologic anatomy of cardiac valve replacement: A study of 224 necropsy patients, Prog. Cardiovasc. Dis. 15:539, 1973.
109. Fishbein, M. C., Roberts, W. C., Golden, A., and Hufnagel, C. A.: Cardiac pathology after aortic valve replacement using Hufnagel trileaflet prostheses: A study of 20 necropsy patients, Am. Heart J. 89:443, 1975.
110. Roberts, W. C., Fishbein, M. C., and Golden, A.: Cardiac pathology after valve replacement by disc prosthesis. A study of 61 necropsy patients, Am. J. Cardiol. 35:740, 1975.
111. Fishbein, M. C., and Roberts, W. C.: Late postoperative anatomic observations after insertion of Hufnagel caged-ball prostheses in descending thoracic aorta, Chest 68:6, 1975.
112. Roberts, W. C., and Hammer, W. J.: Cardiac pathology after valve replacement with a tilting disc prosthesis (Björk-Shiley type): A study of 46 necropsy patients and 49 Björk-Shiley prostheses, Am. J. Cardiol. 37:1024, 1976.
113. Cohn, L. H., Roberts, W. C., Rockoff, S. D., and Morrow, A. G.: Bacterial endocarditis following aortic valve replacement. Clinical and pathologic correlations, Circulation 33:209, 1966.
114. Roberts, W. C., and Morrow, A. G.: Bacterial endocarditis involving prosthetic mitral valves. Clinical and pathologic observations, Arch. Pathol. 82:162, 1966
115. Arnett, E. N., and Roberts, W. C.: Prosthetic valve endocarditis. A

clinicopathologic analysis of 22 necropsy patients with comparison of observations to 74 necropsy patients with active infective endocarditis involving natural left-sided cardiac valves, Am. J. Cardiol. 38:281, 1976.
116. Björk, V. O.: Aortic valve replacement, Thorax 19:369, 1964.
117. Newman, W. H., and Cordell, A. R.: Aspergillus endocarditis after open-heart surgery. Report of a case and review of literature, J. Thorac. Cardiovasc. Surg. 48:652, 1964.
118. Amoury, R. A., Bowman, F. O., Jr., and Malm, J. R.: Endocarditis associated with intracardiac prostheses. Diagnosis, management, and prophylaxis, J. Thorac. Cardiovasc. Surg. 51:35, 1966.
119. Stein, P. D., Harken, D. E., and Dexter, L.: The nature and prevention of prosthetic valve endocarditis, Am. Heart J. 71:393, 1966.
120. Fraser, R. S., Rossall, R. E., and Dvorkin, J.: Bacterial endocarditis occurring after open-heart surgery, Can. Med. Assoc. J. 96:1551, 1967.
121. McConnell, E. M., and Roberts, W. C.: Pathological findings in three cases of fungal endocarditis complicating open-heart surgery, J. Clin. Pathol. 20: 555, 1967.
122. Geraci, J. E., Forth, R. J., and Ellis, F. H.: Postoperative prosthetic valve endocarditis due to *Corynebacterium xerosis*, Mayo Clin. Proc. 42:736, 1967.
123. Cheng, T. O., Kinhal, V., and Tice, D. A.: Fatal thrombosis of the Starr-Edwards mitral valve prosthesis associated with bacterial endocarditis. Diagnostic significance of a disappearing prosthetic click, Chest 57:151, 1970.
124. Hairston, P., and Lee, W. H., Jr.: Management of infected prosthetic heart valves, Ann. Thorac. Surg. 9:229, 1970.
125. Killen, D. A., Collins, H. A., Koenig, M. G., and Goodman, J. S.: Prosthetic cardiac valves and bacterial endocarditis, Ann. Thorac. Surg. 9:238, 1970.
126. Shafer, R. B., and Hall, W. H.: Bacterial endocarditis following open heart surgery, Am. J. Cardiol. 25:602, 1970.
127. Chadhuri, M. R.: Fungal endocarditis after valve replacements, J. Thorac. Cardiovasc. Surg. 60:207, 1970.
128. Gage, A. A., Dean, D. C., Schimert, G., and Minsley, N.: Aspergillus infection after cardiac surgery, Arch. Surg. 101:384, 1970.
129. Block, P. C., DeSanctis, R. W., Weinberg, A. N., and Austen, W. G.: Prosthetic valve endocarditis, J. Thorac. Cardiovasc. Surg. 60:540, 1970.
130. Okies, J. E., Viroslav, J., and Williams, T. W., Jr.: Endocarditis after cardiac valvular replacement, Chest 59:198, 1971.
131. Ostermiller, W. E., Jr., Dye, W. S., and Weinberg, M.: Fungal endocarditis following cardiovascular surgery, J. Thorac. Cardiovasc. Surg. 61:670, 1971.
132. Lawrence, T., Shockman, A. T., and MacVaugh, H., III: Aspergillus infection of prosthetic aortic valves, Chest 60:406, 1971.
133. Robinson, M. J., Greenberg, J. J., Korn, M., and Rywlin, A. M.: Infective endocarditis at autopsy: 1965–1969, Am. J. Med. 52:492, 1972.
134. Levin, S., Balagtas, R., Susmano, A., Edwards, L., and Dainauskas, J.: Meningococcus endocarditis at the site of Starr-Edwards mitral prosthesis, Arch. Intern. Med. 129:963, 1972.
135. Joassin, A., and Edwards, J. E.: Late causes of death after mitral valve replacement, J. Thorac. Cardiovasc. Surg. 65:255, 1973.
136. Vlachakis, N. D., Gazes, P. C., and Hairston, P.: Nocardial endocarditis following mitral valve replacement, Chest 63:276, 1973.
137. Slaughter, L., Morris, J. E., and Starr, A.: Prosthetic valvular endocarditis. A 12-year review, Circulation 47:1319, 1973.
138. Case records of the Massachusetts General Hospital. Weekly clinicopathological exercises. Case 24-1973, N. Engl. J. Med. 288:1290, 1973.
139. Dismukes, W. E., Karchmer, A. W., Buckley, M. J., Austen, W. G., and Swartz, M. N.: Prosthetic valve endocarditis. Analysis of 38 cases, Circulation 48:365, 1973.
140. Jackson, G., and Saunders, K.: Prosthetic valve diphtheroid endocarditis

treated with sodium fusidate and erythromycin, Br. Heart J. 35:931, 1973.

141. Harris, J. A., and Cobbs, C. G.: Serratia endocarditis in patients with a Starr-Edwards valve. Report of a case of bacteriologic cure with antimicrobial therapy, South. Med. J. 66:1117, 1973.

142. Hall, W. J., III: Penicillium endocarditis following open heart surgery and prosthetic valve insertion, Am. Heart J. 87:501, 1974.

143. McAllister, R. G., Samet, J., Mazzoleni, A., and Dillon, M. L.: Endocarditis on prosthetic mitral valves. Fatal obstruction to left ventricular inflow, Chest 66:682, 1974.

144. Madison, J., Wang, K., Gobel, F. L., and Edwards, J. E.: Prosthetic aortic valvular endocarditis, Circulation 51:940, 1975.

145. Wilson, W. R., Jaumin, P. M., Danielson, G. K., Giuliani, E. R., Washington, J. A., and Getaci, J. E.: Prosthetic valve endocarditis, Ann. Intern. Med. 82:751, 1975

146. Rubenstein, E., Noriega, E. R., Simberkoff, M. S., Holzman, R., and Rahal, J. J.: Fungal endocarditis: Analysis of 24 cases and review of the literature, Medicine 54:331, 1975.

147. Robboy, S. J., and Kaiser, J.: Pathogenesis of fungal infection on heart valve prostheses, Hum. Pathol. 6:711, 1975.

148. Kloster, F. E.: Diagnosis and management of complications of prosthetic heart valves, Am. J. Cardiol. 35:872, 1975.

149. Conte, J. E., Cohen, S. N., Roe, B. B., and Elashoff, R. M.: Antibiotic prophylaxis and cardiac surgery. A prospective double-blind comparison of single-dose versus multiple-dose regimens, Ann. Intern. Med. 76:943, 1972.

150. Goodman, J. S., Schaffner, W., Collins, H. A., Battersby, E. J., and Koenig, M. G.: Infection after cardiovascular surgery: Clinical study including examination of antimicrobial prophylaxis, N. Engl. J. Med. 278:117, 1968.

151. Nelson, R. M., Jenson, C. B., Peterson, C. A., and Sanders, B. C.: Effective use of prophylactic antibiotics in open-heart surgery, Arch. Surg. 90:731, 1965.

152. Herr, R., Starr, A., McCord, C. W., and Wood, J. A.: Special problems following valve replacement. Embolus, leak, infection, red cell damage, Ann. Thorac. Surg. 1:403, 1965.

153. Ankeney, J. L., and Parker, R. F., Staphylococcal Endocarditis Following Open Heart Surgery Related to Positive Intraoperative Blood Cultures, in Brewer, L. A. III (ed.), *Prosthetic Heart Valves* (Springfield, Ill.: Charles C Thomas, Publisher, 1969), pp. 719–730.

154. Blakemore, W. S., McGarrity, G. J., Thurer, R. J., Wallace, H. W., MacVaugh, H. III, and Ciriell, L. L.: Infection of air-borne bacteria with cardiopulmonary bypass, Surgery 70:830, 1971.

155. Kammer, R. B., and Utz, J. P.: Aspergillus species endocarditis. The new face of a not so rare disease, Am. J. Med. 56:506, 1974.

156. Wigle, E. D., and Labrosse, C. J.: Sudden, severe, aortic insufficiency, Circulation 32:708, 1965.

157. Wise, J. R., Bentall, H. H., Cleland W. P., Goodwin, J. F., Hallidie-Smith, K. A., and Oakley, C. M.: Urgent aortic-valve replacement for acute aortic regurgitation due to infective endocarditis, Lancet 2:115, 1971.

158. Wise, J. R., Jr., Oakley, C. M., and Goodwin, J. F.: Acute aortic regurgitation in patients with infective endocarditis. The distinctive clinical features and the role of premature mitral valve closure, J. Maine Med. Assoc. 63:273, 1972.

159. Mann, T., McLaurin, L., Grossman, W., and Craige, E.: Assessing the hemodynamic severity of acute aortic regurgitation due to infective endocarditis, N. Engl. J. Med. 293:108, 1975.

160. Yarbrough, J. W., Roberts, W. C., and Reis, R. L.: Structural alterations in tissue cardiac valves implanted in patients and in calves, J. Thorac. Cardiovasc. Surg. 65:364, 1973.

161. Clarkson, P. M., and Barratt-Boyes, B. G.: Bacterial endocarditis following homograft replacement of the aortic valve, Circulation 42:987, 1970.

162. Sande, M. A., Johnson, W. D., Jr., Hook, E. W., and Kaye, D.: Sustained bacteremia in patients with prosthetic cardiac valves, N. Engl. J. Med. 286: 1067, 1972.
163. Weinstein, L.: Infected prosthetic valves: A diagnostic and therapeutic dilemma, N. Engl. J. Med. 286:1108, 1972.
164. Watanakunakorn, C., and Hamburger, M.: Staphylococcus epidermidis endocarditis complicating a Starr-Edwards prosthesis. A therapeutic dilemma, Arch. Intern. Med. 126:1014, 1970.
165. Walker, S. R., Shumway, N. E., and Merigan, T. C.: Management of infected cardiac valve prostheses, JAMA 208:531, 1969.
166. Perlman, B. B., and Freedman, L. R.: Experimental endocarditis. II. Staphylococcal infection of the aortic valve following placement of a polyethylene catheter in the left side of the heart, Yale J. Biol. Med. 44:206, 1971.
167. Durack, D. T., and Beeson, P. B.: Experimental bacterial endocarditis. I. Colonization of a sterile vegetation, Br. J. Exp. Pathol. 53:44, 1972.
168. Koiwai, E. K., and Nahas, H. C.: Subacute bacterial endocarditis following cardiac surgery, AMA Arch. Surg. 73:272, 1956.
169. Denton, C., Pappas, E. G., Uricchio, J. F., Goldberg, H., and Likoff, W.: Bacterial endocarditis following cardiac surgery, Circulation 15:525, 1957.
170. Linde, L. M., and Heins, H. L.: Bacterial endocarditis following surgery for congenital heart disease, N. Engl. J. Med. 263:65, 1960.
171. Yeh, T. J., Anabtawi, I. N., Cornett, V. E., White, A., Stern, W. H., and Ellison, R. G.: Bacterial endocarditis following open heart surgery, Ann. Thorac. Surg. 3:29, 1967.
172. Dalton, J. C., Williams, B., and Atkins, L.: Staphylococcal endocarditis after mitral valvulotomy. Report of three cases, N. Engl. J. Med. 254:205, 1956.
173. Johnson, D. H., Rosenthal, A., and Nadas, A. S.: A forty-year review of bacterial endocarditis in infancy and childhood, Circulation 51:581, 1975.
174. Pankey, G. A.: Subacute bacterial endocarditis at the University of Minnesota Hospital, 1939 through 1959, Ann. Intern. Med. 55:550, 1961.
175. Rodbarb, S.: Blood velocity and endocarditis, Circulation 27:18, 1963.
176. Taussig, H. B., Crocetti, A., Eshaghpour, E., Keinonen, R., Yap, K. N., Bachman, D., Momberger, N., and Kirk, H.: Long-time observations on the Blalock-Taussig operation. III. Common complications, Johns Hopkins Med. J. 129:274, 1971.
177. Buchbinder, N. A., and Roberts, W. C.: Active infective endocarditis confined to mural endocardium, Arch. Pathol. 93:435, 1972.
178. Taniguchi, T., and Murphy, F. D.: Mural bacterial endocarditis produced by Proteus, JAMA 143:427, 1950.
179. Hirsch, E. F.: Septic thrombophlebitis of the leg with mural endocarditis and pulmonary embolism, Ill. Med. J. 114:289, 1958.
180. Clinicopathologic conference. A thirty-eight-year-old woman with overwhelming sepsis, Am. J. Med. 53:233, 1972.

Clinicopathology of Prosthetic Valve Endocarditis

Ernest N. Arnett, M.D.,
and
William C. Roberts, M.D.

Among 450 consecutive patients with one or more rigid-framed prosthetic cardiac valves studied by us at necropsy (1–7), 23 (5%) had infection involving a prosthetic valve. These 23 patients represented 18% of 129 patients diagnosed as having active prosthetic valve endocarditis (PVE) who were studied in this laboratory (8–10). Although numerous reports are available on patients with fatal active infective endocarditis involving natural cardiac valves, surprisingly little information has been available on morphologic features of endocarditis involving prosthetic cardiac valves. This chapter, therefore, will focus on the clinicopathologic features in patients with PVE, comparing them with nonoperated necropsied patients with active infective endocarditis involving natural left-sided cardiac valves.

PATIENTS STUDIED

Clinical and morphologic observations in 23 patients with PVE are summarized in Tables 1 through 5, and special morphologic features in many of them are illustrated in Figures 1 through 12. Certain observations in several of these patients have been published elsewhere (1–3, 11–13). Among the 23 patients, 29 cardiac valves had been replaced: 17 patients

Table 1. Prosthetic endocarditis: type of prosthesis infected

	Aortic	Mitral	Totals
Caged ball*	10	6	16*
Tilting disc†	5	0	5†
Poppet disc	1‡	1§	2
Total	16	7	23

*Starr-Edwards.
†Björk-Shiley.
‡Hufnagel.
§Kay-Shiley.

had one prosthetic valve, and 6, two prosthetic valves. Of the 29 prosthetic valves, 23 were infected (Table 1): aortic in 16 patients and mitral in 7. Clinical evidence of infective endocarditis was present within 2 months after operation in 9 patients (early deaths) (Table 2) and from 3 months to 10 years after valve replacement in 14 patients. In 6 of the latter 14 patients clinical evidence of infection did not appear until more than 1 year after valve replacement. The length of signs and symptoms of infective endocarditis ranged from 14 days to 13 months. In 17 patients, the length of illness was less than 60 days, and in 6 patients, more than 60 days. Predisposing factors to development of PVE were apparent in only 5 of the 14 late deaths: tooth extraction (2 patients), skin-graft infection (1 patient), prolonged use of an intravenous catheter (1 patient), and prolonged use of a transthoracic pacing wire (1 patient). It was presumed that the infection in the 9 early deaths was either incurred at operation or was secondary to a wound infection.

The infecting organisms (cultured from the blood during life in 21 patients) are listed in Table 3. Staphylococcus was the responsible organism in 14 patients, and various other organisms were isolated from each of the other 9 patients. Fungi caused PVE in two patients, and in each of them blood cultures were negative during life. Evidence of prosthetic dysfunction was present clinically in 12 of the 16 patients with infected aortic prostheses (regurgitation in 11 and stenosis in 1), but in none of the 7 patients with infected mitral prostheses. High grade conduction disturbances occurred in 7 patients, all of whom had infected aortic valve prostheses: left bundle branch block in 2 and complete heart block in 5. Fourteen of the 23 patients received appropriate antibiotic therapy

Table 2. Prosthetic endocarditis: clinical observations

Prosthetic infected	No. patients	Age range, yr (avg.)	Sex		Pre-op. lesion		Onset from op.		Length of S+S of infection		No. patients receiving antibiotic <7 days	Conduction disturbance		Prosthetic dysfunction	
			M	F	Stenosis	Pure regurg.	<2 mo	>2 mo	<60 days	>60 days		LBBB	CHB	Regurg.	Stenosis
Aortic	16	37–69 (54)	14	2	12	4	6	10	11	5	10	2	5	11	1
Mitral	7	37–65 (52)	3	4	7	0	3	4	6	1	2	0	0	0	0
Totals	23	37–69 (53)	17	6	19	4	9	14	17	6	12	2	5	11	1

op.: operation (valve replacement); Regurg.: regurgitation; CHB: complete heart block; LBBB: left bundle branch block; S+S: signs and symptoms.

Table 3. Prosthetic endocarditis: infecting organism

Organism	Onset from op. <2 mo	Onset from op. >2 mo	Total
I. Gram-positive bacterium	7	11	18
Staphylococcus epidermidis	4	7	11
Staphylococcus aureus	2	1	3
Streptococcus pneumoniae	0	1	1
Group D Streptococcus	0	1	1
Diphtheroids	1	0	1
Listeria monocytogenes	0	1	1
II. Gram-negative bacterium	1	2	3
Proteus mirabilis	1	0	1
Klebsiella sp.	0	1	1
Serratia marcescens	0	1	1
III. Fungus	1	1	2
Candida sp.	0	1	1
Aspergillus fumigatus	1	0	1
Total	9	14	23

for longer than 7 days. Three patients underwent valve replacement for PVE. The principle causes of death in the 23 patients were congestive heart failure (20 patients), central nervous system embolus (2 patients), and generalized infection (1 patient).

Among the 23 patients, 29 valves were replaced: 1 valve in 17 patients and 2 valves in 6 patients. In each of the 6 patients with 2 prosthetic valves, only the "downstream" valve was infected: the aortic valve in the 4 patients with mitral and aortic prostheses, and the mitral in the 2 patients with tricuspid and mitral prostheses. Twelve of the 16 infected aortic prostheses and 2 of the 7 infected mitral prostheses were either partially or completely detached. In contrast, 5 of the 7 infected mitral prostheses and only two of the 16 infected aortic prostheses were obstructed by vegetative material.

Ring abscesses (Table 4) were present with each of the 23 infected prostheses, but in one the abscess was visible only by histologic examination. The ring abscess involved the entire valve anulus in 15 patients and only portions of the anulus in the other 8 patients. In 14 of the 23 patients the infective process spread to adjacent structures. In 12 of the 16

Table 4. Prosthetic endocarditis: necropsy observations

Prosthetic infected	No. patients	Ring abscess	Ring organisms	Prosthetic detachment (regurgitation)	Prosthetic stenosis
Aortic	16	16	9	12	2
Mitral	7	7	5	2	5
Total	23	23	14	14	7

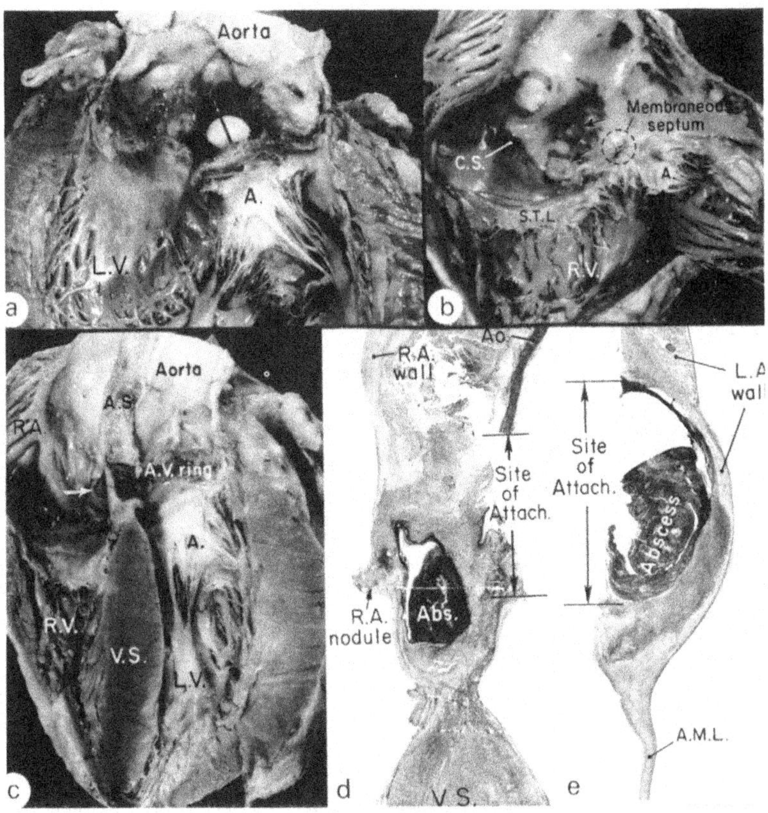

Figure 1. *Staphylococcus epidermidis* prosthetic valve endocarditis in a 49-year-old man (A67-22) who died 3 months after aortic replacement. Symptoms of infection appeared 16 days before death. Despite large doses of antibiotics, complete heart block and wide-open aortic regurgitation developed. *a:* opened aorta, aortic valve, and left ventricle (L.V.) showing a necrotic anulus to which the prosthesis is only partially attached. A.: anterior mitral leaflet. *b:* opened right atrium, tricuspid valve, and right ventricle (R.V.) showing vegetative material (arrows) which had burrowed through the atrial septum from the necrotic aortic valve ring. C.S.: ostium of coronary sinus; S.T.L.: septal tricuspid leaflet; A.: anterior tricuspid leaflet. *c:* longi-

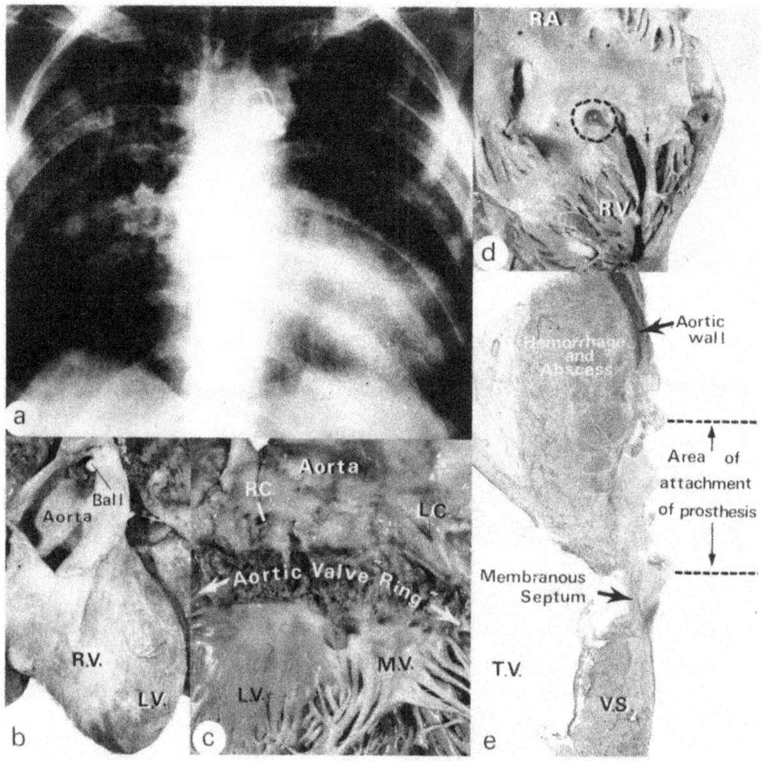

Figure 2. *Staphylocococcus epidermidis* prosthetic aortic valve endocarditis in a 48-year-old man (A64-189). He had been well for 11 months following insertion of the Starr-Edwards prosthesis when, 1 month before death and 6 weeks after dental extraction, shaking chills appeared and blood cultures were positive for *S. epidermidis.* Despite intensive antibiotic therapy, signs of aortic regurgitation appeared, and minutes before death he complained of "feeling funny." *a:* chest roentgenogram immediately postmortem revealed that the prosthesis had dislodged and migrated to the aortic arch. *b:* anterior view of the heart and opened ascending aorta. The detached prosthetic ball is visibly lodged in the transverse aorta. L.V.: left ventricle; R.V.: right ventricle. *c:* opened aorta, aortic valve "ring," and left ventricle showing a totally necrotic aortic anulus. M.V.: anterior mitral leaflet; R.C.: ostium of right coronary artery; L.C.: ostium of left coronary artery. *d:* opened right atrium (R.A.) tricuspid valve and right ventricle showing a ring abscess (dashed circle) which had extended from the aortic prosthetic anulus. *e:* photomicrograph through the aortic valve "ring" showing a large ring abscess, and the necrotic aortic anulus material which extended through the membranous ventricular septum into the right atrium. Hematoxylin and eosin stain: original magnification × 1.2. T.V.: tricuspid valve leaflet; V.S.: ventricular septum.

---

tudinal section of the heart with the anterior portion removed. The necrotic aortic valve (A.V.) ring is again seen and the penetration of the infective process through the atrial septum (A.S.) is apparent. An arrow again designates the vegetation in the right atrium (R.A.). V.S.: ventricular septum. *d* and *e:* histologic sections through the ring abscess. The site of attachment of the prosthesis, which has been removed, is indicated. The infected nodule, an extension of the ring abscess (Abs.), is showing in the right atrium (R.A.) Ao.: aortic wall; L.A.: left atrium; A.M.L.: anterior mitral leaflet.

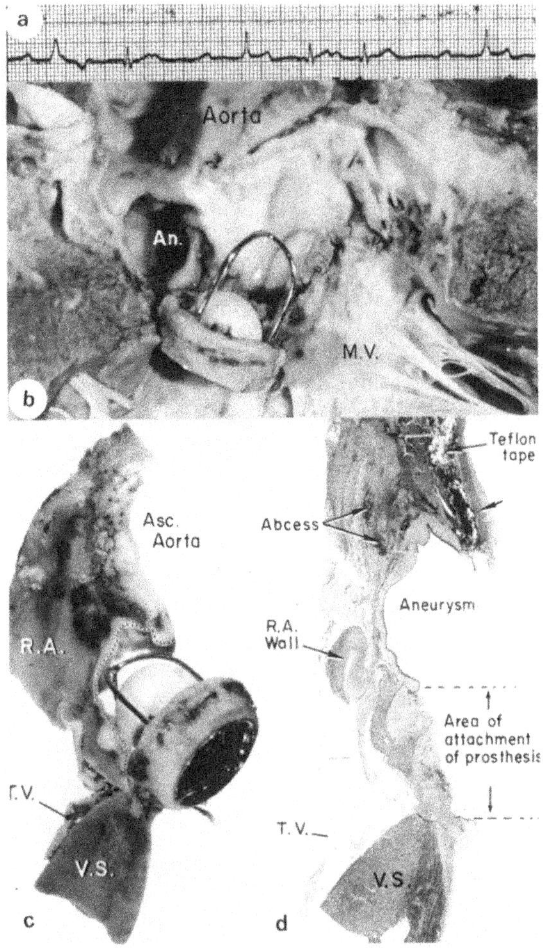

Figure 3. *Staphylococcus epidermidis* prosthetic aortic valve endocarditis in a 55-year-old man (A 63-176). The Starr-Edwards prosthesis was used to replace an infected trileaflet Teflon (Muller) valve 45 days before death. *a:* complete heart block and signs of massive aortic regurgitation appeared despite antibiotic therapy. *b:* opened aorta, aortic valve, and left ventricle. The aortic valve ring is necrotic, and the prosthesis is almost totally detached. The cage of the prosthesis has burrowed into the wall of aorta causing a saccular aneurysm (An.). M.V.: mitral valve. *c:* longitudinal section showing the caged-ball prosthesis burrowing into the ascending (Asc.) aorta, producing the aneurysm. R.A.: right atrium; T.V.: septal tricuspid valve leaflet; V.S.: ventricular septum. *d:* photomicrograph through the same area after prosthesis has been removed. Hematoxylin and eosin stain: original magnification × 1.3.

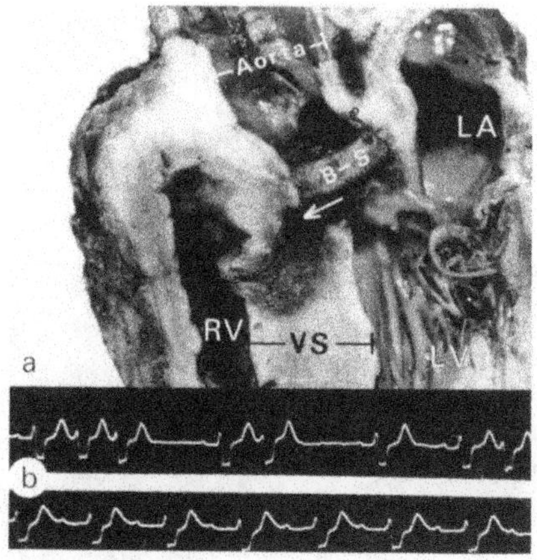

Figure 4. *Staphylococcus epidermidis* prosthetic aortic valve endocarditis in a 51-year-old man (74A-51). His stenotic bicuspid aortic valve had been replaced with a Björk-Shiley prosthesis 83 days before death. Fever was present in the early post-operative period, and shortly before death complete heart block and signs of congestive heart failure appeared. *A:* longitudinal section of the heart with the anterior portion removed. The Björk-Shiley (B-S) prosthesis is partially detached, and the ring abscess (arrow) has burrowed through the ventricular septum (VS) into the right ventricle (RV). LA: left atrium; LV: left ventricle.

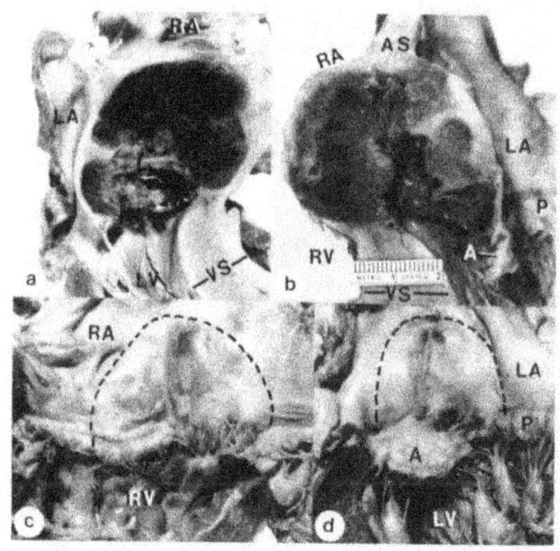

Figure 5. *Diplococcus pneumoniae* aortic prosthetic endocarditis in a 40-year-old man (74A-82). The preoperative hemodynamic lesion was aortic regurgitation which was caused by a previous episode of pneumococcal endocarditis. Evidence of infection was apparent clinically 10 months after valve replacement with a Björk-Shiley prosthesis. When he was brought to the hospital shortly before death, complete heart block and signs of prosthetic valve obstruction were present. *a:* infected hematoma about the aortic prosthesis. This is a view of the anterior half of the heart from the posterior position. The disc of the prosthesis is totally immobilized by the infected thrombus. LA: left atrium; LV: left ventricle; RA: right atrium; VS: ventricular septum. *b:* this is a view of the posterior half of the heart. The prosthesis is not present here. AS: atrial septum; A: anterior mitral leaflet; P: posterior mitral leaflet. *c:* opened right atrium (RA), tricuspid valve, and right ventricle (RV) showing extension of the infected thrombus (dashed half circle) into the right atrium. *d:* opened left atrium (LA), mitral valve, and left ventricle (LV) showing the infected thrombus extending into the left atrium.

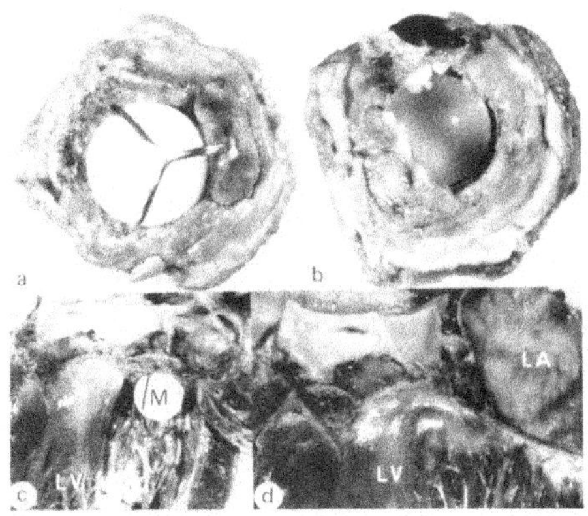

Figure 6. *Serratia marcescens* prosthetic aortic valve endocarditis in a 57-year-old man (A68-33) who became infected 4 months after replacement of both aortic and mitral valves. The apparent source of the infection was an intravenous catheter. Left bundle branch block and signs of aortic regurgitation appeared, and despite massive doses of antibiotics he died 3 months after onset of symptoms of infection. *a:* view of aortic prosthesis from above. Infected thrombus is present on its anulus. *b:* view of prosthesis as it appeared from left ventricle. Some of the infected thrombus became detached during excision of this prosthesis at necropsy. The primary orifice is partially obstructed by the infected material. *c:* opened aortic root, aortic valve, and left ventricle (LV) after removal of the aortic prosthesis. Most of the aortic ring is necrotic. In addition, the portion of mitral (M) prosthesis in direct apposition to the aortic anulus also is infected. *d:* view after excision of the mitral prosthesis showing extension of the aortic annular infection into the junctional area between aortic and mitral anuli. LA: left atrium.

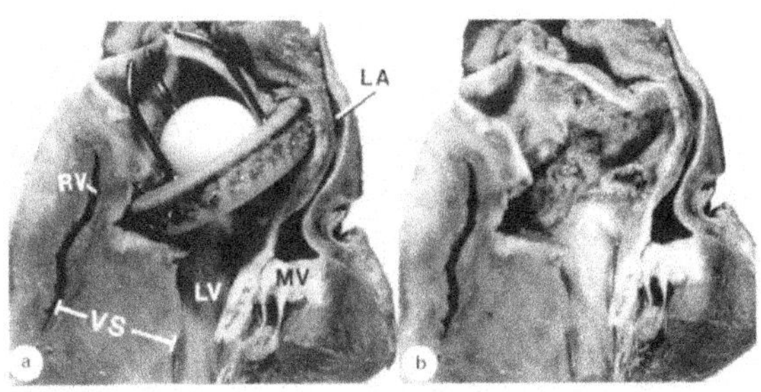

Figure 7. *Staphylococcus epidermidis* endocarditis originally involving a Björk-Shiley aortic valve prosthesis which was excised and replaced with a Magovern prosthesis 28 days before death in a 69-year-old man (A75-200). Fever and signs of aortic regurgitation appeared 7 months after aortic valve replacement with the Björk-Shiley prosthesis. After replacement with the Magovern prosthesis, a murmur of aortic regurgitation reappeared. At necropsy, the sewing ring of the Magovern prosthesis had burrowed deeply into the necrotic anulus, and caused the ball of the prosthesis to strike the non-necrotic portion of aortic wall, probably producing prosthetic aortic stenosis. *a:* longitudinal section of the heart through the aortic anulus with the Magovern prosthesis in place; *b:* after removal of the prosthesis. The frame of the prosthesis has burrowed deeply into the necrotic anulus. VS: ventricular septum; RV: right ventricular cavity; MV: mitral valve; LA: left atrium; LV: left ventricle.

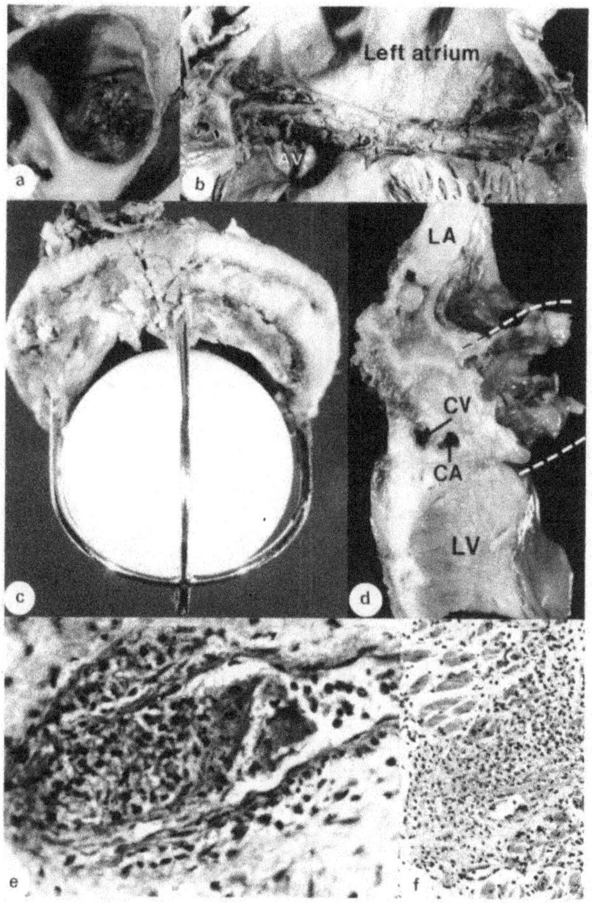

Figure 8. *Staphylococcus aureus* prosthetic mitral valve endocarditis in a 47-year-old man (A65-186) who had the onset of symptoms of infective endocarditis 4 months after valve replacement. He had done well during the first 3 months after operation, but developed symptoms of infection after grafting of a cutaneous ulcer. Signs of prosthetic dysfunction were never detected clinically. *a:* prosthetic mitral orifice obstructed by vegetative material, as viewed from left atrium. *b:* opened left atrium, mitral anulus, and left ventricle after removal of the mitral prosthesis. The entire anulus is necrotic. AV: aortic valve. *c:* mitral prosthesis showing infected thrombus at its base. *d:* longitudinal section through left atrium (LA), mitral anulus, and left ventricle (LV). The former site of attachment of the prosthesis is designated by the dashed lines. The infective process burrowed through the wall of the heart and caused pericarditis. CA: coronary artery; CV: coronary vein in the right atrioventricular sulcus. *e* and *f:* hematoxylin and eosin-stained histologic sections of the left ventricle remote from the infected mitral anulus. *e:* infected embolus in an intramural coronary artery. *f:* microscopic sized myocardial abscess. Original magnifications × 216 (*e*), × 86 (*f*).

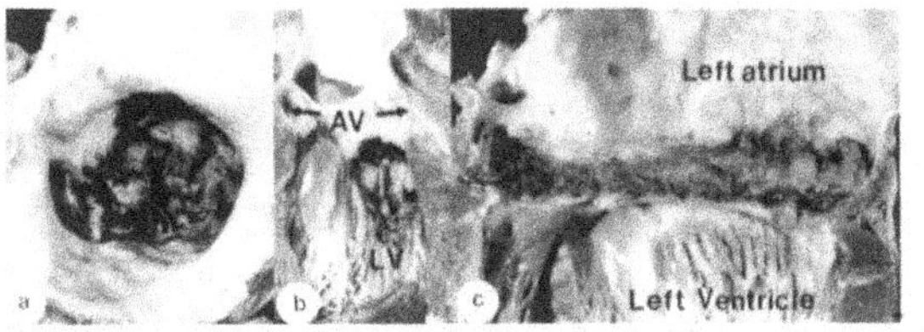

Figure 9. *Staphylococcus epidermidis* prosthetic mitral valve endocarditis in a 46-year-old man (A65-221) who died 16 months after mitral replacement with a Starr-Edwards prosthesis. Eight months postoperatively, when he was asymptomatic, cardiac catheterization disclosed normal left atrial pressure and cardiac output. Signs of infection appeared 15 months after valve replacement. Despite antibiotics, he developed fatal congestive heart failure. *a:* mitral prosthesis as viewed from the left atrium. A large infected thrombus virtually occludes the mitral orifice. *b:* opened aorta, aortic valve, and left ventricle (LV) showing infected thrombus on the cage of the mitral prosthesis. *c:* opened left atrium and ventricle showing a completely necrotic mitral anulus. The prosthesis has been removed.

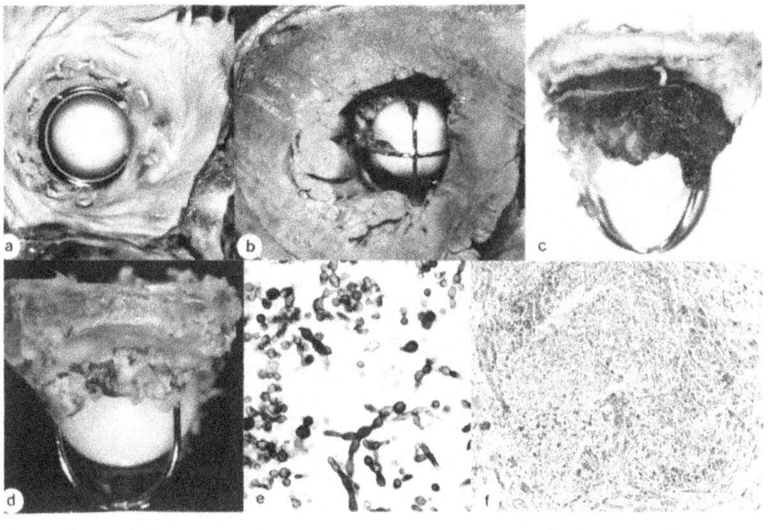

Figure 10. Candida sp. prosthetic mitral valve endocarditis in a 37-year-old woman (A75-242) who had undergone valve replacement 125 months before death because of mitral stenosis (mean mitral gradient 7 mm Hg) and regurgitation. Her tricuspid valve was replaced with a porcine xenograft because of severe tricuspid regurgitation 66 days before death. Postoperatively, she required prolonged use of a transthoracic pacing wire, which was the apparent source of the infection. She died from central nervous system embolism. Necropsy disclosed infection of the mitral prosthesis. *a:* mitral prosthesis viewed from the left atrium; *b:* from the left ventricle. Large vegetations are present on the base and struts of the prosthesis. *c* and *d:* extracted mitral valve prosthesis from two different sides showing large vegetations. *e:* photomicrograph of Candida sp. in the mitral vegetation. Methenemine silver stain; original magnification × 353. *f:* photomicrograph of microabscess in left ventricular myocardium. Hematoxylin and eosin stain: original magnification × 33.

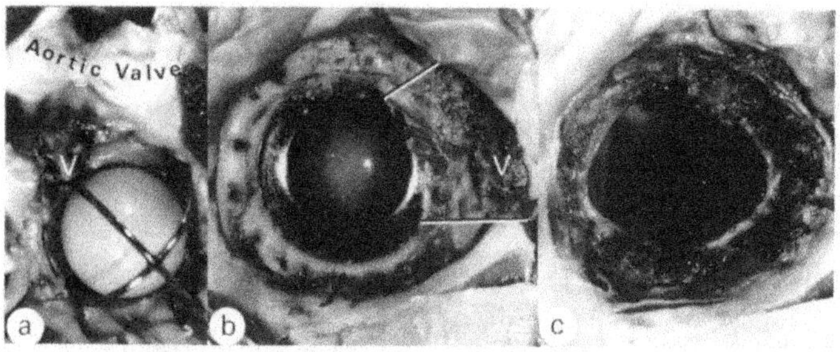

Figure 11. *Staphylococcus epidermidis* prosthetic mitral valve endocarditis in a 59-year-old woman (A74-196). The infection appeared 10 years after replacement of both mitral and tricuspid valves. At necropsy, only the miral prosthesis was infected. *a:* infected mitral prosthesis viewed from the left ventricle. Vegetative material (V) is present on the prosthetic anulus just below the aortic valve. *b:* mitral prosthesis as viewed from left atrium showing vegetations (V) at the junction of the prosthetic and natural valve anuli. *c:* same view after removal of the prosthesis showing even greater extensiveness of the infection at the site of attachment of the prosthesis.

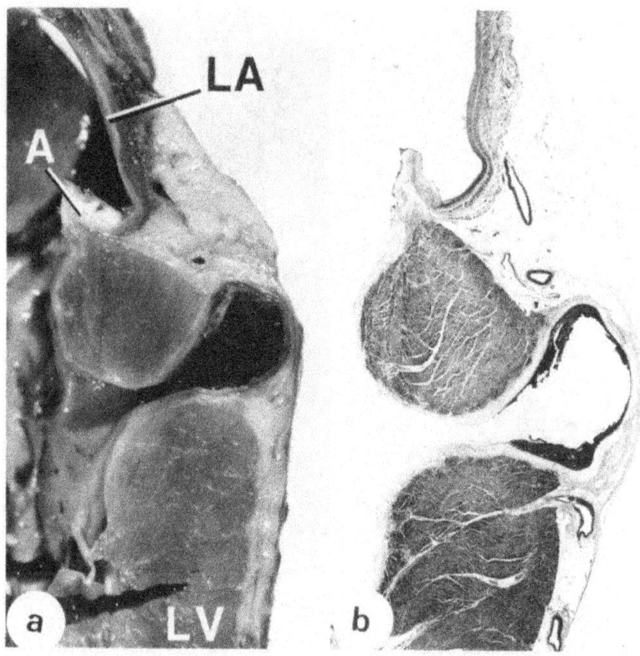

Figure 12. Left ventricular aneurysm simulating prosthetic valve endocarditis in a 46-year-old woman (A75-17). She had almost daily fever after mitral valve replacement 4 months before death and only of many blood cultures grew *Staphylococcus epidermidis* and diphtheroids. The clinical diagnosis was prosthetic valve endocarditis and she was treated with prolonged intravenous antibiotic therapy. She died from central nervous system embolism. At necropsy, an aneurysm was present in the basal portion of the left ventricular free wall. The prosthesis and its anulus were free of signs of infection. *a:* longitudinal cut of the left atrial (LA) wall, mitral anulus (A), and left ventricular (LV) wall through the aneurysm. *b:* histologic section of the aneurysm (Movat strain). Thrombus is present in the aneurysm.

patients with infected aortic prostheses the ring abscess burrowed into adjacent structures: through ascending aorta into the periaortic space (7 patients); through atrial septum into right atrium (10 patients) or into left atrium (2 patients); through ventricular septum into right ventricle (8 patients); and into anterobasal left ventricular wall (2 patients). In 2 patients with infected mitral prostheses the ring abscess burrowed through the atrial wall into the pericardial space. Histologic examination of the infected rings disclosed colonies of organisms in 14 of the 22 patients.

Both arterial emboli and gross organ infarcts were common with both aortic and mitral PVE (Table 5). Of the 23 patients, grossly visible infarcts were present in the spleen in 13, kidney in 7, and brain in 7. Two patients had bowel infarcts, 1 had a pancreatic infarct, and 2 had transmural myocardial infarcts. In addition, mycotic aneurysms were present in the ascending aorta of 3 patients: in 2 patients, aneurysms resulted from jet lesions from the infected prosthesis, and in the third, the cage of the partially detached prosthesis burrowed into the wall of a weakened aorta (from an aortotomy—weeks earlier), causing a sacular aneurysm.

The spleen ranged in weight from 120 to 1,000 g (avg. 460) and in 15 of the 22 patients the spleen weighed more than 300 g. The livers ranged in weight from 1,350 to 2,950 g (avg. 2,070).

COMMENTS

A study of our 23 necropsy patients and analysis of over 150 necropsied patients with PVE reported by others (14–47) allows certain general conclusions regarding this condition. PVE is a devastating complication of cardiac valve replacement, but fortunately it is infrequent. Its exact frequency is uncertain, but it is clearly less than 1% per year among patients with prosthetic cardiac valves (37, 39, 45, 48) (see Chapter 1). Although prospective studies (49, 50) have been inconclusive, retrospective studies

Table 5. Prosthetic endocarditis: organ weights and infarcts

		Organ weight range, g (avg.)		Gross infarcts (no. patients)		
Prosthetic	No.	Spleen	Liver	Spleen	Kidney	Brain
Aortic	16	120–1,000 (480)	1,450–2,950 (2,110)	8	3	3
Mitral	7	170–920 (370)	1,350–2,000 (1,950)	5	4	4
Total	23	120–1,000 (460)	1,350–2,950 (2,070)	13	7	7

(16, 17, 51, 52) have shown a reduction in the frequency of early (less than 2 months after valve replacement) PVE coincident with the use of prophylactic antibiotics. Late infection now appears to be more common than early infection (37, 45), presumably because there are now many persons with prosthetic cardiac valves. Although the mortality rate is high for both groups, early infection from PVE apparently is more often fatal than late infection (37, 39, 45, 48).

Most early infections are either incurred at operation, or result from a wound infection (25, 29, 37, 39, 48) (see Chapter 5). The former appears to result from contamination of the cardiopulmonary bypass equipment (53, 54). Staphylococci are the most frequent organisms cultured from cardiopulmonary bypass equipment and the most frequent cause of early PVE (14, 16–18, 25, 30, 37, 39, 44, 45). When Gram-negative bacteria or fungi cause PVE early, they are usually also recovered from the operating room equipment or from a wound infection (28, 39). Late infections usually result from transient bacteremias (37, 39, 45, 48). Although both staphylococci and streptococci are frequent causes of clinically diagnosed late PVE (37, 39, 45), the former have caused most cases of necropsy-proven late PVE and the latter, relatively few (see Chapter 4). In one of our 23 necropsy patients with PVE the infection was caused by streptococci. Staphylococci were the most common cause of PVE in our patients irrespective of whether the infection occurred early or late.

Among patients with PVE, blood cultures are almost always positive, except when the infections are caused by certain fungi (27, 28, 31, 32, 37, 39, 44, 45, 48) (see Chapter 9). Blood cultures were positive during life in each of our 21 patients with PVE caused by bacteria, and were negative in each of our 2 patients with fungal PVE. Among 39 patients with endocarditis caused by Aspergillus species reviewed by Kammer and Utz (55) blood cultures were positive in only 3.

Signs of prosthetic dysfunction are usually present when the aortic prosthesis is infected, and usually absent when the mitral prosthesis is infected. Clinical signs of aortic regurgitation were present in 11 of our 16 patients with prosthetic aortic infection. In the four patients without clinical signs of aortic regurgitation, no prosthetic detachment was present at necropsy. Among patients with acute aortic regurgitation, however, classic signs of aortic regurgitation may be absent (56–59). Signs of aortic regurgitation were not detected in 3 of 9 necropsy patients with aortic PVE reported by Madison and associates (44), but in each of them prosthetic detachment was present at necropsy.

In contrast, patients with infection involving the mitral prosthesis usually have no clinical signs of mitral prosthetic dysfunction. Clinical signs of mitral prosthetic dysfunction were not detected in any of our seven patients with mitral PVE; yet the prosthesis was significantly obstructed by vegetative material in five of them, and partially detached from the anulus in two (12). McAllister and associates (42) reported two patients with virtual total obstruction of the mitral prosthesis.

The most consistent morphologic feature of prosthetic valve infection in our 23 patients was infection behind the site of attachment of the valve prosthesis, resulting in valve ring abscess. Ring abscess was present in each of our 23 patients, and in two-thirds of them the infection involved the entire circumference of the valve anulus. In several patients, however, only a portion of the circumference of the valve anulus was involved, and in one patient, histologic examination of the anulus disclosed infection which had not been apparent on gross examination. Extension of the ring infection to adjacent cardiac structures was common, especially with aortic prosthetic infection. This extension resulted in the frequent occurrence of both complete heart block or left bundle branch block and of intracardiac fistulas. Among 9 necropsied patients with aortic PVE reported by Madison and associates (44), each had infection at the site of attachment of the prosthesis, and among their entire group of 16 patients with aortic PVE, 7 (44%) developed atrioventricular conduction defects. Obviously, it is the occurrence of the infection behind the site of attachment of the prosthesis which makes reoperation so hazardous. Were the infection limited to the interior portion of the prosthesis, excision of the prosthesis should eliminate the infection. Unfortunately, as demonstrated by our patients and by those reported by others (20, 35, 38, 43, 44, 47), the tissues behind the site of attachment of the prosthesis usually are involved by the infective process.

The occurrence of a grossly necrotic anulus, however, at the time of reoperation for PVE does not mean that valve replacement will be fruitless. Although it may be grossly necrotic, the anulus may be free of colonies of organisms, and cultures of the necrotic anulus may be negative. In 9 of our 23 patients with PVE and ring abscess, no stainable organisms were found in histologic sections from the prosthetic anulus.

One hazard of inserting a prosthesis in a necrotic anulus at the time of valve replacement for PVE is burrowing of the sewing ring of the new prosthesis into the necrotic anulus with resulting impingement on movement of the poppet of the prosthesis by adjacent tissue. This sequence occurred in one of our patients and resulted in prosthetic aortic stenosis from inability of the ball to ascend in the cage (Figure 7).

Although PVE in patients with rigid-framed prostheses, as were present in our 23 patients, usually indicates the presence of infection behind the site of attachment of the prosthesis, i.e., sewing ring, ring abscess may not be so frequent with endocarditis involving tissue valves. Indeed, both experimentally and in humans, the infective process may be limited to the cusps of the tissue valve, just like the situation with infective endocarditis involving natural valves (60, 61). Thus, the chance of cure, either by antibiotics or valve replacement or both when infective endocarditis is superimposed on a homograft or heterograft (porcine valve, for example), is much better than when endocarditis involves a rigid-framed prosthesis (61). This then is an advantage, although a small one, of the tissue valve (porcine) over the rigid-framed prosthesis.

Establishment of the diagnosis of PVE, particularly in the early postoperative period, at times may be difficult, as pointed out by a number of authors (48, 62, 63) (see Chapter 4). Diagnosis in the late postoperative period, in contrast, is usually made quite readily (48, 62, 63). It is worth emphasizing however, that the combination of fever and a positive blood culture in a patient with a prosthetic cardiac valve does not always indicate the presence of PVE. We recently studied a patient at necropsy who was diagnosed during life as having mitral PVE on the basis of fever, cerebral episodes consistent with emboli, and one blood culture which grew *Staphylococcus epidermidis* and diphtheroids. She received antibiotics during most of her 4-month postoperative period and at necropsy no PVE was found. A left ventricular aneurysm, however, was present immediately caudal to the mitral anulus and a sterile thrombus was present in the aneurysm (Figure 12). The latter was the likely source of the cerebral emboli.

There is a general view that PVE can at times be cured by antibiotics. For cure of PVE to be established, however, it is necessary that PVE be confirmed during life, and this unequivocal confirmation can only be obtained by examination of the prosthetic valve and its anulus (site of attachment) at reoperation. In other words, to establish cure of PVE it is necessary to be absolutely positive of the diagnosis of PVE. Although usually not obtained, this confirmation has now been obtained in enough patients to support the view that PVE can indeed be cured with antibiotics in some patients (16, 17, 21, 23, 24, 29, 30, 37, 39, 44, 45, 48, 64, 65).

Comparison of observations in our 23 patients with PVE to those in 74 nonoperated necropsied patients with active infective endocarditis (AIE) involving natural *left-sided* cardiac valves (also studied by us) disclosed certain clear differences (Table 6). 1) Ring abscess was always present in patients with PVE regardless of the site of the prosthesis, but, in contrast, it was present in only 30% of our 74 patients with AIE involving natural left-sided valves, and then, with rare exception, only when the aortic valve was infected. 2) The hemodynamic consequences were different. PVE

Table 6. Comparison between active infective endocarditis (IE) involving prosthetic cardiac valves and natural cardiac valves

	Mitral valve				Aortic valve			
	Prosthetic		Natural		Prosthetic		Natural	
	No.	%	No.	%	No.	%	No.	%
Number necropsy patients	7		22		16		52*	
Age range, yr (avg.)	37–65 (52)		15–74 (43)		37–69 (54)		17–83 (45)	
Sex (ratio of male/female)	3/4		12/10		14/2		41/11	
Underlying valve disease	7	100	7	32	16	100	26	50
Rheumatic			6	27			4	8
Congenital			0	0			12	23
Other			1†	5			10‡	19
None			15	68			26	50
Previous episode IE	1	14	0	0	2	13	3	6
Infecting organism								
Staphylococcus§	4	57	7	32	10	63	13	25
Alpha Streptococcus	0	0	0	0	0	0	9	17
Pneumococcus	0	0	2	9	1	7	6	12
Valve regurgitation (from IE)	2	29	14	64	12	75	36	69
Valve stenosis (from IE)§	5	71	1	5	2	13	1	2
Valve-ring abscess§	7	100	1	5	16	100	21	40
Complete heart block§	0	0	1	5	5	31	4	8
Left bundle branch block§	0	0	0	0	2	13	0	0
Organ infarcts	5	71	17	77	10	63	31/47	66
Spleen >300 g	2/6	33	3	20	13	81	19/38	50

*Eighteen of the 52 also had infection of the mitral valve, but in at least 13 of these the mitral valve infection appeared to be secondary to the aortic valve infection.

†Floppy mitral valve

‡Degenerative, five patients; previous IE which healed, three patients, and uncertain etiology, two patients.

§$P < 0.05$.

caused valve obstruction nearly as often as valvular regurgitation, whereas valvular stenosis from AIE involving natural cardiac valves was extremely rare (10, 66). 3) Spread of a ring abscess was more extensive in patients with PVE than in patients with natural valve AIE, and consequently the frequency of high grade conduction defects was much greater in patients with PVE. 4) The infecting organism in fatal PVE was most commonly Staphylococcus. Alpha Streptococcus, which remains a common cause of fatal AIE in patients with natural cardiac valves, is a rare cause of fatal PVE.

Among patients with infective endocarditis involving native cardiac valves, ring abscesses, when present, almost always (95%) involve the aortic value (67). Among our necropsied patients with active infective endocarditis involving natural aortic valves, 40% had a valve ring abscess, whereas only 5% of patients with endocarditis involving natural mitral values had ring abscesses. In contrast, each of our 23 patients with PVE had a ring abscess. Thus, valve ring abscess is the usual morphologic feature of PVE, regardless of the valve infected.

Ring abscesses in patients with infections involving prosthetic valves are generally more extensive than those in patients with AIE involving natural cardiac valves. This occurrence appears to be a consequence of the rigid nature of the prosthetic frame. Once the prosthesis is loosened by the infection, the rocking-rigid frame promotes spread of the infection. The greater turbulence across the aortic valve prosthesis probably accounts for the generally more extensive nature of ring abscess with aortic PVE than with mitral valve PVE. A consequence of this extension is the greater frequency of complete heart block and left bundle branch block in patients with aortic PVE (31%) compared with patients with natural aortic valve endocarditis (8%).

Staphylococcus (either *aureus* or *epidermidis*) is the most common cause of PVE (61%). Many different organisms cause the remainder of the infections. Although alpha streptococci were the responsible organisms in 17% of our 74 patients with AIE on natural valves, these bacteria were not the causative organisms in any of our 23 patients with PVE.

The hemodynamic consequences of PVE vary with the site of the infected prosthesis. Twelve of the 16 patients (75%) with aortic PVE and 2 of 7 patients with prosthetic mitral valve infection developed valvular regurgitation from the PVE. In contrast, 5 of 7 patients (71%) with mitral PVE and 2 of 16 patients (13%) with aortic PVE developed valvular obstruction from the infection. Among patients with natural left-sided valvular infection, 65% (64% of the mitral and 69% of the aortic patients) developed valvular regurgitation from active infective endocarditis, and relatively few (3%) developed valvular obstruction from the endocarditis (10). Thus, aortic PVE almost always causes valvular regurgitation, and mitral PVE most often causes valvular obstruction.

Splenomegaly (greater than 300 g) is common both in patients with PVE (18%) and in patients with native left-sided valve AIE (37%). Similarly, the frequency of infarcts in other body organs is similar in both PVE (65%) and native valve endocarditis (70%).

SUMMARY

Clinical and morphologic features are described in 23 necropsied patients with endocarditis involving rigid-framed prosthetic valves: aortic in 16 patients, and mitral in 7. The interval from valve replacement to onset of symptoms of prosthetic valve endocarditis was less than 2 months in 9 patients and longer than 2 months in 14 patients. The most frequent infecting organism was Staphylococcus (14 patients). In each of the 23 patients the infection was located behind the site of attachment of the prosthesis to the valve ring, and the infection spread to adjacent structures in 14 patients, 12 of whom had aortic prostheses. Prosthetic detachment causing severe regurgitation occurred in 12 of the 15 patients with infected aortic prostheses, and 2 of the 7 patients with infected mitral prostheses. Prosthetic obstruction by vegetative material occurred in 5 of 7 patients with prosthetic mitral infection and in only 2 of 15 with prosthetic aortic infection. Seven patients with aortic prosthetic valve endocarditis developed high degrees of conduction defects: complete heart block in 5, and complete left bundle branch block in 2.

Comparison of observations in the 23 patients with prosthetic valve endocarditis to those in 74 patients with active infective endocarditis involving natural left-sided cardiac valves showed significant ($P < 0.05$) differences in percentage with ring abscess, hemodynamic consequences of the endocarditis (valve stenosis), frequency of staphylococci as the causative organism, and percentage with complete heart block or left bundle branch block. No significant differences were observed between the two groups when comparing age, sex, type of underlying valve disease, or frequency of organ infarcts or splenomegaly.

LITERATURE CITED

1. Roberts, W. C., and Morrow, A. G.: Anatomic studies of hearts containing caged-ball prosthetic valves. Johns Hopkins Med. J. 121:271–295, 1967.

2. Roberts, W. C., and Morrow, A. G.: Causes of death and other anatomic observations after cardiac valve replacement. Adv. Cardiol. 7:226–247, 1972.
3. Roberts, W. C., Bulkley, B. H., and Morrow, A. G.: Pathologic anatomy of cardiac valve replacement: a study of 224 necropsy patients. Prog. Cardiovasc. Dis. 15:539–587, 1973.
4. Fishbein, M. C., Roberts, W. C., Golden, A., and Hufnagel, C. A.: Cardiac pathology after aortic valve replacement using Hufnagel trileaflet prostheses: a study of 20 necropsy patients. Amer. Heart. J. 89:443–448, 1975.
5. Roberts, W. C., Fishbein, M. C., and Golden, A.: Cardiac pathology after valve replacement by disc prosthesis: a study of 61 necropsy patients. Amer. J. Cardiol. 35:740–760, 1975.
6. Fishbein, M. C., and Roberts, W. C.: Late postoperative anatomic observations after insertion of Hufnagel caged-ball prosthesis in descending thoracic aorta. Chest 68:6–11, 1975.
7. Roberts, W. C., and Hammer, W. J.: Cardiac pathology after valve replacement with a tilting disc prosthesis (Björk-Shiley type). A study of 46 necropsy patients and 49 Björk-Shiley prostheses. Amer. J. Cardiol. 37:1024–1032, 1976.
8. Roberts, W. C., and Buchbinder, N. A.: Right-sided valvular infective endocarditis. A clinicopathologic study of twelve necropsy patients. Amer. J. Med. 53:7–19, 1972.
9. Buchbinder, N. A., and Roberts, W. C.: Left-sided valvular active infective endocarditis: a study of forty-five necropsy patients. Amer. J. Med. 53:20–35, 1972.
10. Arnett, E. N., and Roberts, W. C.: Active infective endocarditis. A clinicopathologic study of 137 necropsy patients. Current Concepts in Cardiology, October, 1976.
11. Cohn, L. H., Roberts, W. C., Rockoff, S. D., and Morrow, A. G.: Bacterial endocarditis following aortic valve replacement: clinical and pathological correlations. Circulation 33:209–217, 1966.
12. Roberts, W. C., and Morrow, A. G.: Bacterial endocarditis involving prosthetic mitral valves: clinical and pathologic observations. Arch. Pathol. 82:164–169, 1966.
13. Arnett, E. N. and Roberts, W. C.: Prosthetic valve endocarditis. a study of 18 patients at necropsy (Abstract). Amer. J. Cardiol. 35:120, 1975.
14. Björk, V. O.: Aortic valve replacement. Thorax 19:369–378, 1964.
15. Newman, W. H., and Cordell, A. R.: Aspergillus endocarditis after open-heart surgery: report of a case and review of literature. J. Thorac. Cardiovasc. Surg. 48:652–660, 1964.
16. Amoury, R. A., Bowman, F. O., Jr., and Malm, J. R.: Endocarditis associated with intracardiac prostheses: diagnosis, management and prophylaxis. J. Thorac. Cardiovasc. Surg. 51:36–48, 1966.
17. Stein, P. D., Harken, D. E., and Dexter, L.: The nature and prevention of prosthetic valve endocarditis. Amer. Heart J. 71:393–407, 1966.
18. Fraser, R. S., Rossall, R. E., and Dvorkin, J.: Bacterial endocarditis

occuring after open heart surgery. Can. Med. Assoc. J. 96:1551–1558, 1967.
19. Leffert, R. C. and Hackett, R. L.: Aspergillus aortitis following replacement of aortic valve. J. Thorac. Cardiovasc. Surg. 53: 866–874, 1967.
20. McConnell, E. M. and Roberts, C.: Pathological findings in three cases of fungal endocarditis complicating open-heart surgery. J. Clin. Pathol. 30:555–560, 1967.
21. Geraci, J. E., Forth, R. I., and Ellis, F. H.: Postoperative prosthetic valve endocarditis due to *Corynebacterium xerosis*. Mayo Clin. Proc. 42:736–743, 1967.
22. Cheng, T. O., Kinhal, V., and Tice, D. A.: Fatal thrombosis of the Starr-Edwards mitral valve prosthesis associated with bacterial endocarditis: diagnostic significance of a disappearing prosthetic click. Chest 57:151–155, 1970.
23. Hairston, P., and Lee, W. H., Jr.: Management of infective prosthetic heart valves. Ann. Thorac, Surg. 9:229–237, 1970.
24. Killen, D. A., Collins, H. A., Koenig, M. G., and Goodman, J. S.: Prosthetic cardiac valves and bacterial endocarditis. Ann. Thorac. Surg. 9:238–246, 1970.
25. Shafer, R. B. and Hall, W. H.: Bacterial endocarditis following open heart surgery. Amer. J. Cardiol. 25:602–607, 1970.
26. Sutton, G. C. and Wright, J. E. C.: Major detachment of aortic prosthetic valves. Br. Heart. J. 32:337–343, 1970.
27. Chaudhuri, M. R.: Fungal endocarditis after value replacements. J. Thorac. Cardiovasc. Surg. 60:207–214, 1970.
28. Gage, A. A., Dean, D. C., Schimert, G., and Minsley, N.: Aspergillus infection after cardiac surgery. Arch. Surg. 101:384–387, 1970.
29. Block, P. C., DeSanctis, R. W., Weinberg, A. N., and Austen, W. C.: Prosthetic valve endocarditis. J. Thorac. Cardiovasc. Surg. 60:540–548, 1970.
30. Okies, J. E., Viroslav, J., and Williams, T. V., Jr.: Endocarditis after cardiac valvular replacement. Chest 59:198–202, 1971.
31. Ostermiller, W. E., Jr., Dye, W. S., and Weinberg, M.: Fungal endocarditis following cardiovascular surgery. J. Thorac. Cardiovasc. Surg. 61:670–675, 1971.
32. Lawrence, T., Shockman, A. T., and Macvaugh, H., III: Aspergillus infection of prosthetic aortic valves. Chest 60:406–414, 1971.
33. Robinson, M. J., Greenberg, J. J., Korn, M., and Rywlin, A. M.: Infective endocarditis at autopsy: 1965–1969. Amer. J. Med. 52:492–498, 1972.
34. Levin, S., Balagtas, R., Susmano, A., Edwards, L., and Dainauskas, J.: Meningococcus endocarditis at the site of Starr-Edwards mitral prosthesis. Arch. Intern. Med. 129:963–966, 1972.
35. Joassin, A. and Edward, J. E.: Late causes of death after mitral valve replacement. J. Thorac. Cardiovasc. Surg. 65:225–263, 1973.
36. Vlachakis, N. D., Gazes, P. C., and Hairston, R.: Nocardial endocarditis following mitral valve replacement. Chest 63:276–278, 1973.

37. Slaughter, L., Morris, J. E., and Starr, A.: Prosthetic valvular endocarditis: 12-year review. Circulation 47:1319–1326, 1973.
38. Case records of the Massachusetts General Hospital: Weekly clinicopathological exercises. Case 24, 1973. New Engl. J. Med. 288: 1290–1296, 1973.
39. Dismukes, W. E., Karchmer, A. W., Buckley, M. J., Austen, W. G., and Swartz, M. N.: Prosthetic valve endocarditis: analysis of 38 cases. Circulation 48:365–377, 1973.
40. Jackson, G. and Saunders, K.: Prosthetic valve diphtheroid endocarditis treated with sodium fusidate and erythromycin. Br. Heart J. 35:931–936, 1973.
41. Harris, J. A. and Cobbs, C. G.: Serratia endocarditis in patients with a Starr-Edwards valve: report of a case of bacteriologic cure with antimicrobial therapy. South. Med. J. 66:1117–1120, 1973.
42. Hall, W. J., III: Penicillium endocarditis following open heart surgery and prosthetic valve insertion. Amer. Heart J. 87:501–506, 1974.
43. McAllister, R. G., Samet, J., Mazzoleni, A., and Dillon, M.L.: Endocarditis on prosthetic mitral valves: fatal obstruction to left ventricular inflow. Chest 66:682–686, 1974.
44. Madison, J., Wang, K., Gobel, F. L., and Edwards, J. E.: Prosthetic aortic valvular endocarditis. Circulation 51:940–949, 1975.
45. Wilson, W. R., Jaumin, P. M., Danielson, G. K., Giuliani, E. R., Washington, J. A., and Geraci, J. E.: Prosthetic valve endocarditis. Ann. Intern. Med. 83:751–756, 1975.
46. Rubenstein, E., Noriega, E. R., Simberkoff, M. S., Holzman, R., and Rahal, J. J.: Fungal endocarditis: analysis of 24 cases and review of the literature. Medicine 54:331–344, 1975.
47. Robboy, S. J. and Kaiser, J.: Pathogenesis of fungal infection on heart valve prostheses. Human Pathol. 6:711–715, 1975.
48. Kloster, F. E.: Diagnosis and management of complications of prosthetic heart valves. Amer. J. Cardiol. 35:872–885, 1975.
49. Conte, J. E., Cohen, S. N., Roe, B. B., and Elashoff, R. M.: Antibiotic prophylaxis and cardiac surgery: a prospective double-blind comparison of single-dose versus mulitple-dose regimens. Ann. Intern. Med. 76:943–949, 1972.
50. Goodman, J. S. Shaffner, W., Collins, H. A., Battersby, E. J., and Koenig, M. E.: Infection after cardiovascular surgery: clinical study including examination of antimicrobial prophylaxis. New Engl. J. Med. 278:117–123, 1968.
51. Nelson, R. M., Henson, C. B., Peterson, C. A., and Saunders, B. C.: Effective use of prophylactic antibiotics in open-heart surgery. Arch. Surg. 90:731–735, 1965.
52. Herr, R., Starr, A., McCord, C. W., and Wood, J. A.: Special problems following valve replacement: embolus, leak, infection, red cell damage. Ann. Thorac. Surg. 1:403–415, 1965.
53. Aakeney, J. L. and Parker, R. F.: Staphylococcal endocarditis following open heart surgery related to positive intraoperative blood cultures. *In* Prosthetic Heart Valves. Edited by L. A. Brewer. Springfield, Illinois, Charles C Thomas, pp. 719–730, 1969.

54. Blakemore, W. S., McGarrity, G. J., Thurer, R. J., Wallace, H. W., MacVaugh, H., III, and Coriell, L. L.: Infection by air-borne bacteria with cardiopulmonary bypass. Surgery 70:830–838, 1971.
55. Kammer, R. B. and Utz, J. P.: Aspergillus species endocarditis: the new face of a not so rare disease. Amer. J. Med. 56:506–521, 1974.
56. Wigle, E. D. and Labrosse, C. J.: Sudden, severe aortic insufficiency. Circulation 32:708–720, 1965.
57. Wise, J. R., Bentall, H. H., Cleland, W. P., Goodwin, J. F., Hallidie-Smith, K. A., and Oakley, C. M.: Urgent aortic-valve replacement for acute aortic regurgitation due to infective endocarditis. Lancet 2:115–121, 1971.
58. Wise, J. R., Jr., Oakley, C. M., and Goodwin, J. F.: Acute aortic regurgitation in patients with infective endocarditis: the distinctive clinical features and the role of premature mitral valve closure. J. Maine Med. Assoc. 63:273–278, 1972.
59. Mann, T., McLaurin, L., Grossman, W., and Craig, E.: Assessing the hemodynamic severity of acute aortic regurgitation due to infective endocarditis. New Engl. J. Med. 293:108–113, 1975.
60. Yarbrough, J. W., Roberts, W. C., and Reis, R. L.: Structural alterations in tissue cardiac valves implanted in patients and in calves. J. Thorac. Cardiovasc. Surg. 65:364–375, 1973.
61. Clarkson, P. M. and Barratt-Boyes, B. G.: Bacterial endocarditis following homograft replacement of the aortic valve. Circulation 42:987–991, 1970.
62. Sande, M. A., Johnson, W. D., Jr., Hook, E. W., and Kaye, D.: Sustained bacteremia in patients with prosthetic cardiac valves. New Engl. J. Med. 286:1067–1070, 1972.
63. Weinstein, L.: Infected prosthetic valves: a diagnostic and therapeutic dilemma. New Engl. J. Med. 286:1108–1109, 1972.
64. Watanakunakorn, C., and Hamburger, M.: *Staphylococcus epidermidis* endocarditis complicating a Starr-Edwards prosthesis: a therapeutic dilemma. Arch. Intern. Med. 126:1014–1018, 1970.
65. Walker, S. R., Shumway, N. E., and Merigan, T. C.: Management of infected cardiac valve prosthesis. JAMA 208:531–533, 1969.
66. Roberts, W. C., Ewy, G. A., Glancy, D. L., and Marcus, F. I.: Valvular stenosis produced by active infective endocarditis. Circulation 36:449–451, 1967.
67. Arnett, E. N. and Roberts, W. C.: Valve ring abscess in active infective endocarditis. Frequency, location, and clues to clinical diagnosis from study of 95 necropsy patients. Circulation 54:140–145, 1976.

QUESTIONS, ANSWERS, AND COMMENTS

Q: (DR. GORDON ARCHER–RICHMOND): Because valvular abscesses appear to be so common, I wonder if you could speculate on where the responsible organisms first arrive?

A: (DR. WILLIAM ROBERTS–BETHESDA): I do not know. I believe

the answer will have to come from experimental observations, because it is difficult to determine the beginning by studying the end. With rigid-framed prostheses, the infection is not established on the prosthesis per se, but rather the invading organism attacks the soft tissues beneath the site of attachment of the prosthesis. Probably, rigid-framed prostheses rock a little during each phase of the cardiac cycle. This movement at the site of attachment, for one reason or another, allows organisms to enter and spread in the adjacent tissues.

Q: (DR. RICHARD DUMA–RICHMOND): Could you tell from the age of the inflammatory response as to perhaps where the infection started; i.e., how the lesion spread in the tissues of the heart? For example, could the presence of a nidus of calcium within the area of endocarditis suggest the original point of spread within the heart?

A: (DR. WILLIAM ROBERTS): I do not know. In none of our patients was there residual calcium at the site of attachment. Most of our patients, however, had had stenotic values excised at the time of valve replacement, and all of them had calcific deposits on the excised leaflets.

Q: (DR. WILLIAM DISMUKES–BIRMINGHAM): You commented on conduction problems. Did you study microscopically the conduction system, and did you think the conduction disturbances were due to invasion of the conduction system by bacteria and inflammatory cells or were they secondary to microemboli? Also, what percentage of patients had emboli to the coronary arteries?

A: (DR. WILLIAM ROBERTS): Several of our patients had microemboli to the intramural coronary arteries. All of our patients with conduction disturbances had aortic valve prosthetic endocarditis. In each, the atrioventricular bundle and/or node area was invaded by the infective process. None of our patients with conduction disturbances had significant coronary arterial disease.

Q: (DR. RICHARD HORNICK–BALTIMORE): In your large series of autopsied patients (not just infected patients) did you have any feeling as to how long it takes the aortic area or mitral area to re-endothelialize? Is this a rapid or slow process? What are the repair processes that occur in those regions?

A: (DR. WILLIAM ROBERTS): I think of it like an acute myocardial infarction. How long does it take to heal an acute myocardial infarction? In general, 2 months, depending on its size. This is the reason I use, like Dr. Wilson and others, the division point between "early" and "late" PVE as 2 months rather than 1 month or some other time. In general, after 2 months there is considerable endothelialization over cloth-covered frames, but again, the process is highly individualized. Some patients with cloth-covered prostheses will re-endothelialize the whole thing within 3 months and some have virtually no covering at all 2 years later.

Q: (DR. ALLEN B. KAISER–NASHVILLE): In your pictures, I noticed how clean the cages looked in the cage-type valves compared to the cloth-type or flexible mitral valves. I wonder in patients with organ infarcts or other evidence of embolization if you can correlate embolic findings with the appearance of the valves?

A: (DR. WILLIAM ROBERTS): The valves often looked awful. They all had vegetations. Thus, most had emboli to one organ or another. The numbers I presented were based just on obvious gross infarcts, i.e., those that might be detected clinically. If gross infarcts are not present, microscopic-sized ones usually are. The bigger the vegetation, the greater the likelihood that a portion of it will dislodge and embolize.

Q: (DR. RICHARD DUMA): In the cage-type prosthesis, are vegetations coming from the anulus? Are they breaking off from that spot or also from the ball and cage?

A: (DR. WILLIAM ROBERTS): Vegetations are not behind the site of attachment of the prosthesis, that is, in the "rotten" area. Vegetations protrude into the lumen.

Q: (DR. WALTER WILSON–ROCHESTER): We also observed in the 24 patients who underwent necropsy that each had abscesses in the areas where the valves were implanted. One thing that you mentioned earlier which intrigued me (as well as mystified me) is that in eight of our patients who underwent replacement of infected valves with late onset symptoms, the surgeons described considerable amounts of necrotic and purulent tissue in areas in which these valves were implanted. Yet six of these eight patients survived, although two of the six required subsequent re-replacement of the prosthesis. I have also been mystified as to why all of the valveş did not dehisce, since they were implanted in an area of necrotic tissue and purulent material. I wonder if you might have any explanation for this or if anyone might have any comments concerning this?

A: (DR. WILLIAM ROBERTS): I have wondered about that also. I think that some of the patients who make it are just lucky. However, not all of those rotten anuli have organisms in them, and several of these patients were treated with antibiotics for a long time. Organisms were absent histologically from the infected anuli in several of our patients.

Q: (DR. WILLIAM DISMUKES): I would like to go back to the observation made earlier that Gram-negative endocarditis occurs early and has a very high mortality, as compared to late onset PVE. Is the pathogenesis different for these entities? Although patients who die have annular involvement, perhaps in the late onset cases infection of more accessible tissue is occurring, such as the struts and the more movable parts, with relative sparing of the anulus. Do you have any comments on this hypothesis?

A: (DR. WILLIAM ROBERTS): I think it boils down to how one defines PVE. Personally, I would hate to defend to the courts the diagnosis of PVE when it has not been confirmed, as Dr. Wilson pointed out, morphologically, either at reoperation or at necropsy. I saw a patient at necropsy recently, in whom mitral replacement had been performed 4 months earlier and postoperatively; several blood cultures were positive. The clinicians who cared for this patient were convinced that she had PVE. At necropsy, however, the mitral prosthesis was clean. An aneurysm containing thrombus, however, was present at the site of excision of the papillary muscles. Probably, at one time, thrombus in this small aneurysm had been infected and the aneurysm served as the source of multiple emboli which occurred in her.

Clinical pathologic conference

A conversation on prosthetic valve endocarditis

Ernest N. Arnett, M.D.*
David G. Kastl, M.D.
A. Julian Garvin, M.D., Ph.D.
William C. Roberts, M.D.
Bethesda, Md.

Dr. Roberts: The starting point for this discussion on prosthetic valve endocarditis will be a description of a patient with this fatal complication of cardiac valve replacement.

Dr. Kastl: This 47-year-old man (J.G. #1123701) was in good health until 11 months before death when symptoms of fatigue and exertional dyspnea appeared four weeks after a dental procedure. Hospitalization four months after onset of symptoms (seven months before death) revealed anemia, a colonic filling defect, periodic fever, and *Streptococcus bovis* in several blood cultures. Penicillin, 20 million units intravenously per day, was administered for six weeks; the fever rapidly disappeared, but murmurs of mitral and aortic regurgitation and signs of congestive heart failure appeared. Digoxin and diuretic therapy resulted in transient improvement of the congestive heart failure, and the colonic mass, which proved to be a benign polyp, was resected. He returned home, but heart failure quickly returned and he was hospitalized, now in functional Class IV (New York Heart Association classification), 55 days before death. Digoxin, furosemide, and aldactone produced a 20 pound weight loss. Subsequently, at cardiac catheterization, the pressures in mm. Hg were: pulmonary artery wedge mean 35, a wave 35, v wave 55; pulmonary artery 60/35 (mean 50); right ventricle 60/15; and right atrial mean 15, a wave 22, and v wave 17. Multiple blood cultures during that hospitalization were negative. He was transferred to the National Heart, Lung and Blood Institute (NHLI) 37 days before death.

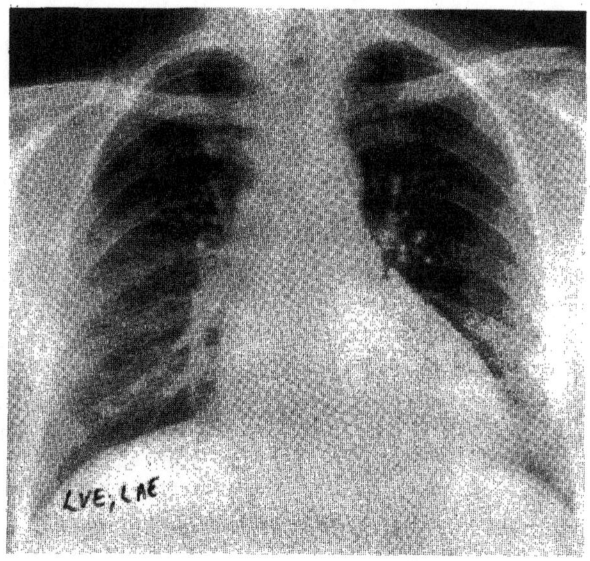

Fig. 1. Posteroanterior chest roentgenogram 4 days before valve replacement.

The blood pressure was 140/70 mm. Hg, cardiac rate, 90 beats per minute, and respiratory rate, 20 breaths per minute. The jugular venous pressure was elevated, and the carotid upstroke was rapid but weak. Basilar râles were present in both lungs. The second heart sound split paradoxically and both third and fourth heart sounds were present. A Grade 3/6 decrescendo diastolic murmur was present along the left sternal border, and a Grade 2/6 holosystolic murmur and a Grade 2/6 middiastolic rumbling murmur were present at the apex. The anteroinferior edge of the liver was palpable 4 cm. below the right costal margin. Chest roentgenograms (Fig. 1) showed marked cardiac enlargement and electrocardio-

From the Pathology Branch and Clinic of Surgery, National Heart, Lung and Blood Institute, and the Laboratory of Pathology, National Cancer Institute, National Institutes of Health, Bethesda, Md.

Received for publication June 9, 1976.

Reprint requests: W. C. Roberts, M.D., Bldg. 10A Rm 3E-30, National Institutes of Health, Bethesda, Maryland 20014.

*Present address: Department of Medicine, The Johns Hopkins Hospital, Baltimore, Maryland.

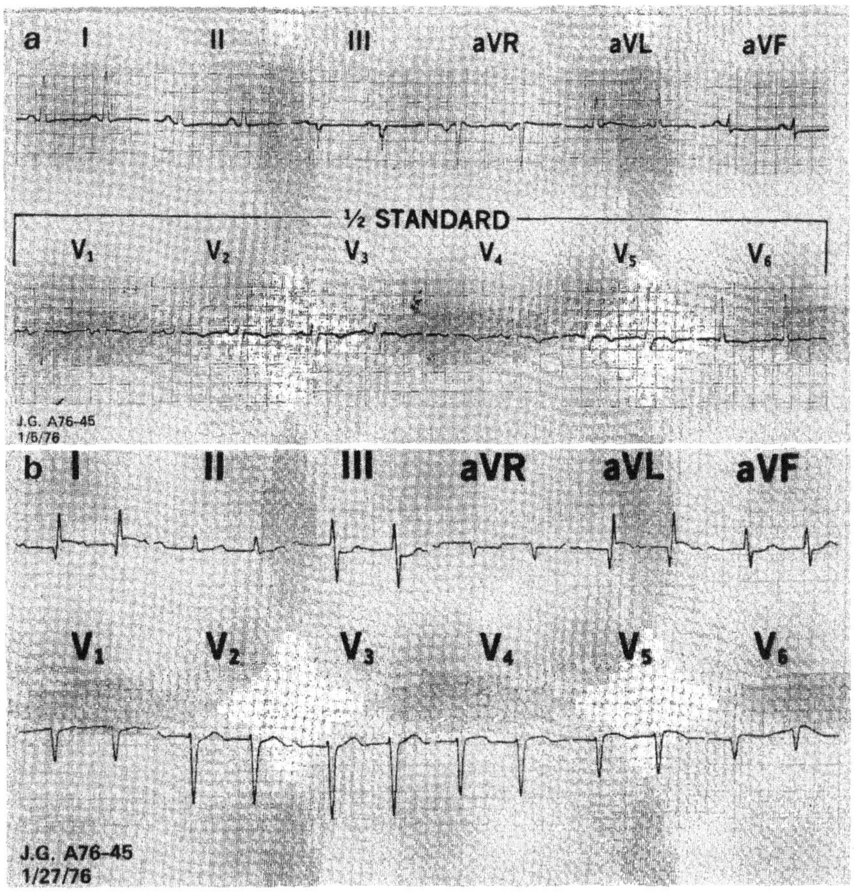

Fig. 2. Electrocardiograms. *a,* Four days before valve replacements showing changes of left ventricular hypertrophy and left atrial enlargement. *b,* Eighteen days postoperatively (10 days before death). Q waves are present in Leads I, aVR, aVL and V_6, the R waves in the precordial leads are of markedly diminished amplitude, and the ST segments are elevated in Leads I, aVL and V_4 through V_6. In addition, the P-R interval is prolonged.

gram (Fig. 2*a*) showed left ventricular hypertrophy. The hematocrit was 37 per cent, and the white blood count 11,900 per cubic millimeter. Simultaneous aortic and left ventricular pressures were 120/50 and 120/30 mm. Hg, respectively. Cineangiography revealed severe aortic and mitral valve regurgitation, but good left ventricular function.

The aortic valve was replaced with a No. 10A model 2320, Starr-Edwards prosthesis and the mitral valve, with a 33 mm. Hancock xenograft 28 days before death. Both the excised aortic valve and the excised mitral valve (Fig. 3) contained one or more perforations in the cusps. Histologic examination of the excised valves revealed no evidence of active infection.

During the first 24 hours postoperatively, excessive bleeding necessitated repeat thoracotomy. Although no specific bleeding sites were found, a large quantity (2,000 ml.) of blood was evacuated from the mediastinum. Oxacillin, 4 Gm. intravenously per day, and streptomycin, 1 Gm. intramuscularly per day, were started at the time of the initial operation and continued for 10 and 7 days, respectively. All chest tubes were removed on the fourth postoperative day. Two days later fever (38.5° C.) was noted but he otherwise appeared to be doing well. Nine days postoperatively ventricular fibrillation occurred, but electroshock was successful in restoring sinus rhythm. Electrocardiograms following this episode showed diffuse nonspecific ST segment and T wave abnormalities. Over the ensuing 4 days, he continued to have frequent ventricular premature beats. On the 17th postoperative day his temperature rose to 39.5° C., the white blood cell

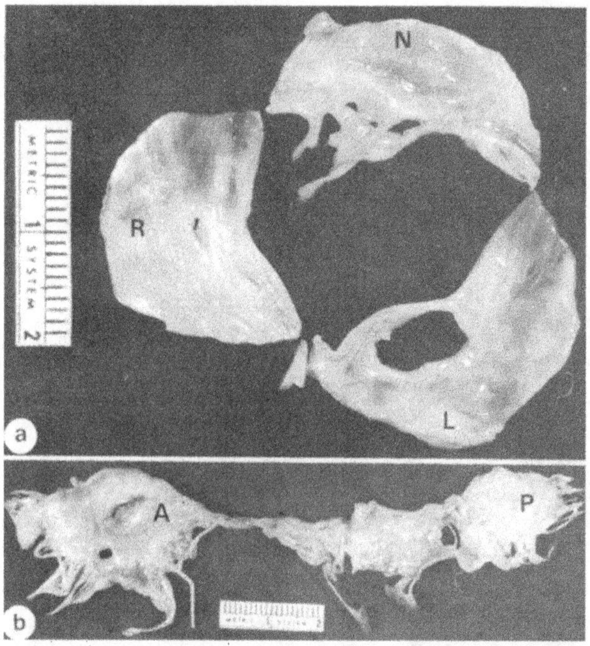

Fig. 3. Operatively excised aortic *(a)* and mitral *(b)* valves. A single perforation is present in the left *(L)* and right *(R)* coronary cusp, and multiple ones are present in the noncoronary *(N)* cusp. A perforation is present in the anterior *(A)* mitral leaflet, and several chordae tendineae from the posterior *(P)* mitral leaflet are absent.

count was 14,500 per cubic millimeter, and blood cultures were positive for *Staphylococcus epidermidis.* Oxacillin, 12 Gm. intravenously per day, was reinstituted. The following day the blood pressure dropped to 95/70 mm. Hg and the electrocardiogram (Fig. 2*b*) showed changes of an acute anterolateral myocardial infarction. On the nineteenth postoperative day, splinter hemorrhages were noted, the white blood cell count was 17,000 per cubic millimeter, and blood cultures again were positive for *S. epidermidis,* resistant to penicillin but sensitive to both oxacillin and cephalosporin. On the twenty-first postoperative day he lost consciousness, his temperature rose to 39° C., and his systolic blood pressure fell to 90 mm. Hg. During insertion of a catheter into a jugular vein, a collection of pus was entered, and Gram stain and culture of the aspirated material disclosed *S. epidermidis.* Exploration of the mediastinum revealed no focal collections of pus. Oxacillin was stopped and cephalosporin, 12 Gm. intravenously per day, was started. Over the next four days consciousness returned, the blood pressure rose to 110/60 mm. Hg, but the white blood count was 27,000 per cubic millimeter, and fever and positive blood cultures continued. On the twenty-seventh postoperative day, his blood pressure suddenly dropped and he died the next day.

Dr. Garvin: Necropsy (A76-45) disclosed no residual pus in the chest. The heart weighed 660 Gm., and the anterolateral left ventricular wall from midportion to apex was necrotic. Large vegetations closed the primary orifice of the aortic valve prosthesis, and a fibrin thrombus was present at the apex of its cage (Fig. 4). Although the aortic prosthesis remained attached, the site of attachment of the prosthesis was necrotic. Necrosis of the valve anulus, however, was apparent only after removal of the prosthesis (Fig. 5). The ring infection extended through the atrial spetum into the right atrium and into the adjacent portion of the prosthetic mitral anulus. Histologic sections from the site of attachment of the aortic prosthesis revealed numerous colonies of Gram-positive cocci. Examination of subserial sections of the extramural coronary arteries revealed total obstruction of the lumen of the left anterior descending coronary artery by a septic embolus (Fig. 6). Sections of myocardium showed numerous foci of suppurating and nonsuppurating inflammation. The lungs were edematous and contained foci of acute inflammation. The walls of the small muscular pulmonary arteries were thick. Both the liver (2,600 grams) and spleen (670 grams) were enlarged, and multiple infarcts were present in the spleen. Focal collections of mononuclear cells were present in the renal interstitium, but otherwise the kidneys were normal.

Dr. Roberts: The above-described patient provides an opportunity to apply information previously derived from a study of 22 necropsy patients with fatal prosthetic valve endocarditis to the present patient.[1] To begin this discourse, Dr. Arnett, how do you define "Prosthetic Valve Endocarditis?"

Dr. Arnett: "Prosthetic valve endocarditis" is an infection involving a prosthetic cardiac valve in a patient in whom no active infective endocarditis was present at the time of prosthetic valve insertion. In other words, the infection was acquired after valve replacement. Although the present patient's valvular disease resulted from infective endocarditis, the infection was healed at the time of valve replacement.

Dr. Roberts: Dr. Kastl, in your presentation of this patient, you mentioned that the cause of

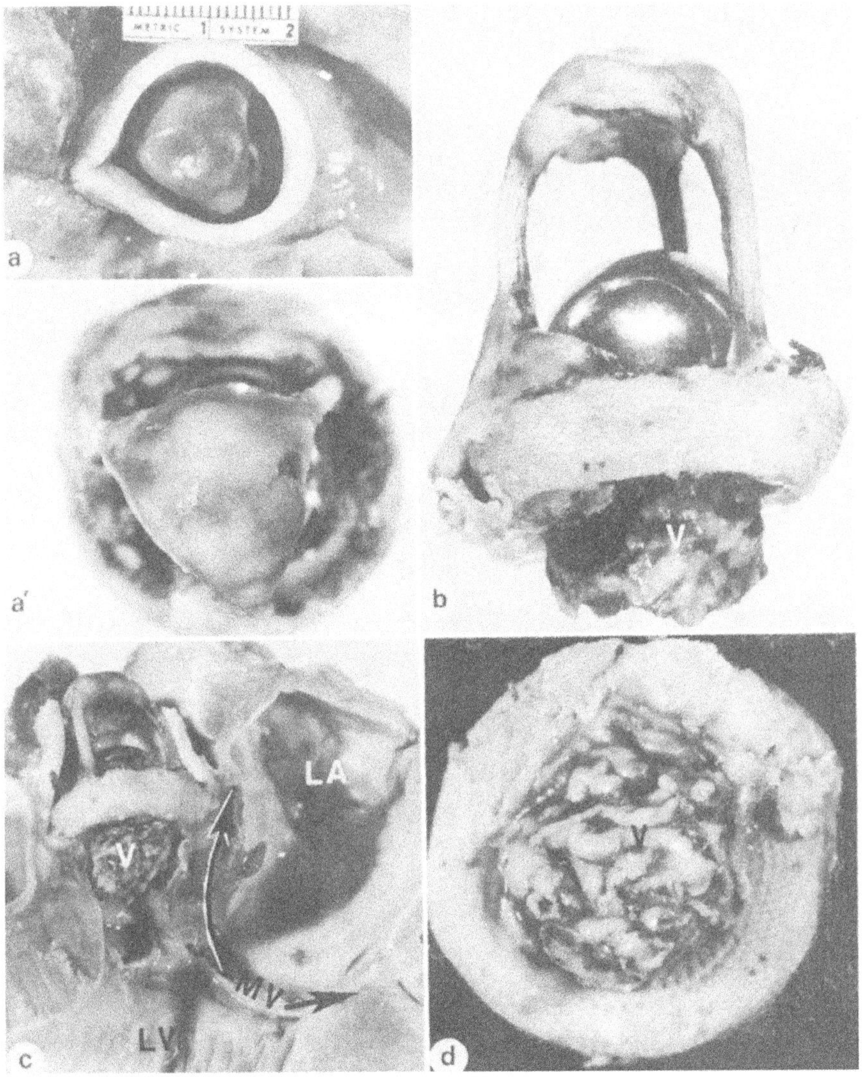

Fig. 4. Infected aortic valve prosthesis. *a,* Prosthesis, viewed from above, in place, and *a'* after removal. Thrombus covers the apex of the cage. *b,* Excised prosthesis viewed laterally. *c,* Longitudinal section showing aortic prosthesis in place. The mitral valve prosthesis has been excised. The aortic "anulus" is necrotic and so is the adjacent portion of mitral anulus. A large vegetation *(V)* is present in the primary orifice of the prosthesis; its obstructive nature is better seen in *d,* a view of the prosthesis from the left ventricular *(LV)* aspect. *LA* = left atrium.

this patient's infective endocarditis, which had involved presumably both anatomically and functionally normal valves, was *Streptococcus bovis.* The cause of the prosthetic valve endocarditis in him, however, was *Staphylococcus epidermidis.* Dr. Arnett, could you summarize the organisms found in our previous 22 patients with prosthetic valve endocarditis?

DR. ARNETT: Among our 22 previous necropsy patients with prosthetic valve endocarditis, *Staphylococcus (epidermidis* in 10 and *aureus* in three) caused the infection in 13 (59 per cent.) In the other nine patients, nine different organisms caused the infection. Of these later nine organisms, three were Gram-negative bacteria, and two were fungi.

DR. ROBERTS: We have found it useful to subdivide patients with prosthetic valve endocarditis into those with early infection, i.e., appearing within two months of valve replacement, and those with infection appearing later, i.e., those with signs of cardiac infection appearing longer than two months after operation. Dr. Arnett, have there been any differences in the types of infecting organisms in patients with early prosthetic valve endocarditis as contrasted to those in

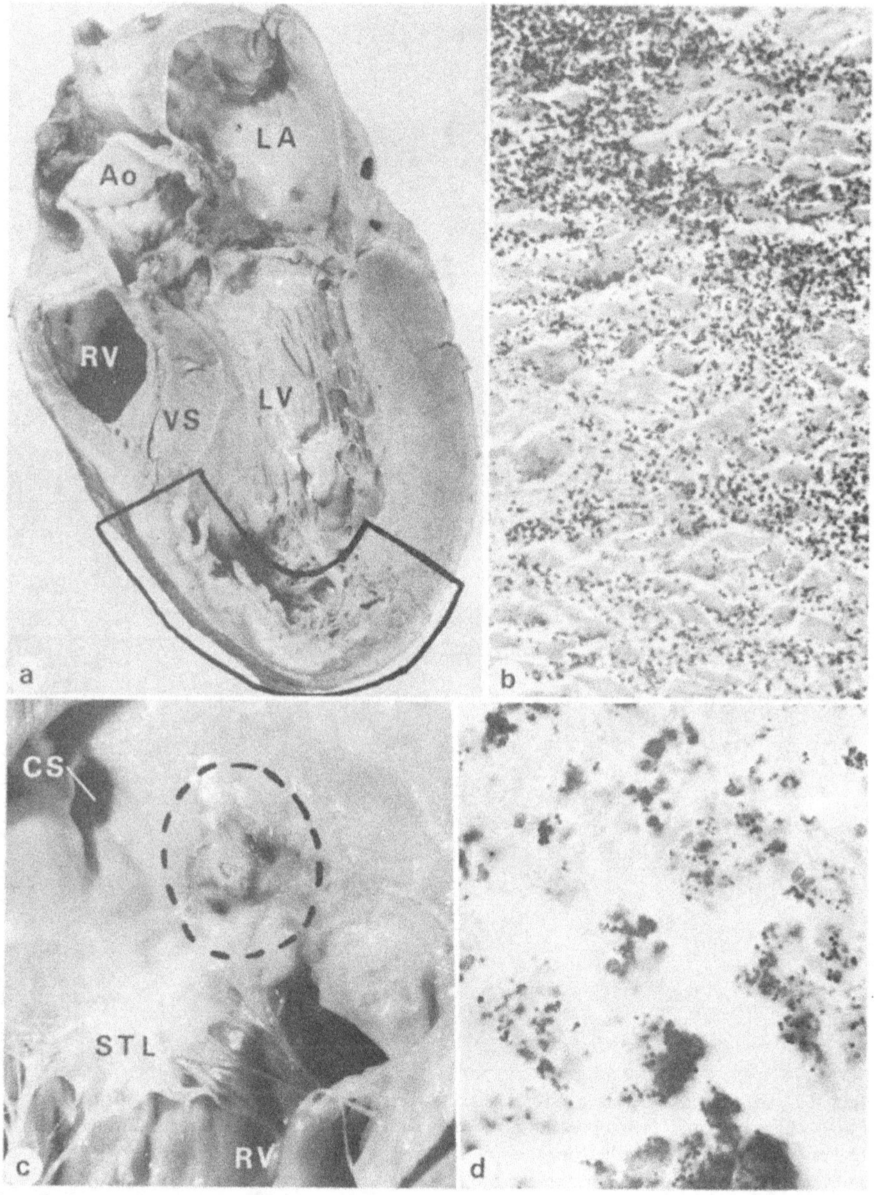

Fig. 5. Ring abscess and acute myocardial infarct. *a,* Longitudinal section of heart showing the ring abscess involving the entire aortic "anulus" and the portion of mitral anulus adjacent to the aortic valve. A large transmural infarct is present in the anterior wall of left ventricle (in brackets). *Ao* = aorta; *LA* = left atrium; *LV* = left ventricle; *RV* = right ventricle; *VS* = ventricular septum. *b,* Histologic section of the anterior left ventricular wall. The myocardial cells are necrotic and numerous polymorphonuclear leukocytes are present. (Hematoxylin and eosin stain; × 330). *c,* Opened right atrium, tricuspid valve, and right ventricle *(RV).* The aortic ring abscess has extended through the adjacent atrial septum and is visible in right atrium *(dashed circle). CS* = ostium of coronary sinus; *STL* = septal tricuspid leaflet. *d,* Histologic section showing colonies of Gram-positive cocci in the necrotic aortic valve anulus (Brown and Brenn stain; × 880).

whom the infection appeared months or years after valve replacement?

Dr. Arnett: Among patients with early prosthetic valve endocarditis, *Staphylococcus epidermidis* has been the most frequent causative organism.[2-4] Among patients with late prosthetic valve endocarditis both staphylococci and streptococci have been frequent causes; however, the former have caused most cases of necropsy-proven late prosthetic valve endocarditis, and the latter, relatively few.

Dr. Roberts: Among patients with early prosthetic valve endocarditis it is presumed that the infection either was incurred at operation or resulted from a wound infection. The former may result from contamination of cardiopulmonary bypass equipment.[5,6] Dr. Arnett, what have been the predisposing factors in patients with late prosthetic valve endocarditis?

DR. ARNETT: Late prosthetic valve endocarditis presumably results from transient bacteremia, and the source of the bacteremia is often obscure.[3,7] Among our previous 22 necropsy patients with prosthetic valve endocarditis, 14 had the onset of symptoms of prosthetic endocarditis longer than two months after operation. Predisposing factors were apparent in only five of them: dental procedures in two, and in one patient each, skin graft infection, prolonged use of an intravenous catheter, and prolonged use of a transthoracic pacing wire.

DR. ROBERTS: Dr. Arnett, you mentioned a similarity between early and late prosthetic endocarditis in regard to the types of infecting organisms. Are there distinct clinical differences between patients with prosthetic valve endocarditis appearing early after operation as contrasted to those with infection appearing late?

DR. ARNETT: Prosthetic valve endocarditis occurring in the early postoperative period is often more difficult to diagnose.[7] Signs of prosthetic infection may be masked by other more common postoperative complications, and transient bacteremia may be attributed to another cause. That was the situation in the present patient: persistent staphylococcal bacteremia was attributed to the known mediastinal infection and the diagnosis of prosthetic valve endocarditis was never established during life. When fever and bacteremia appear suddenly in an otherwise well patient months or years after cardiac valve replacement, however, a diagnosis of prosthetic valve endocarditis is usually made quite readily.

DR. ROBERTS: It is worth emphasizing, however, that the combination of fever and positive blood culture in a patient with a prosthetic cardiac valve, especially in the early postoperative period, does not always indicate the presence of prosthetic valve endocarditis.[8] We recently studied at necropsy a patient who was diagnosed during life as having mitral prosthetic valve endocarditis on the basis of fever, cerebral episodes consistent with emboli, and a blood culture which grew *Staphylococcus epidermidis*. She received antibiotics during most of her four-month postoperative period and, at necropsy, no prosthetic valve endocarditis was found. A left ventricular aneurysm, however, was present immediately

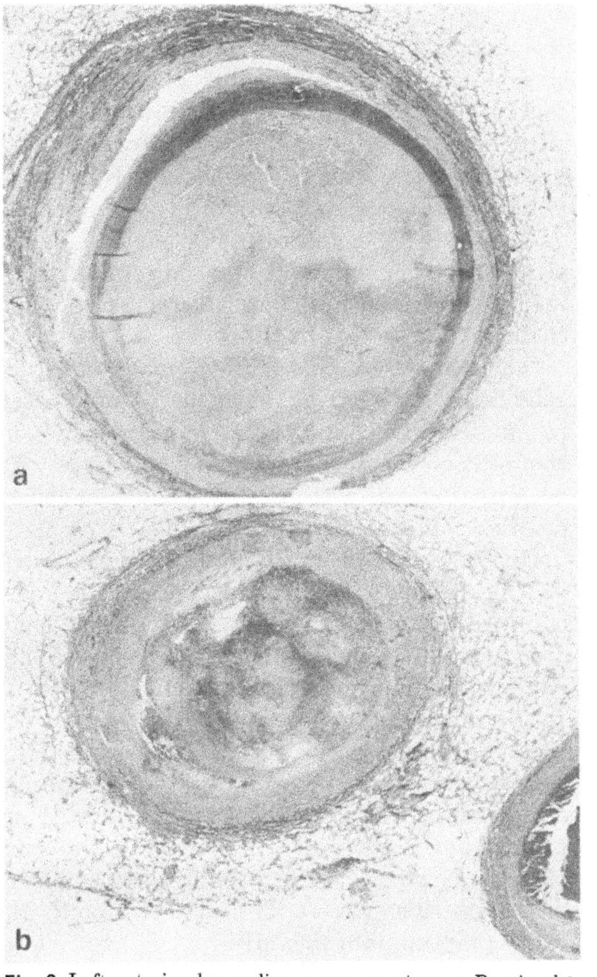

Fig. 6. Left anterior descending coronary artery. *a*, Proximal 1 cm. and *b*, a distal branch. The lumen is totally obstructed by a septic embolus. (*a*, Elastic van Gieson stain; *b*, hematoxylin and eosin stain; both × 12.)

caudal to the mitral anulus and a thrombus, which presumably had been infected at one time, was present in the aneurysm. The latter appeared to have been the source of cerebral emboli.

Although the present patient's aortic valve prosthesis was almost totally obstructed by vegetative material, a diagnosis of endocarditis was never established, presumably because signs of prosthetic dysfunction were absent. Dr. Arnett, do patients with prosthetic valve endocarditis usually have signs of prosthetic dysfunction?

DR. ARNETT: This patient was somewhat unusual. Infection of an aortic valve prosthesis usually results in detachment of the prosthesis, not obstruction, and signs of aortic regurgitation are usually present. Eleven of our previous 15 necropsy patients with aortic prosthetic infection had signs of aortic regurgitation, and in each of them the prosthesis was at least partially detached. Only one previous patient had aortic prosthetic obstruction from infection, and he had clinical signs of aortic valve obstruction. In contrast to aortic prosthetic infection, mitral infection usually causes obstruction of the prosthesis, but signs of mitral obstruction usually are not detected. None of our seven patients with mitral prosthetic endocarditis had clinical signs of prosthetic dysfunction, but at necropsy five of them had large vegetations obstructing the orifice of the prosthesis.

DR. ROBERTS: This patient had infection behind the site of attachment of the prosthesis, i.e., in the valve ring. Dr. Arnett, would you comment on the frequency of ring abscess among necropsy patients with prosthetic valve endocarditis?

DR. ARNETT: Infection behind the sewing ring, or ring abscess, is a consistent morphologic feature of prosthetic valve endocarditis. Ring abscess was present in each of our 22 previous patients, all of whom had rigid-framed prosthesis. In two thirds of them the entire circumference of the valve anulus was necrotic. Extension of the ring infection into adjacent cardiac structures also is common, especially in the patients with an infected aortic prosthesis. In nine of our previous 15 patients with aortic prosthetic valve endocarditis, the ring abscess burrowed through the cardiac septum into ring atrium, just as it did in the present patient.

DR. ROBERTS: Thus ring abscess is to be expected in patients with infection involving rigid-frame prostheses. Indeed, the infection in these patients nearly always involves the site of attachment of the prosthesis, and this is why patients with prosthetic valve endocarditis are so difficult to treat. If the infection was limited to the prosthesis, an infected prosthesis could be excised and replaced with another prosthesis. In the present patient, as in most of the others, the entire valve anulus was necrotic, and although he had received appropriate antibiotic therapy, intravenously for four weeks, numerous colonies of viable-appearing Gram positive cocci were present in the valve ring at necropsy. This patient developed prolongation of the PR interval, presumably from extension of the aortic ring abscess into the cephalad portion of the ventricular septum. Dr. Arnett, how common are atrioventricular conduction defects in patients with aortic prosthetic endocarditis?

DR. ARNETT: Among our previous 15 patients with aortic valve prosthetic endocarditis, five developed complete heart block and two others developed left bundle branch block. In each of these patients the ring abscess had extended into the basal portion of the ventricular septum.

DR. ROBERTS: The present patient had multiple infarcts in the spleen as well as a transmural acute myocardial infarct. Are systemic emboli common in patients with prosthetic valve endocarditis?

DR. ARNETT: Fourteen of our 22 previous necropsy patients (64 per cent) had gross infarcts in other organs. The organs most frequently involved were: spleen (12 patients), kidney (7 patients), and brain (7 patients). Only one of the previous 22 patients, however, had a transmural acute myocardial infarct from a coronary arterial embolus.

DR. ROBERTS: We have not touched on the frequency of prosthetic valve endocarditis. We have examined at necropsy approximately 450 patients in whom one or more cardiac valves had been replaced by prostheses. Twenty-three of them (5 per cent), including the patient described herein, had infection involving a prosthetic valve. Thus, although prosthetic valve endocarditis is a devastating complication of cardiac valve replacement, fortunately, it is infrequent. Although its exact frequency is uncertain, it may be less than 1 per cent per year among patients with prosthetic cardiac valves. In the early days of cardiac valve replacement, prosthetic infection in the early postoperative period was more common than in the late postoperative period. Now, however, it is likely that infection occurring late is more common than that occurring early, simply because there are large numbers of patients with prosthetic valves.

Dr. Arnett and I have studied 74 patients with active infective endocarditis involving natural left-sided cardiac valves. Dr. Arnett, would you summarize the major differences between our patients with prosthetic endocarditis and those with natural valve infective endocarditis.

DR. ARNETT: Comparison of observations in the 22 patients with prosthetic valve endocarditis to those in the 74 patients with active left-sided valvular endocarditis revealed two major differences. *Ring abscess* was present in each of the patients with prosthetic valve endocarditis, regardless of the site of the prosthesis. Among the patients with natural valve endocarditis, ring abscess was common only in patients with aortic valve infection.[9] Because heart block in patients with infective endocarditis is usually due to extension of ring abscess into the ventricular septum, it is more frequent in patients with prosthetic endocarditis than in patients with natural valve endocarditis.

The second major difference between patients with prosthetic endocarditis, and those with natural valve endocarditis is the frequency of *valvular obstruction* from infective endocarditis. The hemodynamic consequence of natural valve endocarditis is almost always regurgitation; valvular obstruction is rare.[10, 11] The hemodynamic consequence of prosthetic valve infection often is obstruction, especially when a mitral prosthesis is infected.

REFERENCES

1. Arnett, E. N., and Roberts, W. C.: Prosthetic valve endocarditis. A clinico pathologic analysis of 22 necropsy patients with comparison of observations to 74 necropsy patients with active infective endocarditis involving natural left-sided cardiac valves, Am. J. Cardiol. **38**:281, 1976.
2. Slaughter, L., Morris, J. E., and Starr, A.: Prosthetic valvular endocarditis. A 12-year review, Circulation **47**:1319, 1973.
3. Dismukes, W. E., Karchmer, A. W., Buckley, M. J., Austen, W. G., and Swartz, M. N.: Prosthetic valve endocarditis. Analysis of 38 cases, Circulation **48**:365, 1973.
4. Wilson, W. R., Jaumin, P. M., Danielson, G. K., Giuliani, E. R., Washington, J. A., and Geraci, J. E.: Prosthetic valve endocarditis, Ann. Intern. Med. **82**:751, 1975.
5. Ankeney, J. L., and Parker, R. F.: Staphylococcal endocarditis following open heart surgery related to positive intraoperative blood cultures, *in* Prosthetic heart valves, edited by Brewer, L. A., III, Springfield, Ill., 1969, Charles C Thomas, Publisher, pp. 719-730.
6. Blakemore, W. S., McGarrity, G. J., Thurer, R. J., Wallace, H. W., MacVaugh, H., III, and Coriell, L. L.: Infection by air-borne bacteria with cardiopulmonary bypass, Surgery **70**:830, 1971.
7. Kloster, F. E.: Diagnosis and management of complications of prosthetic heart valves, Am. J. Cardiol. **35**:872, 1975.
8. Sande, M. A., Johnson, W. D., Jr., Hook, E. W., and Kaxe, D.: Sustained bacteremia in patients with prosthetic cardiac valves, N. Engl. J. Med. **286**:1067, 1972.
9. Arnett, E. N., and Roberts, W. C.: Valve ring abscess in active infective endocarditis. Frequency, location, and clues to clinical diagnosis from study of 95 necropsy patients, Circulation **54**:140, 1976.
10. Roberts, W. C., Ewy, G. A., Glancy, D. L., and Marcus, F. I.: Valvular stenosis produced by active infective endocarditis, Circulation **36**:449, 1967.
11. Arnett, E. N., and Roberts, W. C.: Active infective endocarditis. A clinico pathologic analysis of 137 necropsy patients. Current Concepts in Cardiology (In press, October, 1976 issue).

Echocardiographic Observations in Opiate Addicts With Active Infective Endocarditis

Frequency of Involvement of the Various Valves and Comparison of Echocardiographic Features of Right- and Left-Sided Cardiac Valve Endocarditis

JOSEPH J. ANDY, MD
MAZHAR U. SHEIKH, MD
NAYAB ALI, MD, FACC
BOISEY O. BARNES, MD
LAY M. FOX, MD, FACC
CHARLES L. CURRY, MD, FACC
WILLIAM C. ROBERTS, MD, FACC

Washington, D.C. and Bethesda, Maryland

Echocardiographic observations are described in 25 opiate addicts with active infective endocarditis involving apparently previously normal valves. Infective endocarditis was isolated to the tricuspid valve in 11 patients, involved both right- (tricuspid valve) and left-sided valves in 7 and was isolated to the left-sided valves in 7 (mitral valve in 6). Twenty patients (80 percent) had tricuspid valve regurgitation, 12 had mitral regurgitation, 3 had aortic regurgitation and none had pulmonary valve regurgitation. Considering the 75 cardiac valves (excluding the pulmonary) in the 25 patients, echocardiographic abnormalities consistent with active infective endocarditis were detected in 26 (74 percent) of the 35 clinically incompetent valves but in none of the 40 competent valves. Comparison of the 20 incompetent tricuspid valves with the 12 incompetent mitral valves indicated that (1) the echocardiogram was less sensitive in detecting tricuspid valve lesions, (2) rupture of tricuspid valve chordae tendineae was absent or not detectable, and (3) tricuspid valve vegetations tended to be larger.

Echocardiographic manifestations of cardiac valve vegetations were described for the first time in 1973.[1,2] Subsequently, other reports[3-10] confirmed and extended the initial observations. The following general conclusions from these studies appear justified: (1) there are echocardiographic features indica ive of vegetations in many patients with active infective endocarditis, (2) these echocardiographic features occur mainly in the sickest patients, that is, those requiring valve replacement, and (3) the echocardiogram may be useful in the initial diagnosis of active infective endocarditis in patients with negative blood cultures.

The reported echocardiographic observations have mainly concerned patients with active infective endocarditis involving the left-sided cardiac valves: aortic in 33 patients and mitral in 25 patients.[1-10] To our knowledge, echocardiographic observations have been reported in only four patients with active infection involving a right-sided cardiac valve.[2,10] During a recent 19 month period, we studied with echocardiography 25 opiate addicts with active infective endocarditis. Because endocarditis in these patients usually involves previously normal valves, the resulting echocardiographic abnormalities can reasonably be attributed to the infective endocarditis rather than to a combination of underlying valve scarring plus superimposed valve infection. A high percent of patients have active infective endocarditis involving the tricuspid valve. This study describes the echocardiographic features in the 25 opiate addicts, focusing on the echocardiographic features produced by the tricuspid valve infection and comparing them with those produced by infection involving the mitral valve.

From the Departments of Medicine of the District of Columbia General Hospital and the Howard University Hospital, Washington, D.C. and the Pathology Branch, National Heart, Lung, and Blood Institute, National Institutes of Health, Bethesda, Maryland. Manuscript received November 23, 1976; revised manuscript received January 10, 1977, accepted January 11, 1977.

Address for reprints: William C. Roberts, MD, Building 10A, Room 3E-30, National Institutes of Health, Bethesda, Maryland 20014.

Material and Methods

Criteria for inclusion in this study included: (1) typical clinical features of active infective endocarditis (Table I); (2) regurgitation of at least one cardiac valve; (3) the recording of at least one echocardiogram during the period of active infective endocarditis; and (4) a history of recent opiate addiction (Table II). The 25 patients ranged in age from 21 to 49 years (average 29 years); 11 were women and 14 men. All were studied between October 1974 and May 1976 at either the District of Columbia General Hospital (17 patients) or the Howard University Hospital (8 patients). During this period, echocardiograms were obtained from all patients with active infective endocarditis whose presence was known to the cardiology staffs of either hospital.

Clinical diagnostic features (Tables I and II): All 25 patients had fever (more than 100° F), 22 had clinical evidence of pulmonary (17 patients) or systemic (3 patients) infarcts or both (2 patients) and all 25 had precordial murmurs of the regurgitant type.

Tricuspid regurgitation was diagnosed when a dominant *V* wave was observed in neck veins and when a blowing systolic murmur heard along the lower left sternal border increased in intensity with inspiration or leg raising, or both. Of the 20 patients with such a murmur, 18 also had clinical evidence of pulmonary infarction and these 18 were considered to have tricuspid regurgitation on the basis of infective endocarditis of the triscuspid valve; the remaining 2 patients (Cases 21 and 24) with a murmur of tricuspid regurgitation but no clinical evidence of pulmonary infarction were considered to have tricuspid regurgitation on a "functional" basis, that is, secondary to pulmonary hypertension from severe mitral regurgitation.

Mitral regurgitation was diagnosed when a blowing pansystolic murmur was heard loudest over the cardiac apex and with radiation into the left axilla. This murmur did not increase with inspiration and in addition was louder in intensity than the murmurs considered to represent tricuspid regurgitation. Twelve of the 25 patients were considered to have a murmur of mitral regurgitation: In 6 this was the only precordial murmur; the remaining 6 also had a murmur of tricuspid regurgitation, and 1 had a murmur of aortic regurgitation as well. Six of these 12 patients with mitral regurgitation

TABLE I

Clinical Observations in 25 Opiate Addicts With Active Infective Endocarditis

	Patients (no.)	
Positive blood cultures	24	
Fever (>100° F)	25	
Valve regurgitation	25	
Isolated right-sided	11	
Tricuspid (TV) only		11
Right- and left-sided	9*	
TV + mitral (MV)		7*
TV + aortic (AV)		1
TV + MV + AV		1
Isolated left-sided	7	
MV only		6
AV only		1
Emboli with infarcts	22	
Pulmonary (P)		17
Systemic (S)		3
P + S		2

* In two of these patients the murmur of tricuspid regurgitation was considered to be of functional origin secondary to pulmonary hypertension and not caused by infective endocarditis involving the tricuspid valve.

TABLE II

Clinical and Echocardiographic Observations in the 25 Opiate Patients With Active Infective Endocarditis

Case no.	Age (yr) & Sex	Regurgitant Murmur			Vegetation by Echo			Vegetation at Necropsy			Infecting Organism	Clinical Infarcts	
		TV	MV	AV	TV	MV	AV	TV	MV	AV		P	S
1	24M	+	0	0	+	0	0	+*	–	–	S aureus	+	0
2	26M	+	0	0	+	0	0	+	0	0	S aureus	+	0
3	34M	+	0	0	+	0	0	–	–	–	S aureus	+	+
4	28M	+	0	0	–	0	0	–	–	–	S aureus	+	0
5	45M	+	0	0	0	0	0	–	–	–	S aureus	+	0
6	29F	+	0	0	+	0	0	–	–	–	α-strep	+	0
7	21F	+	0	0	+	0	0	–	–	–	No growth	+	0
8	26F	+	0	0	0	0	0	–	–	–	S aureus	+	0
9	30M	+	0	0	–	0	0	–	–	–	S aureus	+	0
10	23M	+	0	0	0	0	0	–	–	–	S aureus	+	0
11	23F	+	0	0	+	0	0	–	–	–	S aureus	+	0
12	40M	+	+	0	+	0	0	–	–	–	S aureus	+	0
13	28F	+	+	0	+	+	0	–	–	–	S aureus	+	0
14	25F	+	+	0	+	+	0	–	–	–	S aureus	+	0
15	33F	+	+	0	+	+	0	–	–	–	S aureus	+	+
16	26M	+	+	0	+	+	0	–	–	–	S aureus	+	0
17	38F	+	0	+	+	0	+	–†	–†	–†	S aureus	+	0
18	27M	+	+	+	0	+	+	–†	–†	–†	Strep sp	+	0
19	23F	0	+	0	0	+	0	–	–	–	Enterococcus	0	0
20	24M	0	+	0	0	+	0	–	–	–	S aureus	0	+
21	36M	+‡	+	0	0	+	0	0	+	0	Enterococcus	0	+
22	29F	0	+	0	0	+	0	–	–	–	α-strep	0	0
23	21M	0	+	0	0	+	0	–	–	–	α-strep	0	0
24	25F	+‡	+	0	0	+	0	0	+	0	α-strep	0	+
25	49M	0	0	+	–	0	+	+§	0	+	S aureus	+	0

* Confirmed at time of cardiac operation. Patient alive.
† Died but no necropsy.
‡ Tricuspid regurgitation was mild and probably secondary to right ventricular systolic hypertension resulting from severe mitral regurgitation.
§ Vegetation small (<1 cm in diameter) and attached entirely to chordae tendineae of tricuspid valves, not to its leaflets.
AV = aortic valve; echo = echocardiography; MV = mitral valve; P = pulmonary; S = systemic; S aureus = Staphylococcus aureus; sp = species; strep = streptococcus; TV = tricuspid valve.
+ = present or positive; 0 = absent or negative; – = not applicable or no information available.

had clinical evidence of pulmonary infarction, and each of these 6 also had a murmur of tricuspid regurgitation that was attributable to infective endocarditis involving the tricuspid valve. Of the remaining six patients with a murmur of mitral regurgitation but no pulmonary infarct, four had only this murmur; the other two also had a murmur of tricuspid regurgitation that was considered of functional origin because neither patient had pulmonary infarcts or echocardiographic evidence of vegetations on the tricuspid valve leaflets.

Aortic regurgitation was diagnosed in three patients (Cases 17, 18 and 25) on the basis of a diastolic blowing murmur over the base of the heart or along the left sternal border. The

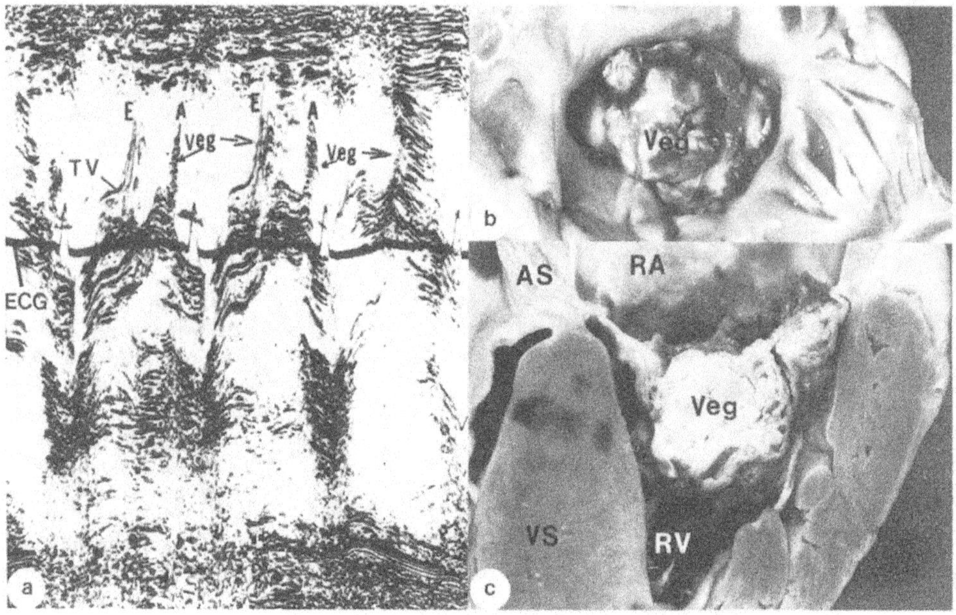

FIGURE 1. Case 2. This man had clinical signs and symptoms of active infective endocarditis for about 84 days. This echocardiogram **(a)** was recorded 5 days before death. Masses of echoes (veg) fill most of the space encompassed by the tricuspid valve (TV) leaflets in diastole. The E and A points of the tricuspid valve echoes are shown. **b,** the tricuspid valve orifice, as viewed from the right atrium, is completely occupied by vegetation (veg). **c,** longitudinal section of heart showing the space between the tricuspid valve leaflets completely occupied by vegetative material. AS = atrial septum; ECG = electrocardiogram; RA = right atrium; RV = right ventricle; VS = ventricular septum.

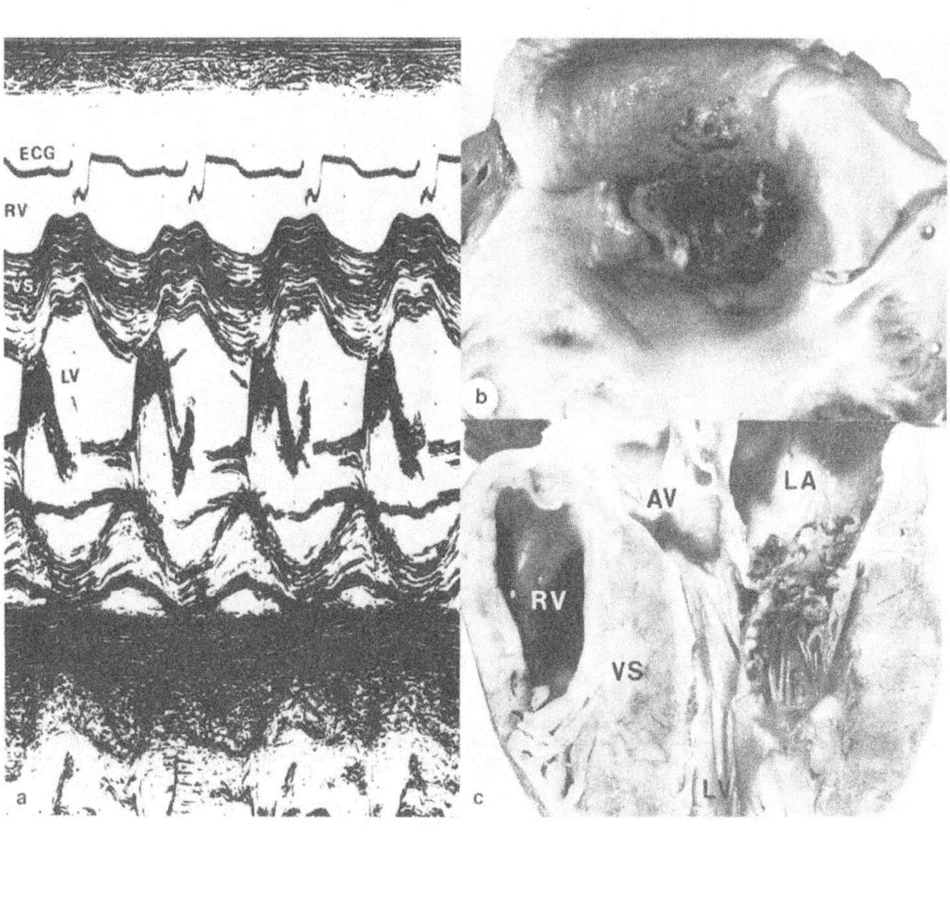

FIGURE 2. Case 21. This man had clinical signs and symptoms of active infective endocarditis for about 30 days. **a,** echocardiogram recorded 7 days before death showing marked thickening of the mitral leaflets **(arrows).** The motion of the ventricular septum (VS), posterior left ventricular (LV) wall and anterior mitral leaflet is exaggerated. Prolapse of the mitral valve leaflet into the left atrium also was recorded (not shown). The right ventricle (RV) is dilated. A small posterior echo-free space indicating pericardial effusion also is present. **b,** view of mitral valve as seen from the left atrium. A tongue of the anterior mitral leaflet protrudes into this cavity and a jet lesion is present on the left atrial wall. **c,** longitudinal view of the heart showing prolapse of a portion of the anterior mitral valve leaflet into the left atrium (LA). The tongue of the prolapsed anterior leaflet contacts the mural endocardium of the left atrium at the site of the jet lesion. Although the ventricular septum appears to be thicker than the ventricular free wall, the cut of the septum is not completely perpendicular to it. Other cuts showed the septum to be no thicker than the left ventricular free wall. AV = aortic valve; ECG = electrocardiogram.

murmur was considered of aortic rather than of pulmonary valve origin because each of the three patients had a cuff diastolic blood pressure of less than 60 mm Hg, bounding systemic arterial pulses and echocardiographic evidence of vegetations on the aortic valve cusps. Pulmonary valve regurgitation was not diagnosed clinically (or with echocardiography) in any of the 25 patients.

Sites of valve vegetations: Determination of these sites was based on the presence of precordial murmurs typical of regurgitation involving one or more of the various cardiac valves (Table I). Eighteen patients had a murmur typical of regurgitation of only one valve: tricuspid in 11, mitral in 6 and aortic in 1; the other 7 had murmurs indicative of regurgitation of more than one valve. Seven patients had evidence of regurgitation limited to a left-sided cardiac valve; only one of these (Case 25) had pulmonary changes compatible with infarction and, at necropsy, this patient was found to have a small vegetation on the chordae tendineae of the tricuspid valve in

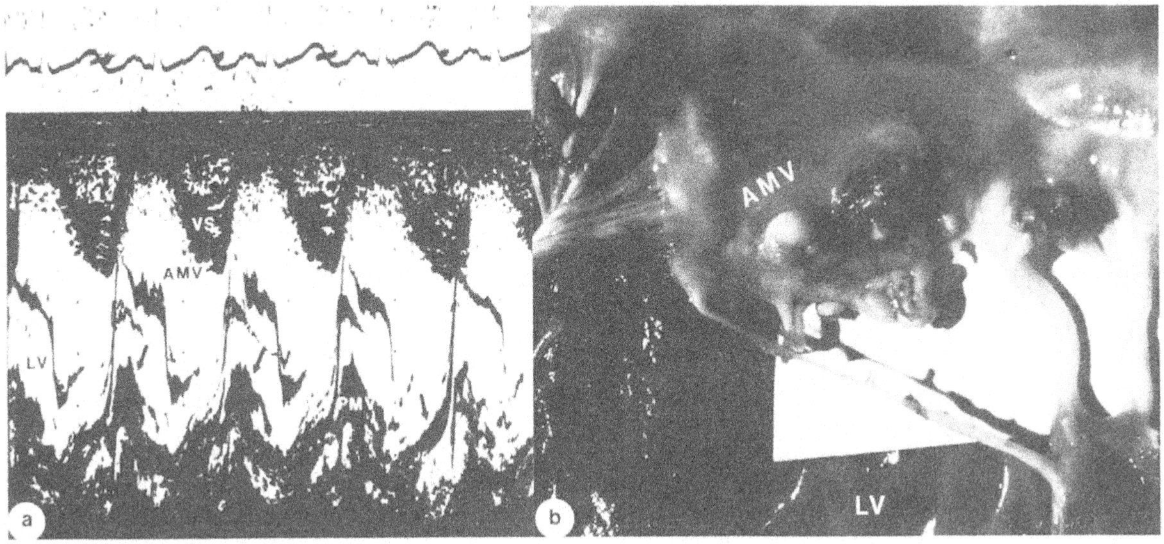

FIGURE 3. Case 24. This woman had signs and symptoms typical of active infective endocarditis for 60 days before death. **a,** echocardiogram recorded 3 days before death showing irregular thickening **(arrows)** of the mitral valve leaflets and erratic opening motion of the anterior mitral leaflet (AMV). The posterior mitral leaflet (PMV) moves anteriorly in early diastole and slightly posteriorly in early systole. Motion of the ventricular septum (VS) is greatly exaggerated. These changes are compatible with rupture of mitral chordae tendineae due to active infective endocarditis. **b,** opened mitral valve showing a vegetation on the atrial aspect of the posterior half of the anterior leaflet. Most of the chordae have ruptured at this site. LV = left ventricle.

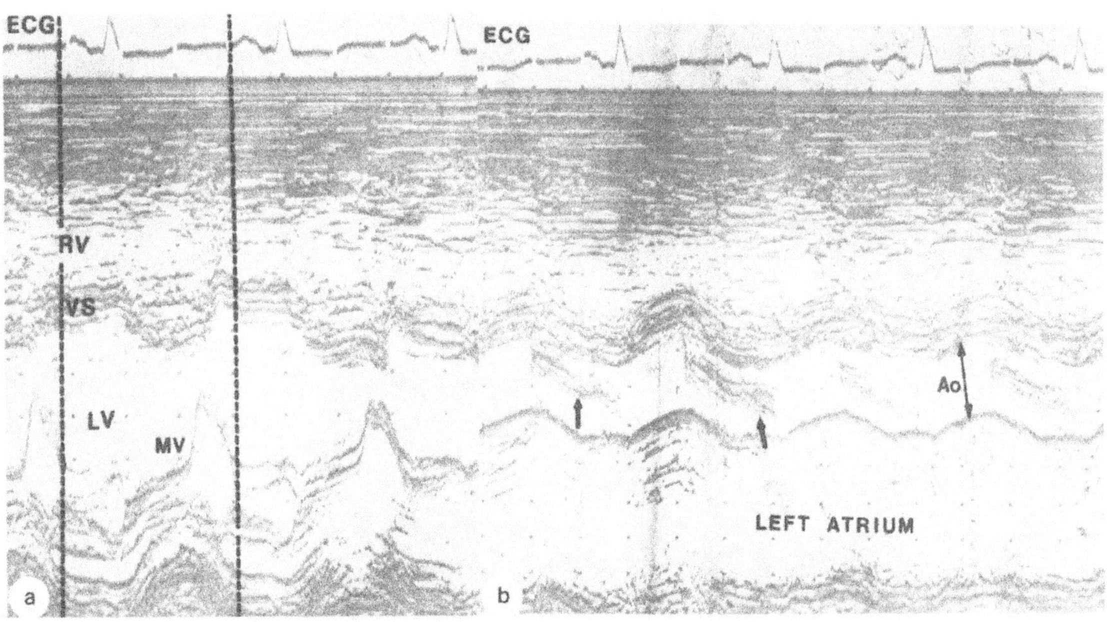

FIGURE 4. Case 17. Echocardiogram obtained 2 days before death. Clinically, the patient had evidence of both severe tricuspid and severe aortic valve regurgitation. **a,** there is diastolic fluttering of the mitral leaflets. **b,** fine diastolic fluttering **(arrows)** of aortic valve cusps, thickened presumably by vegetative material. The fluttering of these cusps and the premature closure of the mitral leaflets, which developed 2 days before death, are indicative of aortic valve cuspal perforation or tear, or both. Ao = aorta; ECG = electrocardiogram; LV = left ventricle; MV = mitral valve; RV = right ventricle; VS = ventricular septum.

addition to vegetations on the aortic valve. The other 18 patients had evidence of tricuspid valve regurgitation that was isolated in 11 and associated with left-sided regurgitation in the other 7; all 18 had radiographic changes consistent with pulmonary infarction, presumably secondary to dislodgment of vegetative material from the tricuspid valve. None of the 25 patients had historical or recorded evidence of a precordial murmur before the onset of active infective endocarditis, and none had a history of rheumatic fever or clinical evidence of valve stenosis.

Necropsy findings (Table II): Six of the 25 patients died from consequences of the active infective endocarditis, and necropsy was performed in 4; an additional patient (Case 1) underwent successful operative excision of the tricuspid valve. The other 18 patients recovered and were discharged from the hospital. Studies at necropsy or operation confirmed that the clinical diagnosis of involvement of one or more valves by the infective process was correct in all five patients so examined. In Case 25, however, necropsy disclosed a single small vegetation on several chordae tendineae of the tricuspid valve although evidence of tricuspid valve dysfunction had not occurred during life. In Case 1 cardiac operation confirmed that each of the tricuspid valve leaflets had large vegetations that appeared to prevent proper coaptation of the leaflets during ventricular systole. The tricuspid valve anulus was dilated. In Case 2 necropsy disclosed huge vegetations on each of the three tricuspid valve cusps. In Case 25, a single large vegetation on the aortic valve at the junction of the right and noncoronary cusps caused detachment of both of these cusps at, and adjacent to, their commissural attachment. The detachment resulted in severe aortic regurgitation. In addition, the aortic vegetation extended through the membraneous ventricular system to appear on the right side of the heart on the underside of the junction of the septal and anterior tricuspid valve leaflets. As mentioned earlier, a small vegetation encircled several chordae tendineae attached to the tricuspid valve leaflets.

Echocardiograms: A total of 55 echocardiograms were recorded in the 25 patients. Tracings are illustrated from three of the five patients whose sites of cardiac valve vegetations were confirmed morphologically (Fig. 1 to 3) and from two additional patients with echocardiographic confirmation of vegetations on each of two cardiac valves (Fig. 4 and 5).

Two types of echocardiographic recorders were used: (1) a Unirad 100 series (D.C. General) or (2) a Honeywell 1856 strip-chart recorder (Howard). Each machine utilized a 0.5 inch (1.27 cm) diameter, 2.25 megahertz transducer with a repetitive rate of 1,000 pulses/sec. Recordings were made in the standard fashion[11] with the patient supine at an inclination of 45°. Each valve studied was continuously scanned. Echocardiographic criteria utilized as indicative of lesions resulting from active infective endocarditis are defined in Table III.[1-10,12,13]

TABLE III

Echocardiographic Characteristics of Cardiac Valve Lesions Resulting From Active Infective Endocarditis

Anatomic Lesion	Applicable Cardiac Valve	Echocardiographic Characteristics
1. Valve vegetations	TV, MV, AV	Irregular ("shaggy") thickening of valve echoes
2. Torn or perforated valve cusp	TV	Uncertain
	MV	Uncertain
	AV	Fine diastolic "fluttering" of the cusps; diastolic separation of the cusps; prolapse of cusp into left ventricular outflow tract
3. Ruptured chordae tendineae	TV, MV	Atrioventricular valve echoes in the atria; coarse, erratic diastolic opening movements of anterior leaflet (either TV or MV); prolapse of atrioventricular leaflet(s); diastolic thickenings of the valvular leaflets
4. Ring abscess	TV, MV, AV	Uncertain

AV = aortic valve; MV = mitral valve; TV = tricuspid valve.

Results

Four valve lesions occurring during active infective endocarditis are recognized:[14-17] (1) vegetations; (2)

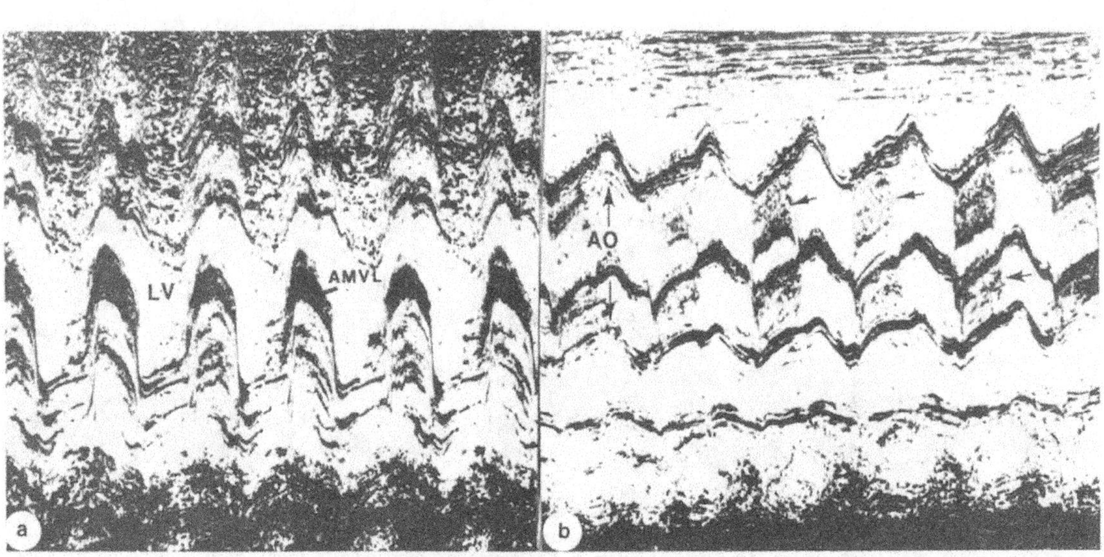

FIGURE 5. Case 18. **a,** echocardiogram showing irregular thickening of the anterior mitral valve leaflet (AMVL) and coarse erratic opening motion of the mitral leaflets. The motion of the ventricular septum is exaggerated. **b,** there are masses of echoes (**arrows**) on the aortic valve cusps. AO = aorta; LV = left ventricle.

TABLE IV

Frequency of Echocardiographic Detection of Cardiac Valve Lesions of Active Infective Endocarditis (IE) in 25 Opiate Addicts

	Valves (no.)	Valves Adequately Seen by Echo (no.)	Valve by Echo: Abnormal (no.)	Valve by Echo: Normal (no.)
Tricuspid	20	18	12	6
Vegetation		18	12	–
Torn or perforated cusp		18	0	–
Ruptured chordae tendineae		18	0	–
Ring abscess		18	0	–
Mitral	12	12	11	1
Vegetation		12	11	–
Torn or perforated cusp		12	0	–
Ruptured chordae tendineae		12	3	–
Ring abscess		12	0	–
Aortic	3	3	3	0
Vegetation		3	3	–
Torn or perforated cusp		3	2	–
Ruptured chordae tendineae		–	–	–
Ring abscess		3	0	–
Totals	35	33	26	7

cuspal tears or perforations; (3) ruptured chordae tendineae, and (4) ring abscess. The number of valves in the 25 patients with echocardiographic demonstration of these four lesions are summarized in Table IV.

The mitral and aortic valves were well visualized with the echocardiogram in all 25 patients and the tricuspid valve was well seen in 22 (Table II). Echocardiograms disclosed lesions indicative of active infective endocarditis in one valve (14 patients) or two or three valves (6 patients) in 20 of the 25 patients (80 percent). No valve lesions were evident in five patients (20 percent) (Fig. 1 to 5). However, in each of these five patients, the infective endocarditis clinically was limited to the tricuspid valve, and in two of these the tricuspid valve leaflets were not recorded at all in the echocardiogram. Auscultatory evidence of regurgitation in one valve (16 patients) or more (9 patients) was present in all 25 patients. Of all 75 valves (excluding the pulmonary valves) in the 25 patients, 35 were incompetent and 40 were functionally normal. Of the 35 incompetent valves, 33 were adequately visualized with the echocardiogram; in 26 (79 percent) of these 33 cases, the echocardiogram disclosed lesions indicative of active infective endocarditis; in the remaining 7 (21 percent) findings were normal (Table IV). Of the 20 incompetent tricuspid valves, 18 were adequately visualized with the echocardiogram, which disclosed lesions consistent with active infective endocarditis in 12 (67 percent) and showed normal findings in 6 (33 percent). There were 12 clinically incompetent mitral valves; in 11 cases (92 percent) the echocardiogram disclosed valve lesions indicative of active infective endocarditis and no valve lesions in the remaining case (8 percent) (Table IV). In all three cases of aortic valve regurgitation, the echocardiogram revealed valve lesions indicative of active infective endocarditis.

In none of the 25 patients nor in any of the 75 valves (pulmonary valve excluded) were valve lesions indicative of underlying disease detected with the echocardiogram, and none of the five patients with morphologic confirmation had underlying valve disease.

Comments

Previous necropsy studies of patients with right-sided active infective endocarditis[14,17,18] and of opiate addicts with either left- or right-sided infective endocarditis have shown that the involved valves were nearly always anatomically normal before the onset of the cardiac infection.[17,19] All 25 patients in our study were opiate addicts, none had documented evidence of a precordial murmur before the onset of infective endocarditis and none had a history of rheumatic fever; of the 5 patients studied at necropsy (4 patients) or at cardiac operation (1 patient), none had evidence of previous or chronic cardiac valve disease. Thus, it is reasonable to believe that the active infective endocarditis in our 25 patients involved previously normal valves and that the changes observed in their echocardiograms are attributable to infective endocarditis. In our 25 patients, all 40 competent valves (excluding the pulmonary valve) were normal on echocardiography and echocardiographic abnormalities consistent with infective endocarditis were detected in 26 (74 percent) of the 35 incompetent valves.

Tricuspid versus mitral regurgitant valves: Comparison of the 20 regurgitant tricuspid valves in our 25 patients with the 12 regurgitant mitral valves disclosed several differences: (1) The echocardiogram was less sensitive in detecting lesions resulting from infective endocarditis in the tricuspid than in the mitral valve; (2) the echocardiogram detected on the tricuspid valve only one of the four recognized valve lesions (Table IV) resulting from active infective endocarditis (vegetations), whereas it detected both vegetations and ruptured chordae tendineae on the mitral valve; (3) the vegetations detected with echocardiography on the tricuspid valve generally appeared larger than those detected on the mitral valve.

Aortic regurgitant valves: Although it does not appear appropriate to compare atrioventricular with semilunar valves, two of our three patients with an incompetent aortic valve secondary to active infective endocarditis had echocardiographic evidence of torn or perforated cusps, whereas none of the 20 patients with an incompetent tricuspid valve had such evidence. This difference is understandable in view of necropsy studies showing the infrequency of tears or perforations in the tricuspid valve leaflets and the frequency of these lesions in the aortic valve cusps.[17]

Our 25 opiate addicts with active infective endocarditis had unusually infrequent evidence of aortic regurgitation. Only 3 of the 35 valves with clinical evidence of regurgitation were aortic. Previous echocardiographic studies[1–10] and a recent necropsy study[17] showed that the aortic valve was the valve most frequently involved in active infective endocarditis.

Accuracy of echocardiographic diagnosis: Among the 20 clinically recognized incompetent tricuspid valves in our 25 patients, 18 had adequate echocardiographic visualization of the tricuspid valve leaflets and only 12 of these (67 percent) showed echocardiographic abnormalities indicative of active infective endocarditis. In contrast, echocardiographic features indicative of active infective endocarditis were recognized in 11 (92 percent) of 12 incompetent mitral valves and in 3 of 3 incompetent aortic valves.

Tricuspid versus mitral valve vegetations and chordal rupture: Necropsy studies[14,15,17] have demonstrated that vegetations on the tricuspid valve tend to be larger than those on other valves, and in our 25 patients the largest vegetations assessed with echocardiography were located on the tricuspid valve. The explanation for this observation is uncertain. The average anular circumference of the tricuspid valve is larger than that of the mitral valve (11 versus 9 cm); therefore, a tricuspid valve vegetation has a larger area within which to grow. The smaller systolic pressure in the right ventricle (compared with the left ventricle) may also be a factor. Rupture of tricuspid valve chords is infrequent, whereas mitral chordal rupture in infective endocarditis is frequent. The greater incidence of chordal rupture with mitral infection may be due to the greater left ventricular systolic pressure. The infrequency of chordal rupture on the tricuspid valve may delay development of significant tricuspid regurgitation and allow the right-sided vegetations to grow larger before valve dysfunction ensues.

To our knowledge, no echocardiographic investigation has detected the occurrence of a valve ring abscess from active (or healed) infective endocarditis. However, these abscesses rarely involve the tricuspid valve and occur frequently only in patients with infective endocarditis involving the aortic valve[16]; only 3 of our 25 patients had infection involving the aortic valve.

Pulmonary valve involvement: In none of our 25 patients and in none reported has echocardiography detected lesions of active infective endocarditis on the pulmonary valve. The echocardiogram of the pulmonary valve was recorded in 12 of our patients. Only 3 of the 25 patients, however, had auscultatory evidence of regurgitation in a semilunar valve and in each it was clear that aortic rather than pulmonary valve regurgitation was present. Furthermore, infection of a pulmonary valve is extremely rare except in patients with congenital heart disease; in previous studies of opiate addicts studied at necropsy,[17,18] involvement of the tricuspid valve by vegetation was more than 10 times as common as involvement of the pulmonary valve.

References

1. **Spangler RD, Johnson ML, Holmes JH, et al:** Echocardiographic demonstration of bacterial vegetations in active infective endocarditis. J Clin Ultrasound 1:126–128, 1973
2. **Dillon JC, Feigenbaum H, Konecke LL, et al:** Echocardiographic manifestations of valvular vegetations. Am Heart J 86:698–704, 1973
3. **Lee C-C, Ganguly SN, Magnisalis K, et al:** Detection of tricuspid valve vegetations by echocardiograhy. Chest 66:432–433, 1974
4. **Gottlieb S, Khuddus SA, Balooki H, et al:** Echocardiographic diagnosis of aortic valve vegetations in candida endocarditis. Circulation 50:826–830, 1974
5. **Martinez EC, Burch GE, Giles TD:** Echocardiographic diagnosis of vegetative aortic bacterial endocarditis. Am J Cardiol 34: 845–849, 1974
6. **DeMaria AN, King JF, Salel AF, et al:** Echography and phonography of acute aortic regurgitation in bacterial endocarditis. Ann Intern Med 82:329–335, 1975
7. **Wray TM:** Echocardiographic manifestations of flail aortic valve leaflets in bacterial endocarditis. Circulation 51:832–835, 1975
8. **Wray TM:** The variable echocardiographic features in aortic valve endocarditis. Circulation 52:658–663, 1975
9. **Roy P, Tajik AJ, Giuliani ER, et al:** Spectrum of echocardiographic findings in bacterial endocarditis. Circulation 53:474–482, 1976
10. **Wann LS, Dillon JC, Weyman AE, et al:** Echocardiography in bacterial endocarditis. N Engl J Med 295:135–139, 1976
11. **Feigenbaum H:** Echocardiography. Philadelphia, Lea & Febiger, 1973, p 239
12. **Sweatman T, Selzer A, Kamagaki M, et al:** Echocardiographic diagnosis of mitral regurgitation due to ruptured chordae tendineae. Circulation 46:580–586, 1972
13. **Giles TD, Burch GE, Martinez EC:** Value of exploratory "scanning" in the echocardiographic diagnosis of ruptured chordae tendineae. Circulation 49:678–681, 1974
14. **Roberts WC, Buchbinder NA:** Right-sided valvular infective endocarditis. A clinico-pathologic study of twelve necropsy patients. Am J Med 53:7–19, 1972
15. **Buchbinder NA, Roberts WC:** Left-sided valvular active infective endocarditis. A study of forty-five necropsy patients. Am J Med 53:20–35, 1972
16. **Arnett EN, Roberts WC:** Valve ring abscess in active infective endocarditis. Frequency, location, and clues to clinical diagnosis from study of 95 necropsy patients. Circulation 54:140–145, 1976
17. **Arnett EN, Roberts WC:** Active infective endocarditis: a clinicopathologic analysis of 137 necropsy patients. Curr Concepts Cardiol 1:1–76, 1976 (Oct)
18. **Banks T, Fletcher R, Ali N:** Infective endocarditis in heroin addicts. Am J Med 55:444–451, 1973
19. **Buchbinder NA, Roberts WC:** Alcoholism, an important but unemphasized factor predisposing to infective endocarditis. Arch Intern Med 132:689–692, 1973

Trichinosis Causing Extensive Ventricular Mural Endocarditis with Superimposed Thrombosis

Evidence That Severe Eosinophilia Damages Endocardium

JOSEPH J. ANDY, M.D.*
JOSEPH P. O'CONNELL, M.D.
ROBERT C. DADDARIO, M.D.
WILLIAM C. ROBERTS, M.D.
Bethesda, Maryland

Clinical and morphologic observations are described in a 46 year old woman with fatal trichinosis. Attention is called to the occurrence of extensive ventricular endocardial damage with superimposed thrombosis. Evidence is presented to indicate that the most likely cause of the endocardial damage is the associated eosinophilia. The mechanism by which eosinophils damage endocardium, however, remains obscure.

Trichinosis, once a common disorder but always an uncommon cause of death, today is rarely observed clinically and even more rarely encountered in its acute form at necropsy [1]. Recently we studied a patient with fatal acute trichinosis who was found at necropsy to have extensive ventricular endocardial damage with superimposed thrombosis. Stimulated by this patient, previous reports on necropsy patients with acute trichinosis were reviewed. Observations in our patient and in those previously described are summarized in this report, which also calls attention to the probable detrimental effect of large numbers of eosinophils on the ventricular endocardium.

CASE REPORT

A 46 year old white female nurse (NIH 101-20-63-18) was asymptomatic until 13 days before death (on August 5, 1973) when she noted fever (temperature 100° to 102°F), headache, neck stiffness, myalgias, dizziness and pleuritic chest pain. These symptoms thereafter progressed, and 10 days later she was admitted to Suburban Hospital. She had been well until age 44 (March 1971) when, on routine examination, signs of hypothyroidism were noted and she was treated with thyroid extract (120 mg/day). In November 1972 a routine employment examination showed no abnormalities by physical examination. The blood hematocrit value, however, was 34 per cent and the white blood cell count 3,300/mm^3. The erythrocyte indices were consistent with a hypochromic microcytic anemia and iron therapy was begun. Tuberculin skin test (purified protein derivative) was positive and isoniazid therapy (300 mg daily) was begun. From November 1972 until June 1973 monthly leukocyte counts ranged from 2,900 to 5,900/mm^3. The blood hematocrit value gradually increased to 45 per cent. Monthly serum glutamic oxaloacetate and glutamic phosphate transaminase levels during this period also were normal.

On admission three days before death, she appeared acutely ill. Her temperature was 100°F, blood pressure 100/70 mm Hg and pulse rate 120 beats/min. The neck was rigid, and the proximal limb muscles were markedly tender. The neck veins were normal. The heart sounds were normal and precordial murmurs were absent. Lymph nodes and abdominal organs were

From the Pathology Branch, National Heart, Lung and Blood Institute, National Institutes of Health, and the Departments of Pathology and Medicine, Suburban Hospital, Bethesda, Maryland. Requests for reprints should be addressed to Dr. William C. Roberts, Building 10A, Room 3E-30, National Institutes of Health, Bethesda, Maryland 20014.
Manuscript accepted September 24, 1976.

* Work done while on leave from Howard University, Washington, D.C. Present address: Faculty of Health Sciences, University of Ife, Ile-Ife, Nigeria.

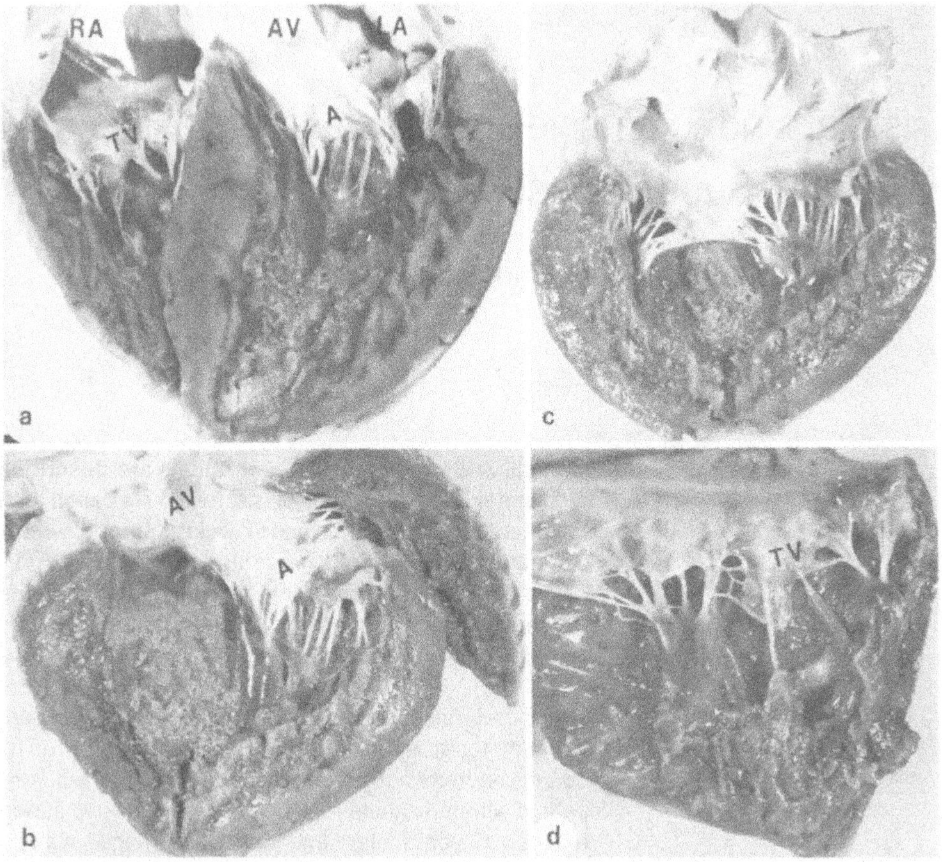

Figure 1. *Heart in the patient described.* ***a,*** *the anterior half has been excised and here is shown the posterior half. The endocardium of the left ventricle is diffusely covered by thrombus and much of the right ventricle is similarly involved. A = anterior mitral leaflet; AV = aortic valve; LA = left atrium; RA = right atrium; TV = tricuspid valve.* ***b,*** *opened aortic valve and left ventricle. In addition to the superimposed thrombus, the endocardium is hemorrhagic. The latter is probably the result of the severe thrombocytopenia.* ***c,*** *opened left atrium, mitral valve and left ventricle.* ***d,*** *opened tricuspid valve and right ventricle showing thrombus on the endocardium. TV = tricupid valve leaflet.*

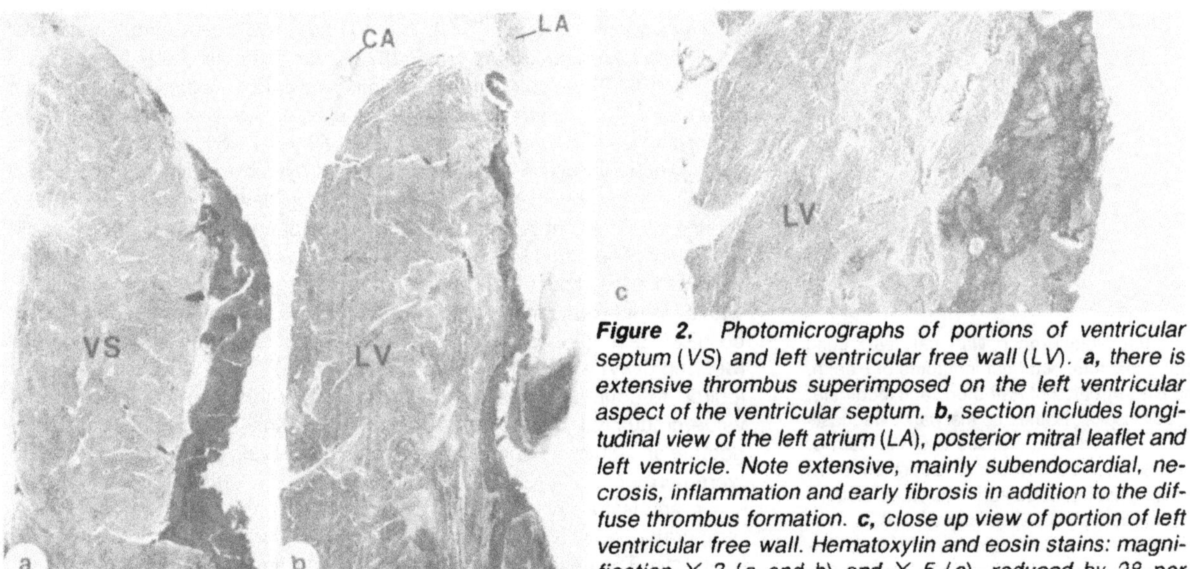

Figure 2. *Photomicrographs of portions of ventricular septum (VS) and left ventricular free wall (LV).* ***a,*** *there is extensive thrombus superimposed on the left ventricular aspect of the ventricular septum.* ***b,*** *section includes longitudinal view of the left atrium (LA), posterior mitral leaflet and left ventricle. Note extensive, mainly subendocardial, necrosis, inflammation and early fibrosis in addition to the diffuse thrombus formation.* ***c,*** *close up view of portion of left ventricular free wall. Hematoxylin and eosin stains: magnification × 3 (a and b) and × 5 (c), reduced by 28 per cent.*

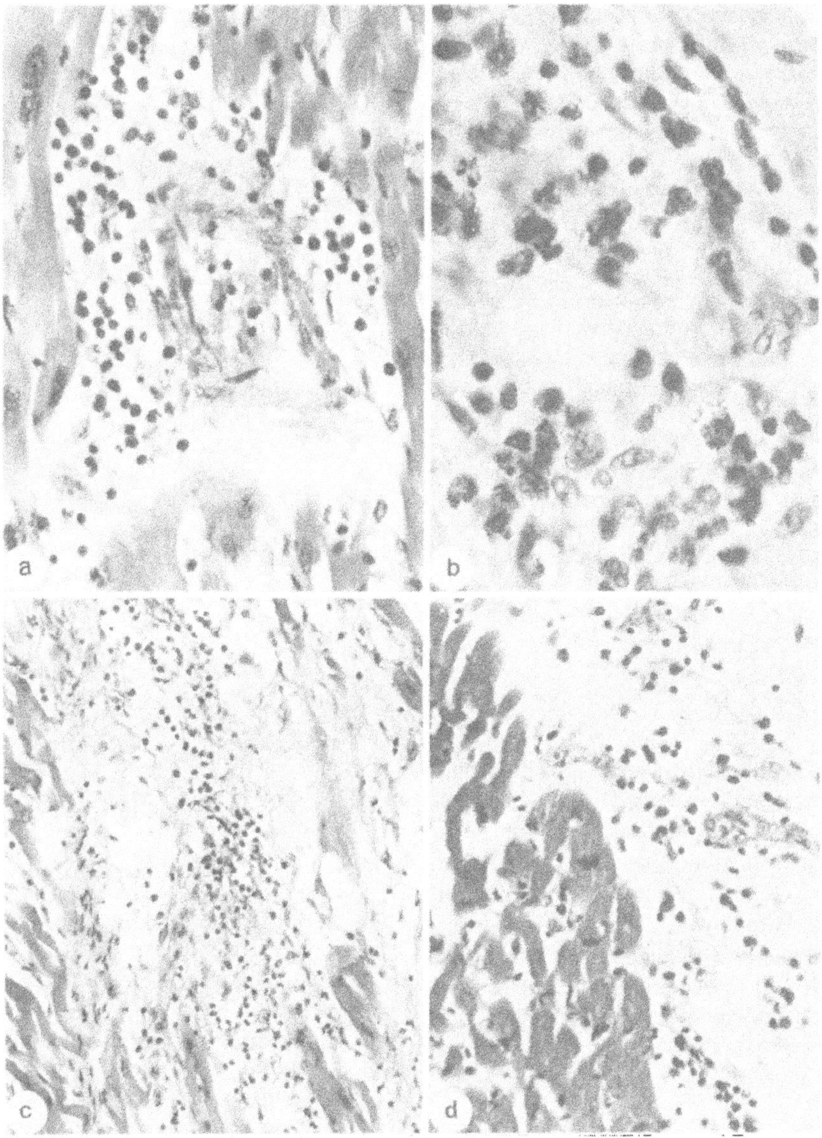

Figure 3. *Photomicrographs showing myocardial (a, b, c) and epicardial (d) inflammation.* ***a,*** *many inflammatory cells surround a vessel in the left ventricular wall. The cells are both mononuclear and polynuclear* ***b,*** *close-up of the interstitial myocardial inflammatory cells, most of which are eosinophils.* ***c,*** *inflammatory cells in an area of loose fibrous tissue.* ***d,*** *inflammatory cells in epicardial fat. All stains are hematoxylin and eosin; original magnification X 400 (a), X 860 (b), X 330 (c) and X 220 (d), reduced by 28 per cent.*

not palpable, and subcutaneous edema was absent. Other than nuchal rigidity, the neurologic examination disclosed no abnormal findings. The blood hematocrit value was 42 per cent and the white blood cell count 11,000/mm^3, blood smear examination showed 38 per cent eosinophils and decreased numbers of platelets. The erythrocyte sedimentation rate was 1 mm in 1 hour. A lupus erythematosus preparation, a serologic test for syphilis and an infectious mononucleosis spot test yielded negative results. The electrocardiogram and chest roentgenogram disclosed no abnormalities. The cerebrospinal fluid pressure, appearance and chemical composition were normal. Cultures of urine blood and cerebrospinal fluid showed no growth.

During hospitalization, headache, myalgias, pleuritic chest pains and tachycardia persisted; dermal petechiae and splenomegaly appeared. The per cent of eosinophils on peripheral blood smear rose to 43 per cent and the platelet count decreased to 23,000/mm^3. Aspiration of bone marrow disclosed excessive numbers of eosinophils and marked diminution in numbers of megakaryocytes. Although the patient felt and looked better, she was found dead in bed on the third hospital day.

After death, it was learned that the patient often had eaten raw meat, particularly raw hamburger and steak, and that another person who had purchased meat from the same market also had trichinosis (nonfatal).

At necropsy, excess amounts of serous fluid were present in the pleural spaces (about 600 ml each) and pericardial sac (about 100 ml). The heart weighed 260 g; the cavities were of normal size and the ventricular walls of normal thickness. The endocardium of both ventricles was covered by fibrin deposits within which were numerous erythrocytes (Figures 1 and 2). The extramural coronary arteries, cardiac valves and pericardium were normal.

Histologically, the ventricular myocardium and overlying mural thrombus contained many eosinophils (Figure 3), and foci of necrotic myocardium were present in left ventricular wall, mainly the subendocardium. Thromboembolic material, similar to that on the ventricular endocardium, was present in a few intramural coronary arteries. No trichina larva was seen in five large sections of myocardium. Numerous encysted trichinella larvae, however, were found in the diaphragm and tongue (Figure 4) associated with eosinophilic myositis. Rare alveolar pulmonary hemorrhages were present, and one minute focus of eosinophils was present in the pulmonary interstitium (five sections examined). The kidneys were normal. The liver (weight = 1,260 g) showed mild peripheral fatty change. The spleen (200 g) contained numerous eosinophils and increased numbers of plasma cells. The brain was normal.

COMMENTS

The evidence is good that the patient described had trichinosis: (1) trichina cysts surrounded by inflammatory cells, including many eosinophils, were present in the tongue and diaphragm; (2) the patient was known to frequently eat raw meat, and raw hamburger had been ingested shortly before the onset of the present illness; (3) an illness compatible with trichinosis and occurring simultaneously with that in our patient occurred in a person who also ate raw hamburger meat purchased from the same butcher; and (4) the clinical illness was compatible, including myalgias, neck stiffness, fever and eosinophilia.

Review of findings in 41 previously described necropsy patients with fatal acute (active) trichinosis disclosed three major causes of death [2–35]: (1) myocarditis, (2) encephalitis and (3) pneumonitis (Figure 5). Myocarditis was by far the most common cause of death. Of the 41 previously descibed necropsy patients with acute trichinosis, myocarditis was present in 32 (94 per cent) [2–12,14–17,18,21,22,24,25,27,28,30,31,33,34], absent in two [13,26], and observations on the heart were not described in seven [17,19,20,23,29,32,35]. The myocarditis was most commonly eosinophilic in type. Eosinophilic myocarditis occurred with or without peripheral blood eosinophilia.

The occurrence of mural endocarditis with or without superimposed thrombosis, as occurred in our patient, however, is rare in patients with fatal acute trichinosis. Although focal mural endocardial "edema" [2], "coagulation" [3] and "hyalin thickening" [4] have been described in each of three patients, diffuse ventricular mural endocarditis with superimposed thrombosis has been described, to our knowledge, in only one other patient with fatal acute trichinosis. That patient, reported on twice [4,5], was a 39 year old woman who died during the fifth week of illness; she also had "eosinophilia."

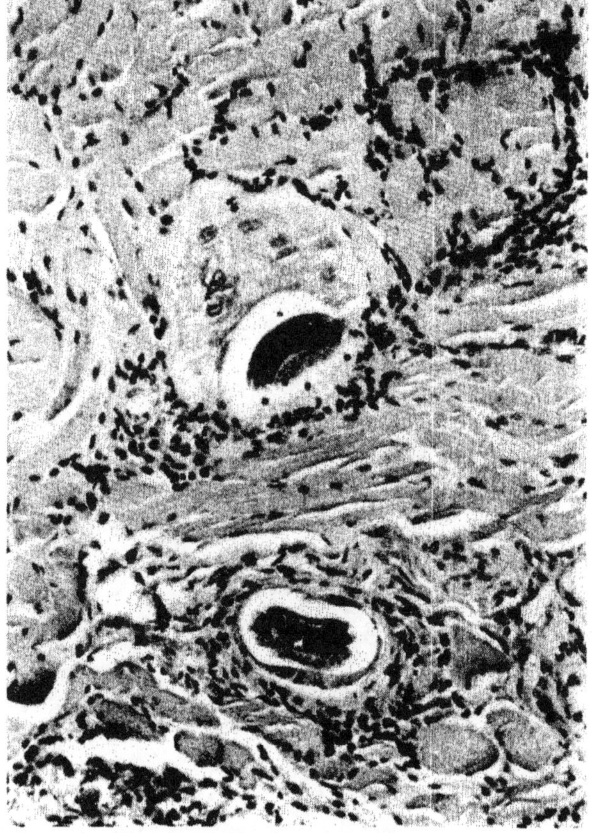

Figure 4. *Photomicrograph of section of tongue showing two encysted trichina larvae associated with many inflammatory cells, most of which are eosinophils. Hematoxylin and eosin stain; magnification X 220.*

Extensive right and left ventricular endocardial damage with or without superimposed thrombosis has

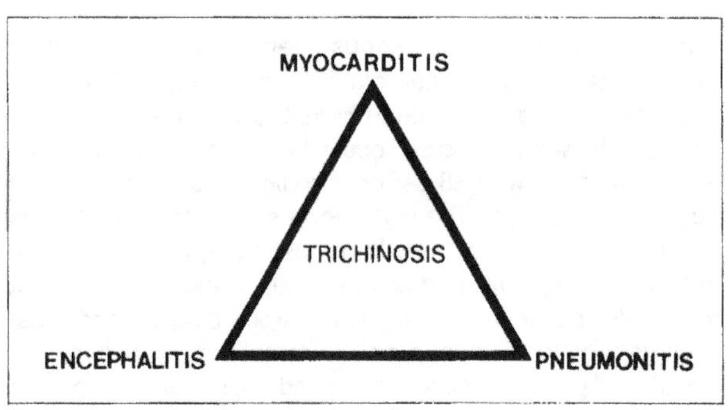

Figure 5. *Diagram showing the three major causes of death in acute trichinosis.*

been reported in other conditions associated with severe eosinophilia. Löffler's fibroplastic parietal endocarditis is the classic example [36–39]. Death in these subjects results usually from congestive cardiac failure, and the ventricular endocardium in its inflow portion is extensively damaged [37–39]. "Eosinophilic leukemia" [37–39] and "disseminated eosinophilic collagen disease" [40], both of which are associated with severe blood eosinophilia and extensive ventricular endocardial damage with or without superimposed thrombosis, are probably forms of Löffler's endocarditis simply seen at differing stages in the disease process [38]. Extensive eosinophilic infiltration of the ventricular endocardium was found in the one necropsy patient with Löffler's pneumonia with blood eosinophilia [41]. Davies' endomyocardial fibrosis of the African also often is associated with blood eosinophilia [42,43]. At necropsy, these patients have severe ventricular endocardial damage, primarily in the inflow tracts, and usually mild eosinophilia. It is possible, however, that the degree of blood eosinophilia was considerably higher in the earlier (preclinical) stage of the disease process. Löffler mentioned in his original paper on this subject that the blood eosinophilic count falls, sometimes to normal levels, in the later stages of the illness [36].

That mural endocardial disease was infrequently reported in the previously described patients with trichinosis, however, cannot be used as evidence that eosinophilia is not a producer of endocardial damage. Of the 41 previously described patients with fatal acute trichinosis, eosinophilia (>6 per cent) was reported in only nine [4,7,12,15,19,24,25,27,29]. In two [19,29] of the nine patients, however, the heart was not examined at all, and in three others [24,25,27] the endocardium was not mentioned. Furthermore, the per cent of eosinophils in peripheral blood smear was greater than 30 per cent in only two patients [12,19] and the heart was not examined in one of them [19].

REFERENCES

1. Barr R: Human trichinosis: report of four cases with emphasis on central nervous system involvement, and a survey of 500 consecutive autopsies at the Ottowa Civic Hospital. Can Med Assoc J 95: 912, 1966.
2. Terplan K, Kraus R, Barnes S: Eosinophilic meningoencephalitis with predominantly cerebellar changes caused by trichinella infection. J Mount Sinai Hosp (N.Y.) 24: 1293, 1957.
3. McCabe ES, Zatuchni J: Fulminating trichiniasis. Am J Dig Dis 18: 205, 1951.
4. Zoller H: Uber die herzmuskelentzundung im verlauf der trichinose. Virchow Arch [Pathol Anat] 265: 430, 1927.
5. Gruber GB, Gamper E: Uber gehirnveranderungen bei menschlicher trichinose. Verh Dtsch Ges Pathol 22: 219, 1927.
6. Zenker FA: Ueber die trichinen-krahnheit des menschen. Virchow's Arch [Pathol Anat] 18: 561, 1860.
7. Chase GO: Death due to eosinophilic myocarditis related to trichinosis. JAMA 165: 1826, 1957.
8. Fey LD, Moore AM: Fulminating trichinosis with myocarditis. Northwest Med 53: 701, 1954.
9. Terry LL, Work JL: Trichinosis of the myocardium. Report of a case with autopsy findings. Am Heart J 19: 478, 1940.
10. Spink WW: Cardiovascular complications of trichinosis. Arch Intern Med 56: 238, 1935.
11. Frothingham C Jr: A contribution to the knowledge of the lesions caused by Trichina spiralis in man. J Med Res 15: 483, 1906.
12. Horlick SS, Bicknell RE: Trichiniasis with widespread infestation of many tissues. N Engl J Med 201: 816, 1929.
13. Reimann HA, Price AH, Herbut PA: Trichinosis and periarteritis nodosa. JAMA 122: 274, 1943.
14. Weller CV, Shaw M: Myocardial failure due to trichinosis. Preliminary Report. Trans Assoc Am Physicians 47: 41, 1932.
15. Gordon MB, Cares R, Kaufman B: Encephalitis and myocarditis in a fatal case of trichinosis. J Pediatr 6: 667, 1935.
16. Stryker WA: The intestinal phase of human trichinosis. Am J Pathol 23: 819, 1947.
17. Kratz F: Die trichinenepidemie zu hedersleben, Leipzig, Engelmann, 1866, p. 125.
18. Sobel IP: Sporadic trichinosis in children. Am J Dis Child 51: 367, 1936.
19. Cummins WT, Carson GR: A case of trichinosis with embryo in the spinal fluid. JAMA 66: 1856, 1916.
20. Van Cot JM, Lintz W: Trichinosis. JAMA 62: 680, 1914.
21. Gauttery JM, Milne J, House R: Observations on hepatic and renal dysfunction in trichinosis. Anatomic changes in these organs occurring in cases of trichinosis. Am J Med 21: 567, 1956.
22. Pund ER, Mostseller R: Trichinosis: Demonstration of the parasites in the brain. JAMA 102: 1220, 1934.
23. Most H, Abeles MM: Trichinosis involving the nervous system: A clinical and neuropathologic review with report of two cases. Arch Neural Psychiat 37: 589, 1937.
24. Hassin GB, Diamond IB: Trichinosis encephalitis. A pathologic study. Arch Neurol Psychiat 15: 34, 1926.
25. Houston JC, Ross L: Trichiniasis with cerebral symptoms. Report of two cases. Lancet 2: 397, 1941.
26. Bovaird D Jr: On sporadic trichinosis. NY Med J 83: 436, 486, 1906.
27. Carter LF: Plasma cell hyperplasia and hyperglobulinemia in trichinosis; The duration of laviposition. Am J Pathol 25: 309, 1949.
28. Walker AT: Trichiniasis: report of an outbreak caused by eating trichinous bear meat in the form of "jerky." JAMA 98: 2051, 1932.
29. Murphy FD, James HD, Rossetter JW: Trichinosis, study of 23 cases. Am J Med Sci 199: 328, 1940.
30. Vance BM, Ryder M: Three rapidly fatal cases with trichinosis with autopsy findings. Proc NY Pathol Soc 22: 97, 1922.
31. Howard WT Jr: Report of a fatal case of trichinosis without eosinophilia, but with large numbers of eosinophilic cells in the muscle lesions; with remarks on the origin of eosinophilic cells in trichinosis. Philadelphia Med J 4: 1085, 1899.
32. Bloch L, Hassin GB: Trichinosis complicated by encephalitis. A clinical and histopathological report. Med Rec 91: 537, 1917.
33. Simmonds M: Ueber Myocarditis trichinosa. Zentralbl Allg Pathol 30: 1, 1919.
34. Cohnheim J; Todtliche trichinose mit parenchymatoser de-

generation von leber, herz und nieren. Virchow's Arch [Pathol Anat] 33: 447, 1865.
35. Ehrhardt O; Zur Kenntniss der muskelveränderungen bei der trichinose des menschen. Beitr Pathol 20: 43, 1896.
36. Löffler W: Endocarditis parietalis fibroplastica mit bluteosinophile. Schweiz Med Wchnschr 66: 817, 1936.
37. Roberts WC, Leigler DG, Carbone PP: Endomyocardial disease and eosinophilia. A clinical and pathologic spectrum. Am J Med 46: 28, 1969.
38. Roberts WC, Buja LM, Ferrans VJ: Löffler's fibroplastic parietal endocarditis, eosinophilic leukemia, and Davies' endomyocardial fibrosis: the same disease at different stages? Pathol Microbiol 35: 90, 1970.
39. Roberts WC, Ferrans VJ: Pathologic anatomy of the cardiomyopathies. Idiopathic dilated and hypertrophic types, infiltrative types and endomyocardial disease with and without eosinophilia. Hum Pathol 6: 287, 1975.
40. Engfeldt B, Zetterstrom R: Disseminated eosinophilic "collagen disease." Acta Med Scand 153: 337, 1956.
41. Bayley EC, Lindberg DON, Baggenstoss AH: Löffler's syndrome: Report of a case with pathologic examination of the lungs. Arch Pathol 40: 376, 1945.
42. Davies JNP: Endocardial fibrosis in Africans. East African M J 25: 10, 1948.
43. Ive FA, Willis AJP, Ikeme AC, et al.: Endomyocardial fibrosis and filariasis. Q J Med 36: 495, 1967.

Healed Left-Sided Infective Endocarditis: A Clinicopathologic Study of 59 Patients

WILLIAM C. ROBERTS, MD, FACC
NEIL A. BUCHBINDER, MD*

Bethesda, Maryland

Clinical and morphologic observations are described in 59 patients who had a history of active left-sided infective endocarditis that had been eradicated by antibiotic therapy. Of the 59 patients, 42 were from a group of 584 necropsy patients with fatal cardiac valve disease of various types; the remaining 17 were from a group of 79 patients who had undergone mitral or aortic valve replacement, or both, because of severe mitral or aortic regurgitation, or both. Examination of the heart at necropsy (42 patients) or at valve replacement (17 patients) disclosed that 30 (51 percent) had anatomic lesions that could readily be attributed to the active infective endocarditis that healed: cuspal perforations in 16 patients, rupture of chordae tendineae in 15 and aneurysms at or near the involved valve in 3. Unequivocal residua of the valve infection were more common in the purely incompetent than in the stenotic cardiac valves. Comparison of observations in the 42 necropsy patients with healed left-sided infective endocarditis with observations previously reported in 74 necropsy patients with active left-sided infective endocarditis showed that among the patients with healed endocarditis the infection more commonly involved a previously abnormal valve, the causative organism was more likely to be alpha streptococcus and recognized predisposing factors (opiate addiction, alcoholism, immunodeficiencies, operative procedures) were less frequent.

Although there are many reports describing various morphologic observations in patients with *active* infective endocarditis, reports describing cardiac morphologic changes in patients with healed infective endocarditis are rare. One reason is that healing of active infective endocarditis became possible, for practical purposes,[1,2] only in 1944 when penicillin began to be used for this condition. Although antibiotic agents often "cure" patients with active infective endocarditis, residual valve damage obviously may be a consequence of the infection. This report describes certain clinical and morphologic observations in 59 patients with a history of active infective endocarditis whose infection was cured with antibiotic therapy.

Patients Studied and Methods

The observations in this report are based on examination of both clinical records and cardiac valves from two groups of patients. All patients had severe left-sided valve disease; the cardiac status of each patient was judged to be either moderately or severely compromised (New York Heart Association classification[3]) immediately before death or valve replacement; all were over 14 years of age; and none had valve disease on the basis of papillary muscle dysfunction. The cardiac valves were examined for lesions consistent with healed infective endocarditis (to be described later).

The first group consisted of 584 necropsy patients with fatal valve disease (Table I), of whom 42 had a history of healed infective endocarditis. The hearts of all 584 patients were examined by one of us (WCR) and classified according

From the Pathology Branch, National Heart, Lung, and Blood Institute, National Institutes of Health, Bethesda, Maryland 20014. Manuscript received April 25, 1977; revised manuscript received June 9, 1977, accepted June 12, 1977.
* Present address: Department of Cardiology, Cedars of Lebanon Hospital, Los Angeles, California 20029.
Address for reprints: William C. Roberts, MD, Building 10A, Room 3E30, National Heart, Lung, and Blood Institute, National Institutes of Health, Bethesda, Maryland 20014.

TABLE I

Types of Valve Lesions Observed at Necropsy or Operation in 59 Patients With a History of Healed Infective Endocarditis

Type of Valve Dysfunction at Necropsy or Operation	Patients (no.) Total	With History of Healed IE	With CP	With RCT	With CP + RCT	With RA	With CT Only	Total With Anatomic Evidence of Healed IE
Necropsy Patients								
Stenosis								
Aortic stenosis (AS)	195	11 (6%)	2	—	—	3*	6	5
Mitral stenosis (MS)	99	5 (5%)	0	2	0	0	3	2
AS + MS	76 }385	2 (3%) }18(5%)	0	0	0	0	2	0 } 7(39%)
Tricuspid stenosis (TS) + MS	3	0 (0%)	0	0	0	0	0	0
AS + MS + TS	12	0 (0%)	0	0	0	0	0	0
Regurgitation								
Aortic regurgitation (AR)	65	7 (11%)	5*	—	0	0	2	5
Mitral regurgitation (MR)	58 }148	7 (12%) }21(14%)	0	4	2	0	1	6 }15(71%)
AR + MR	25	7 (28%)	1*	1	2	0	3	4
Stenosis and regurgitation								
AS + MR	16	3 (19%)	0	0	0	0	3	0
AR + MS	35 } 51	0 } 3(6%)	0	0	0	0	0	0
Subtotal	584	42 (7%)	8	7	4	3	20 (48%)	22 (52%)
Nonnecropsy (Valve Replacement) Patients								
Regurgitation								
AR	44	10 (23%)	4†	—	—	—	6	4
MR	32	5 (16%) }17(21%)	0	3	0	—	2	3 } 8(47%)
AR + MR	5	2	0	1	0	—	1	1
Subtotal	81	17 (21%)	4	4	0	—	9 (53%)	8 (47%)

* One also had a healed focal aneurysm, probably the result of a mycotic aneurysm, in the tubular portion of ascending aorta.
† Two also had cuspal indentations.
CP = cuspal perforation; CT = cuspal thickening; IE = infective endocarditis; RA = ring aneurysm (residuum of ring abscess); RCT = ruptured chordae tendineae.

to the functional valve lesion (Table I). The 584 patients ranged in age from 15 to 88 years (average 45); 374 (64 percent) were male and 210 (36 percent) were female.

The second group consisted of 79 patients who underwent replacement of either the aortic (44 patients) or the mitral (30 patients) valve, or both (5 patients), because of *pure valve regurgitation* (Table I); 17 of these had a history of healed infective endocarditis. Seventy-two of the 79 patients survived operation; in the 7 patients who did not, necropsy was not performed. The 79 patients at the time of valve replacement ranged in age from 21 to 69 years (average 42); 50 (63 percent) were men and 29 (37 percent) were women.

Results

Of the 584 necropsy patients, 42 (7 percent) had had a history of active infective endocarditis that had healed; 26 of the 42 had had replacement of one or more cardiac valves with a

TABLE II

Relation of Clinical Features of Active Infective Endocarditis (IE) to Anatomic Evidence of Healed Infective Endocarditis

Clinical Features of Active IE Obtained by History After IE Had Healed	Patients (no.) Total	With Anatomic Evidence of IE	With No Anatomic Evidence of IE
+ BC, + PS + CHF	8	7	1
+ BC, + PS	6	3	3
+ BC, + CHF	7 } 26	4 }15 (58%)	3 }11 (42%)
+ BC only	5	1	4
0 BC, + PC, + CHF	3	2	1
0 BC, + PS, 0 CHF	0 } 5	0 } 2	0 } 3
0 BC, 0 PS, − CHF	2	0	2
− BC, + PS, + CHF	4	3	1
− BC, + PS, 0 CHF	2	0	2
− BC, 0 PS, + CHF	13 }28	6 }13 (46%)	7 }15 (54%)
− BC, − PS, − CHF	9	4	5
Totals	59	30 (51%)	29 (49%)

0 = negative or absent; + = positive or present; − = not done or no information available.
BC = blood culture; CHF = congestive heart failure appearing for the first time or, if present previously, worsening during the active infection.
PS = one or more peripheral signs consisting of palpable spleen, dermal petechiae, splinter hemorrhages, clubbing, Osler's nodes and clinically diagnosed systemic embolus or infarct.

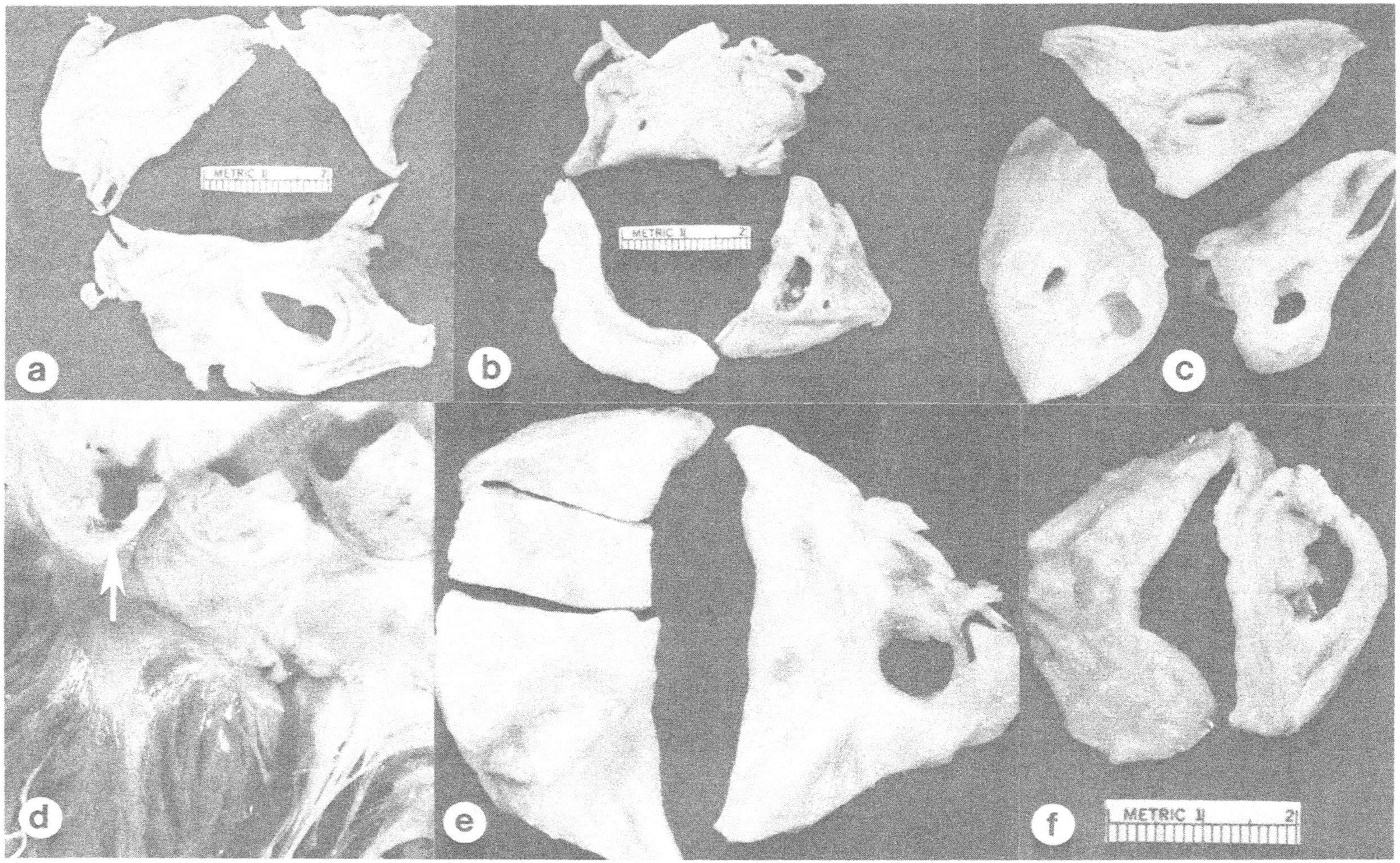

FIGURE 1. *Purely incompetent aortic valves with perforations from six patients with healed infective endocarditis.* **a** to **c, e** and **f** are operatively excised valves and **d** is an opened aortic valve at necropsy. **a,** from a 34 year old man (A64-92) with ventricular septal defect and prolapse of the largest cusp, the one with the perforation, into the defect. He died 1 day after operative closure of the defect and replacement of the aortic valve with a prosthesis. The patient had an episode compatible with active infective endocarditis at age 21, thirteen years before death. **b,** from a 44 year old man (S64-3239) who had active infective endocarditis at age 37. He too had a ventricular septal defect with prolapse of two of the three cusps into the defect. Perforations are present in each of the two prolapsed cusps, and small calcific deposits, probably the residua of vegetations, border the largest cuspal perforation. **c,** from a 30 year old man (S63-2226) who had historical evidence of active infective endocarditis on two occasions, at ages 19 and 20. He too had an associated ventricular septal defect. A single perforation is present in each of the three cusps. **d,** from a 58 year old woman (A70-96) with aplastic anemia. She had Staphylococcus epidermidis endocarditis 6 months before death. She had no precordial murmur before the episode of bacterial endocarditis. A perforation, or more correctly an indentation **(arrow),** is present in the right anterior cusp. The valve appears to have been both functionally and anatomically normal before the episode of active infective endocarditis. **e,** a congenitally bicuspid valve from a 49 year old man (GT69A-577) who had an episode compatible with active infective endocarditis at age 41. He died from prosthetic thrombosis at age 51, eighteen months after valve replacement. **f,** congenitally bicuspid valve from a 45 year old man (S66-3582) who had active infective endocarditis at age 39. A large perforation is present in one cusp.

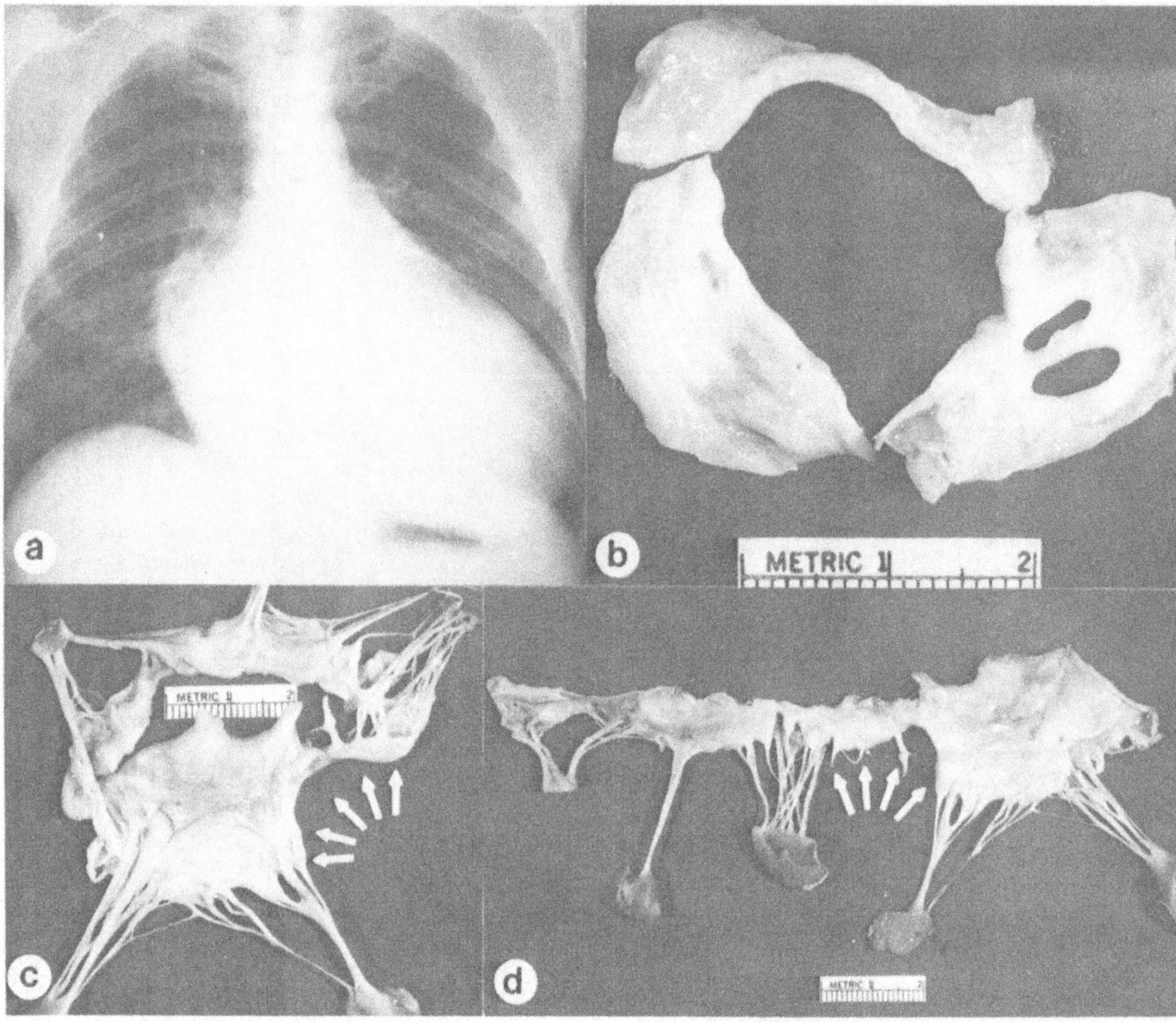

FIGURE 2. *Chest roentgenogram* **(a)** *and operatively excised aortic* **(b)** *and mitral valves* **(c** *and* **d)** *in a 45 year old man* (A68-22) (S68-167) *with pure aortic and mitral regurgitation.* He was said to have had acute rheumatic fever when 4 years old and active infective endocarditis at age 31. He died 10 days after double valve replacement. **a,** the heart is huge. It weighed 1,090 g. **b,** aortic valve with two perforations in one of the three cusps. **c,** unopened mitral valve showing loss of the chordae tendineae on the margin of the anterior and posterior leaflets adjacent to the anterolateral commissure **(arrows). d,** opened mitral valve. The **arrows** again indicate the absent chordae tendineae. The unruptured chordae are delicate.

TABLE III

Relation of Type of Mitral or Aortic Valve Hemodynamic Lesion to the Frequency of Lesions Indicative of Healed Infective Endocarditis (73 dysfunctional valves in 59 patients with healed infective endocarditis)

Type of Valve Dysfunction at Death or Operation	Valves (no.)	Valves With Perforation no.	%	Valves With Ruptured Chordae Tendineae no.	%	Valves With Healed Ring Abscess no.	%
Aortic stenosis*	16	2†	12	0		3	19
Aortic regurgitation	26	12	46	0		0	
Mitral stenosis*	7	0		2	30	0	
Mitral regurgitation	24	2‡	8	13	54	0	
Totals	73	16	22	15	48	3	4

* With or without valve regurgitation.
† Despite the perforations, simultaneous left ventricular to systemic arterial peak systolic pressure gradient in one patient was 15 and in the second, 20 mm Hg.
‡ Chordae tendineae in both valves were also ruptured.

prosthesis and had died subsequently. Of the 79 operative (nonnecropsy) patients, 17 (22 percent) had had a history of active infective endocarditis that had healed (Table I). Thus, of the total of 663 patients analyzed, 59 (9 percent) had had a history of active infective endocarditis that had healed. All 59 patients were stated to have had "subacute bacterial endocarditis" or "an infection in their heart" or "an infection of a heart valve" for which they were hospitalized, treated with antibiotic agents and discharged from the hospital. The details of the histories are summarized in Table II. Although some patients had better documentation of past active infective endocarditis than did others, the frequency of positive anatomic evidence of healed infection was similar in those with a clear-cut history and in those with less clear-cut clinical evidence (58 percent and 46 percent) (Table II).

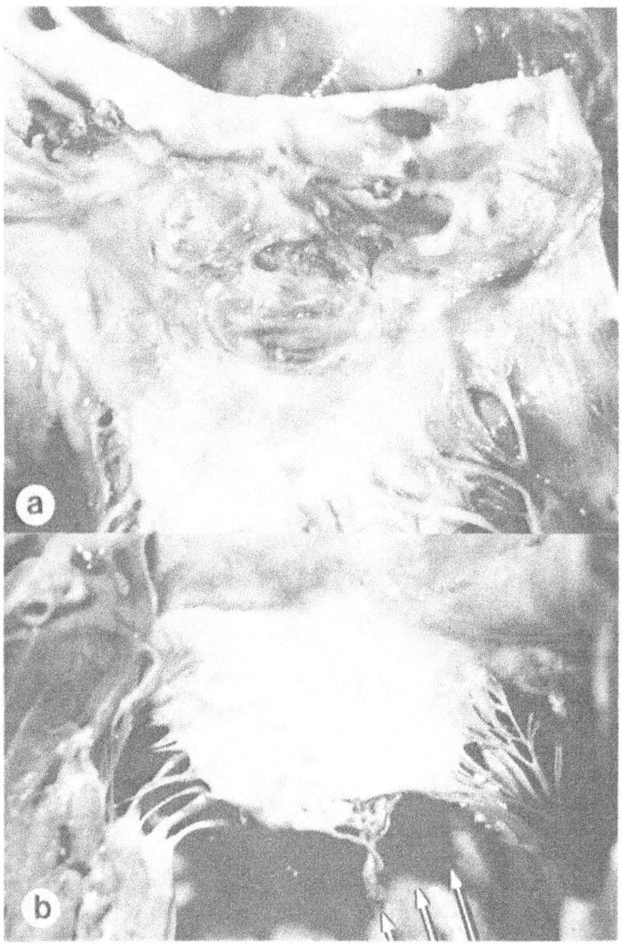

FIGURE 3. *Opened aortic valve* **(a)** *and mitral valve* **(b)** *in a 39 year old man* (A69-254) *who had an episode of active infective endocarditis at age 24 and died suddenly at age 39 while playing golf.* A minimal amount of aortic regurgitation was worsened by the episode of infective endocarditis. When the patient was studied 2 months before death, simultaneous left ventricular and brachial arterial pressures were 140/20 and 140/38 mm Hg, respectively, and the cardiac index was 2.8 liter/min per m^2. Angiography with injection of contrast material into the ascending aorta revealed severe aortic regurgitation and, with injection into the left ventricle, mild mitral regurgitation. The heart was huge (1,010 g). **a,** the aortic valve is congenitally malformed, consisting of two nearly equal-sized cusps and one rudimentary cusp (called bicuspid); a perforation is present in each of the two developed cusps. Calcific deposits border the perforations. **b,** several chordae tendineae from the posterior half of the anterior mitral leaflet are ruptured (**arrows**).

Valve lesions considered indicative of healed infective endocarditis: These included *cuspal perforations* (Fig. 1 to 5), *ruptured chordae tendineae* (Fig. 2, 3 and 6 to 8) and *aneurysms at or near sites of attachment of valve cusps* (the residua of ring abscesses) (Fig. 4, 9 and 10). Of the 59 patients with a history of active infective endocarditis that healed, 30 (51 percent) had one or more of the three anatomic lesions indicative of previous active infective endocarditis (Table I): Cuspal perforations occurred in 16 patients, rupture of chordae tendineae in 15 and aneurysms at or near the involved valve in 3. Other cardiac lesions also almost surely the consequence of healed active infective endocarditis are illustrated in Figures 7, 8, 11 and 12. Figure 13 shows an aortic valve in a woman who had three well documented episodes of active infective endocarditis and diffuse fibrous thickening of the aortic valve cusps as the only residuum.

Valve dysfunction: Among the 59 patients with a history of healed infective endocarditis, the mitral or aortic valve, or both, was either stenotic or purely incompetent at the time of necropsy or valve replacement: 28 patients had isolated aortic valve dysfunction, 17 isolated mitral valve dysfunction and 14 combined aortic and mitral dysfunction. Of the 59 aortic valves in the 59 patients, 16 were stenotic, 26 purely incompetent and 17 functionally normal; of the 59 mitral valves, 7 were stenotic, 24 purely incompetent and 28 functionally normal. Thus, a total of 73 valves in the 59 patients functioned abnormally (Table III). Valve lesions indicative of healed infective endocarditis were more common in the 38 patients with purely incompetent valves than in the 21 patients with stenotic or mixed valve lesions: Anatomic evidence of healed infective endocarditis was present in 7 (30 percent) of the 23 stenotic valves; and in 25 (50 percent) or the 50 purely incompetent valves. Fourteen of the 16 patients with valve perforations had purely incompetent valves as did 13 of the 15 patients with ruptured chordae tendineae. In contrast, none of the three patients with a healed ring abscess had purely incompetent valves. Valve lesions indicative of healed infective endocarditis were present in 15 (48 percent) of the 31 dysfunctioning mitral valves and in 17 (40 percent) of 42 dysfunctioning aortic valves (Table III). Anatomic evidence of healed infective endocarditis was present in 15 (58 percent) of 26 patients with positive blood cultures during active endocarditis, in 2 of 5 with negative blood cultures and in 13 (46 percent) of 28 in whom the clinical events during active endocarditis were not known (Table II). Eleven (38 percent) of the 29 patients without anatomic evidence of infective endocarditis were known to have had positive blood cultures during the active stage.

All 23 stenotic valves (in 21 patients) at operation or at necropsy were diffusely fibrotic and 19 of them contained calcific deposits (extensive in 16 [14 patients]). Of the 50 purely incompetent valves (in 41 patients), the valve leaflets were diffusely fibrotic in 37 and focally fibrotic in 13; 9 of these valves (in 9 patients) contained calcific deposits but in each the deposits were focal and small.

Etiology of valve disease: From examination of both the clinical records and the cardiac valves, it appeared likely that the left-sided cardiac valves *before* the onset of active infective endocarditis had been both anatomically and functionally normal in 9 (15 percent) and abnormal in 50 (85 percent) of the 59 patients. The most likely origins of the underlying valve disease in the latter 50 patients were: *rheumatic* (24 patients, 41 percent; mitral valve in all)[4]; *congenital* (17 patients, 29 percent; bicuspid aortic valve in 12 [20 percent], unicuspid aortic valve in 1 [2 percent][6,7] and aortic regurgitation associated with ventricular septal defect in 4 [7 percent]); *degenerative* (4 patients, 7 percent; aortic valve in all[8]); the *Marfan*

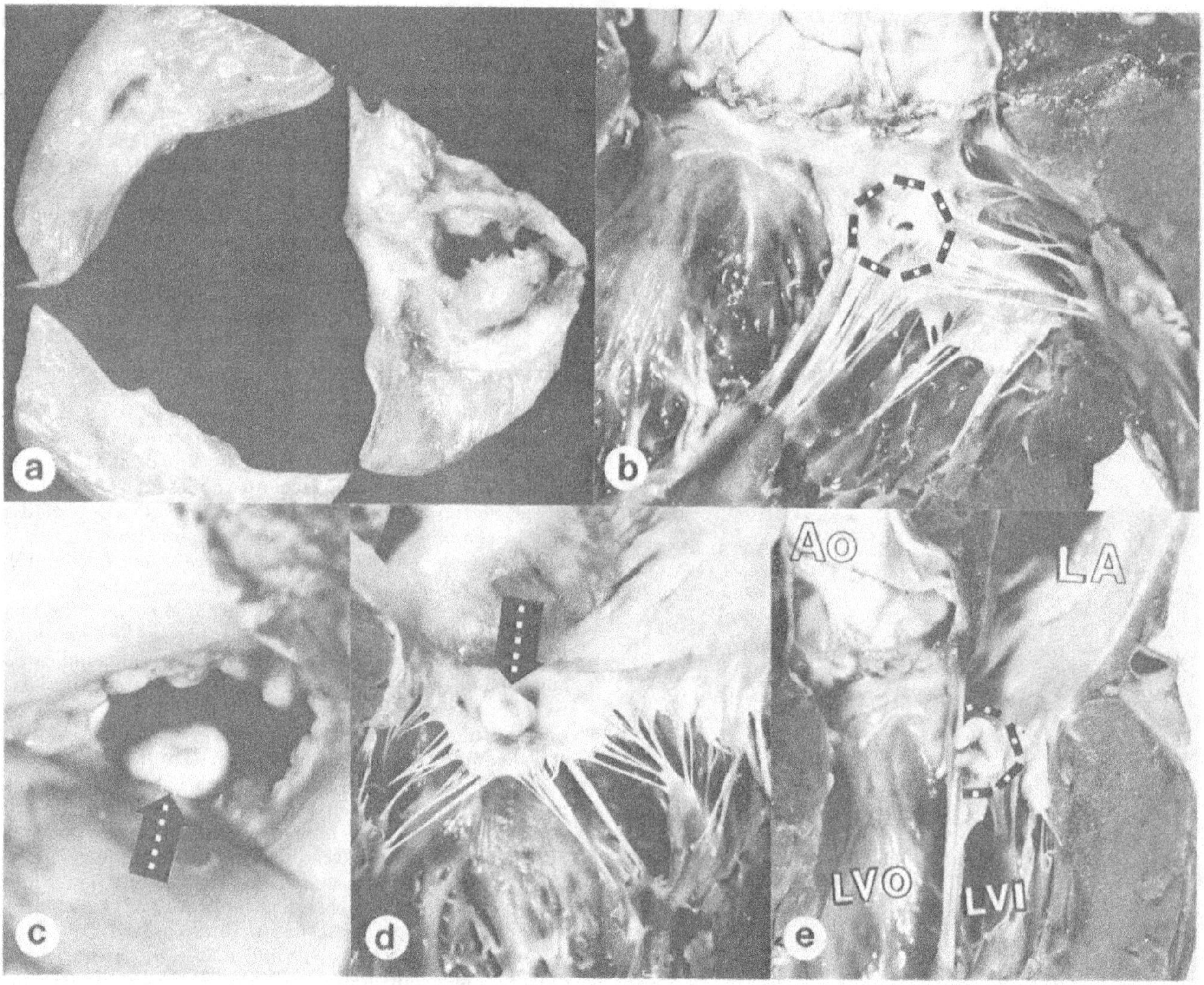

FIGURE 4. *Aortic and mitral valves in a 45 year old man* (A70-227) *who had nonhemolytic streptococcal endocarditis 2 years earlier with the onset of mitral and aortic regurgitation at that time.* He died 5 days after double valve replacement. It is believed that both valves were functionally and anatomically normal before the onset of infective endocarditis. **a,** excised aortic valve showing a perforation in two of the three cusps. **b,** opened left ventricular outflow tract showing a small opening **(dashed circle)** in the anterior mitral leaflet. **c,** mitral valve orifice as seen from left atrium showing an aneurysm **(arrow)** on the atrial aspect of the anterior mitral leaflet. **d,** opened left atrium, mitral valve and left ventricle showing the aneurysm **(arrow)** on the anterior leaflet. **e,** longitudinal cut of aorta (Ao), left ventricle, mitral valve and left atrium (LA) showing the aneurysm (enclosed by **dashes**) on the anterior leaflet. The mitral leaflet aneurysm as well as the aortic cuspal perforation is the result of the active infective endocarditis that healed. LVI and LVO = left ventricular inflow and outflow tract, respectively.

syndrome (2 patients, 3 percent)[9]; and *uncertain* etiology (2 patients, 3 percent).

Valve stenosis antedating active infective endocarditis: Of the 21 patients (among the 59) with valve stenosis at necropsy or operation, valve stenosis had been diagnosed *before* the episode of active infective endocarditis in only 3. Fourteen of the remaining 18 patients had considerable stenosis (aortic valve peak systolic pressure gradient more than 70 mm Hg or mean diastolic mitral valve gradient more than 7 mm Hg shortly before death or valve replacement) and short intervals (less than 2.5 years) from active infective endocarditis to death or operative valve excision. Therefore, in these 14 patients the stenosis almost certainly had been present before the active infective endocarditis. Each of the remaining four patients had small (12 to 20 mm Hg) simultaneous peak systolic pressure gradients across the aortic valve and long intervals between the episode of active infective endocarditis and valve replacement or death. It is probable that the mild aortic stenosis in each of these four patients resulted in whole or in part from the valve infection.

Clinical features: Of the 59 patients with a history of active infective endocarditis that healed, 41 (69 percent) were male and 18 (31 percent) female. At the time of active infective endocarditis, the patients ranged in age from 7 to 63 years (average 26), and at necropsy or valve replacement their ages ranged from 15 to 69 years (average 42). The interval from active infective endocarditis to death or cardiac operation (Table IV) ranged from 3 months to 34 years (average 7). Six patients had had more than one episode of active infective endocarditis. Factors predisposing to active infective endocarditis were present in 18 (31 percent) of the 59 patients. Blood cultures were positive during active infective endocarditis in 26 of the 31 patients in whom this information was available (Table V). Congestive heart failure was present during active infective endocarditis in 37 of the 40 patients in whom this information was available: In at least 27 of the

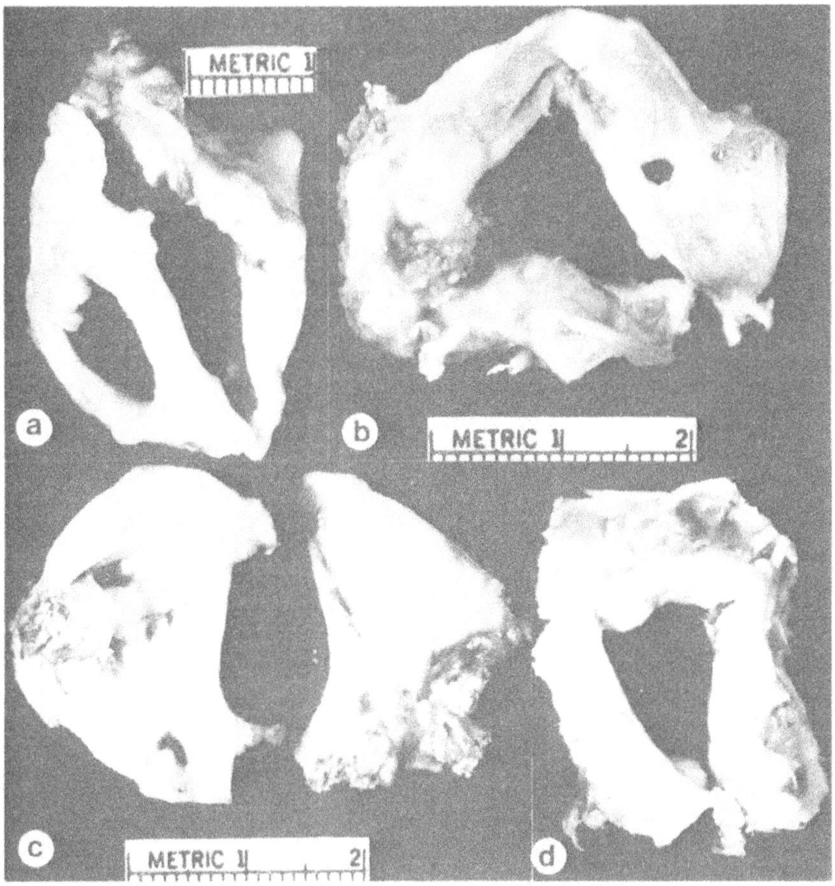

FIGURE 5. *Operatively excised, mildly stenotic* (12 to 20 mm Hg peak systolic pressure gradients), *calcified aortic valves from four patients, each of whom had a history of healed infective endocarditis.* **a**, congenitally bicuspid aortic valve from a 52 year old man (A70-54) who had active infective endocarditis at age 40 with severe aortic regurgitation thereafter. A large perforation is present in one of the two cusps. **b**, tricuspid aortic valve from a 42 year old man (A70-57) who had streptococcal endocarditis at age 32. A small perforation is present in one of the three cusps. **c**, congenitally bicuspid aortic valve from a 53 year old man (A69-27) who had alpha streptococcus endocarditis 5 months before valve excision. **d**, tricuspid aortic valve from a 69 year old man (A67-29) who had active infective endocarditis at age 50. No definite anatomic residua of endocarditis are apparent in the valves shown in **c** and **d**.

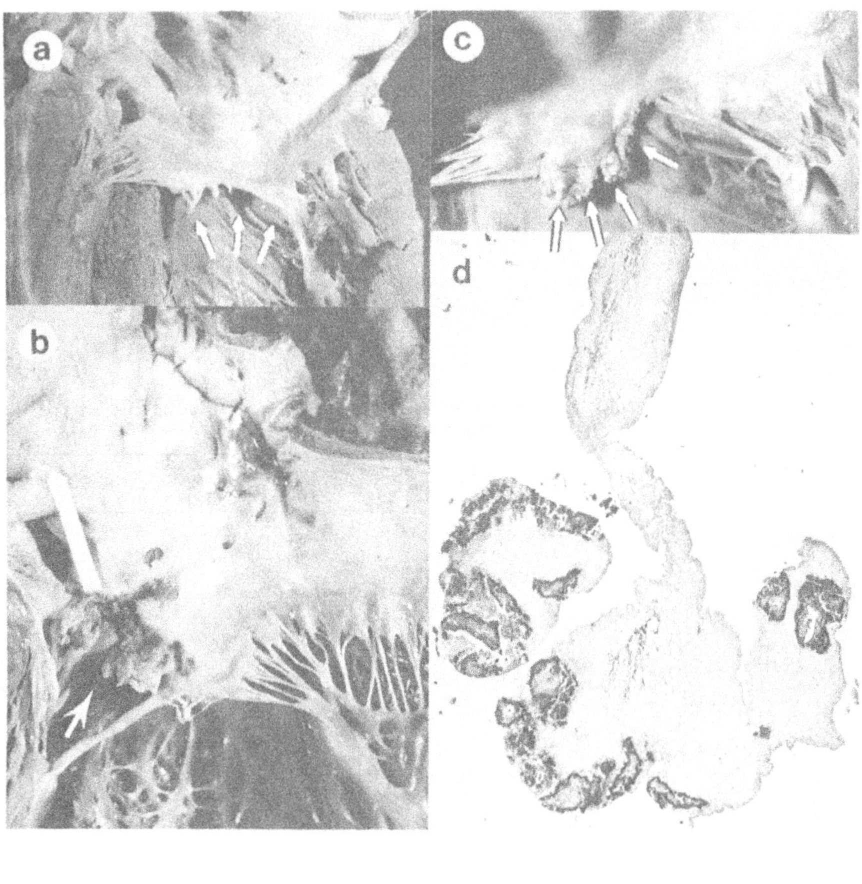

FIGURE 6. *Ruptured chordae tendineae* (**arrows**) *of the mitral valve from three patients with a history of healed infective endocarditis.* **a**, opened left atrium, mitral valve and left ventricle of a 29 year old woman (A63-97) who had Staphylococcus albus endocarditis at age 24 with severe mitral regurgitation subsequently. **b**, from a 19 year old woman (A61-221) who had streptococcus Group D endocarditis 16 months earlier with severe mitral regurgitation subsequently. **c**, from a 24 year old woman (A62-19) who had enterococcus endocarditis 5 months earlier. Calcific deposits are present at the sites of the previous vegetations and these are better shown in **d**. This case illustrates that calcific deposits are consequences of healing of active infective endocarditis and that the calcific deposits can form fairly rapidly. Each of the three patients shown here had active infective endocarditis on a previously normal mitral valve and each also had a normal aortic valve.

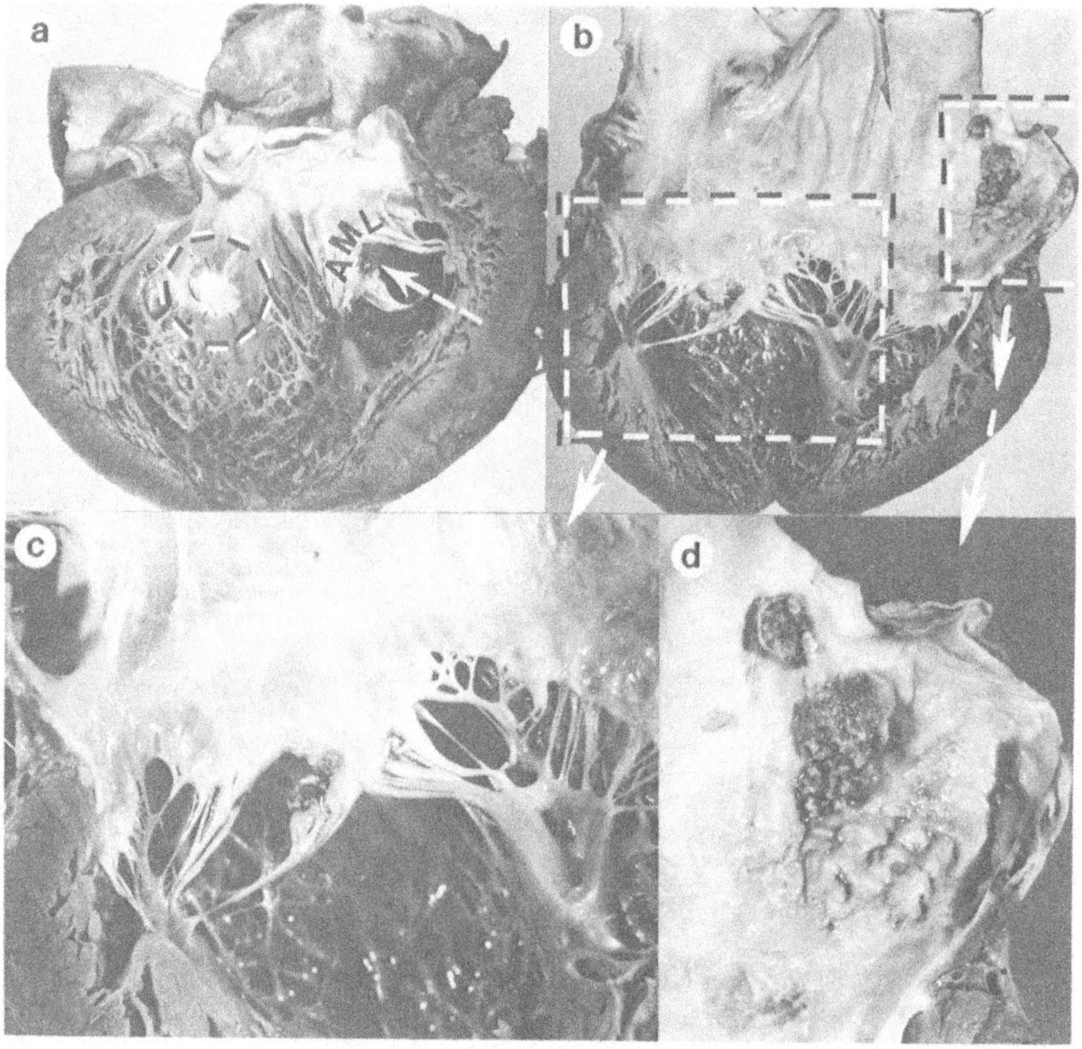

FIGURE 7. *Heart of a 25 year old woman* (A71-252) *who had Staphylococcus aureus endocarditis at age 7 with mitral regurgitation thereafter.* At age 18, she had a second well documented episode of infective endocarditis, this time due to alpha streptococcus. She died from severe congestive cardiac failure. **a,** opened aortic valve and left ventricle showing a jet lesion **(dashed circle)** corresponding to the indentation **(arrow)** in the anterior mitral leaflet (AML). **b,** opened left atrium, mitral valve and left ventricle. **c,** close-up of large area in brackets in **b.** There is an identation and ruptured chordae tendineae on the anterior half of the anterior mitral leaflet. Small calcific deposits border the indentations. **d,** close-up of small area in brackets in **b.** These calcific deposits on the posterior wall of left atrium represent healed vegetations that apparently developed during one or both periods of active infective endocarditis.

TABLE IV

Relation of Interval Between Active Infective Endocarditis to Presence or Absence of Anatomic Evidence of Infective Endocarditis at Operation or Necropsy (59 patients with a history of infective endocarditis)

Interval (yr) Between Active Infective Endocarditis and Valve Replacement or Death	Patients (no.) Total	With Anatomic Evidence of Infective Endocarditis
<2	15	8
2–5	16	7
>5–10	12	8
>10	16	7
Totals	59	30 (51%)

TABLE V

Organisms Causing Active Infective Endocarditis (31 patients with available information)

Organism	Patients no.	%
Streptococcus species		
Alpha hemolytic	16	52
Micro-aerophilic	2	6
Enterococcus	1	3
Total	19	61
Staphylococcus species		
Unspecified	4	13
Aureus	1	3
Epidermidis	1	3
Total	6	19
Diplococcus pneumoniae	1	3
Unknown	5	17

37 patients, cardiac failure was not present before active infection and in 10 it was present before, but worse during, the infection. All 59 patients had congestive heart failure before death or valve replacement. The causes of death in the 42 necropsy patients are summarized in Table VI.

Histologic findings: Extensive histologic examination of the heart was carried out in the 16 patients in whom cardiac operation was never performed. Fifteen (94 percent) had microscopic-sized foci of myocardial fibrosis: In five it was confined to left ventricular papillary muscle, in four, to the left ventricular free wall; in 6 it was in both the free wall and papillary muscle. Only 3 of 16 had significant (greater than 75 percent in cross-sectional area) coronary arterial luminal narrowing. Three patients had microscopic-sized foci of necrosis in left ventricular papillary muscle, but each of them had had severe congestive cardiac failure before death.

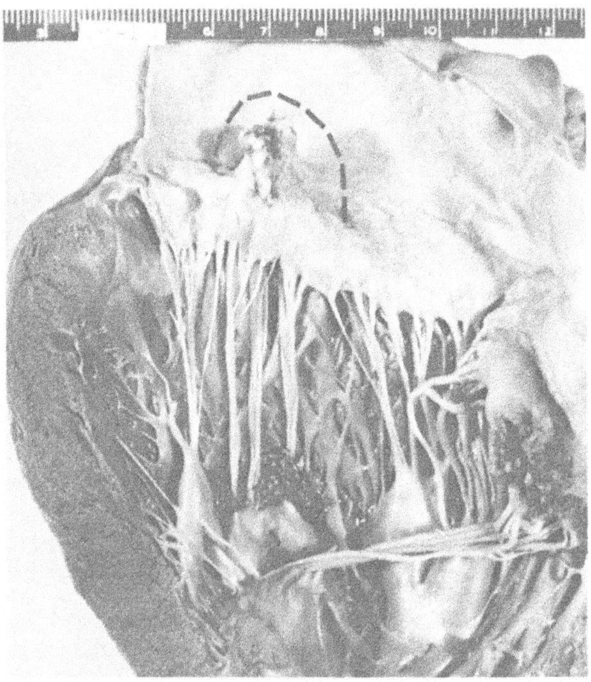

FIGURE 8. *Opened posterier mitral leaflet in a 30 year old man* (A56-132) *who had alpha streptococcus endocarditis 2 years earlier.* He had typical clinical features of the Marfan syndrome with aortic regurgitation in addition to mitral regurgitation. Shown here is a calcified protrusion (enclosed by **dashes**) on the atrial aspect of the posterior mitral leaflet. This protrusion probably represents a healed vegetation. The mitral chordae tendineae are elongated, and several from the anterior leaflet are ruptured.

Comments

Previous studies of causes of death after healed infective endocarditis: Successful therapy for active infective endocarditis with the introduction of penicillin for this condition in 1944 represents one of the great successes in the treatment of heart disease. Overnight this condition changed from a virtually universally fatal condition[2] to one that could be cured. However, despite the use of penicillin, and, later, other antibiotic agents, a number of patients so treated nevertheless died.[10-28] Table VII summarizes the reported results of therapy with penicillin for active infective endocarditis in a total of 1,357 patients.[10-28] Of this number, 450 (33 percent) died during the period of active infective endocarditis, and approximately another 33 percent of patients, although cured of the infection, were left with cardiac dysfunction as a consequence of the valve damage produced by the infection. Only about one third of the total patients with active infective endocarditis or one half of the survivors of the active infection were free of valve damage or at least valve damage sufficient

TABLE VI

Mode of Death in Patients with History of Healed Infective Endocarditis (IE) (42 necropsy patients)

	Patients Operated On		Patients Not Operated On		Totals	
Mode of Death	no.	%	no.	%	no.	%
Cardiovascular	19	73	13	81	32	76
Congestive failure	3	12	10	63	13	31
Sudden death	9	34	2	12	11	26
Prosthetic dysfunction	5	19	0		5	2
Operative accident	2	8	0		2	5
Recurrent active IE	0		1	6	1	2
Cerebrovascular	4	15	0		4	10
Other	3	12	3	19	6	14
Totals	26	100	16	100	42	100

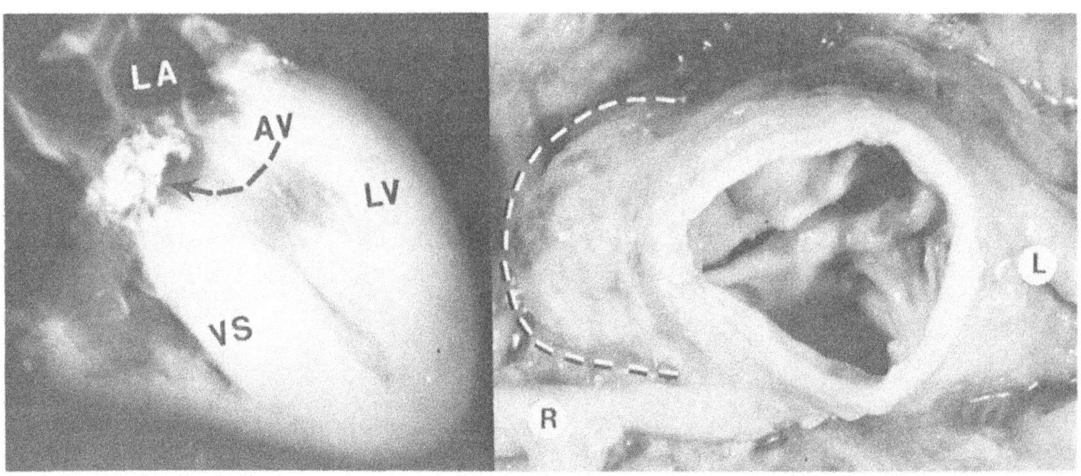

FIGURE 9. *Radiograph of heart* **(left)** *and aortic valve from above* **(right)** *from a 52 year old man* (A63-179) *with a known precordial murmur since age 42 and microacrophilic streptococcus endocarditis 10 months before death.* The aortic valve (AV) is heavily calcified and stenotic (85 mm Hg peak systolic pressure gradient). A "mycotic" aneurysm outlined by **dashed lines (right)** is the residuum of the infection. LA = left atrium; LV = left ventricle; R and L = right and left coronary arteries, respectively; VS = ventricular septum.

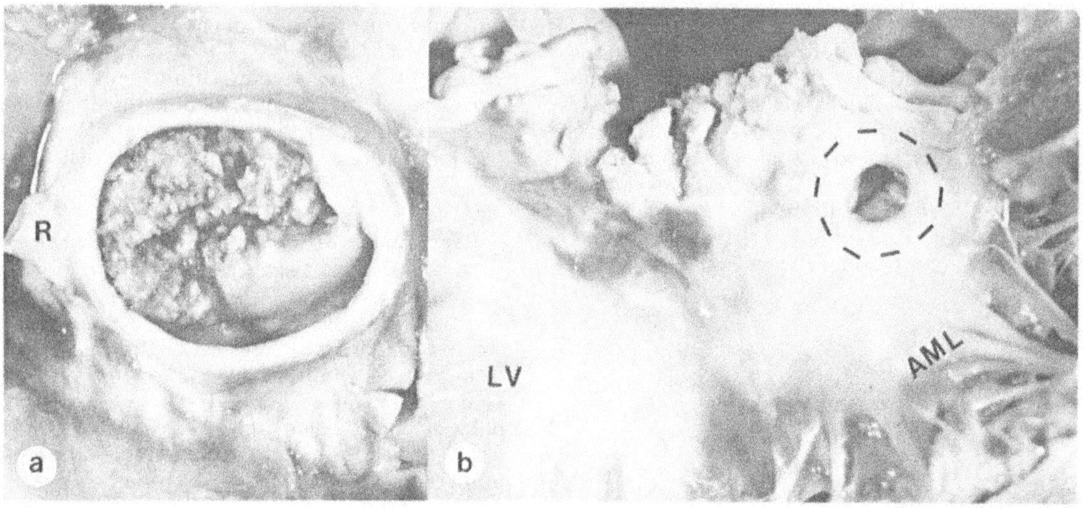

FIGURE 10. *Congenitally unicuspid unicommissural, calcified aortic valve from above* **(a)** *and when opened* **(b)** *from a 32 year old woman* (A61-281) *with a known precordial murmur since age 5 and alpha streptococcus endocarditis at age 29.* A 90 mm Hg peak systolic pressure gradient was present between the left ventricle and the systemic artery. In **b,** a perforation (enclosed by **circle**) is present just below the aortic valve; it is considered the result of the infective endocarditis. AML = anterior mitral leaflet; LV = left ventricle; R = right coronary artery.

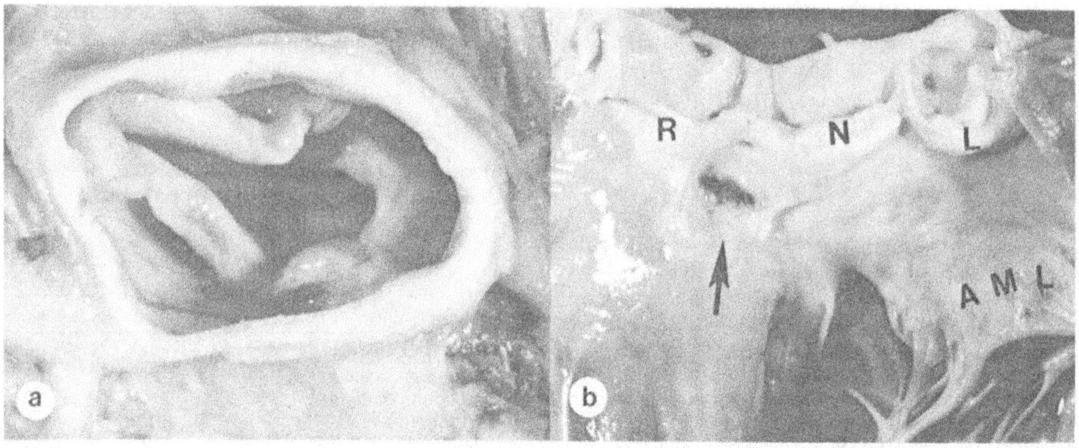

FIGURE 11. *Aortic valve from above* **(a)** *and when opened* **(b)** *from a 24 year old man* (A63-201) *who had acute rheumatic fever at age 9 and alpha streptococcus endocarditis at age 23, one year before death.* Each of the three aortic valve cusps is diffusely thickened and retracted by fibrous tissue. An oval-shaped area of fibrous thickening **(arrow)** between the right (R) and noncoronary (N) cusps probably represents the residuum of infective endocarditis. The anterior mitral leaflet (AML) is diffusely thickened. L = left aortic valve cusp.

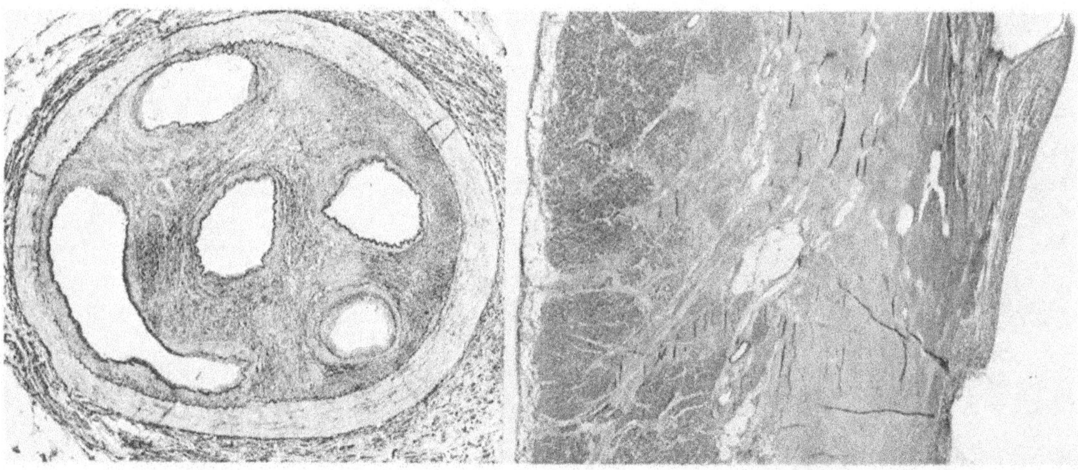

FIGURE 12. *Coronary arterial embolism with healed myocardial infarction in a 26 year old man* (A63-170) *who had active infective endocarditis on a congenitally bicuspid aortic valve 3 years earlier.* At the time of the infection, the patient had a large anterior wall acute myocardial infarction. Examination of the coronary arteries 3 years later disclosed that the right, left main and left circumflex arteries were normal and that the distal left anterior descending (shown here) contained several channels. It is likely that a portion of the aortic valve vegetation dislodged and embolized to the coronary artery at the time of the active infection and that the embolus subsequently recanalized. A section of the healed myocardial infarction is shown at the **right.** Elastic tissue stain ×46 **(left)** and hematoxylin-eosin stain ×10 **(right),** reduced by 22 percent.

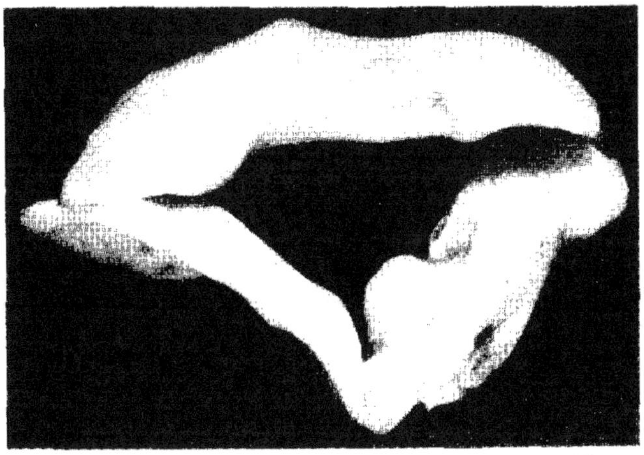

FIGURE 13. *Operatively excised tricuspid aortic valve from a 23 year old woman (S63-3352) who had three well documented episodes of active infective endocarditis* at ages 18, 19 and 21 and yet no anatomic changes in the valve that can unequivocally be attributed to the infection. Each of the three cusps is thickened by fibrous tissue, but no perforations are present.

to produce cardiac dysfunction. Thus, of patients with active infective endocarditis treated with penicillin and reported on from 1950 to 1965,[10-28] one third died during the active infection, one third were left with sufficient damage to one or more valves to cause cardiac dysfunction and one third had either no residual valve damage or insufficient valve damage to produce cardiac dysfunction.

Among patients whose active infective endocarditis was cured with penicillin therapy but who later died, the most common cause of death was congestive heart failure, the result usually of valve damage either initiated or worsened by the active infective endocarditis. Among the survivors of active infective endocarditis whose data are summarized in Table VII, 199 died 2 to 156 months after eradication of the infection by penicillin. Of them, 148 (74 percent) died from a cardiac cause and in 126 of them congestive heart failure was the major cardiac problem; only 24 of the 199 patients clearly died from noncardiac causes.

Few observations at necropsy in patients who died late after healing of active infective endocarditis are available. As Table VII indicates, among the 199 patients who died late after healing of the endocarditis, necropsy was reported in only 30 patients of whom 10 had cardiac lesions that could be attributed to results of the active infection; cuspal perforations were found in all 10 and aneurysm of the anterior mitral leaflet in 2 (possibly as many as 4). None of these reports described the residual valve lesions in detail and, indeed, rupture of chordae tendineae or perianular aneurysm (evidence of healed ring abscess) were not mentioned.

Valve lesions attributable to consequences of active infective endocarditis: The present study is different from any of the previous studies summarized in Table VII. The earlier studies each began with a population of patients with active infective endocarditis who were treated with penicillin. The patients surviving the period of active infection were followed up thereafter for various periods to determine how many later had, or continued to have, cardiac dysfunction despite eradication of the valve infection. The starting point in the previous studies, therefore, was active infective endocarditis. In our study, the starting point was examination of a severely dysfunctioning cardiac valve, either at necropsy or at valve replacement, in a group of patients with historical evidence of active infective endocarditis treated with, and the cardiac infection eradicated by, antibiotic drugs. Among these patients we sought to determine the frequency of anatomic lesions that were clearly attributable to consequences of the active infective endocarditis. Thus, among 584 necropsy patients who died of severe valve disease, 42 (7 percent) had a history of active infective endocarditis that healed and 22 (52 percent) of them had anatomic cardiac lesions readily attributable to the earlier valve infection; among 79 patients who underwent cardiac valve replacement because of severe aortic or mitral regurgitation, or both, 17 (22 percent) had a history

TABLE VII

Summary of Previous Reports of Consequences of Active Infective Endocarditis (IE) Treated With Antibiotics

Reference: First Author	Year	Patients: Total With Active IE Therapy	Dying During Active IE: no.	Dying During Active IE: %	Surviving Active IE and Later Dying: no.	Follow-Up Interval (mo)	Cause of Late Death: Cardiac: CHF	Cardiac: Other	Non-cardiac	Un-known	Necropsies in Late Deaths	Cuspal Per-foration
Pillsbury[10]	1950	31	3	10	7	9–48 (35)	6	0	1	0	—	—
Gorlin[11]	1950	38	11	29	7	12–72	4	3	0	0	—	—
Cates[12]	1951	408	171	42	24	>6	19	0	0	5	—	—
Correll[13]	1951	36	15	42	4	2–24	4	0	0	0	—	—
Donzelot[14]	1953	202	49	24	21	3–84	17	2	0	2	—	—
Newman[15]	1954	39	12	31	9	. . .	9	0	0	0	—	—
Priest[16–18]	1955	34	12	35	6	13–120	5	1	0	0	—	—
Henriksen[19]	1955	19	7	37	2	44–80	2	0	0	0	—	—
Mendelson[20–22]	1956	20	3	15	7	8–102	5	1	0	1	—	—*
Hall[23]	1957	32	15	47	7	6–72	5	1	1	0	3	1
Wedgewood[24]	1957	29	8	28	3	20–114 (40)	3	0	0		—	—
Morgan[25]	1959	175	56	32	50	60–120	21	6	13	10	17	8†
Bunn[26]	1962	64	17	27	14	12–156	7	2	5	0	7	1
Blount[27]	1965	89	18	20	19	2–108 (25)	7	5	3	4	3	—
Rabinovich[28]	1965	141	53	38	19	<60	12	1	1	5	—	—
Totals		1357	450	33	199	2–156	126 (63%)	22 (11%)	24 (12%)	27 (14%)	30	10

* Illustrated case of healed aneurysm of anterior mitral leaflet (Case 14) and another of healed aneurysm plus perforation of anterior mitral leaflet (Case 9) (Mokotoff et al.[20]).

† Two patients also had healed aneurysms of the anterior mitral leaflet.

CHF = congestive heart failure.

TABLE VIII

Relation of Healed Cuspal Perforation and Ruptured Chordae Tendineae to Infective Endocarditis (IE) (607 patients* with severe valve disease)

Dysfunctioning Valve	Total	Patients With Ruptured Chordae Tendineae		Patients With Cuspal Perforation (no.)	
		Total	With History of IE	Total	With History of IE
Aortic (A)	278	. . .	. . .	11†	11 (100%)
Mitral (M)	175	35	10 (29%)	2	2 (100%)
A & M	154	8	5 (62%)	3‡	3‡ (100%)
Totals	607	43	15 (35%)	16	16 (100%)

* This number is 607 rather than 665 as stated in Table I because 58 patients with active infective endocarditis were excluded.
† Two patients with aortic valve perforations were excluded because historical data were insufficient to determine presence or absence of a history of infective endocarditis.
‡ The perforations in each patient involved the aortic valve only.

of active infective endocarditis that healed and 8 (47 percent) of them had anatomic cardiac lesions readily attributable to an earlier valve infection.

Cardiac lesions produced by infective endocarditis on regurgitant versus stenotic valves: Study at necropsy of patients with fatal active infective endocarditis has indicated that *cuspal perforations* (or indentations), *ruptured chordae tendineae, ring abscesses* and *mycotic aneurysms* are cardiac lesions most commonly the consequence of infective endocarditis.[29,30] Among our 59 patients with a history of active left-sided infective endocarditis that healed, 16 had cuspal perforations, 29 had ruptured mitral chordae tendineae, 3 had perianular aneurysms (healed ring abscess) and 1 had a small aortic aneurysm considered to be of infective origin. Although 30 of the 59 patients had cardiac lesions attributable to consequences of infective endocarditis, these lesions were far more common among the patients with purely incompetent valves (immediately before death or valve replacement) than among the patients with stenotic valves. Of the 385 patients with valve stenosis at necropsy, 18 (5 percent) had a history of active infective endocarditis that healed and 7 (39 percent) of them had anatomic cardiac lesions indicative of infective endocarditis; in contrast, of 229 patients with pure valve regurgitation at necropsy or valve replacement, 38 (17 percent) had a history of active infective endocarditis that healed and 23 (61 percent) of them had anatomic cardiac lesions indicative of infective endocarditis. Among the 7 patients with anatomic lesions of infective endocarditis and valve stenosis, the anatomic lesion in 3 was healed ring abscess, and cuspal perforations and ruptured chordae tendineae occurred in each of 2 patients; in contrast, among the 23 patients with anatomic lesions indicative of infective endocarditis and pure valve regurgitation, none had healed ring abscess, 14 (61 percent) had cuspal perforations and 13 (57 percent) had ruptured chordae tendineae (4 of the latter 13 were among the 14 with cuspal perforations). Thus, infective endocarditis superimposed on a previously stenotic valve may not leave evidence of further cuspal damage and, because the chordae tendineae are thick when the mitral valve is stenotic, rupture of a thickened chorda tendinèa is infrequent. The previously normal valve or the purely incompetent valve is easy prey to cuspal destruction by infection because it is not thickened; similarly, the chorda tendinea that is not thickened readily can be ruptured by infection.

Correlation of history of infective endocarditis and anatomic findings: Although anatomic lesions clearly indicative of previous infective endocarditis occurred in half of our patients with a history of active infective endocarditis, the other half had no lesions readily attributable to infective endocarditis. This difference cannot be explained on the basis of better historical evidence of active infective endocarditis in the former group. Anatomic evidence of infective endocarditis was found in 17 (55 percent) of the 31 patients with a "good" history and in 13 (46 percent) of the 26 patients with a "less good" history of active infective endocarditis that healed. Cuspal perforations, ring abscess and ruptured chordae tendineae thus are not inevitable consequences of active infective endocarditis. Although cuspal perforations and ring abscesses in our experience are always indicative of infective endocarditis at some time, ruptured chordae tendineae unassociated with vegetations are not always indicative of past infective endocarditis (Table VIII). Among 16 patients with cuspal perforations unassociated with vegetations studied by us at necropsy, all had a good history of infective endocarditis that healed (Table VIII). In contrast, of 43 patients with ruptured chordae tendineae unassociated with vegetations and studied by us at necropsy, only 15 (35 percent) had a history of past infective endocarditis (Table VIII). Nevertheless, rupture of chordae tendineae is the most common anatomic lesion observed on the mitral valve during active infective endocarditis[29,30] and consequently in patients with a history of healed infective endocarditis and ruptured

TABLE IX

Distinguishing Features of Fatal Left-Sided Infective Endocarditis (IE) (active compared with healed state)

	Active IE (% of 74 patients)	Healed IE (% of 42 patients)
Underlying status of involved valve		
Anatomically normal	55	15
Anatomically abnormal	45	85
Causative organism		
Staphylococcus or pneumococcus	48	19
Alpha hemolytic streptococcus	12	52
Predisposing factors	60	27
Opiate addiction	14	0
Alcoholism	23	2
Immunodeficiencies	9	5
Manipulative procedures (dental, surgical, obstetric)	14	20

chordae tendineae it is most reasonable to attribute the chordal rupture to the infection.

Necropsy findings in patients who die during active infection versus findings in patients who die after healing: Certain differences have been noted at necropsy between patients who died during active left-sided infective endocarditis and those who died after healing of the active infection. Three major differences, summarized in Table IX, have been noted. Among our 74 necropsy patients with fatal active left-sided infective endocarditis,[30] 55 percent had the infection on a previously anatomically and functionally normal valve; in contrast, of our 42 necropsy patients with healed left-sided infective endocarditis, only 25 percent were considered to have had anatomically and functionally normal valves before the infection. Thus, the thicker the valve before the infection, the greater the chance of survival during the infection. The causative organism was quite different: Staphylococcus or pneumococcus was the responsible organism in 48 percent of our 74 necropsy patients with fatal active infective endocarditis, and it was responsible in only 19 percent of our 42 necropsy patients with healed infective endocarditis. In the latter group, alpha streptococcus was the most common infecting organism (52 percent) whereas it was the offending organism in only 12 percent of our patients with fatal active infective endocarditis. Finally, recognized predisposing factors to infective endocarditis were common (60 percent) among our patients who died during the active infection and were less frequent (27 percent) among our patients who died after healing of the valve infection.

Acknowledgment

Secretarial assistance was provided by Ms. Exa M. Murray, Linda B. DeVinney and Ann G. Horn. Technical assistance was provided by Ms. Filippina Giacometti, Carol L. Schurtz and Barbara E. Winterrowd. The gross photographs were taken by Mr. L. Kenzie Edwards and James R. Banks, Jr.

References

1. **Libman E:** A study on the endocardial lesions of subacute bacterial endocarditis, with particular reference to healing or healed lesions: with clinical notes. Am J Med Sci 144:313–327, 1912
2. **Kelson SR, White PD:** Notes on 250 cases of subacute bacterial (streptococcal) endocarditis studied and treated between 1927 and 1939. Ann Intern Med 22:40–60, 1945
3. Criteria Committee of the New York Heart Association: Nomenclature and Criteria for Diagnosis of Diseases of the Heart and Great Vessels, seventh edition. Boston, Little, Brown, 1973, p 286
4. **Roberts WC, Perloff JK:** Mitral valvular disease. A clinicopathologic survey of the conditions causing the mitral valve to function abnormally. Ann Intern Med 77:939–975, 1972
5. **Roberts WC:** The congenitally bicuspid aortic valve. A study of 85 autopsy cases. Am J Cardiol 26:72–83, 1970
6. **Roberts WC, Morrow AG:** Congenital aortic stenosis produced by a unicommissural valve. Br Heart J 27:505–510, 1965
7. **Falcone MW, Roberts WC, Morrow AG, et al:** Congenital aortic stenosis resulting from a unicommissural valve. Clinical and anatomic features in twenty-one adult patients. Circulation 44: 272–280, 1971
8. **Roberts WC, Perloff JK, Costantino T:** Severe valvular aortic stenosis in patients over 65 years of age. A clinicopathologc study. Am J Cardiol 27:497–506, 1971
9. **Roberts WC, Dangel JC, Bulkley BH:** Non-rheumatic valvular cardiac disease: a clinicopathologic survey of 27 different conditions causing valvular dysfunction. Cardiovasc Clin 5:333–446, 1973
10. **Pillsbury PL, Fiese MJ:** Subacute bacterial endocarditis. Follow-up study of thirty patients treated with penicillin. Arch Intern Med 85:675–690, 1950
11. **Gorlin R, Favour CB, Emery FJ:** Long-term follow-up study of penicillin-treated subacute bacterial endocarditis. N Engl J Med 242:995–1001, 1950
12. **Cates JE, Christie RV:** Subacute bacterial endocarditis. A review of 442 patients treated in 14 centres appointed by the Penicillin Trials Committee of the Medical Research Council. Q J Med 20: 93–130, 1951
13. **Correll HL, Lubitz JM, Lindert MCF:** Bacterial endocarditis: clinicopathologic studies of untreated, treated and cured patients. Ann Intern Med 35:45–58, 1951
14. **Donzelot E, Le Bozec J-M, Kaufmann H, et al:** Le pronostic de l'endocardite infectieuse subaiguë traitée par les antibiotiques. Resultats du traitement de 202 cas. Arch Mal Coeur 46:97–107, 1953
15. **Newman W, Torres JM, Guck JK:** Bacterial endocarditis. An analysis of fifty-two cases. Am J Med 16:535–542, 1954
16. **Priest WS, Smith JM, McGee CJ:** Penicillin therapy of subacute bacterial endocarditis. A study of the end results in thirty-four cases, with particular reference to dosage, methods of administration, criteria for judging adequacy of treatment and probable reasons for failures. Arch Intern Med 79:333–359, 1947
17. **Hildebrand E, Priest WS:** Cardiac lesions in subacute bacterial endocarditis treated with penicillin. Report of nine cases. Am J Clin Pathol 17:345–364, 1947
18. **Priest WS, Smith JM:** The effect of healed subacute bacterial endocarditis on cardiac dynamics. Arch Intern Med 95:646–652, 1955
19. **Henriksen E, Neukirch F:** The treatment of subacute bacterial endocarditis. Dan M Bull 2:208–213, 1955
20. **Mokotoff R, Brams W, Katz LN, et al:** The treatment of bacterial endocarditis with penicillin. Results of 17 consecutive unselected cases. Am J Med Sci 211:395–416, 1946
21. **Kaplan SR, Rosenman RH, Katz LN, et al:** Healed subacute bacterial endocarditis. A new entity. JAMA 141:114–116, 1949
22. **Mendelson CE, Cahue A, Katz LN, et al:** Long-term outlook for healed subacute bacterial endocarditis. JAMA 160:437–441, 1956
23. **Hall B:** Long-term follow-up of patients with healed bacterial endocarditis. Ann Intern Med 47:880–888, 1957
24. **Wedgewood J:** Prognosis in subacute bacterial endocarditis. Lancet 2:922–925, 1957
25. **Morgan WL, Bland EF:** Bacterial endocarditis in the antibiotic era. With special reference to the later complications. Circulation 19:753–763, 1959
26. **Bunn P, Lunn J:** Late followup of 64 patients with subacute bacterial endocarditis treated with penicillin. Am J Med Sci 279:549–556, 1962
27. **Blount JG:** Bacterial endocarditis. Am J Med 38:909–922, 1965
28. **Rabinovich S, Evans J, Smith IM, et al:** A long-term view of bacterial endocarditis. 337 cases 1924 to 1963. Ann Intern Med 63: 185–198, 1965
29. **Buchbinder NA, Roberts WC:** Left-sided valvular active infective endocarditis. A study of forty-five necropsy patients. Am J Med 53:20–35, 1972
30. **Arnett EN, Roberts WC:** Active infective endocarditis: a clinicopathologic analysis of 137 necropsy patients. Curr Probl Cardiol 1:1–76, October, 1976

Characteristics and Consequences Of Infective Endocarditis (Active or Healed or Both) Learned from Morphologic Studies

Despite antibiotics and, more recently, cardiac valve replacement, infective endocarditis (IE) continues to be a devastating cardiac disease, and therefore it is frequently seen at necropsy. During the past 16 years my colleagues and I have studied, at necropsy, over 150 patients with either active or healed IE.[1-19] This chapter will summarize certain facts and principles learned about IE from these studies, and it will also review certain observations of others on this subject.

TERMINOLOGY

The word "endocarditis" is used relatively loosely today. Strictly, it means "inflammation of endocardium" and this means the presence of inflammatory cells within endocardium. A number of conditions affecting endocardium are associated with inflammatory cells in this portion of the heart. Thus, in patients with an infection involving endocardium, the word "endocarditis" must be preceded by another word to indicate its infective nature. Through the years this preceding word has usually been "bacterial." However, the patient with endocarditis secondary to a fungus or a parasite does not have "bacterial endocarditis." Therefore, the word "infective" is a better general term to describe this type of endocarditis. When the specific infecting organism is known it is best to apply its name as the immediate preceder of the word "endocarditis;" for example, *Staphylococcus aureus* endocarditis or *Candida albicans* endocarditis.

The words "acute" or, more commonly, "subacute" often are used as diagnostic phrases applied to patients with IE. These terms arose in the preantibiotic era when all or virtually all patients with IE died, and they referred to the time periods between onset of symptoms or signs of IE and death: "acute" indicated time courses of less than 6 weeks and "subacute" time courses of greater than 6 weeks. Antibiotics, obviously, change these time courses, and therefore these terms no longer are proper. "Acute" and "subacute" also have been used to indicate the type of organism responsible for the IE: the alpha streptococcus causing the subacute variety and the staphylococcal, pneumoccal and Gram-negative organisms, etc., the acute variety. Because the virulence of certain organisms is altered by antibiotic and chemotherapeutic agents, the term "acute" is no longer proper to refer to infection caused by so-called nonvirulent organisms.

The terms "active" and "healed" are more useful than the terms "acute" and "subacute." The term "active" can be applied to the infective process from the time of its beginning until it is completely healed. During the pretreatment phase of the active period the patient would be expected to have signs of infection; during the treatment phase of the active period, the signs of IE, hopefully, disappear.

It is also desirable to precede the terms "infective endocarditis" by the terms "valvular" or "mural" because the infective process may be limited to the wall or valve. Although it most commonly is secondary to either direct spread or "jet-stream" extension of valvular IE, mural IE may occur without associated valvular IE.[10] Clinically, however, the two are quite different: IE limited to mural endocardium is virtually never diagnosed clinically, whereas IE involving valvular endocardium is usually diagnosed clinically.

Finally, the term "endocarditis" has been applied to patients with "vegetations" on cardiac valvular leaflets but without inflammatory cells or stainable organisms within the vegetations or adjacent valvular leaflets. This condition has been called "nonbacterial thrombotic or verrucal endocarditis," "marantic endocarditis," or simply "nonbacterial endocarditis." The terms which use the word "nonbacterial" are inappropriate because fungal or parasitic endocarditis is nonbacterial. The term "marantic" also has defects because not all patients with this condition are wasted or emaciated. I have used the term "noninfective endocarditis" for this condition; the term "endocarditis" in this setting, however, is not entirely appropriate because there are no inflammatory cells in the vegetative material or in an adjacent valvular leaflet. The term "endocardiopathy" might avoid this "itis" problem, but the disadvantage of this term appears greater than its advantage.

ACTIVE INFECTIVE ENDOCARDITIS

In this presentation IE is divided into two major types: *active* and *healed*. The patients with active IE are subdivided into seven major groups: (1) IE involving native right-sided cardiac valve(s) with or without involvement of left-sided valve(s); IE limited to native left-sided cardiac valve(s); (3) IE involving a prosthetic valve(s); (4) IE after valvulotomy or valvuloplasty; (5) IE with congential subaortic stenosis; (6) IE complicating congenital cardiac disease with a shunt, and (7) IE limited to mural endocardium in the absence of ventricular septal defect.

Active IE Involving Native Right-Sided Cardiac Valves With or Without involvement of Left-Sided Valves (Figs. 2-1–2-4)

The study at necropsy of 24 patients with right-sided active IE[11,16] and the review of reports of others disclosed several principles applicable to IE at this site: (1) right-sided IE is considerably less frequent than is left-sided IE; (2) the clinical presentation is primarily (90 percent) that of acute pneumonia (septic pulmonary infarction), not cardiac disease; (3) a precordial murmur(s), particularly one of tricuspid or pulmonic valve origin, often is absent or of low intensity; (4) an obvious predisposing factor to IE is virtually always indentifiable (most frequently, opiate addiction, habitual alcoholism, indwelling catheter, or chemotherapy for a malignant neoplasm); (5) the IE nearly always is caused by a highly virulent organism (*Staphylococcus aureus* or *Diplococcus pneumoniae* in 75 percent of the patients); (6) the involved right-sided cardiac valve is nearly always both anatomically and functionally normal before the onset of IE; (7) of the two right-sided cardiac valves, the tricuspid one is involved in 95 percent of the patients, the pulmonic in 5 percent, and, to my knowledge, there are no reports describing active IE involving both tricuspid and pulmonic valves in the same patient; (8) about 50 percent of necropsy patients with right-sided active IE also have active IE involving one or both left-sided cardiac valves, but when both right- and left-sided IE is present, acute "pneumonia" is still nearly always the presenting feature, suggesting that the right-sided IE preceded the left-sided IE; (9) associated acute meningitis is fairly common (30 percent); (10) ring abscess is infrequent (17 percent); (11) associated acute myocarditis is frequent (67 percent); and (12) death is most commonly the consequence of "pulmonary insufficiency" secondary to repeated septic emboli from dislodged vegetative material.

FREQUENCY

In 1856, Rokitansky[20] wrote that the frequency of right-sided IE was rare compared to the frequency of left-sided IE. Osler,[21] in 1885, reported vegetations on right-sided cardiac valves in about 15 percent of over 200 necropsy patients with IE, but in only one-third of them were the vegetations limited to right-sided cardiac valves. In the early 1900s Preble,[22] Clawson,[23] and Thayer[24] found vegetations on right-sided cardiac valves in 5–10 percent of necropsy patients with IE; in 1942 Goldburgh et al.[25] found right-sided vegetations in 53 (8 percent) of 646 necropsy patients with IE. Following the introduction of penicillin in 1943, however, Wilson, in 1963,[26] found a statistically significant increase in the frequency of right-sided IE. The author has found right-sided cardiac vegetations in 24 of 100 necropsy patients with active IE involving unoperated native cardiac valves.

Two major reasons have been advanced to explain the lower frequency of right-sided compared to left-sided IE: (1) the lower pressure in the right side of the heart, and (2) the lower frequency of underlying valvular disease affecting the tricuspid and pulmonic valves compared to the mitral and aortic valves. Among patients with active IE involving unoperated native cardiac valves, the percentage with vegetations on a right-sided valve is similar to the normal right ventricular systolic pressure divided by the normal left ventricular systolic pressure, namely 22/110 mm Hg, or 20 percent.[27] Deformed valves are particularly prone to be sites of vegetations, and the tricuspid and pulmonic valves are far less frequently deformed than are their left-sided counterparts.[28]

PRESENTATION WITH ACUTE PNEUMONIA

Patients with right-sided valvular IE usually present with acute pneumonia rather than with symptoms of cardiac disease.[11,25] Of our 24 patients with vegetations on right-sided cardiac valves, 21 had pulmonary infiltrates on chest roentgenogram, and septic pulmonary infarcts were present in the lung at necropsy in 20 of them. Only 8 (33 percent) of the 24 patients had precordial murmurs from right-sided valvular dysfunction. In each of these 8 patients, the IE caused destruction of the tricuspid-valve leaflets and rupture of several chordae tendineae. Although the infection was caused by highly virulent organisms in 15 of the other 16 patients, none had extensive damage to the valvular apparatus. The lower pressures in the right side of the heart probably also account for the lower frequency of severe leaflet destruction in right-sided compared to left-sided IE.[18]

ORGANISMS INVOLVED

Right-sided IE is usually caused by a highly virulent organism, and circumstances associated with an increased risk of developing IE are almost always present.[11,29] Opiate addiction, a well-recognized predisposing factor to infection on either side of the heart,[30-41] was present in 6 (25 percent) of the 24 necropsy patients with right-sided vegetations. *Staphylococcus aureus,* the most frequent cause of IE among opiate addicts,[18] caused the infection in each. Of 62 opiate addicts with fatal IE reviewed by Sapira,[33] *S. aureas* was the causative organism in 9 of 13 patients with isolated right-sided vegetations. In 1958 Bain and associates[29] reported 23 necropsy patients with right-sided IE observed at the Mayo Clinic between 1910 and 1955; *S. aureus* was the infecting organism in all 11 of their 19 patients in whom the organism was identified. Among 104 patients with staphylococcal endocarditis reviewed by Dowling et al.[42] 25 percent had vegetations on right-sided cardiac valves.

Of the 24 patients we studied with right-sided IE, 9 were habitual alcoholics and *Diplococcus pneumoniae* caused the infection in each;[11,13] 7 of the 9 patients presented with acute pneumococcal meningitis, and in 4 it was fatal. Preble,[22] in 1904, reviewed 141 cases of pneumococcal meningitis and found vegetations on right-sided cardiac valves in 19 percent of them. He calculated that pneumococci infected the tricuspid valve 20 times more often than all other organisms combined. Among 646 necropsy patients with IE studied at the Philadelphia General Hospital, Goldburgh and associates[25] found vegetations on right-sided cardiac valves in 53 (8 percent); in 62 patients the infection was caused by pneumonococci, and in 9 (15 percent) of them vegetations were limited to the tricuspid valve. Straus and Hamburger[43] reported 15 patients with pneumonococcal endocarditis seen at the Cincinnati General Hospital; 3 (20 percent) had involvement of the tricuspid valve. Of their 15 patients, 13 (87 percent) also had pneumonococcal meningitis. Of the 141 patients reported by Preble,[22] 60 percent also had pneumococcal meningitis.

VEGETATION ON TRICUSPID VALVE

Patients with right-sided IE almost always have vegetations on the tricuspid valve;[11,17] the involved valve is, with rare exception, anatomically and functionally normal before the onset of IE[11,17] (Figs.2-1–2-4). In 23 (96 percent) of our 24 patients, vegetations were present on the tricuspid valve, and in only 1 on the pulmonic valve. In each of the 24 patients, the involved valve as well as the uninvolved valves were normal before the onset of IE. Of 54 patients with active *Staphylococcus aureus* endocarditis (82 percent) reported by Pankey,[44] 34 (67 percent) had no underlying cardiac disease, and in 29 percent the tricuspid valve was involved. Rheumatic tricuspid valve disease is uncommon; when it is present the

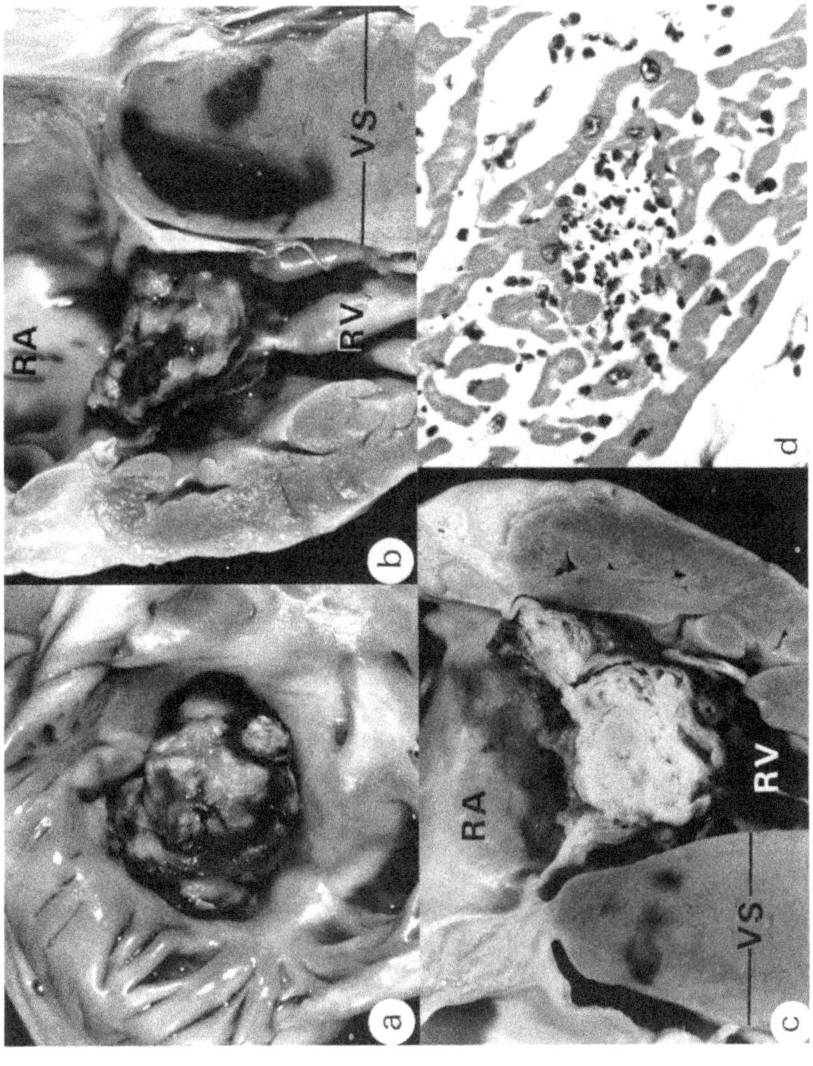
a
b
c
d
RA
RV
VS
RA
RV
VS

Fig. 2–1. Tricuspid valve endocarditis due to *Staphylococcus aureus* and *Enterobacter cloacae* in a 26-year-old male heroin addict. He was hospitalized $4^1/_2$ months before death with fever (104°F), malaise, dyspnea, proteinuria (up to 14 g/24 hours), multiple pulmonary infiltrates, and a grade 3/6 holosystolic murmur which increased in intensity with inspiration. Following 6 weeks of intravenous antibiotic therapy he was discharged, but returned to the hospital 43 days later, just hours before death, with severe dyspnea and massive edema. (A) Tricuspid valve viewed from right atrium. (B) Posterior portion of a longitudinal cut through right atrium (RA), tricuspid valve, and right ventricle (RV). (C) Anterior portion. A huge vegetation virtually fills the tricuspid valve orifice. A hemorrhagic abscess is present in the cephalad portion of the ventricular septum (VS). (D) Microscopic-sized abscess in left ventricular myocardium. Hematoxylin–eosin. × 450.

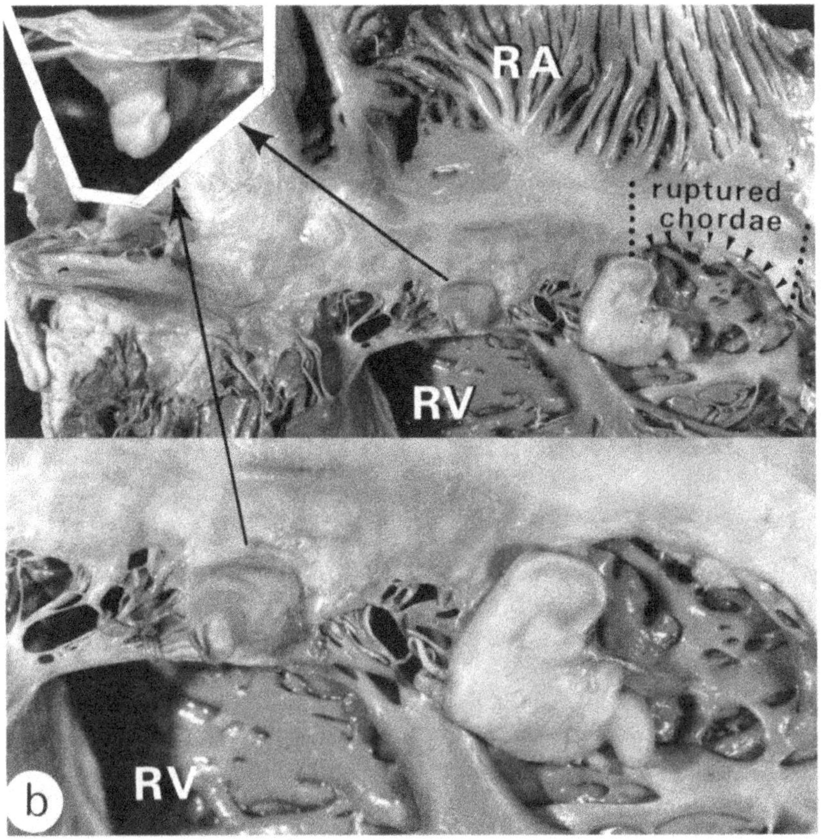

Fig. 2–2. *Diplococcus pneumoniae* tricuspid valve endocarditis in a 56-year-old female chronic alcoholic who had been treated for pneumococcal meningitis 3 months earlier. She was brought to the hospital 3 days before death because of mental confusion. She was febrile and dehydrated, and had a murmur of tricuspid regurgitation. Chest roentgenogram revealed multiple pulmonary infiltrates and blood cultures were positive. (A) Opened right atrium (RA), tricuspid valve, and right ventricle (RV). Two vegetations are present. The inset shows one vegetation as it would appear from right atrium. (B) Close-up of tricuspid valve. The ruptured chordae are apparent.

mitral valve is always stenotic, and usually the aortic valve also is scarred.[45] IE rarely involves hearts with deformed right- and left-sided valves, and when it does it almost always attacks one or both left-sided valves and spares the right-sided valves. Infection of congenitally malformed right-sided cardiac valves is rare.[46–48]

VEGETATION ON LEFT-SIDED CARDIAC VALVES

Patients with infection of right-sided cardiac valves frequently also

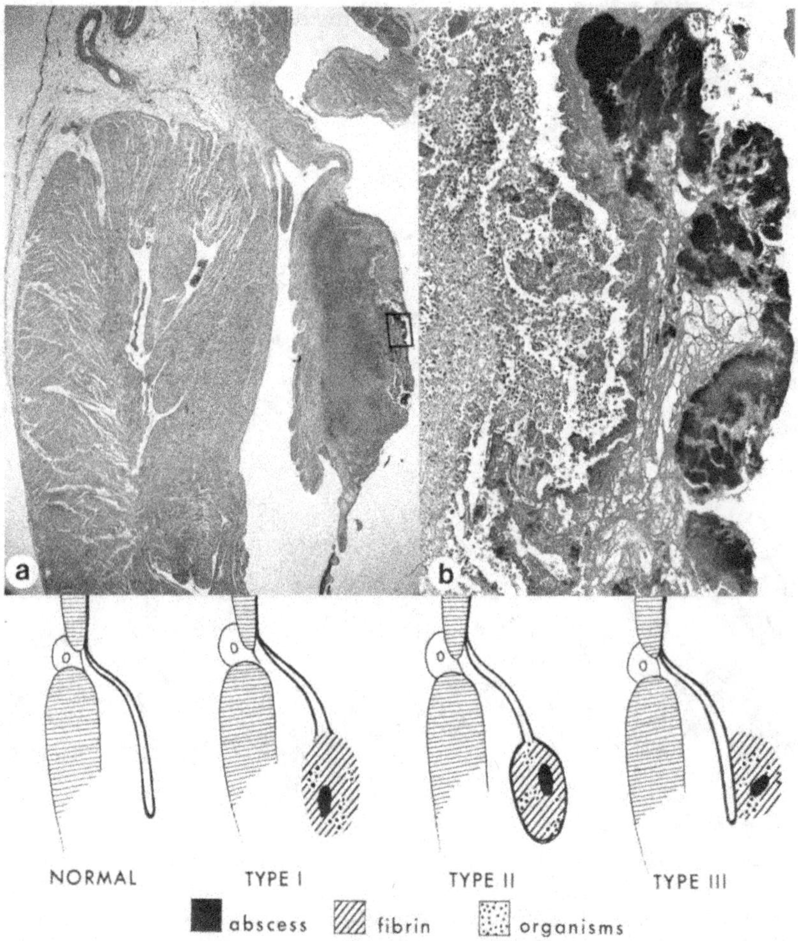

Fig. 2–3. Histologic features of active IE involving the tricuspid valve. Section of tricuspid valve in a 31-year-old female opiate addict who developed acute pneumonia, probably from septic emboli, about 35 days before death. Pulmonary abscesses were present on chest roentgenogram when she was hospitalized 13 days before death. A grade 3/6 blowing precordial systolic murmur was audible and the liver pulsated. She died of congestive cardiac failure. At necropsy, several vegetations were present on the tricuspid valve leaflets. (A) Photomicrograph of section through right atrium, tricuspid valve, and right ventricle. The vegetation more or less is superimposed on the leaflet (type III) as shown in the diagram. (B) Close-up of the area in brackets. The dark areas represent colonies of organisms. The diagram shows three forms vegetations on the tricuspid valve may take. In type I, the vegetations destroy the distal portion of the leaflet. In type II, the normal endocardium of the leaflet is preserved and the vegetative material occupies the central core of the leaflet. In type III, the vegetation appears to be attached simply to the surface of the leaflet. Hemotoxylin–eosin. (A) × 5, (B) × 108.

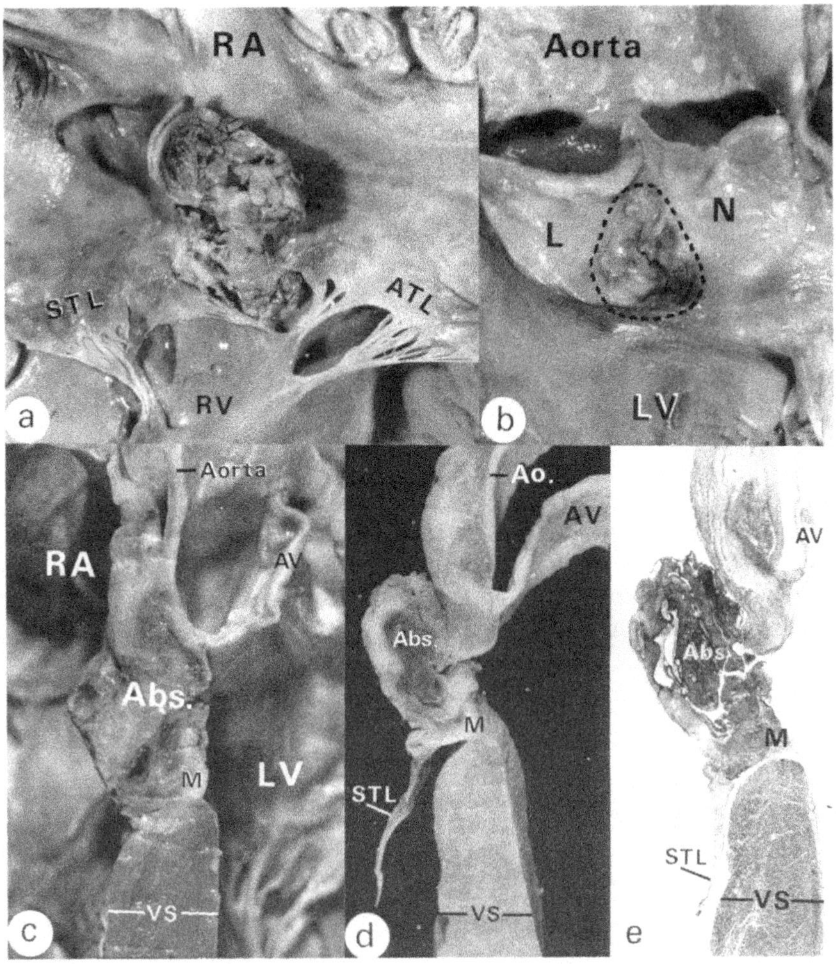

Fig. 2-4. *Staphylococcus aureus* tricuspid valve endocarditis with ring abscess in a 77-year-old male chronic alcoholic. He was hospitalized 3 weeks before death for open reduction of a fractured femur. Postoperatively, he developed fever and positive blood cultures. In spite of intravenous antibiotic therapy he died several days later. (A) Opened right atrium (RA), tricuspid valve, and right ventricle (RV). A large vegetation is present on the septal tricuspid leaflet (STL). ATL, anterior tricuspid valve leaflet. (B) Opened aortic valve. The infection has burrowed through the membranous ventricular septum (circle) and is visible between the right (R) and noncoronary (N) aortic valve cusps. LV, left ventricle. (C), (D) Longitudinal cuts through the atrial septum, aortic valve (AV) cusp, septal tricuspid leaflet (STL), and membranous (M) and muscular ventricular septum (VS). The vegetation has extended cephalad from the base of the septal tricuspid leaflet producing a large abscess (Abs) in the membranous (M) ventricular septum. (E) Histologic section of (D). The dark stained material is composed of fibrin, leukocytes, and colonies of gram-positive cocci. Movat. × 2.

have vegetations on left-sided cardiac valves[11,17] (Fig.2-4). Of the 24 patients with right-sided vegetation studied by the author, 10 (42 percent) also had left-sided valvular infection, and among these patients signs of left-sided valvular infection predominated;[11,17] 7 had signs of left-sided valvular dysfunction and left ventricular failure, and 4 had systemic emboli with gross infarcts in other organs.

SPLENOMEGALY

Splenomegaly is as common in patients with isolated right-sided vegetations as it is in patients with left-sided vegetations. Splenomegaly (> 300) was present at necropsy in 9 of our 24 patients in whom the splenic weight was known, including 6 of the 14 patients with isolated right-sided vegetations. Infection appears to be a more important cause of splenomegaly than congestive cardiac failure. Arnett,[49] in 1922, analyzed the frequency of splenomegaly among 286 necropsy patients dying from either active IE nonendocardial streptococcal infections, or congestive heart failure due to causes other than IE. He found that, while splenomegaly was most frequent among the patients with active IE, it was more frequent among patients with nonendocardial streptococcal infections than among patients with congestive cardiac failure from causes other than IE.

Active IE Limited to Native Left-Sided Cardiac Valves (Figs. 2-5–2-18)

The study at necropsy of 74 patients with active IE limited to one or both left-sided cardiac valves and the review of reports of others disclosed several principles applicable to IE at this site: (1) isolated left-sided IE is about four times more frequent than either isolated right-sided IE or right- plus left-sided IE; (2) the initial clinical presentation is primarily that of a systemic infection, not cardiac disease; (3) a precordial murmur almost always is present, but the murmur is not necessarily indicative of valvular damage or destruction by vegetative material; (4) an obvious predisposing factor to infection is usually (70 percent) present; (5) the IE involves previously anatomically and functionally normal valves in over half the patients and previously functionally normal but anatomically abnormal valves in another 20 percent; (6) IE involving the aortic valve is now more frequent than IE involving the mitral valve; (7) ring abscess is common only when IE involves the aortic valve; (8) pericarditis in patients with IE is primarily a complication of infection involving the aortic valve; (9) staphylococci are more common than streptococci as the infecting organism among necropsy patients with isolated left-sided IE; (10) whereas right-sided IE is usually a complication of infection elsewhere in the body (i.e., secondary), isolated left-sided IE is a primary infection in over 95 percent of patients; (11) associated acute meningitis and pneu-

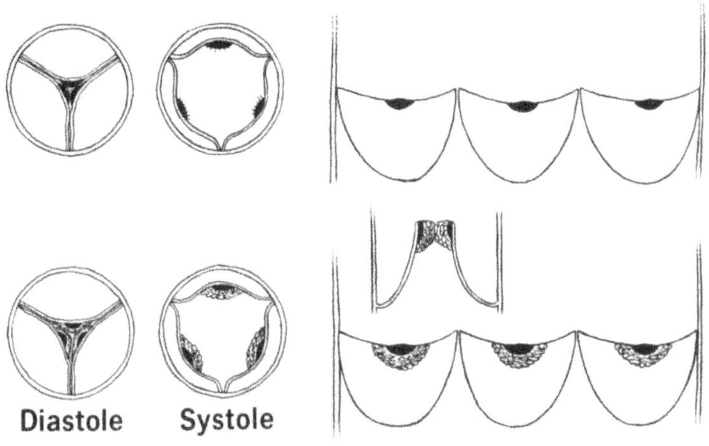

Fig. 2–5. Most common location of vegetations on the aortic valve, i.e., on the ventricular aspects of each cusp, central portion, at the distal margin. It is at this site that fibrous bumps (nodules of Arantii) develop from contact of the cusps with one another during ventricular diastole. Although the vegetations probably begin on only one cusp, they probably spread quickly to the other cusps. The cuspal bumps are not present in childhood; their absence in this age group may be responsible for the relative infrequency of IE in childhood.

monitis is much less frequent than in right-sided IE; and (12) death is most commonly (about 60 percent) the result of cardiac dysfunction rather than the result of the systemic infection or emboli.

Many morphologic observations concerning IE were made in patients dying in the preantibiotic era when IE was a uniformly fatal disease. Since the introduction of antibiotic therapy, however, a number of important changes have occurred:[26,50–52] (1) the frequency of rheumatic heart disease as an underlying condition has declined,[53–55] and consequently the etiologies of the underlying valve diseases in patients with IE have changed; (2) frequency of IE in patients with normal cardiac valves has increased;[12,17] (3) the frequency and mortality of alpha-hemolytic streptococcal endocarditis has increased;[12,17] (4) the frequency of aortic valve infection has increased, and that of mitral valve infection has decreased;[12,17] and (5) congestive heart failure has replaced infection as the leading cause of death among patients with IE.[12,17]

UNDERLYING VALVE DISEASE

To emphasize the change in the types of underlying valve disease observed today compared to earlier periods, among our 74 patients, including 22 with isolated mitral valve vegetations, only 10 (13 percent) had rheumatic valvular disease. Of the 52 patients with aortic valve vegetations, 12 (23 percent) had congenitally malformed valves (bicuspid in 9) (Fig. 2-6). Only in recent years has it been recognized that isolated aortic-valve disease rarely is caused by rheumatic fever.[53-55] Consequently, it is likely that many infected scarred aortic valves in earlier reports were congenital rather than rheumatic in origin. Of our 5 patients with aortic valve vegetations who were over 65 years of age, 4 had degenerative aortic valve disease and 1 had previously normal valves except for aging changes. In 1949 Traut and associates[56] reported on 94 necropsy patients with IE over 45 years of age. They found that 46 (49 percent) had isolated aortic valve vegetations and 5 (11 percent) had underlying degenerative aortic valve disease. Among 41 necropsy patients with IE over 60 years of age reported by Thell and associates[57] in 1975, 6 (14 percent) had degenerative aortic valve disease. A floppy mitral valve, which increases the risk of developing IE,[58] was present in 2 of our patients. In contrast, among 399 necropsy patients with IE summarized from several studies[23,59,60-62] in the preantibiotic era, 258 (65 percent) were stated to have underlying rheumatic valvular disease. Among 424 patients with IE studied clinically by Christian[63] and by Kelson and White,[64] 381 (90 percent) had underlying rheumatic valvular disease. The declining frequency of rheumatic heart disease, the lowered frequency of IE in patients with rheumatic valvular disease, and the increasing age of patients with IE appear to account for these changes.[65,66]

INVOLVEMENT OF PREVIOUSLY NORMAL VALVES

IE occurring on previously normal valves (Figs. 2-7, 2-10, 2-11, and 2-13–2-17) has been considered unusual. Of 1056 necropsy patients with IE summarized from several studies,[23,24,26,51,56,62,67,68-71] 26 percent had previously normal valves. Among our 74 patients with active left-sided valvular endocarditis, however, 41 (55 percent) had anatomically normal valves before the onset of IE, and 4 of the 33 with anatomically abnormal valves and functionally normal valves before the onset of IE. Thus, 67 percent of our 74 patients had functionally normal valves before the onset of IE. Morgan and Bland,[51] Wilson,[26] Uwaydah and Weinberg,[72] and Lerner and Weinstein[67] noted an increasing number of patients with IE involving previously functionally normal valves. The mortality from IE is considerably higher among patients with previously normal valves than among patients with previously abnormal valves.[12,16] Rabinovich and associates[73] found IE to be fatal in 83 percent (10 of 12) of their patients with IE involving previously normal valves, and in 48 percent (61 of 129) of their patients with IE involving previously abnormal valves. Of the 51 patients with fatal active IE reported by Pankey,[44] 63 percent had had previously normal cardiac valves.

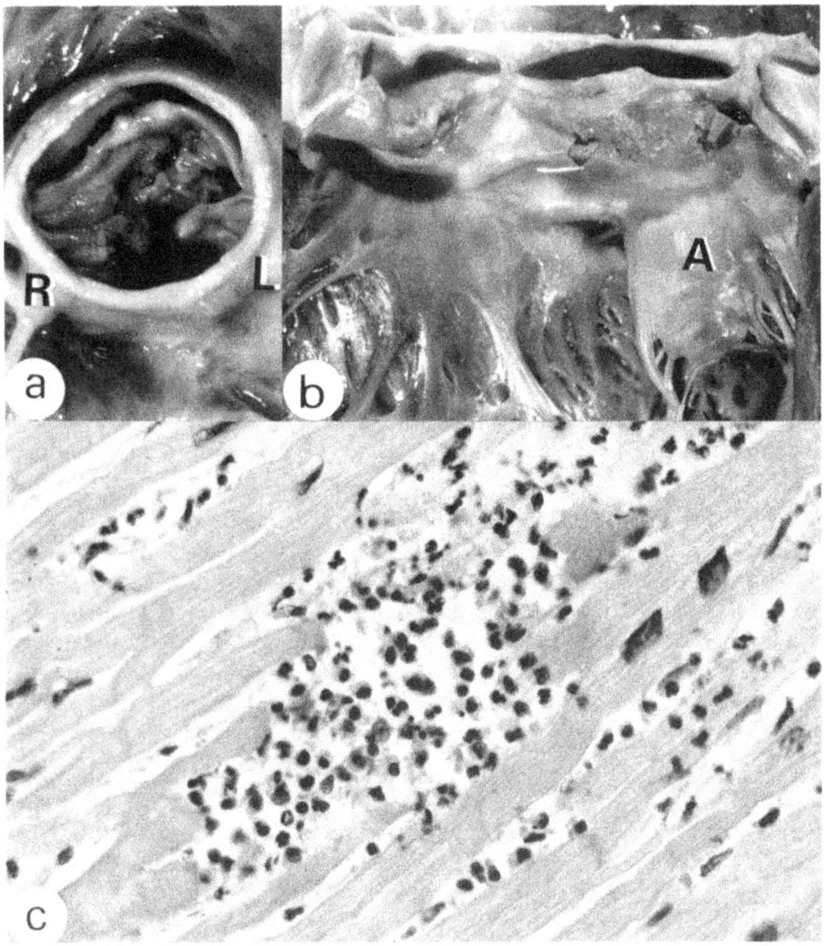

Fig. 2-6. *Staphylococcus aureus* endocarditis involving a congenitally bicuspid aortic valve in a 55-year-old woman. She had never had symptoms of cardiac disease when chillls, fever, and mental confusion appeared 4½ months before death. Blood cultures were positive for *S. aureus*, and penicillin, 40 million units/day intravenously for 4 weeks, followed by 24 million units/day intramuscularly for 2 weeks, was given. A grade 4/6 early diastolic blowing murmur appeared, and the diastolic blood pressure fell to 20 mm Hg. Six days after penicillin was stopped she had a shaking chill and blood cultures were again positive for *S. aureus*. Over the next 3 months she was treated with various combinations of penicillin, methicillin, cephalothin, and vancomycin but each time antibiotics were withdrawn blood cultures again grew *S. aureus*. Signs of congestive cardiac failure increased progressively, the diastolic pressure rose to 60 mm Hg, and the aortic regurgitation became almost inaudible several days before death. (A) Bicuspid aortic valve viewed from above. Both the right (R) and left (L) coronary

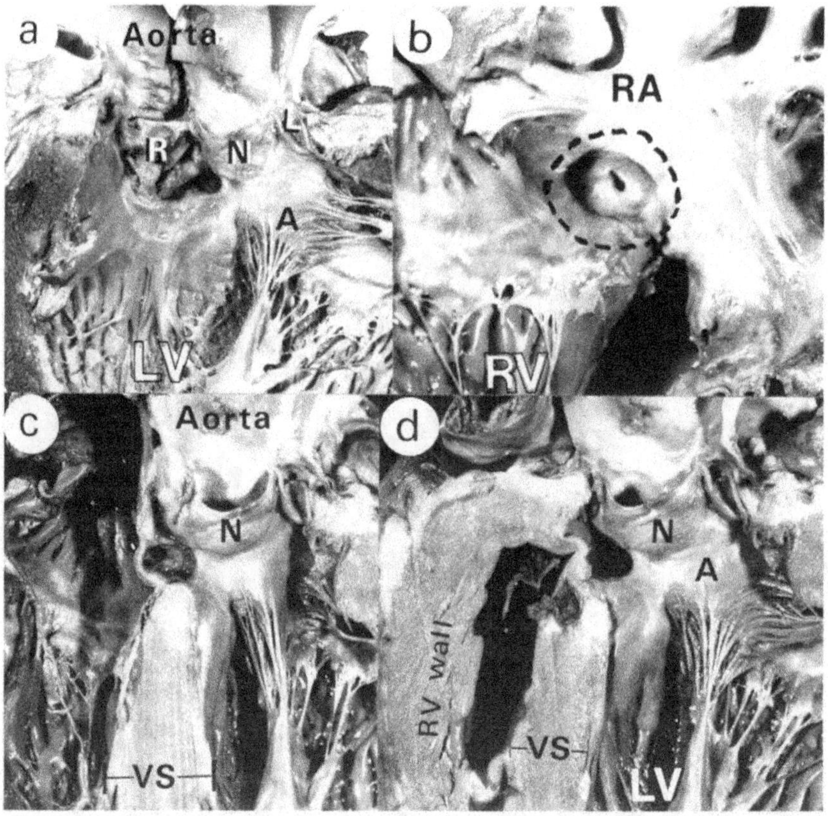

Fig. 2–7. *Staphylococcus epidermidis* aortic valve endocarditis in a 17-year-old boy. Massive aortic regurgitation and right bundle branch block developed during the infection and he died 28 days after the onset of symptoms. (A) Opened aortic valve and left ventricle. The right (R) coronary cusp is destroyed by the infection and a ring abscess is present behind this cusp. N and L, non- and left coronary cusps; A, anterior mitral leaflet; LV, left ventricle. (B) Opened right atrium (RA), tricuspid valve, and right ventricle (RV) showing a bulging membranous ventricular septum (dashed circle) with a perforation in its center. (C) Longitudinal section through the aneurysm in the ventricular septum (VS). (D) Longitudinal section anterior to (C) showing a ring abscess in the muscular portion of the ventricular septum.

---

arteries arise from the anterior sinus. (B) Opened aortic valve and left ventricle. Perforations are present in both cusps. A, anterior mitral leaflet. (C) Histologic section showing microabscess in left ventricular wall. Hematoxylin–eosin stain. × 400.

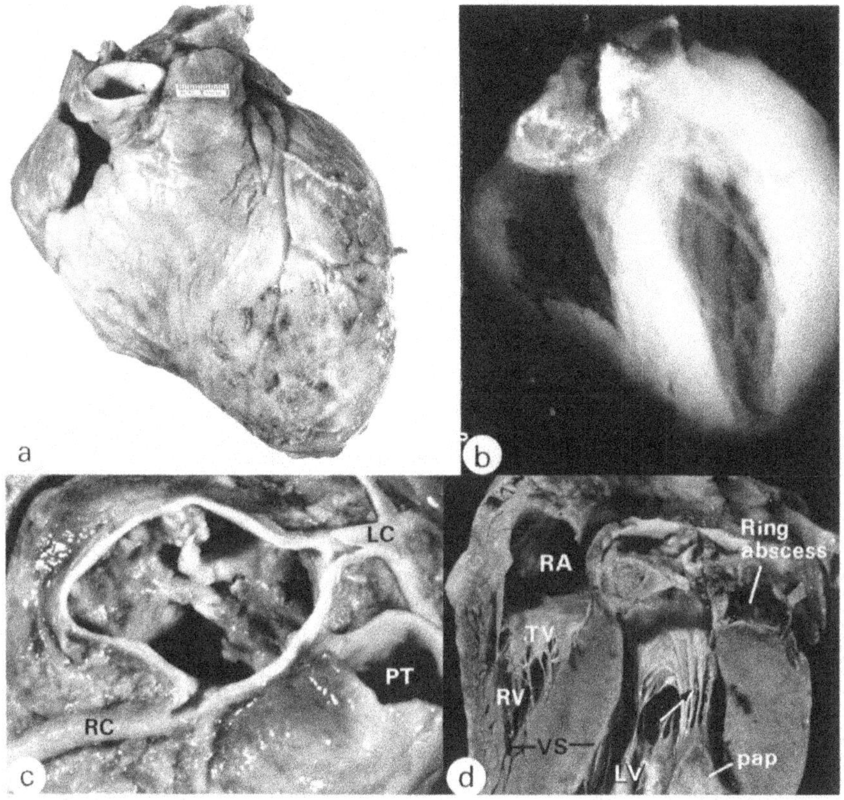

Fig. 2–8. Alpha streptococcus endocarditis involving a calcified, stenotic, congenitally bicuspid aortic valve in a 54-year-old man. Fever and syncope occurred several weeks after tooth extraction and blood cultures were positive. Despite antibiotic therapy, signs of left ventricular failure increased, and he died 23 days after the onset of symptoms of infection. (A) Anterior view of the heart showing focal fibrinous pericarditis. (B) Postmortem roentgenograph of the heart. A large amount of calcium is present in the aortic valve. (C) Bicuspid aortic valve viewed from above. RC, right coronary artery; LC, left coronary artery; PT, pulmonary trunk. (D) Longitudinal section through the aortic valve, right atrium (RA), tricuspid valve (TV), right ventricle (RV), ventricular septum (VS), and left ventricle (LV). A large ring abscess is present. Vegetations also are present on several mitral valve chordae tendineae (arrow). The tip of the papillary muscle (Pap) is necrotic. The pericarditis probably resulted from rupture of the right abscess into the pericardial space.

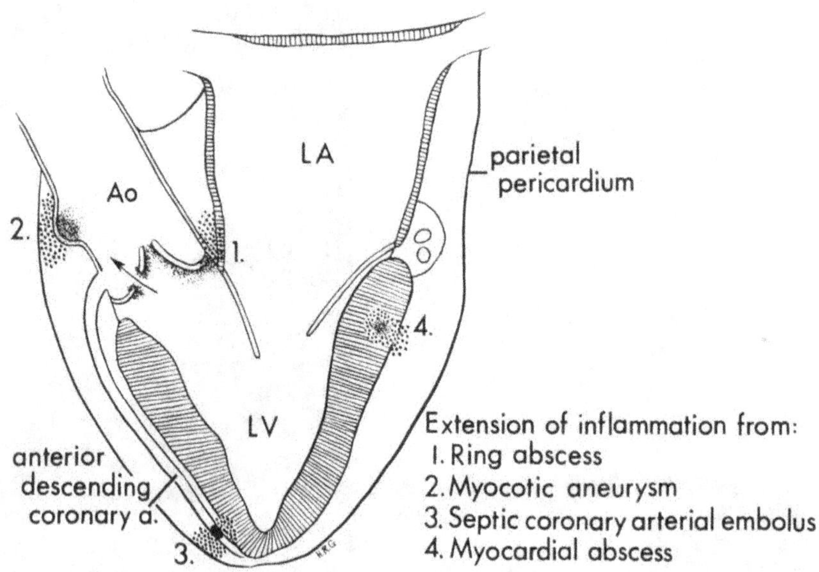

Fig. 2–9. Mechanisms by which pericarditis can develop in patients with active IE.

ORGANISMS INVOLVED

When an anatomically normal valve is the site of infection, the causative organism is usually a highly virulent one. Thayer[24] noted IE on previously normal valves in 63 percent of 70 patients with staphylococcal or pneumococcal endocarditis and in only 20 percent of patients with IE caused by α-hemolytic streptococcus. Finland and Barnes[74] found functionally normal valves in 185 (68 percent) of 271 episodes of IE caused by organisms other than α-hemolytic streptococcus or *Staphylococcus epidermidis*. Among 22 (54 percent) of our 41 patients with previously normal valves, the infection was caused by *Staphylococcus aureus* in 11 patients, *Diplococcus pneumoniae* in 5, and by *Streptococcus faecalis* in 6. Alpha-hemolytic streptococcus was the most frequent causative organism among our patients with previously abnormal valves, but accounted for only 7 (21 percent) of the infections in these 33 patients. Highly virulent bacteria generally cause a more acute illness, and mortality is higher both among patients with infection caused by a highly virulent bacterium[73,75] and among patients with shorter duration of symptoms before diagnosis.[73,76]

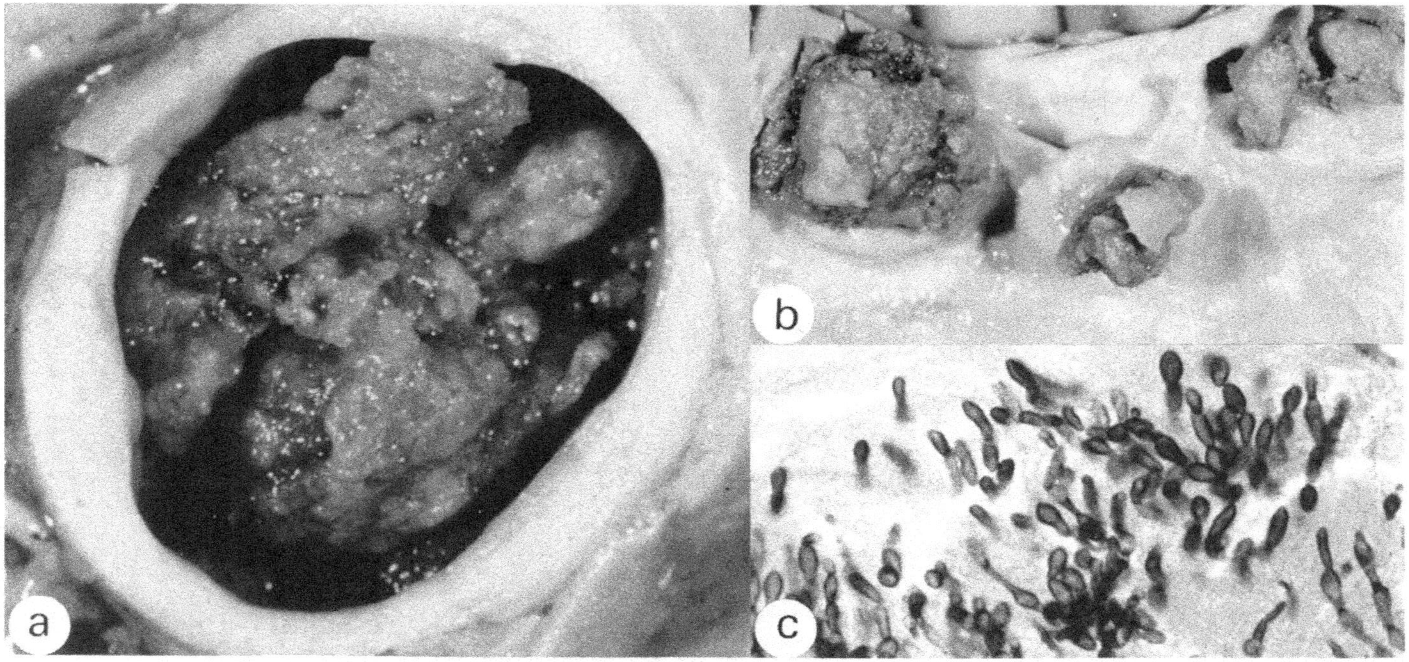

Fig. 2–10. *Candida parapsilosis* endocarditis involving the aortic valve of a 26-year-old male heroin addict. This patient lived for 8 months after initial symptoms and signs of IE appeared. He had an embolus to the left anterior descending coronary artery with a huge transmural acute myocardial infarct 2 months before death. (A) aortic valve viewed from above. The large vegetations appear to obstruct the valve orifice. (B) Opened valve showing vegetations on each cusp. (C) Photomicrograph of vegetation showing pseudomycelia of (C) *parapsilosis*. Methenamine silver. × 775.

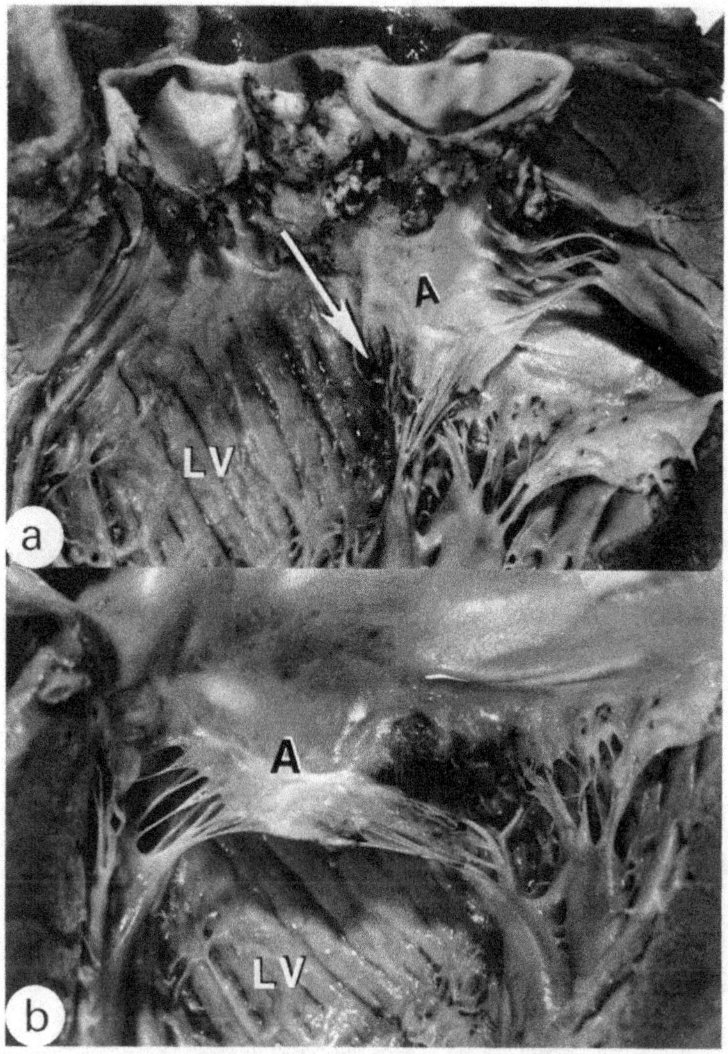

Fig. 2–11. *Streptococcus faecalis* endocarditis involving both aortic and mitral valves in a 61-year-old man. Symptoms and signs of endocarditis appeared 3 weeks after catheterization of his urinary bladder. Both aortic and mitral valves were probably normal before they became sites of infection. (A) Opened left ventricle (LV) and aortic valve. The vegetations have partially destroyed each cusp, causing severe aortic regurgitation. Vegetation on the left ventricular outflow endocardium, mitral leaflet, and chordae tendineae almost certainly resulted from retrograde spread of the aortic vegetations by the aortic regurgitant stream (arrow). A, anterior mitral leaflet. (B) Opened mitral valve showing vegetations at the posteromedial commissure. A number of chordae tendineae are ruptured.

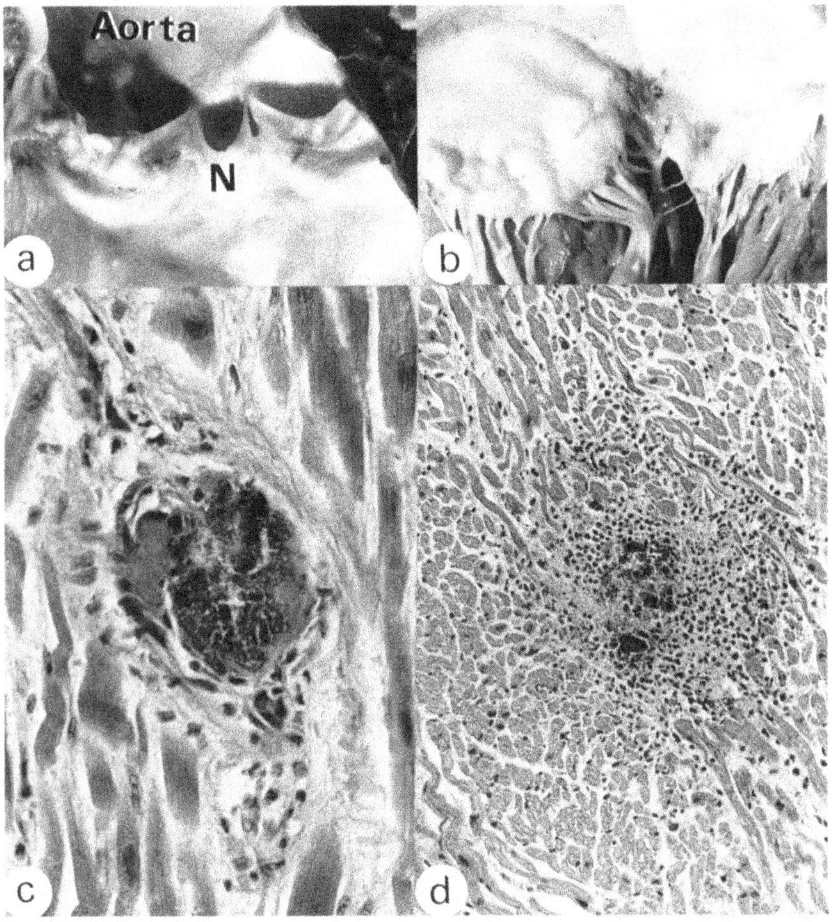

Fig. 2–12. *Staphylococcus aureus* endocarditis in a 36-year-old man with mycosis fungoides. Pneumonia, septicemia, and renal failure occurred in the terminal phase of his chronic illness, but signs of cardiac dysfunction were never present. (A) Opened aorta and aortic valve. The noncoronary (N) cusp is much smaller than the other two cusps, each of which contains vegetations. (B) Opened left atrium, mitral valve, and left ventricle. Small vegetations are present at the posteromedial commissure, but there is no valvular destruction. (C) Histologic section of left ventricular myocardium showing a septic embolus in the lumen of an intramural coronary artery. Hematoxylin–eosin. × 400. (D) Section of myocardium showing a microscopic-sized abscess. Hemotoxylin–eosin. × 160. The dark material in both C and D represents colonies of organisms.

AORTIC VERSUS MITRAL VALVE INFECTION

Among necropsy patients with IE occurring after the introduction of antibiotic therapy, the frequency of aortic valve infection has increased and the frequency of mitral valve infection has decreased.[12,16,26] Of our 74 patients, 52 (70 percent) had infection of the aortic valve, and 36 (49 percent) had infection of the mitral valve. Of the latter 36 patients, however, 18 also had aortic valve infection, and in at least 13 (72 percent) of them the mitral infection appeared to be secondary to the aortic valve IE[16] In a study of 656 patients with IE seen at the Columbia Presbyterian Medical Center between 1938 and 1967, Cherubin and Neu[77] found a progressive increase in aortic valve involvement and a decline in mitral valve infection over the three decades. Of 28 necropsy patients with IE who died in 1969 in Kampala, Uganda, 15 (54 percent) had isolated aortic valve vegetation.[78]

CONGESTIVE HEART FAILURE

Congestive heart failure has replaced infection as the leading cause of death among patients with IE, and damage to the aortic valve is the most common cause of the failure in patients with IE.[12,16,67] Of our 74 patients, 45 (61 percent), including 33 with aortic valve vegetations, died from congestive heart failure, and in each of them the IE had caused severe valve destruction. In a study by Robinson and Ruedy,[79] congestive heart failure was the cause of death in only 6 percent of patients with IE in the pre-antibiotic era, but caused death in 61 percent of those with fatal IE after the introduction of antibiotic therapy. The increased frequency of congestive heart failure resulted from the increased frequency of valve destruction by the vegetations: 16 percent of patients with fatal IE in the preantibiotic era and 45 percent in the antibiotic era had cuspal perforations. In nearly all patients in both eras, the perforations involved the aortic valve. Among 33 patients with IE studied by Cohen and Freedman,[80] damage to the aortic valve was the most common cause of death. Of 14 patients with acute aortic regurgitation from IE reported by Fowler and associates,[81] 10 developed severe congestive heart failure within 4 months of the onset of IE, and 9 of them died.

HEMODYNAMIC CONSEQUENCES

The hemodynamic consequence of IE is almost always regurgitation. IE caused aortic regurgitation in 36 (69 percent) of our 52 patients with aortic valve vegetations and mitral regurgitation in 14 (64 percent) of our 22 patients with isolated mitral vegetations. It also caused mitral regurgitation in 9 of the 52 patients with aortic valve vegetations. Massive vegetations caused valvular stenosis in 1 patient with IE involving the aortic valve and in 1 patient with IE involving the mitral valve.[8]

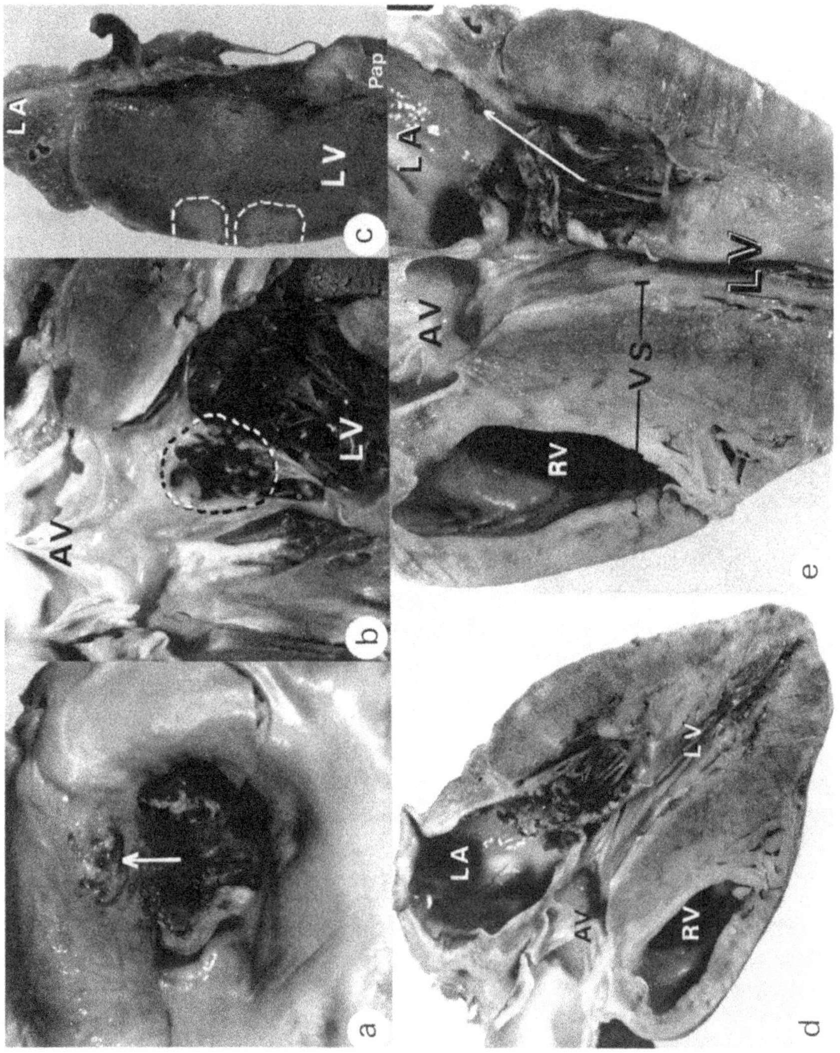
a
b
AV
LV
c
LA
LV
Pap
d
LA
AV
RV
LV
e
RV
VS
AV
LA
LV

Fig. 2–13. *Streptococcus faecalis* mitral valve endocarditis in a 36-year-old male heroin addict. Five months before death he presented with fever and a precordial murmur, and blood cultures were positive. He was treated with antibiotics intravenously, but 4 months later symptoms of congestive heart failure appeared, and blood cultures were again positive for *S. faecalis*. An echocardiogram showed mitral valve vegetations and ruptured chordae tendineae. Despite a second course of intravenous antibiotics, he died from progressive congestive heart failure. (A) Mitral valve viewed from left atrium. Vegetations are present both on the valve and on the left atrial endocardium (arrow). (B) Opened aortic valve (AV) and left ventricle (LV). A perforation (circle) is present in the anterior mitral leaflet. (C) Longitudinal cut including portions of left atrial wall (LA), posterior mitral leaflet, and left venticular free wall. A portion of the leaflet curls toward the left atrium. The tip of the papillary muscle (Pap) is necrotic, and abscesses (dashed lines) are present in the left ventricular wall. (D) Longitudinal cut of the heart. There is extensive destruction of the mitral valve, and a portion of the leaflets as well as several ruptured chordae are prolapsed into left atrium (LA). The papillary muscle is partially necrotic, and multiple abscesses are present in the left ventricular wall. The left atrial cavity is of normal size and the right ventricular (RV) wall is thick, suggesting the presence of pulmonary hypertension. (E) Close-up of the mitral valve showing the ruptured chordae and the left atrial mural (jet) vegetations (arrow).

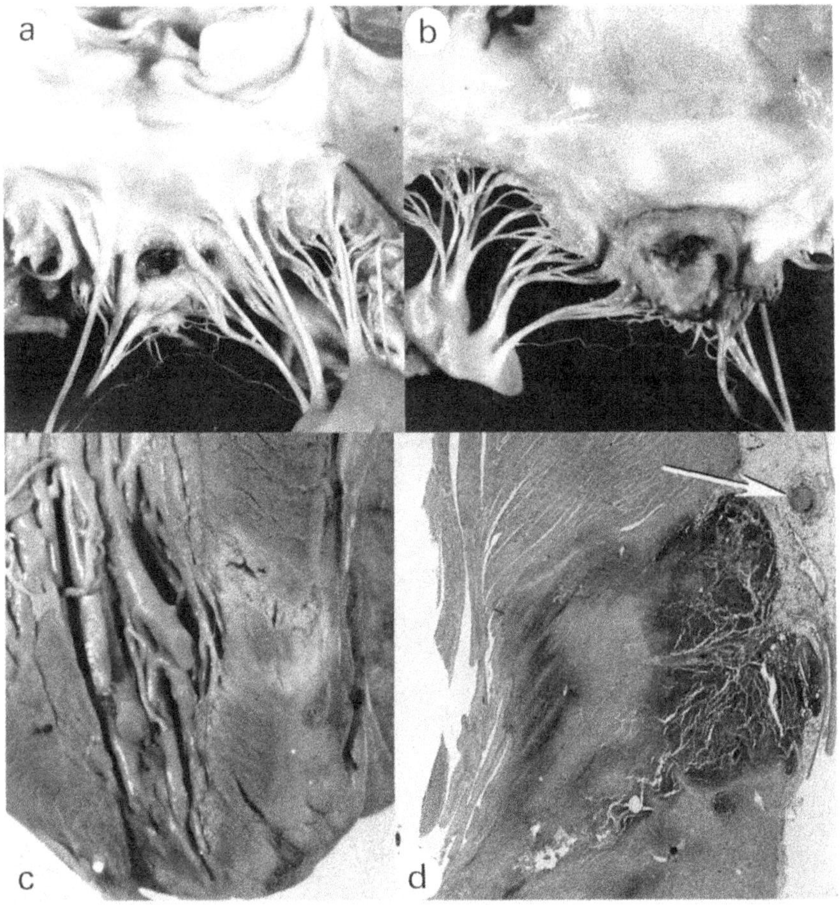

Fig. 2-14. Pneumococcal mitral valve endocarditis in a 43-year-old male chronic alcoholic. Two weeks before death he was hospitalized because of acute pneumonia and acute meningitis. He never had signs of cardiac dysfunction and died of gastrointestinal hemorrhage. (A) Opened left ventricle showing a small vegetation on the ventricular surface of the anterior mitral leaflet. (B) Atrial aspect of anterior mitral leaflet showing a single large vegetation. The valve cusps are otherwise normal. (C) Longitudinal section showing transmural necrosis of the left ventricular wall. (D) Photomicrograph of area in (C) showing extensive myocardial necrosis. An extramural coronary artery (arrow) is occluded by vegetative material. Hematoxylin–eosin. × 2.5.

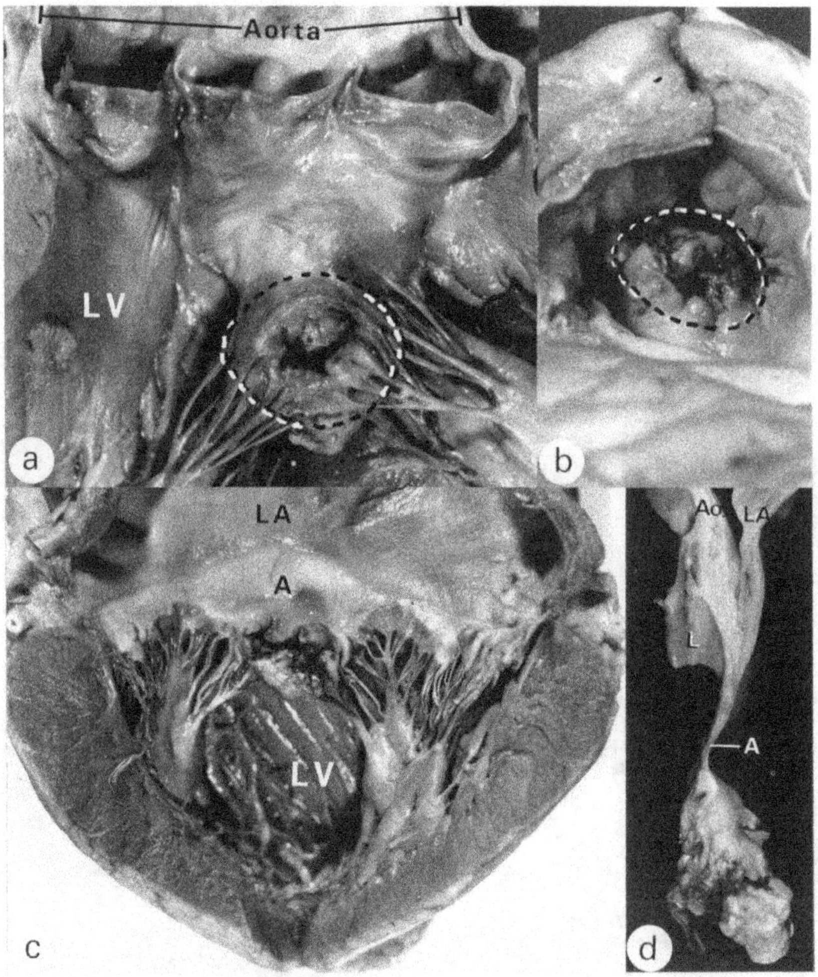

Fig. 2-15. *Serratia marcescens* mitral valve endocarditis in a 59-year-old male chronic alcoholic. He was hospitalized 16 days before death because of fever and leg pain of sudden onset. Examination disclosed an apical systolic murmur, and an echocardiogram revealed a density between the anterior and posterior mitral valve leaflets. Clinical and roentgenographic signs of acute pneumonia appeared shortly after admission and sputum cultures were positive for *S. marcescens*. Blood cultures were negative until the time of death, but postmortem cultures of the mitral valve vegetation grew *S. marcescens*. (A) Opened aorta, aortic valve, and left ventricle (LV). A large perforation (circle) is present in the anterior mitral leaflet. (B) Mitral valve with vegetation (dashed circle) viewed from left atrium. (C) Opened left atrium (LA), mitral valve, and left ventricle. The large vegetation on the anterior mitral leaflet (A) is apparent. (D) Longitudinal section through aorta (Ao), left atrial wall (LA), left coronary cusp (L) of aortic valve, and anterior mitral leaflet (A) showing the large mitral valve vegetation.

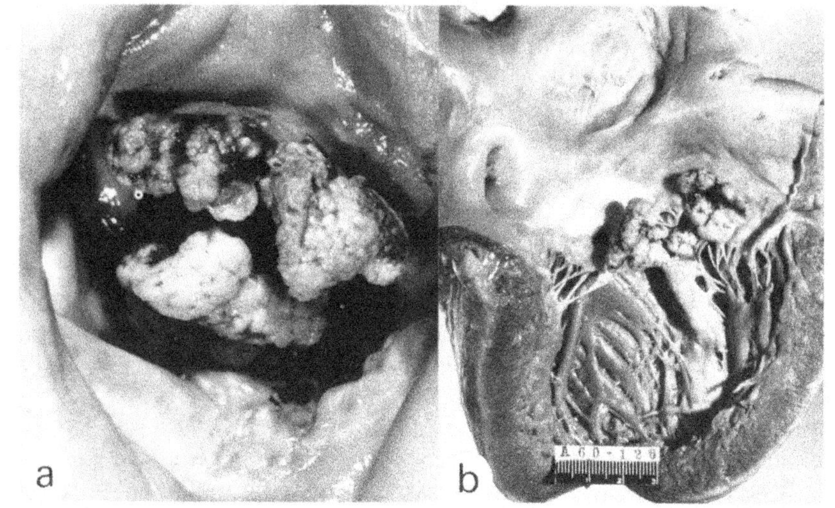

Fig. 2-16. *Candida parapsilosis* endocarditis on a previously normal mitral valve of a 68-year-old man with chronic lung disease and coronary heart disease. Five months before death he had fever, and 45 days later he was hospitalized. A grade 2/6 apical systolic murmur was present. Despite amphotericin B therapy, blood cultures remained positive, and he died of congestive heart failure. A large embolus to the left common iliac artery occurred. (A) Mitral valve viewed from left atrium showing large vegetations on both leaflets. (B) Opened left ventricle showing large vegetations on both leaflets.

RING ABSCESS

Valve ring abscess (Figs. 2-7–2-9 and 2-17) is frequent in patients with IE involving the aortic valve and rare in patients with IE of the mitral valve.[14] Valve ring abscess was present in 24 (32 percent) of our 74 patients; in 22 (92 percent) the ring abscess involved the aortic valve and in only 2 (8 percent), the mitral valve. One of the latter 2 patients had isolated mitral valve infection with ring abscess; the other had aortic valve vegetations and infection of a heavily calcified mitral valve anulus.[82,83] Each of the 24 patients with valve ring abscess had valvular regurgitation from IE.

PERICARDITIS AND ATRIOVENTRICULAR BLOCK

Pericarditis and atrioventricular block in patients with IE almost always is the result of ring abscess, and therefore usually complicates aortic valve infection.[14] Pericarditis was present in 16 (22 percent) of our 74 patients, and in 15 of them vegetations were present on the aortic valve. In 11 of the 16 patients, the pericarditis resulted from rupture of an aortic valve ring abscess into the pericardial space. Rokitansky,[20] in 1856, recognized that ring abscess may be associated with pericarditis and myocarditis, and that it may cause a cardiac aneurysm which may rupture into a cardiac chamber or pericardial space. Ponfick,[84] in 1873, again noted the association of IE with pericarditis, and Osler,[21] in 1885, noted the tendency of valve ring abscess to burrow into adjacent structures. Of 43 consecutive necropsy patients with IE studied by Beck,[85] 8 (16 percent) had pericarditis, and 5 of them had an aortic valve ring abscess with perforation into the pericardial space. McColl[86] reported a patient with pericarditis due to myocotic aneurysm from IE, and concluded from review of previously reported cases that perforation of an aortic valve ring abscess was the most frequent cause of pericarditis in patients with IE. A similar observation was made by Buchbinder and Roberts.[12] Among 38 patients with aortic valve IE reported by Utley and Mills,[76] 15 had ring abscess, and 5 of them had pericarditis. Thus, the occurrence of a pericardial friction rub or pericardial effusion during the course of IE is highly suggestive of ring abscess.

Either complete heart block or a high degree of heart block appearing suddenly in a patient with IE is highly suggestive of the presence of a ring abscess, that has extended into the area of the atrioventricular node or bundle.[14] Of our 6 patients with either complete (5 patients) or Mobitz type II atrioventricular block, 5 had a ring abscess, 4 of which involved the aortic valve. In addition, the appearance of complete right or left bundle branch block during IE is also highly suggestive of the presence of a ring abscess with extension into the most cephalad portion of the muscular ventricular septum.[14] Although only 1 of our patients developed complete right bundle branch block and none developed complete left bundle branch block, the latter has been reported in aortic valve endocarditis by Roberts and Somerville.[87]

MYOCARDIAL INFLAMMATORY LESIONS

Myocardial inflammatory lesions (Figs. 2-6-2-9-2-12- and 2-14) are frequent in patients with IE. Clawson,[23] Buchbinder and Saphir,[88] Saphir,[89] and Perry and associates[69] each observed myocardial lesions in 88 –100 percent of 187 patients with IE studied by them at necropsy. Myocardial inflammatory lesions were observed in 56 (85 percent) of our 66 patients in whom numerous histologic sections of myocardium were examined. The significance of myocardial lesions in patients with IE has been debated. Clawson[23] and Correl and associates[90] considered the lesions to be a major cause of congestive heart failure in patients with active IE. de Navasquez[91] and Perry and associates,[69] however, believed that congestive heart failure in patients with IE was rarely the result of myocardial lesions. In none of our patients did we attribute congestive cardiac failure to the myocardial inflammatory lesion.

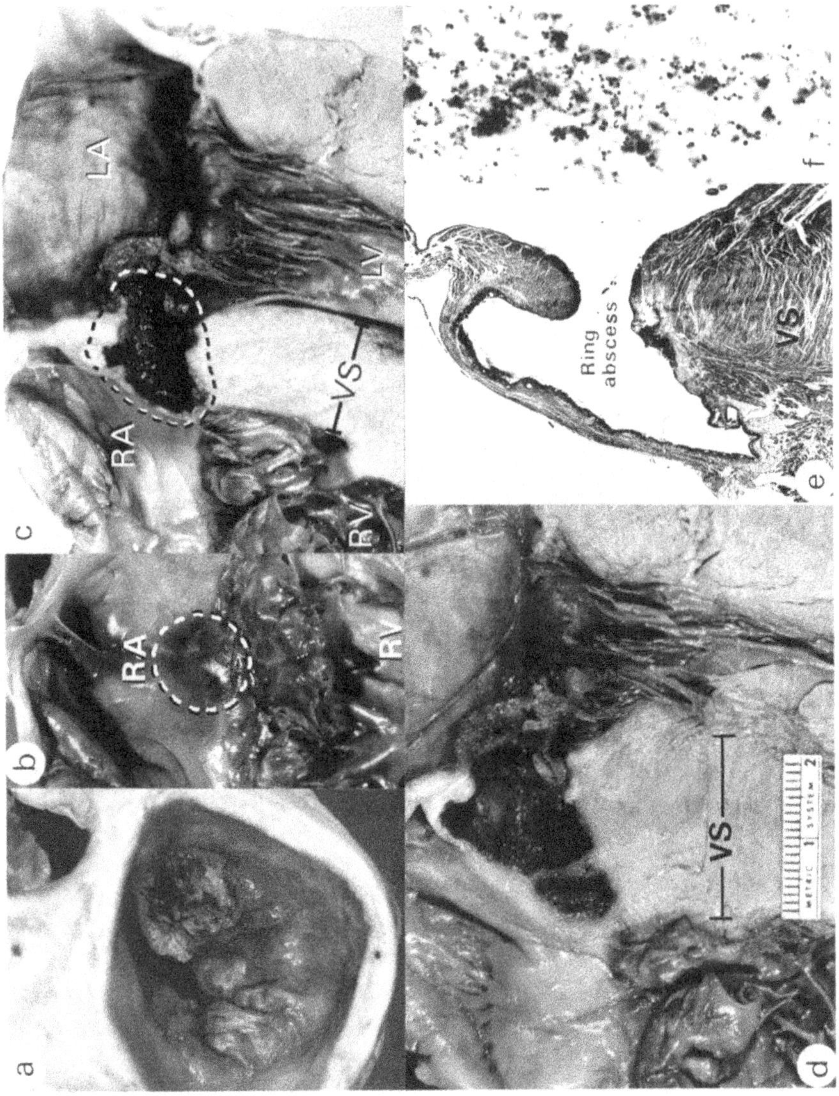
a
b
c
d
e
f
RA
RV
LA
LV
VS
Ring abscess

Fig. 2–17. *Staphylococcus aureus* mitral valve endocarditis with ring abscess in a 66-year-old diabetic man. During hospitalization for treatment of an infected foot, fever developed and blood cultures were positive. Complete heart block and a murmur of mitral regurgitation appeared and he died soon thereafter. (A) Mitral valve viewed from left atrium. Vegetations are present in the region of the posteromedial commissure. (B) Opened right atrium (RA), tricuspid valve, and right ventricle (RV). An abscess (dashed circle) is visible in the area of the membranous septum. (C) Longitudinal section through the four cardiac chambers and both atrioventricular valves. The mitral ring abscess (dashed circle) involves both atrial and ventricular septa. RA, right atrium; RV, right ventricle; LA, left atrium; LV, left ventricle; VS, ventricular septum. (D) Longitudinal section posterior to C showing the abscess in the ventricular septum. (E) Histologic section of the ring abscess. Movat. × 4. (F) Histologic section showing gram-positive cocci in the ring abscess. Brown and Brenn. × 880.

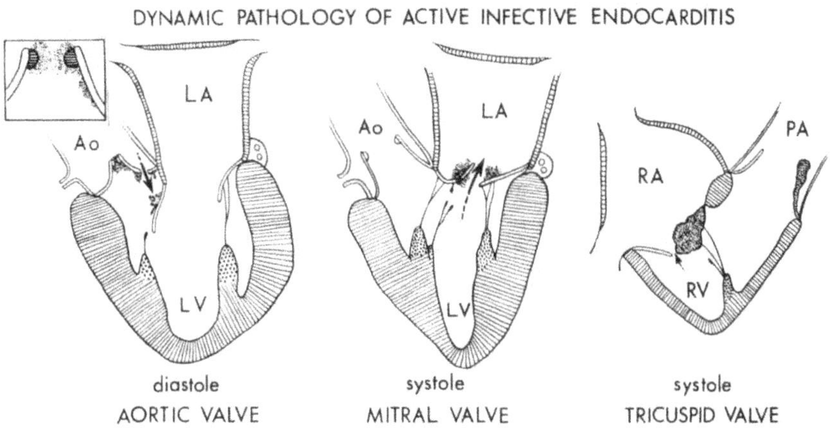

Fig. 2–18. Dynamic pathology of IE. Aortic valve vegetations occur initially on nodules of Anantii with subsequent involvement of more cuspal surface. Resultant perforation of aortic valve cusps may allow regurgitant flow to carry vegetative material onto the ventricular surface of the anterior mitral leaflet. Dotted areas in papillary muscles represent necrosis. When the mitral valve is the initial focus of IE, the vegetations begin on the atrial aspects of the leaflets. Subsequent extension may involve the chordae tendineae, which, if ruptured, cause mitral regurgitation. In right-sided IE the vegetations often involve the cores of the cusps and their surfaces may remain relatively smooth.

PAPILLARY MUSCLE NECROSIS

Papillary muscle necrosis (Figs. 2–8, 2–13, and 2–18) is common in patients with fatal IE with or without associated coronary arterial narrowing.[92] Foci of necrosis were observed in the left ventricular papillary muscles in 39 (59 percent) of our 66 patients in whom sections of both left ventricular papillary muscles were examined. Only 13 of the 39 patients had significant coronary arterial narrowing: by emboli to intramural coronary arteries in 5, by emboli to both intramural and extramural coronary arteries in 5,[93] and by severe (more than 75 percent cross-sectional area luminal narrowing) atherosclerosis in 3, 1 of whom also had coronary arterial emboli. The significant correlation ($p < 0.02$) between papillary muscle necrosis and valve dysfunction resulting in congestive heart failure[12,92] suggests that the necrosis results from poor arterial perfusion associated with the congestive heart failure because the papillary muscles are the last portion of myocardium to be supplied by arterial blood.[94,95] Despite papillary muscle necrosis, no patient had mitral regurgitation in the absence of destruction of mitral leaflets or ruptured chordae tendineae.

Active IE Involving Prosthetic Cardiac Valves (Figs. 2-19–2-22)

The study at necropsy of 23 patients with prosthetic valve endocarditis (PVE)[5–7,15–17,19,96–102] and the review of reports of others disclosed several principles applicable to IE involving rigid-framed prosthetic cardiac valves: (1) PVE is infrequent, its frequency probably being less than 1 percent per year among patients with prosthetic cardiac valves; (2) PVE is now more frequently a late (onset more than 2 months after valve replacement) than an early complication of valve replacement; (3) most early-onset cases result from intraoperative infection or wound infection; (4) staphylococci are the most frequent offending organisms and streptococci are the least frequent; (5) unless the PVE is caused by a fungus, blood cultures are virtually always positive; (6) signs of prosthetic valve dysfunction are usually present when the aortic valve prosthesis is infected, and are usually absent when the mitral prosthesis is infected; (7) in virtually all patients with PVE the infection involves the site of attachment of the prosthesis, or in other words, ring abscess is almost always present; (8) because the infective process often extends to adjacent tissues, associated complete heart block or left bundle branch block or intracardiac fistulae are common; (9) diagnosis of PVE in the early postoperative period may be difficult, whereas it is usually easy in the late postoperative period; (10) prognosis in patients with PVE is usually dismal; and (11) certain clear morphologic differences exist between patients with PVE involving one or both left-sided cardiac valves and patients with active IE involving native cardiac valves.

PVE AS COMPLICATION OF VALVE REPLACEMENT

Although a devastating complication of cardiac valve replacement, PVE fortunately is an infrequent complication of valve replacement. Its exact frequency is uncertain but it is clearly less than 1 percent per year among patients with prosthetic cardiac valves.[15] Although prospective studies[103,104] have been inconclusive, retrospective studies[105,106] have shown a reduction in the frequency of early (less than 2 months after valve replacement) PVE coincident with the use of prophylactic antibiotics. Late infection now appears to be more common than early infection,[15,107,108] presumably because there are now so many persons with prosthetic cardiac valves. Although the mortality rate is high for both groups, early infection from PVE apparently is more often fatal than late infection.[107,108]

ORIGINS OF EARLY INFECTIONS

Most early infections are either incurred at operation or result from a wound infection.[15] The former most often appears to result from contam-

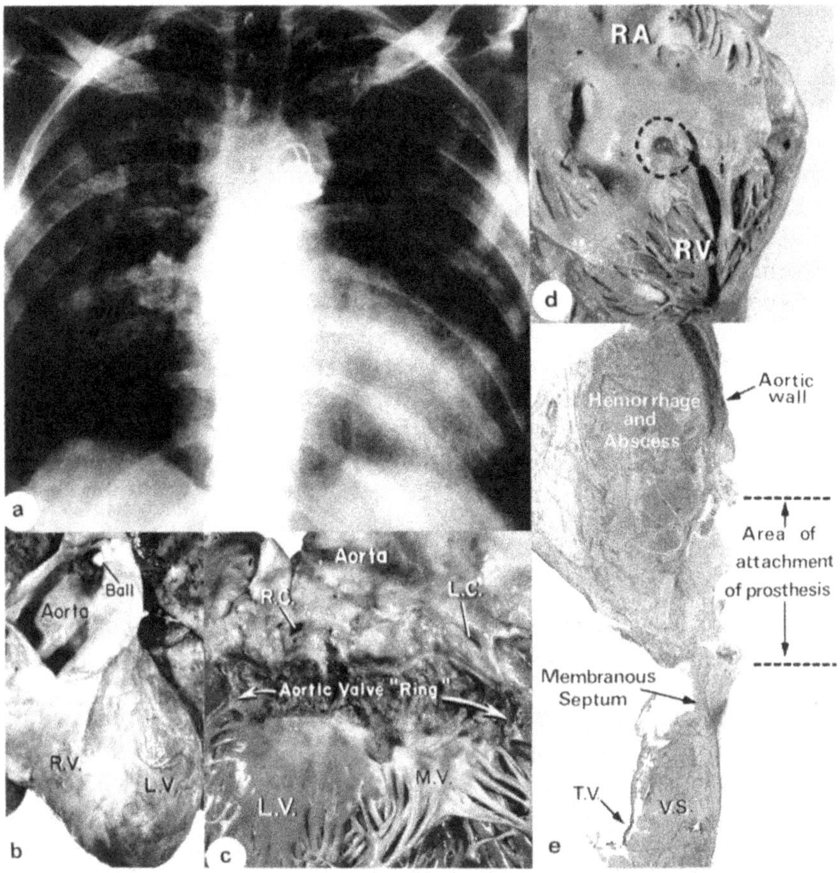

Fig. 2–19. *Staphylococcus epidermidis* prosthetic aortic valve endocarditis in a 48-year-old man. He had been well for 11 months following insertion of the Starr-Edwards prosthesis when, 1 month before death and 6 weeks after dental extraction, shaking chills appeared and blood cultures were positive for *S. epidermidis*. Despite intensive antibiotic therapy, signs of aortic regurgitation appeared, and minutes before death he complained of "feeling funny." (A) Chest roentgenogram immediately postmortem revealed that the prosthesis had dislodged and migrated to the aortic arch. (B) Anterior view of the heart and opened ascending aorta. The detached prosthetic ball is visible in the transverse aorta. LV, left ventricle; RV, right ventricle. (C) Opened aorta, aortic valve ring, and left ventricle showing a totally necrotic aortic anulus. MV, anterior mitral leaflet; RC, ostium of right coronary artery; LC, ostium of left coronary artery. (D) Opened right atrium (RA), tricuspid valve, and right ventricle showing a ring abscess (dashed circle) that had extended from the aortic prosthetic anulus. (E) Photomicrograph through the aortic valve ring showing a large ring abscess and the necrotic aortic anular material that extended through the membranous ventricular septum into the right atrium. TV, tricuspid valve leaflet; VS, ventricular septum. Hematoxylin–eosin. × 2.

ination of the cardiopulmonary bypass equipment.[109] Staphylococci are the most frequent organisms cultured from cardiopulmonary bypass equipment, and staphylococci are the most frequent cause of early PVE.[15,107,108] When gram-negative bacteria or fungi cause PVE early, they are usually also recovered from the operating room equipment or from a wound infection.[110] Late infections usually result from transient bacteremia.[108,110] Staphylococci are the most common cause of PVE and were the most common cause of PVE in our patients irrespective of whether the infection occurred early or late. In none of our 23 necropsy patients with PVE was the infection caused by streptococcus.

Among patients with PVE, blood cultures are almost always positive, except when the infections are caused by certain fungi.[111-117] Blood cultures were positive during life in each of our 21 patients with PVE caused by bacteria, and were negative in each of our 2 patients with fungal PVE. Among 39 patients with endocarditis by *Aspergillus* species reviewed by Krammer and Utz,[118] blood cultures were positive in only 3.

INVOLVEMENT OF AORTIC VERSUS MITRAL PROSTHESIS

Signs of prosthetic dysfunction are usually present when the aortic prosthesis is infected, and usually absent when the mitral prosthesis is infected.[15] Clinical signs of aortic regurgitation were present in 11 of our 15 patients with prosthetic aortic infection. In the 4 patients without clinical signs of aortic regurgitation, no prosthetic detachment was present at necropsy. Among patients with acute aortic regurgitation, however, classic signs of aortic regurgitation may be absent.[119] Signs of aortic regurgitation were not detected in 3 of 9 necropsy patients with aortic PVE reported by Madison and associates,[120] but in each of them prosthetic detachment was present at necropsy. In contrast, patients with infections involving the mitral prosthesis usually have no clinical signs of mitral prosthetic dysfunction.[15] Clinical signs of mitral prosthetic dysfunction were not detected in any of our 7 patients with mitral PVE, yet the prosthesis was significantly obstructed by vegetative material in 5 of them, and was partially detached from the anulus in 2. McAllister and associates[121] reported 2 patients with virtual total obstruction of the mitral prosthesis by infected thrombus.

RING ABSCESS

The most consistent morphologic feature of PVE in our 23 patients was infection behind the site of attachment of the valve prosthesis, resulting in valve ring abscess[15] (Figs. 2-19–2-22). Ring abscess was present in each of our 23 patients, and in two-thirds of them the infection involved the entire circumference of the valve anulus. In several patients, however, only a portion of the circumference of the valve anulus was in-

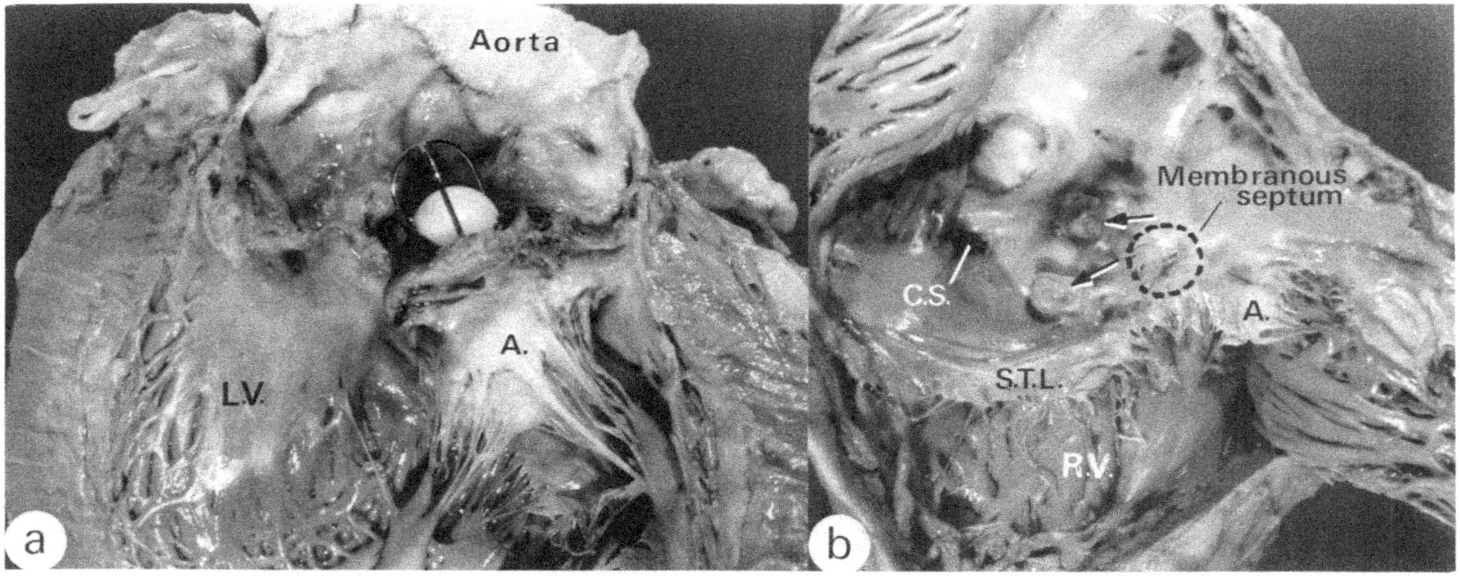

Fig. 2–20. *Staphylococcus epidermidis* prosthetic valve endocarditis in a 49-year-old man who died 3 months after aortic replacement. Symptoms of infection appeared 16 days before death. Despite antibiotics, complete heart block and wide-open aortic regurgitation developed. (A) Opened aorta, aortic valve, and left ventricle (LV) showing a necrotic anulus to which the prosthesis is only partially attached. A, anterior mitral leaflet. (B) Opened right atrium, tricuspid valve, and right ventricle (RV) showing vegetative material (arrows) that had burrowed through the atrial septum from the necrotic aortic valve ring. CS, ostium of coronary sinus; STL, septal tricuspid leaflet; A, anterior tricuspid leaflet. (C) Longitudinal section of the heart with the anterior portion removed. The necrotic aortic valve (AV) ring is again seen and the penetration of the infective process through the atrial septum (AS) is apparent. An arrow again designates the vegetation in the right atrium (RA). VS, ventricular septum. (D), (E) Histologic sections through the ring abscess. The site of attachment (attach) of the prosthesis, which has been removed, is indicated. The infected nodule, an extension of the ring abscess (Abs), is showing in the right atrium (RA.). Ao, aortic wall; LA, left atrium; AML, anterior mitral leaflet. Hematoxylin-eosin. (D) × 2.5. (E) × 4.

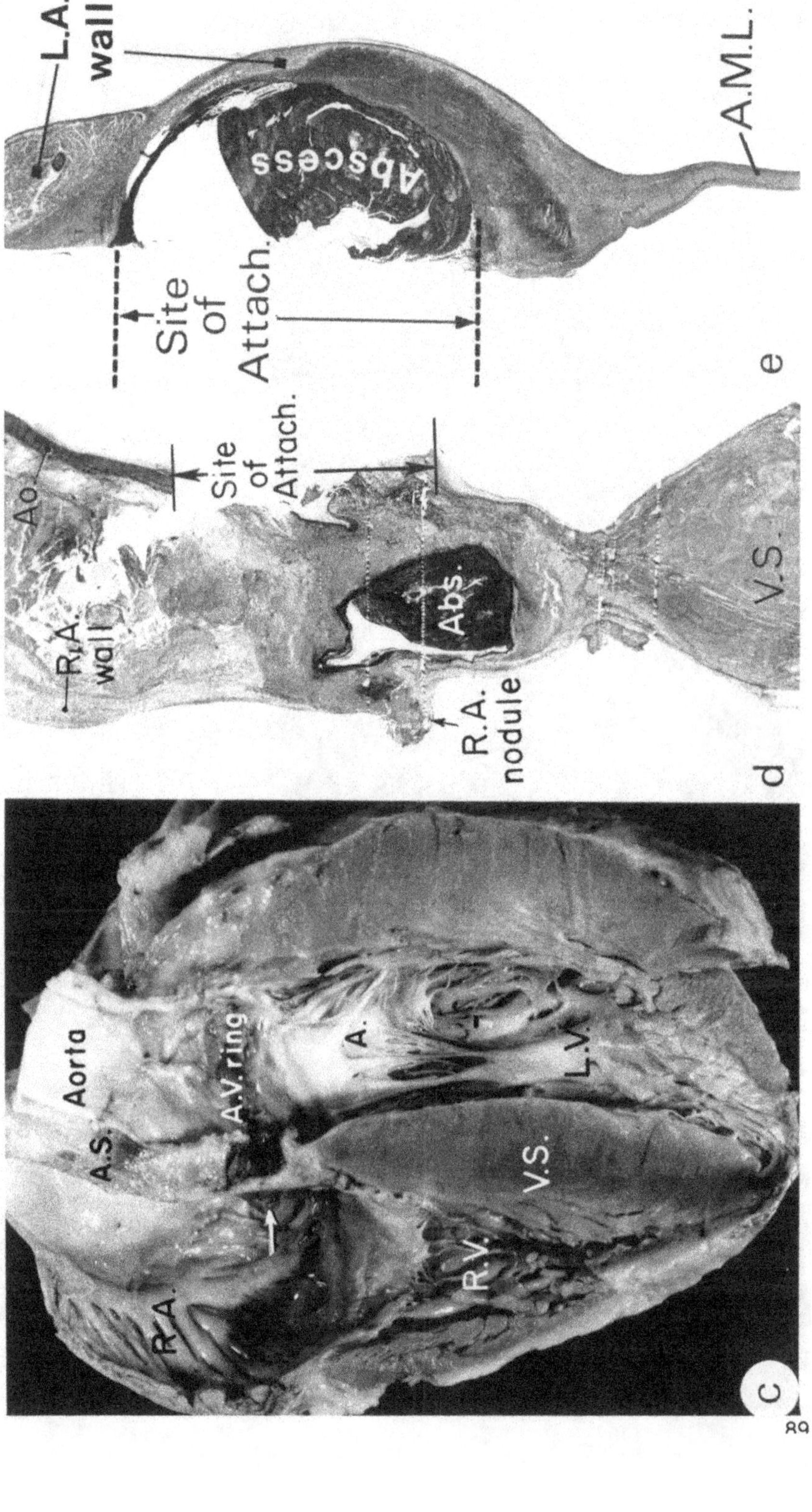
c
R.A.
A.S.
Aorta
A.V. ring
A.
R.V.
V.S.
L.V.
d
R.A. nodule
R.A. wall
Ao
Site of Attach.
Abs.
V.S.
e
Site of Attach.
Abscess
L.A. wall
A.M.L.

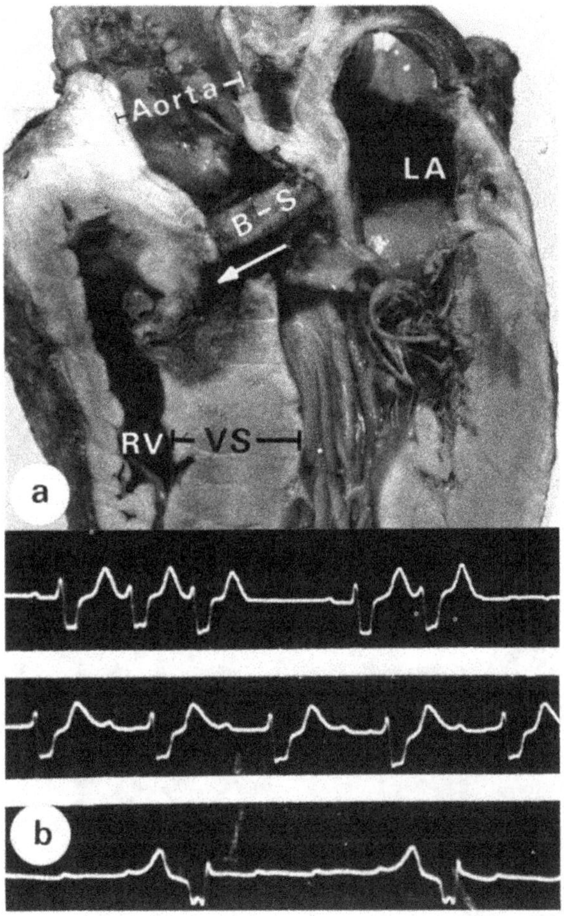

Fig. 2–21. *Staphylococcus epidermidis* prosthetic aortic valve endocarditis in a 51-year-old man. His stenotic bicuspid aortic valve had been replaced with a Bjork-Shiley prosthesis 83 days before death. Fever was present in the early postoperative period, and shortly before death complete heart block and signs of congestive heart failure appeared. (A) Longitudinal section of the heart with the anterior portion removed. The Bjork-Shiley (B-S) prosthesis is partially detached, and the ring abscess (arrow) has burrowed through the ventricular septum (VS) into right ventricle (RV). LA, left antrium; LV, left ventricle. (B) Electrocardiogram showing complete heart block.

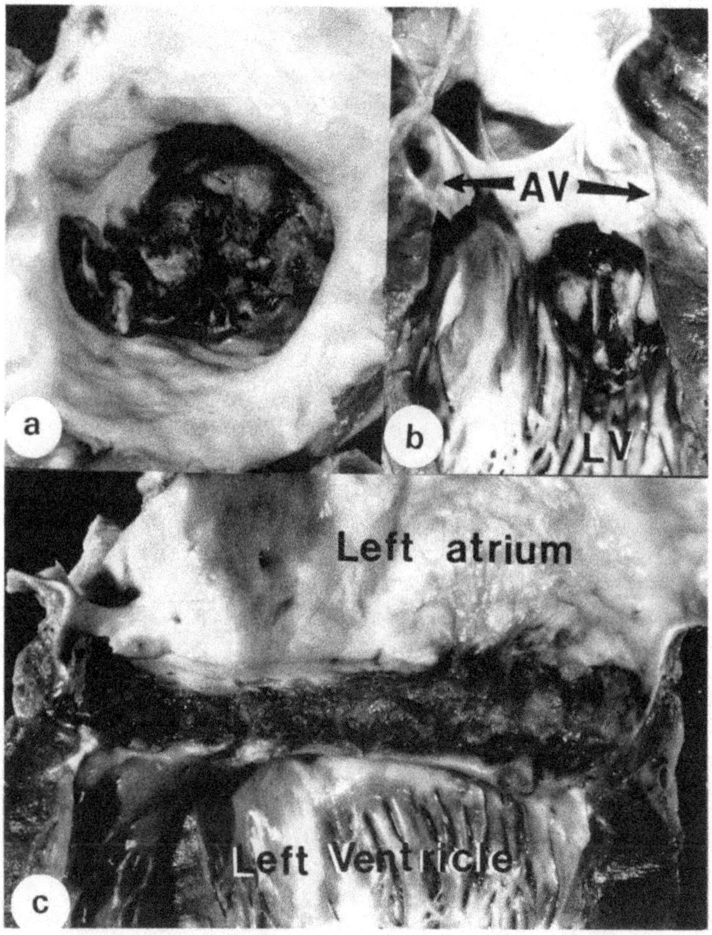

Fig. 2–22. *Staphylococcus epidermidis* prosthetic mitral valve endocarditis in a 46-year-old man who died 16 months after mitral replacement with a Starr-Edwards prosthesis. Eight months postoperatively, when asymptomatic, cardiac catheterization disclosed normal left atrial pressure and cardiac output. Signs of infection appeared 15 months after valve replacement. Despite antibiotics, he developed fatal congestive heart failure. (A) Mitral prosthesis as viewed from the left atrium. A large infected thrombus virtually occludes the mitral orifice. (B) Opened aorta, aortic valve (AV), and left ventricle (LV) showing infected thrombus on the cage of the mitral prosthesis. (C) Opened left atrium and ventricle showing a completely necrotic mitral anulus. The prosthesis has been removed.

volved, and in 1 patient histologic examination of the anulus disclosed infection that had not been apparent on gross examination. Extension of the ring infection to adjacent cardiac structures was common, especially with aortic prosthetic infection. This extension resulted in the frequent occurrence of both complete heart block or left bundle branch block and of intracardiac fistulae. Among 9 necropsy patients with aortic PVE reported by Madison and associates,[120] each had infection at the site of attachment of the prosthesis, and among their entire group of 16 patients with aortic PVE, 7 (44 percent) developed atrioventricular conduction defects. Obviously, it is the occurrence of the infection behind the site of attachment of the prosthesis which makes reoperation so hazardous. Were the infection limited to the interior portion of the prosthesis, excision of the prosthesis should eliminate the infection. Unfortunately, as demonstrated by our patients and by those reported by others, the tissues behind the site of attachment of the prosthesis usually are involved by the infective process.

NECROTIC ANULUS

The occurrence of a grossly necrotic anulus, however, at the time of reoperation for PVE does not mean that valve replacement will be fruitless. Although it may be grossly necrotic, the anulus may be free of colonies of organisms and cultures of the necrotic anulus may be negative. In 9 of our 23 patients with PVE and ring abscess, no stainable organisms were found in histologic sections from the prosthetic anulus. One hazard of inserting a prosthesis in a necrotic anulus at the time of valve replacement for PVE is burrowing of the sewing ring of the new prosthesis into the necrotic anulus with resulting impingement on movement of the poppet of the prosthesis by adjacent tissue. This sequence occurred in one of our patients and resulted in prosthetic aortic stenosis from inability of the ball to ascend in the cage.

TISSUE VALVE ENDOCARDITIS

Although PVE in patients with rigid-framed prostheses, as were present in our 23 patients, usually indicates the presence of infection behind the site of attachment of the prosthesis (i.e., sewing ring), ring abscess may not be so frequent with endocarditis involving tissue valves. Indeed, both experimentally and in humans, the infective process may be limited to the cusps of the tissue valve, just like the situation with IE involving natural valves.[122] Thus, the chance of cure, either by antibiotics or valve replacement or both when IE is superimposed on a homograft or heterograft (porcine valve) is much better than when IE involves a rigid-framed prosthesis. This then is an advantage, although a small one, of the tissue valve (porcine) over the rigid-framed prosthesis.

DIAGNOSIS

Establishment of the diagnosis of PVE, particularly in the early postoperative period, may be difficult at times.[123,124] Diagnosis in the late postoperative period, in contrast, is usually made quite readily.[123,124] It is worth emphasizing, however, that the combination of fever and a positive blood culture in a patient with a prosthetic cardiac valve does not always indicate the presence of PVE. We studied a patient at necropsy who was diagnosed during life as having mitral PVE on the basis of fever, cerebral episodes consistent with emboli, and one blood culture which grew *Staphylococcus epidermidis* with diphtheroids. She received antibiotics during most of her 4-month postoperative period and at necropsy no PVE was found. A left ventricular aneurysm, however, was present immediately caudal to the mitral anulus and a sterile thrombus was present in the aneurysm. The latter was the likely source of the cerebral emboli.

ANTIBIOTIC CURE

There is a general view that PVE can at times be cured by antibiotics. For cure of PVE to be established, however, it is necessary that PVE be confirmed during life, and this unequivocal confirmation can only be obtained by examination of the prosthetic valve and its anulus (site of attachment) at reoperation. In other words, to establish cure of PVE it is necessary to be absolutely positive of the diagnosis of PVE. Although usually not obtained, this confirmation has now been obtained in enough patients to support the view that PVE can indeed be cured in some patients.[106-108,110,120,124]

Comparison of observations in our 23 patients with PVE to those in our 74 nonoperated necropsy patients with active IE involving natural *left*-sided cardiac valves disclosed certain clear differences:[15] (1) Ring abscess was always present in patients with PVE regardless of the site of the prosthesis; in contrast, it was present in 32 percent of our 74 patients with active IE involving native left-sided valves, and then, with rare exception, only when the aortic valve was infected. (2) The hemodynamic consequences were different: PVE caused valve obstruction nearly as often as valvular regurgitation, whereas valvular stenosis from active IE involving native cardiac valves was extremely rare. (3) Spread of ring abscess was more extensive in patients with PVE than in patients with natural valve IE, and, consequently, the frequency of high-grade conduction defects was much greater in patients with PVE. (4) The infecting organisms in fatal PVE were most commonly staphylococci and rarely alpha streptococci, whereas the latter remain a common cause of fatal active IE affecting native cardiac valves.

Among patients with IE involving native cardiac valves, *ring abscess*, when present, almost always (95 percent) involves the aortic valve.

Among our necropsy patients with active IE involving native aortic valves, 40 percent had a ring abscess, whereas only 5 percent of patients with IE involving native mitral valves had a ring abscess. In contrast, each of our 23 patients with PVE had a ring abscess. Thus, valve ring abscess is the usual morphologic feature of PVE, regardless of the valve infected. Ring abscesses in patients with PVE are generally more extensive than those occurring in patients with IE involving native cardiac valves. This occurrence appears to be a consequence of the rigid nature of the prosthetic frame. Once the prosthesis is loosened by the infection, the rocking rigid frame promotes spread of the infection. The greater turbulence across the aortic valve prosthesis probably accounts for the generally more extensive nature of ring abscess in patients with aortic PVE than in those with mitral PVE. A consequence of this extension is the greater frequency of complete heart block and left bundle branch block in patients with aortic PVE (32 percent) compared to patients with IE involving native aortic valves (8 percent).

ORGANISMS INVOLVED

Staphylococcus (either *aureus* or *epidermidis*) is the most common cause of PVE (59 percent). Many different organisms cause the remainder of the infections. Although alpha streptococci were the responsible organisms in 17 percent of our 74 patients with IE on native valves, this bacterium was not the causative organism in any of our 23 patients with PVE.

HEMODYNAMIC CONSEQUENCES

The hemodynamic consequences of PVE vary with the site of the infected prosthesis. Twelve of the 15 patients (80 percent) with aortic PVE and 2 of the 7 patients with prosthetic mitral valve infection developed valvular regurgitation from PVE. In contrast, 5 of the 7 patients (71 percent) with mitral PVE and 1 of the 15 patients (7 percent) with aortic PVE developed valvular obstruction from the infection. Among patients with IE involving native left-sided valves, 65 percent (64 percent of the mitral and 69 percent of the aortic patients) developed valvular regurgitation from active IE, and relatively few (3 percent) developed valvular obstruction from the IE.[8] Thus, aortic PVE almost always causes valvular regurgitation, and mitral PVE most often causes valvular obstruction.

SPLENOMEGALY

Splenomegaly (> 300 g) is common both in patients with PVE (64 percent) and in patients with native left-sided valve IE (37 percent). Similarly, the frequency of infarcts in other body organs is similar (70 percent) in both PVE and in IE affecting native cardiac valves.

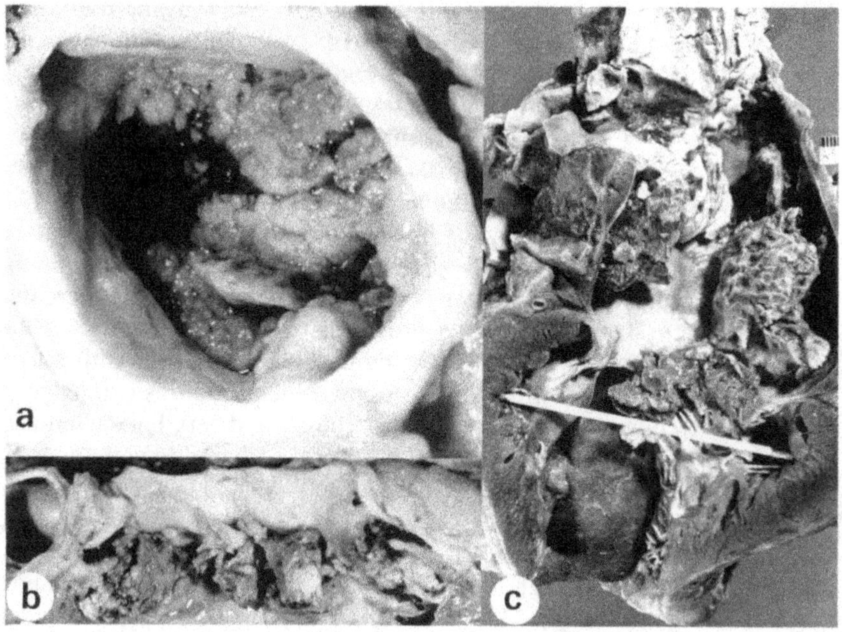

Fig. 2–23. IE after cardiac valve commissurotomy. (A), (B). Aortic valve from a 48-year-old man who developed *Candida guillermondi* endocarditis of the aortic valve after transaortic valvulotomy. He died 5 months after the cardiac operation. The *Candida* organisms were cultured from the heart-lung machine after operation. Aortic valve as seen from above is shown in (A) and after opening in (B). (C) Opened left atrium, mitral valve, and left ventricle from a 45-year-old man who underwent mitral valvulotomy 3 months before death. One month postoperatively, he had fever and sweats, and when reexamined 5 weeks before death he had evidence of congestive cardiac failure. Blood cultures at this time grew *Candida parapsilosis;* these organisms also had been cultured from the heart–lung machine at operation. He died of progressive worsening of the congestive cardiac failure. At necropsy, large vegetations containing *Candida* organisms were present on the mitral valve and in the left atrium.

Active IE Involving a Native Cardiac Valve Previously Treated by Valvulotomy or Valvuloplasty (Fig. 2-23)

Although direct trauma to cardiac valves is a means of producing IE experimentally, IE after valvular operations (excluding replacement) is uncommon.[1,2,125–129] of 1333 patients with open-heart operations for valvular heart disease reported by Koiwai and Nahas,[125] 11 (1 percent) developed IE postoperatively. Of 1889 patients undergoing nonreplacement valvular operations reported by Denton and associates,[126] 19 (1 percent) developed IE postoperatively. Shafer and Hall[129] reported IE in 13 of 2288 patients (0.5 percent) surviving open-heart operations at the University of Minnesota Hospitals. We observed 4 patients with IE after valve commissurotomy among our 137 necropsy patients with active IE.

Among patients undergoing open-heart operations, the frequency of IE is lower in those in whom no prosthetic materials are used. Yah and associates[128] reported IE in 18 of 400 patients (5 percent) following open-heart operations; 14 of the 18 infections, however, occurred among 242 patients in whom prosthetic material was used, and only 2 among 158 patients in whom no prosthetic material was used.

When IE follows commissurotomy or valvuloplasty procedures, the operated valve is generally the site of the infection. In each of our 4 patients, 3 of whom had multivalvular disease, vegetations were limited to the operated valve, mitral in 3 and aortic in 1. Of 2 necropsy patients with IE following mitral valvulotomy reported by Dalton and associates,[130] the vegetations were limited to the mitral valve in each. In 3 of our 4 patients *Candida* species was the offending organism.[1]

Active IE In Patients with Subaortic Stenosis (Figs. 2-24 and 2-25)

It is important to separate patients with IE complicating subaortic stenosis because IE in this group presents different clinical and morphologic features than those observed in other patients with IE. Among patients with *discrete* subaortic stenosis the infection, at least initially, is almost always located on the aortic valve[131–134] (Figs. 2-24 and 2-25). This valve is traumatized by blood ejected through the subaortic obstruction under high pressure and velocity. When infected in this circumstance, the aortic cusps are rapidly destroyed. In patients with destroyed aortic valve cusps and no subaortic stenosis the consequence is severe aortic regurgitation with progressive dilatation and, finally, failure of the left ventricle. However, in patients with destroyed aortic valve cusps associated with subaortic stenosis, at least of the discrete variety, severe aortic regurgitation is prevented by the subaortic obstruction, and, therefore, the aortic or systemic arterial diastolic pressure does not fall significantly despite an anatomically destroyed aortic valve. As a consequence, the left ventricle does not dilate and congestive cardiac failure may be absent. Diagnosis of active IE in these patients may be difficult. Since the aortic valve cusps are previously traumatized by the jet of blood transversing the subaortic stenosis, the infection complicates a previously abnormal valve. In this situation the most common infecting organisms are alpha streptococci, organisms of relatively low virulence that are compatible with active IE over a long period (many months) without antibiotic treatment.

Although we have studied at necropsy only 2 patients with active IE complicating discrete subaortic stenosis, this congenital malformation, on a percentage basis, may be the one most prone to be complicated by active IE; its complication by IE is that of the congenitally bicuspid or unicuspid aortic valve, the prolapsed aortic valve associated with ventricular septal defect, or the floppy mitral valve. The narrow jet of blood contacting one or more aortic valve cusps under high pressure and velocity provides the ideal circumstance for IE to develop. We have studied 8 Newfoundland dogs who also had discrete subaortic stenosis: of the 5 who died naturally, at necropsy 4 had active IE, which was the cause of death.[134] Furthermore, 4 of the 42 patients with healed IE whom we studied at necropsy (to be discussed later) also had discrete subaortic stenosis.

Active IE Complicating Congenital Cardiac Disease with a Shunt (Fig. 2-26)

The study at necropsy of 6 patients with active IE complicating congenital heart disease with a shunt and the review of reports of others disclosed several principles applicable to IE in this circumstance: (1) patients with congenital cardiac malformations clearly have an increased risk of developing IE; (2) the congenital malformations associated with the greatest risk of developing either IE or infective endarteritis are ventricular septal defect, with or without associated obstruction to right ventricular outflow or aortic valve prolapse, and patent ductus arteriosus; (3) in patients with cardiovascular shunts and IE, the vegetations are usually located on the low-pressure side of the defect; and (4) in the antibiotic era, staphylococci appear to be the most frequent causative organisms.

RISK OF IE

Patients with congential heart disease have an increased risk of developing IE. Of 453 necropsy patients of all ages with congenital heart disease studied by Gelfman and Levine[46] in the preantibiotic era, 35 (7 percent) developed IE; of their 181 necropsy patients older than 2 years of age, however, 30 (17 percent) had IE. In a study of IE in infants and children, Johnson and associates[135] found an absolute increase in the number of hospital admissions for IE in each decade from 1943 to 1972; this increase appeared to result from a growing population of older patients with congenital heart disease.

Among patients with congenital heart disease, those with ventricular septal defect, with (tetralogy of Fallot) or without right ventricular outflow obstruction or aortic valve prolapse, and patent ductus arteriosus have the greatest risk of developing IE. Of 164 necropsy patients with ventricular septal defect of all sizes reported by Gelfman and Levine,[46] 17

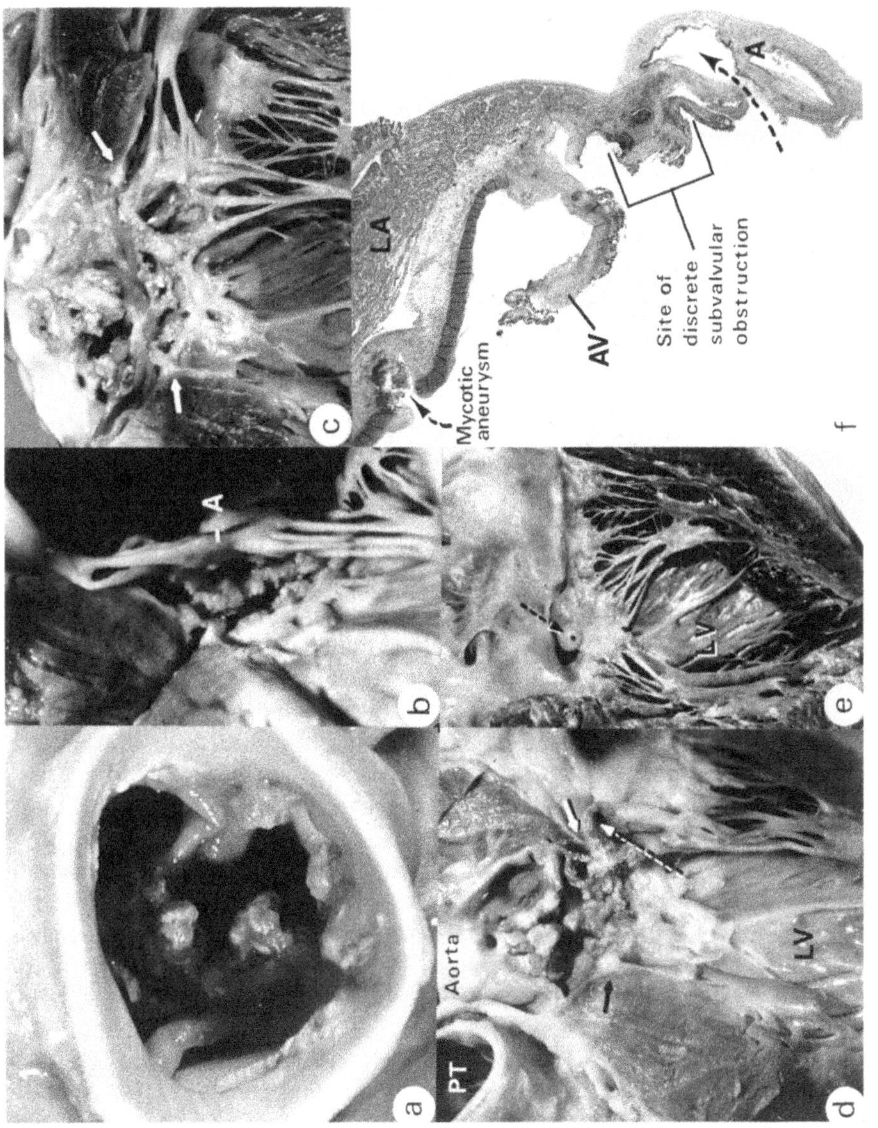
a
b
A
c
PT
Aorta
LV
d
LV
e
LA
Mycotic aneurysm
AV
Site of discrete subvalvular obstruction
A
f

Fig. 2–24. Alpha-hemolytic streptococcus endocarditis complicating congenitally discrete subaortic stenosis in a 28-year-old man. Evidence of infection appeared about 9 months before death. (A) Aortic valve as viewed from above. (B) Left ventricular outflow tract viewed from below showing vegetative material on the subvalvular "membrane" adjacent to the anterior mitral leaflet (A). (C) Opened left ventricular outflow tract showing vegetations on each aortic cusp and on the subvalvular "membrance" (between the solid arrows) and ventricular surface of the anterior mitral leaflet. (D) Longitudinal section showing the left ventricular outflow tract. The area of subaortic stenosis is clearly seen (between the solid arrows), and a mycotic aneurysm (dashed arrow) is seen in the anterior mitral leaflet. The mitral aneurysm is in the high-pressure portion of the left ventricle (LV), i.e., below the discrete subvalvular obstruction. PT, pulmonary trunk. (E) Opened mitral valve showing the atrial aspect of the mycotic aneurysm (dashed arrow) on the anterior leaflet. (F) Photomicrograph of section through aorta, left atrium (LA), aortic valve (AV) cusp, subvalvular "membrane," and anterior mitral leaflet (A). A mycotic aneurysm is present in the ascending aorta as well as in the anterior mitral leaflet (dashed arrow). Vegetations are present on the aortic valve cusp and on the subvalvular membrane. Hematoxylin–eosin. × 3.2.

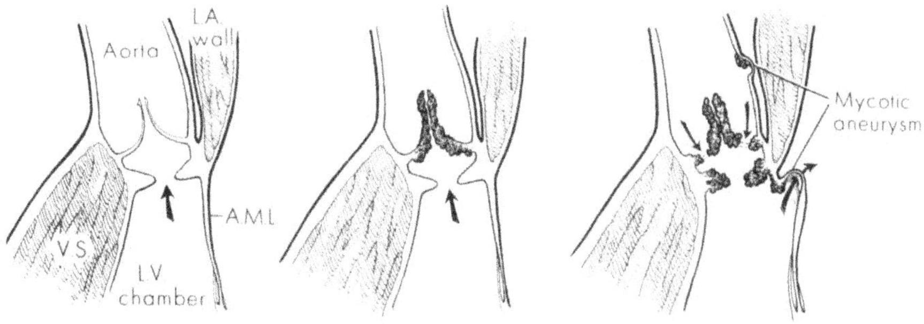

Fig. 2–25. Aortic valve region of the patient shown in Figure 24 illustrating the course of the pathologic process suggested by the necropsy findings. The left diagram shows the discrete subvalvular obstruction before the development of infective endocarditis. At this time, the valve was traumatized by the jet of blood from below. The central diagram depicts the initial formation of bacterial vegetations, exclusively on the aortic valve cusps. As this process progressed, the cusps ruptured (right diagram); the infection then extended to the discrete subvalvular fibrous band and anterior mitral leaflet (AL), where a mycotic aneurysm formed immediately below the membrane where systolic pressure was highest. A second aneurysm in the wall of the ascending aorta resulted from the effects of a systolic jet through the valve. LA, left atrium; VS, ventricular septum; LV, left ventricle.

Fig. 2–26. Alpha-hemolytic streptococcus endocarditis in a 5-year-old girl with ventricular septal defect (VSD). Pneumonia and anemia developed 4 months before death, and 2 months later a grade 2/6 murmur of aortic regurgitation was noted for the first time. Death resulted from a cerebral embolus. Vegetations probably formed initially on the jet lesion in the right ventricular outflow tract. Dislodgment of portions of the right ventricular vegetation produced septic pulmonary emboli which presented clinically as "acute pneumonia." The exact mechanism of involvement of the aortic valve by the infective process is uncertain. (A) Location of the vegetative material. Calcific deposits developed in the aortic valve vegetations during the 4-month course. RA, right atrium; RV, right ventricle; PT, pulmonary trunk; LA, left atrium; A, aneurysm with orifice just below aortic valve. (B) View of opened right atrium, tricuspid valve, and right ventricle showing the large vegetations (enclosed by dashed circle) in the right ventricular outflow tract adjacent to the small VSD. (C) View of opened left ventricle, aortic valve, and aorta showing partial but extensive destruction of the aortic valve cusps by vegetative material. The borders of the VSD are free of vegetation. (D) Photomicrograph of a section through the VSD including a portion of aorta, aortic valve (AV) cusp, and ventricular septum (VS). The endocardium bordering the VSD and that in the right ventricular outflow tract is thick. CA, coronary artery. Elastic van Gieson. × 8.

(10 percent) developed IE; among the 44 in whom the defect was small, IE developed in 23 percent. Two (12 percent) of their 16 patients with tetralogy of Fallot and 4 (3 percent) of their 134 patients with patent ductus arteriosus developed IE. Among 38 patients with congenital heart disease and either IE or infective endarteritis reported by Volger and Dorney,[48] 15 (39 percent) had ventriculr septal defect, 7 (19 percent) had tetralogy of Fallot, and 7 had patent ductus arteriosus. Of our 6 patients, 2 had isolated ventricular septal defect, 2 had tetralogy of Fallot, and 2 had persistent truncus arteriosus.

Patients with ventricular septal defect and aortic regurgitation have a particularly high incidence of IE involving the prolapsed cusp(s) of the aortic valve. Of 6 patients with ventricular septal defect and aortic regur-

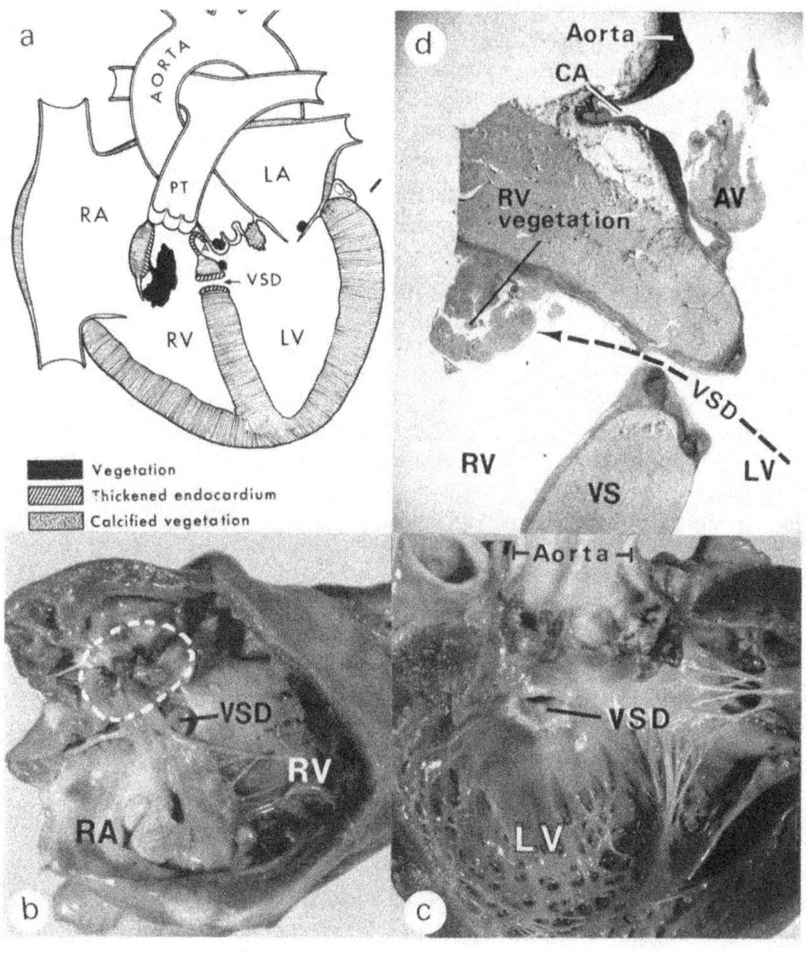

gitation whom we studied at necropsy, 2 had healed perforations in the prolapsed cusp—a finding indicative of active IE in the past.

LOCATION OF VEGETATIONS

In patients with congenital cardiovascular shunts and IE, the vegetations are usually located on the low-pressure side of the defect, which usually is the site of endocardial trauma.[46,69] Patients with isolated ventricular septal defect and IE usually have vegetations on the right ventricular mural endocardium or tricuspid valve, or both, in apposition to the defect. When IE or endarteritis occurs in nonoperated patients with tetralogy of Fallot, vegetations usually occur on the arterial side of the stenotic pulmonic valve. In patients with patent ductus arteriosus or tetralogy of Fallot with an operative systemic–pulmonary arterial shunt, the vegetations usually occur on the pulmonary side of the shunt.

ORGANISMS INVOLVED

Staphylococci have become a frequent cause of IE among patients with congenital heart disease. Among 141 patients under 25 years of age with IE between 1933 and 1972, Johnson and associates[135] found that the frequency with which staphylococci caused the IE rose from 22 percent during the first 2 decades to 33 percent during the later 2 decades. Staphylococci were the most frequent cause (34 percent) of IE among the 38 patients with congenital heart disease reported by Volger and Dorney.[48] In 3 of our 6 patients, the endocarditis was due to *Staphylococcus* species.

Active IE Confined to Mural Endocardium in the Absence of Ventricular Septal Defect (Figs. 2-27–2-29)

The study at necropsy of 8 patients[10,16] with active IE limited to mural (nonvalvular) endocardium and unassociated with ventricular septal defect disclosed several principles applicable to IE at this site: (1) IE confined to mural endocardium in the absence of ventricular septal defect is rare; (2) it is virtually limited to patients with a debilitating disease, particularly those treated with chemotherapeutic agents; (3) the mural endocardial vegetations are nearly always secondary to an infection in an organ other than the heart; (4) the mural endocardial vegetations usually represent either an extension of a myocardial abscess onto endocardium or an extension of an infectious process involving the intrapulmonary veins with extension into the left atrium; (5) the causative organism is usually a fungus; (6) mural endocarditis by itself is rarely fatal; and (7) it is rarely diagnosed clinically.

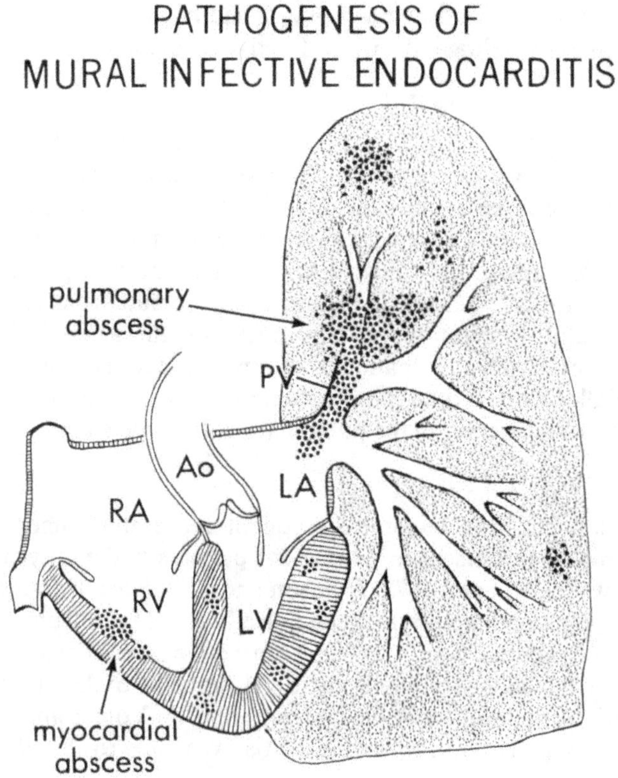

Fig. 2-27. Two mechanisms by which mural infective endocarditis, unassociated with ventricular septal defect, comes about: (1) by extension of a myocardial abscess into endocardium, and (2) by extension of a pulmonary abscess into left atrial (LA) endocardium via a pulmonary vein (PV). RA, right atrium; RV, right ventricle; LV, left ventricle; Ao, aorta.

Of our 8 patients with active IE confined to mural endocardium, all had leukemia or lymphoma. Each had received cytotoxic drugs. A fungus caused the IE in each. None had symptoms or signs of cardiac disease and IE was not suspected clinically in any of them. The endocardial vegetations resulted from extension of an infective process arising elsewhere. In 5 patients, the vegetations were confined to ventricular endocardium and each had underlying multiple myocardial abscesses (Figs. 2-27 and 2-28). In the other 3 patients, pulmonary mycosis extended into atrial endocardium via the pulmonary veins (Figs. 2-27 and 2-29).

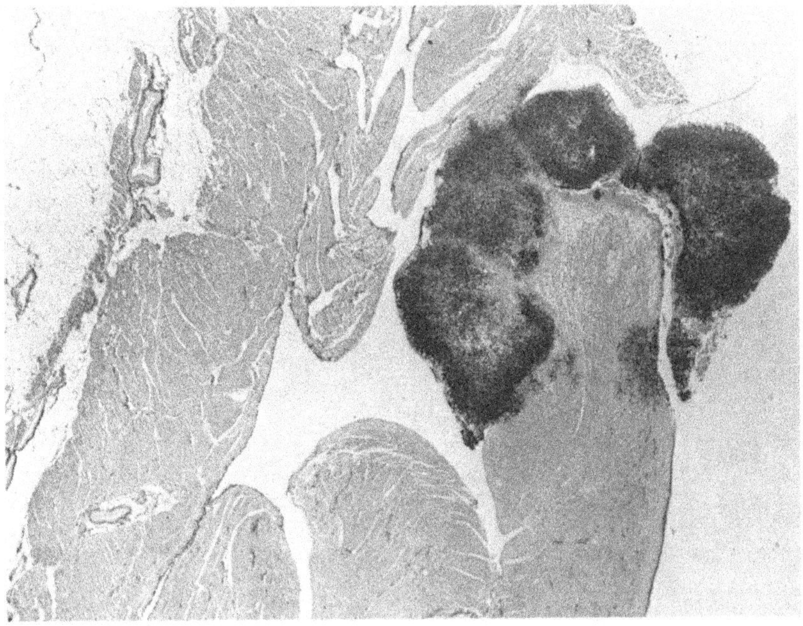

Fig. 2–28. IE limited to mural endocardium. A large fungal ball (*Candida* species) is on the apex of a right ventricular papillary muscle in a 65-year-old man with chronic myelocytic leukemia for 1 year. PAS. × 5.

HEALED INFECTIVE ENDOCARDITIS

General Comments

Although there are many reports describing various morphologic observations in patients with *active* IE, reports describing cardiac morphologic changes in patients with *healed* IE are rare. One reason is that healing of active IE became possible, for practical purposes, only when the use of penicillin for this condition began in 1944. Although antibiotics often "cure" patients with active IE, residual valvular damage obviously may be a consequence of the infection. This section will be a summary of certain clinical and morphologic observations in 42 necropsy patients with histories of active IE in whom the infection was cured by antibiotic therapy.[136]

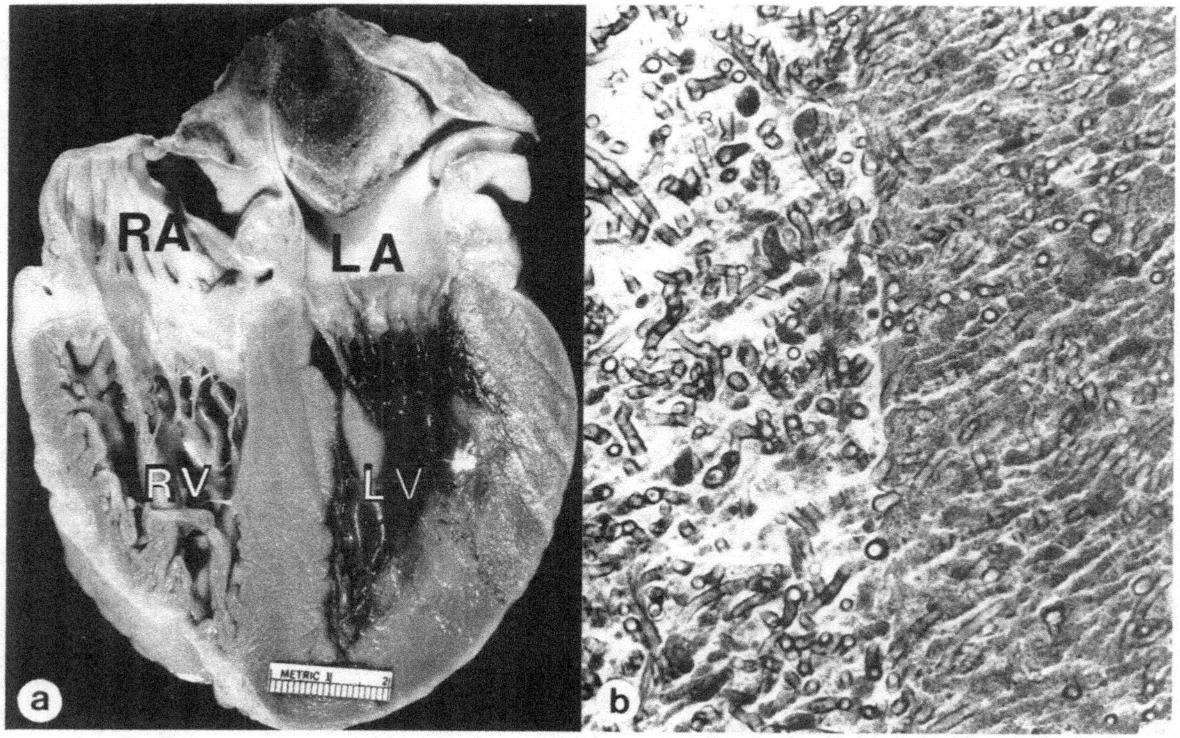

Fig. 2–29. IE limited to mural endocardium. (A) Large fungal mass (*Mucor* species) in a right pulmonary vein and in the left atrium (LA) in a 15-year-old boy with acute myelocytic leukemia of 6 months' duration. One month before death, bilateral acute pneumonia developed and it was found to result from *Mucor* species. The pulmonary fungal mass extended into the left atrium via the right pulmonary veins. LV, left ventricle; RA, right atrium; RV, right ventricle. (B) Photomicrograph of the *Mucor* organisms. Methenamine silver. × 400.

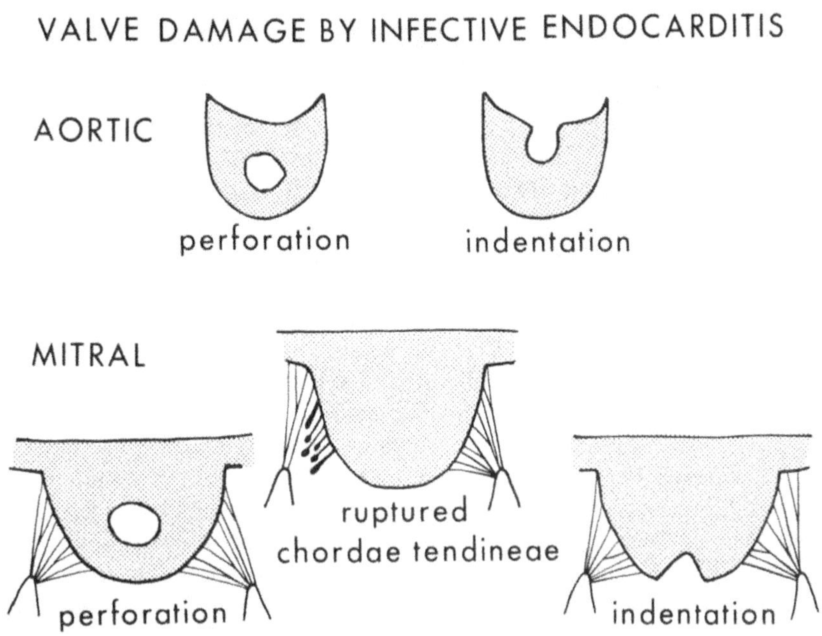

Fig. 2-30. Two most common anatomic residua of active IE "cured" by antibiotic therapy: (1) perforations or identations in one or more valvular cusps, and (2) rupture of chordae tendineae.

Healed IE Involving Native Right-Sided Cardiac Valves

There are no data available on healed IE involving right-sided cardiac valves. Focal fibrous thickening of one or more tricuspid valve leaflets has been observed at necropsy in patients who had had life styles (opiate addiction or chronic alcoholism[13]) that predisposed them to IE, but because episodes of active IE have not been well documented, it can only be suspected that the ieaflet scarring was the residua of IE.

Healed IE Limited to One or Both Left-Sided Cardiac Valves (Figs. 2-31–2-36)

The study at necropsy of 42 patients and operatively excised purely incompetent mitral or aortic valves from 17 patients[136] with histories of IE that was "cured" by antibiotic therapy and the review of reports of others disclosed certain principles applicable to these patients: (1) of patients with active IE treated with penicillin, about one-third, die during the active infection, another third are left with cardiac dysfunction as a consequence of the valvular damage produced by the infection, and only one-third are really cured without residual consequence; (2) among patients with active IE "cured" by penicillin therapy, the most common cause of death is congestive cardiac failure; (3) cardiac lesions that are attributable to results of active IE which healed are cuspal perforations or indentations, rupture of chordae tendineae, perianular aneurysm (evidence of healed ring abscess), and cuspal or aortic aneurysm (evidence of healed "mycotic" aneurysm); (4) of patients with healed IE and clinical evidence of cardiac dysfunction after healing, about 50 percent have one or more of the above lesions indicative of active IE which healed; and (5) these anatomic lesions are far more common among patients with purely incompetent valves than among patients with stenotic cardiac valves.

Successful therapy for active IE by the introduction of penicillin for this condition in 1944 represents one of the great successes in the treatment of heart disease. Overnight this condition went from being virtually universally fatal to curable.[137] Despite penicillin, and later other antibiotics, it soon became apparent that a number of patients so treated still died.[90,138-155] Of 1357 previously reported patients with active IE treated with penicillin,[90,138-155] 450 (33 percent) died during the period of active IE; approximately another 33 percent of the patients, although cured of the infection, were left with cardiac dysfunction as a consequence of the valvular damage produced by the infection. Only about one-third of the total patients with active IE, or one-half of the survivors of active IE, were free of valvular damage, or at least valvular damage sufficient to produce cardiac dysfunction. Thus, among patients with active IE treated with penicillin and reported from 1950 to 1965[90,138-155] one-third died during the active IE, one-third were left with sufficient damage to one or more valves to cause cardiac dysfunction, and one-third had either no residual valve damage or insufficient valve damage to produce cardiac dysfunction.

CONGESTIVE CARDIAC FAILURE

Among patients with active IE cured by penicillin therapy, the most common cause of death is congestive cardiac failure, usually the result of valvular damage either initiated or worsened by the active IE. Among the 907 survivors of active IE[90,138-155] 199 subsequently died 2–156 months after eradication of the infection by penicillin: 148 (74 percent) died from a cardiac cause, and in 126 of these congestive cardiac failure was the major cardiac problem; only 24 of the 199 patients died from noncardiac causes.

Few observations at necropsy in patients dying late after healing of active IE are available. Among the 199 patients dying late after healing of the IE,[90,138–155] necropsies were reported in only 30 patients. Cardiac lesions which could be attributed to results of the active IE were described in 10 of these patients: cuspal perforations in all 10 and aneurysm of the anterior mitral leaflet in 2 (possibly in as many as 4). None of these reports described the residual valve lesions in detail, and rupture of chordae tendineae or perianular aneurysm (evidence of healed ring abscess) were not mentioned.

The study at this laboratory was different from previous studies.[90,138–155] The earlier studies each began with a population of patients with active IE, all of whom were treated with penicillin. The patients surviving the period of active IE were followed for varying periods to determine how many developed, or continued to have, cardiac dysfunction despite eradication of the valvular infection. The starting point in the previous studies, therefore, was active IE. In our study[136] the starting point was examination of a severely dysfunctioning cardiac valve, either at necropsy or at valve replacement, in a group of patients with historical evidence of active IE treated and eradicated by antibiotic therapy. Among these patients the frequency of anatomic lesions which clearly could be attributable to consequences of the active IE was sought. Thus, among 584 necropsy patients who died of severe valvular heart disease, 42 (7 percent) had histories of active IE that healed; of these 42, 22 (52 percent) had anatomic cardiac lesions readily attributable to the earlier valvular infection. Among 79 patients in whom cardiac valve replacement was performed because of severe aortic regurgitation or mitral regurgitation or both, 17 (22 percent) had histories of active IE that healed; of these 17, 8 (47 percent) had anatomic cardiac lesions readily attributable to an earlier valvular infection.

LESIONS RESULTING FROM IE

Study of necropsy of patients with fatal active IE had indicted that cuspal perforation (or indentations) (Figs. 2-31–2-34, and 2-36), ruptured chordae tendineae (Figs. 2-31, 2-35, and 2-36), ring abscess, and mycotic aneurysm (Fig. 2-34) are the cardiac lesions most commonly the consequence of IE.[1-19] Among our 59 patients with histories of active left-sided IE that healed, 16 had cuspal perforations, 29 had ruptured mitral chordae tendineae, 3 had perianular aneurysms (healed ring abscess), and 1 had a small aortic aneurysm considered to be of infective origin. Although 30 of the 59 patients had cardiac lesions attributable to consequencies of IE, these lesions were far more common among the patients with purely incompetent valves (immediately before death or valve replacement) than

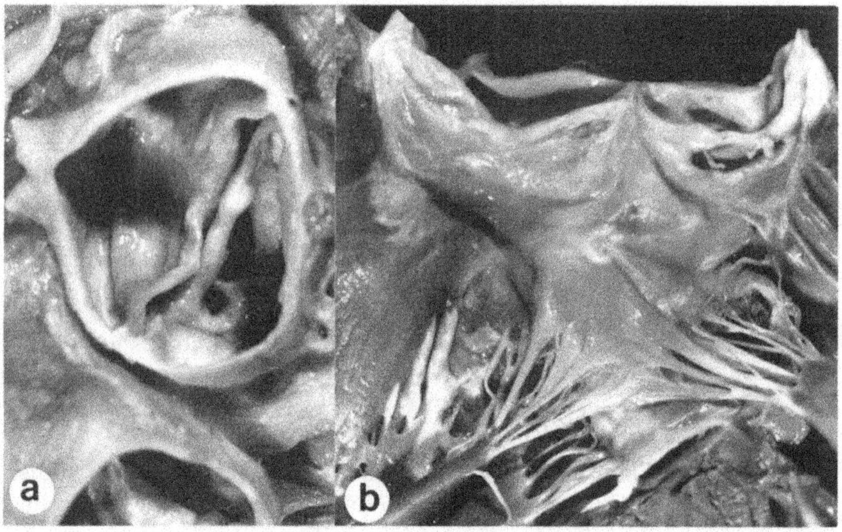

Fig. 2–31. Healed IE of a congenitally bicuspid aortic valve in a 47-year-old man who died from a kick in the head by a horse. In the distant past he had an episode of active IE which was cured by antibiotics. (A) Aortic valve showing a large perforation in the left cusp. (B) Opened aortic valve again showing a perforation in the left cusp. An aortic regurgitant jet is present on the mural endocardium of the left ventricular outflow tract.

among the patients with stenotic valves. Of the 385 patients with valvular stenosis at necropsy, 18 (5 percent) had histories of active IE that healed, and 7 of these 18 (39 percent) had anatomic cardiac lesions indicative of IE. In contrast, of 229 patients with pure valvular regurgitation at necropsy or valve replacement, 38 (17 percent) had histories of active IE that healed, and 23 of these 38 (61 percent) had anatomic cardiac lesions indicative of IE. Among the 7 patients with anatomic lesions of IE and valve stenosis, the anatomic lesions in 3 was healed ring abscess and cuspal perforations, and ruptured chordae occurred in each of 2 patients; in contrast, among the 23 patients with anatomic lesions indicative of IE and pure valvular regurgitation, 13 (57 percent) had ruptured chordae tendineae (4 of the latter 13 were among the 14 with cuspal perforations). Thus, IE superimposed on a previously stenotic valve may not leave evidence of further cuspal damage; as the chordae tendineae are thick when the mitral valve is stenotic, rupture of a thickened chordae tendineae is infrequent. The previously normal valve or the purely incompetent valve is easy prey to cuspal destruction by infection because it is not thickened; similarly, the chordae tendineae which is not thickened can readily be ruptured by infection.

Although anatomic lesions clearly indicative of previous IE occurred in half the patients we studied with histories of active IE, the other half had no lesions readily attributable to IE. This difference cannot be explained on the basis of better historical evidence of active IE in the former group. Anatomic evidence of IE was found in 17 (55 percent) of

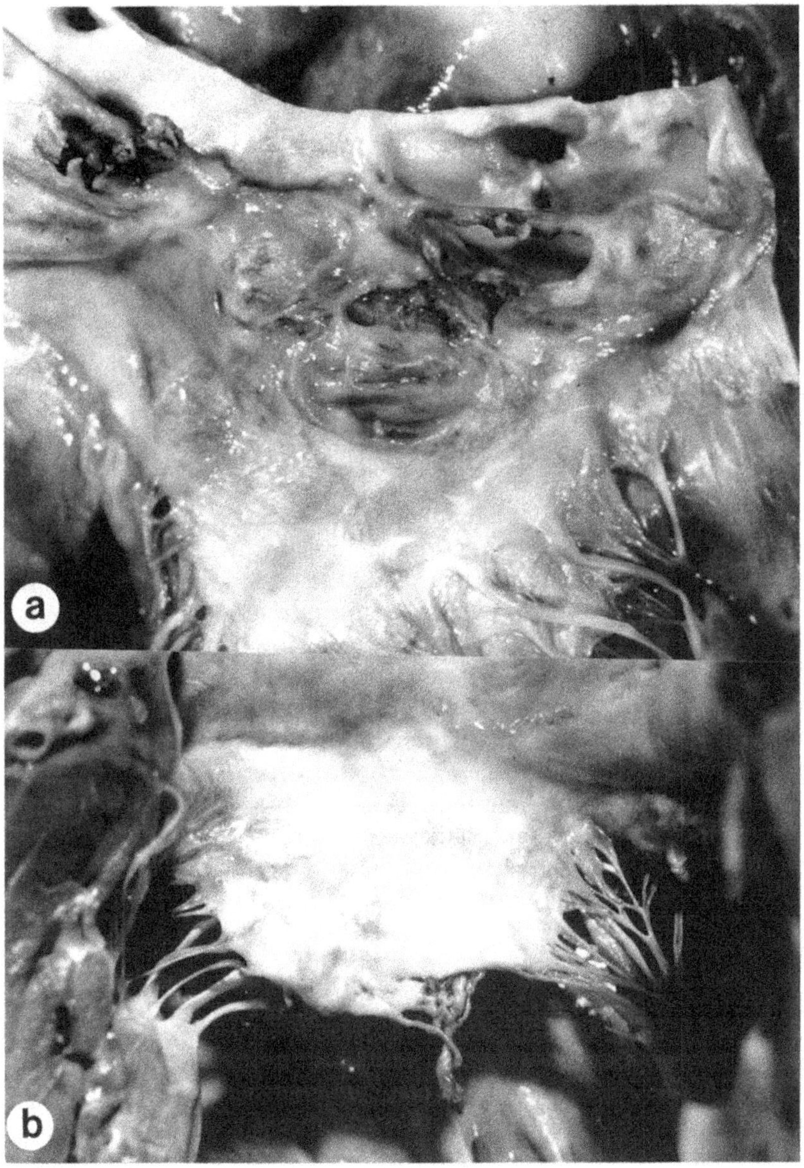

the 31 patients with "good" histories and in 13 (46 percent) of the 26 patients with "less good" histories of active IE that healed. It is clear that cuspal perforations, ruptured chordae tendineae, and ring abscess, however, are not inevitable consequences of active IE. Although cuspal perforations and ring abscesses in my experience always are indicative of IE at some time, ruptured chordae tendineae unassociated with vegetations are not always indicative of IE in the past. Among 16 patients with cuspal perforations unassociated with vegetations whom we studied at necropsy, all had good histories of IE which healed. In contrast, of 43 patients with ruptured chordae tendineae unassociated with vegetations who we studied at necropsy, only 15 (35 percent) had histories of IE in the past. Nevertheless, rupture of chordae tendineae is the most common anatomic lesion observed on the mitral valve during active IE, and thus in patients with histories of healed IE and ruptured chordae tendineae it is most reasonable to attribute the chordal rupture to the infection.

DEATH DURING VERSUS POSTINFECTION

Certain differences at necropsy are apparent between patients dying during active left-sided IE compared to patients dying after healing of the active infection. Three major difference have been noted. Among our 74 necropsy patients with fatal active left-sided IE, 55 percent had the infection on a previously anatomically and functionally normal valve; in contrast, of our 42 necropsy patients with healed left-sided IE, only 15 percent were considered to have had anatomically and functionally normal valves before the infection. Thus, the thicker the valve before the infection, the greater the chance of survival during the infection. The causative organism was quite different: staphylococci or pneumococci were the responsible organisms in 48 percent of our 74 necropsy patients with fatal active IE, and they were responsible in only 19 percent of our 42 necropsy patients with healed IE. In the latter group, alpha streptococcus was the most common infecting organism (52 percent), whereas it was the offend-

Fig. 2–32. Opened aortic and mitral valves in a 39-year-old man who had an episode of active IE at age 24 and died suddenly at age 39 while playing golf. A minimal amount of aortic regurgitation was worsened by the episode of IE. When studied 2 months before death, simultaneous left ventricular and brachial arterial pressures were 140/20 and 140/38 mm Hg, respectively, and the cardiac index was 2.8 liters/min/m^2. Angiography with injection of contrast material into the ascending aorta showed severe aortic regurgitation, and into the left ventricle, mild mitral regurgitation. The heart was huge (1010 g). (A) The aortic valve is congenitally malformed, consisting of two nearly equal sized cusps and one rudimentary cusp; a perforation is present in each of the two developed cusps. Calcific deposits border the perforations. (B) Several chordae tendineae from the posterior half of the anterior mitral leaflet are ruptured.

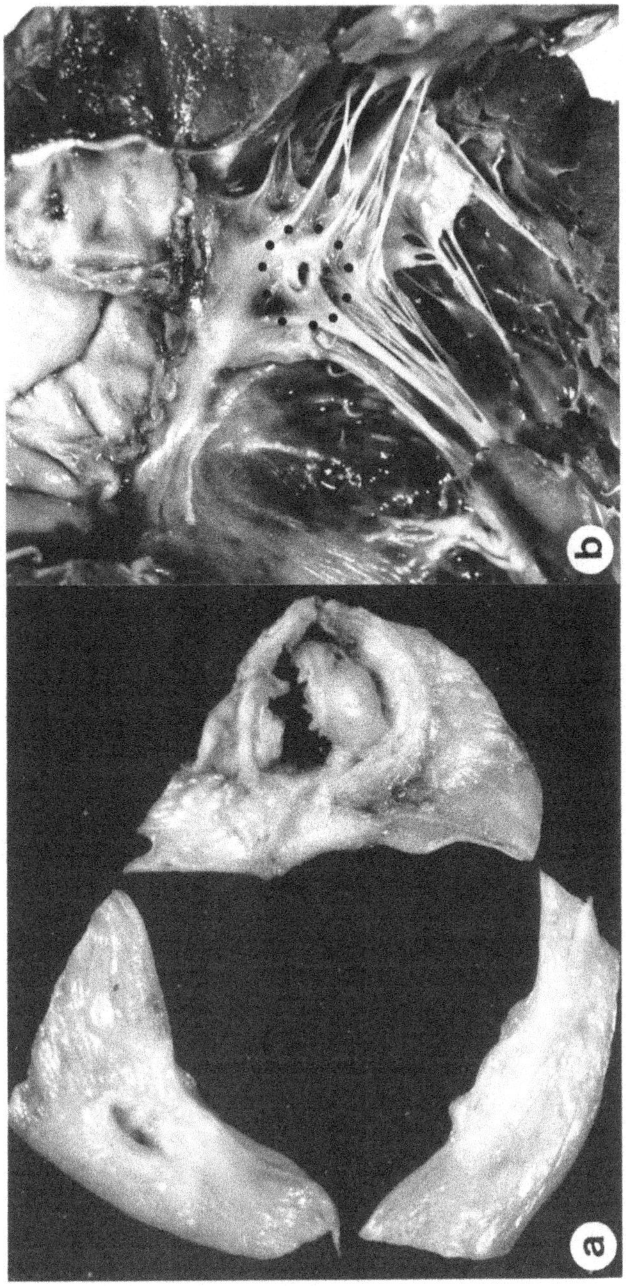
b
a

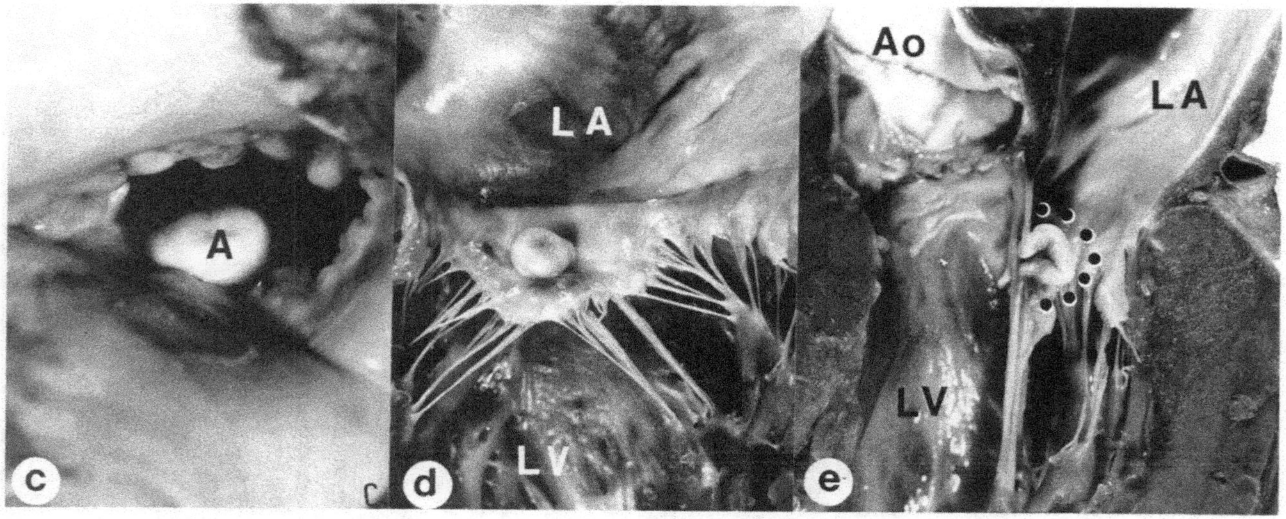

Fig. 2–33. Aortic and mitral valves in a 45-year-old man who had nonhemolytic streptococcal endocarditis 2 years earlier, with the onset of mitral and aortic regurgitation at that time. He died 5 days after double-valve replacement. It is believed that both valves were functionally and anatomically normal before the onset of IE. (A) Excised aortic valve showing a perforation in two of the three cusps. (B) Opened left ventricular outflow tract showing a small opening (dashed circle) in the anterior mitral leaflet. (C) Mitral valve orifice as seen from left atrium showing an aneurysm (A) on the atrial aspect of the anterior mitral leaflet. (D) Opened left atrium (LA), mitral valve, and left ventricle (LV) showing the aneurysm on the anterior leaflet. (E) Longitudinal cut of aorta (Ao), left ventricle, mitral valve, and left atrium (LA) showing the aneurysm (enclosed by dashes) on the anterior leaflet. The mitral leaflet aneurysm and the aortic cuspal perforation were the result of the active IE that healed.

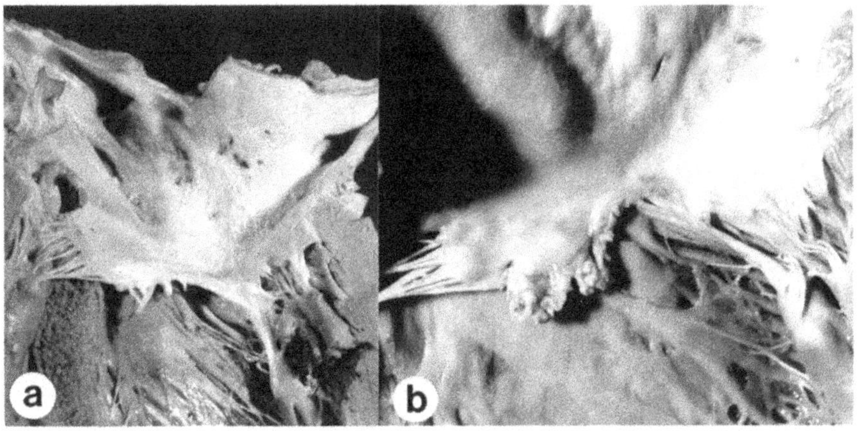

Fig. 2–34. Ruptured chordae tendineae of the mitral valve from two different patients with histories of healed IE. (A) Opened left atrium, mitral valve, and left ventricle of a 29-year-old woman who had *Staphylococcus epidermidis* endocarditis at age 24 with subsequent severe mitral regurgitation. (B) Mitral valve of a 19-year-old woman who had streptococcal group D endocarditis 16 months earlier with subsequent severe mitral regurgitation. Each of the two patients had active IE on previously normal mitral valves and each had normal aortic valves.

ing organism in only 12 percent of our patients with fatal active IE. Finally, recognized predisposing factors to IE were common (60 percent) among our patients who died during the active infection and were less frequent (27 percent) among our patients who died after healing of the valvular infection.

Active IE Complicating Healed IE

An occasional patient with active IE cured by antibiotics months or years later has one or more additional bouts of active IE. Indeed, a cardiac valve damaged once by IE probably has a marked susceptibility to reinfection. Despite this likely increased susceptibility, no published information is available regarding morphologic observations on necropsy patients with more than one documented episode of active IE. We have studied 2 patients, each with two separate episodes of active IE. In each, new vegetations were located at borders of cuspal perforations caused by the first bout of active IE, and in each the new vegetations were small. Examination of the affected valves (mitral in 1, aortic in 1) indicated that the initial bout of IE almost certainly involved a previously normal valve. It is reasonable to believe that healed IE in itself is a predisposing factor to active IE. Of 606 reported patients with active IE cured by antibiotics,

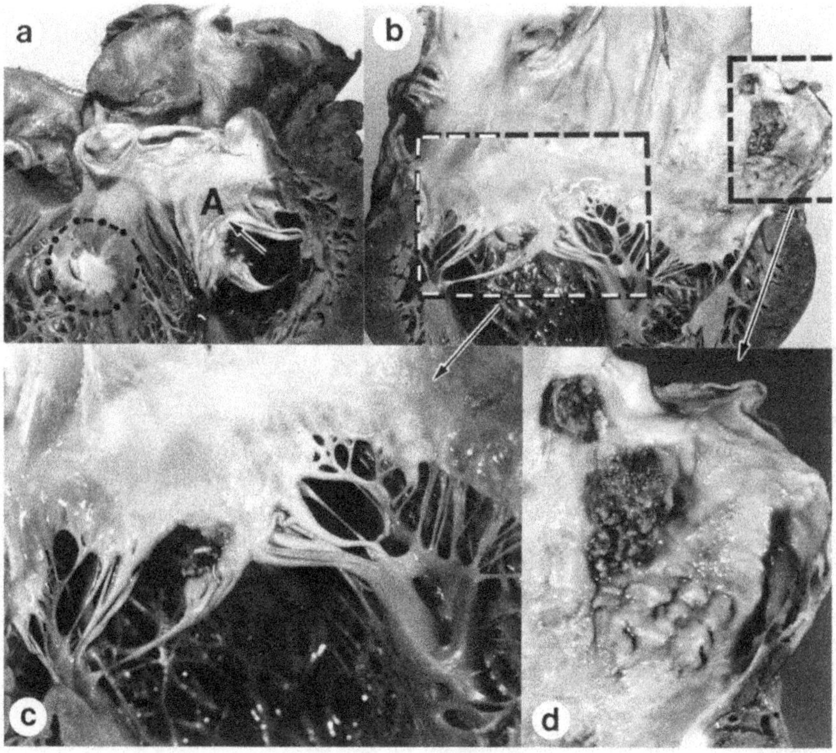

Fig. 2–35. Heart of a 25-year-old woman who had *Staphylococcus aureus* endocarditis at age 7 with mitral regurgitation thereafter. At age 18, she had a second well-documented episode of IE, this time due to alpha streptococcus. She died from severe congestive cardiac failure. (A) Opened aortic valve and left ventricle showing a jet lesion (dashed circle) corresponding to the indentation (arrow) in the anterior mitral leaflet (A). (B) Opened left atrium, mitral valve, and left ventricle. (C) Close-up of area in brackets in (B). There are an indentation and ruptured chordae tendineae on the anterior half of the anterior mitral leaflet. Small calcific deposits border the indentations. (D) Close-up of area in brackets in (B). These calcific deposits on the posterior wall of the left atrium represent healed vegetations that apparently occurred during one or both periods of active IE.

50 (8 percent) developed a second bout of active IE.[48,90,140,150–152,154] The outcome of the second bout of active IE was known in only 18 of the 50 patients: 4 died of congestive heart failure during the second episode of active IE,[90,152,154] and the remaining 13 were alive up to 5 years after cure of the second episode of active IE.[48,90,152] For none of the 50 patients was the status of the valve before the initial episode of active IE commented upon.

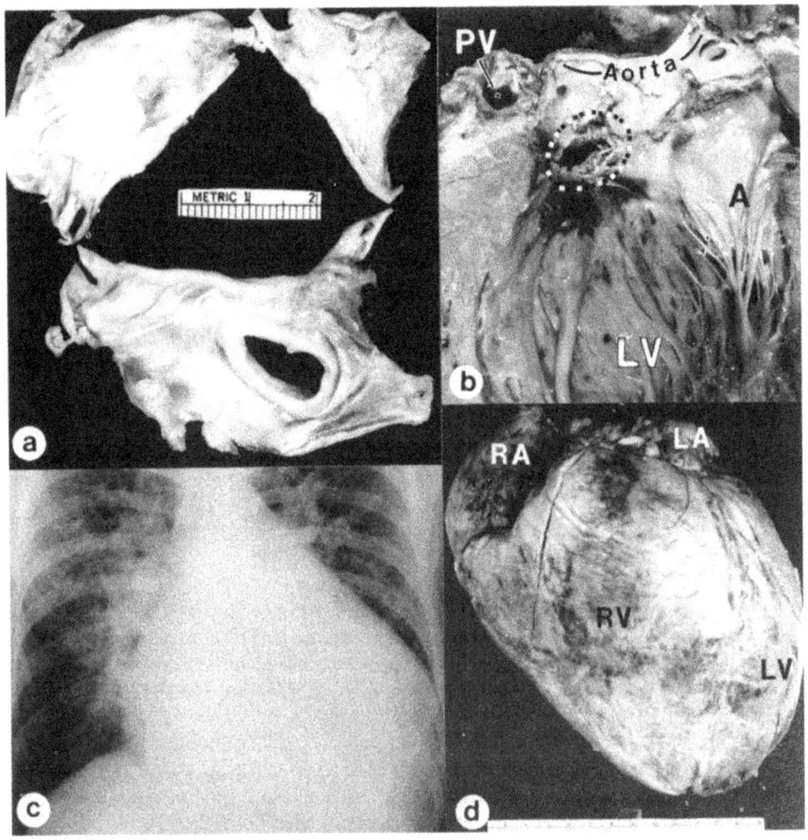

Fig. 2–36. Healed IE in a 34-year-old man with ventricular septal defect and aortic regurgitation. He died 1 day after operative closure of the defect and replacement of the aortic valve with a prosthesis. He had had an episode of active IE at age 21, 13 years before death. (A) Operatively excised aortic valve showing a large perforation in the largest cusp, i.e., the one that had prolapsed into the ventricular septal defect. (B) Opened left ventricle (LV) and aorta showing the location of the ventricular septal defect (enclosed by dashed circle). A, anterior mitral leaflet; PV, pulmonic valve. (C), (D) The heart in this patient was massively enlarged; it weighed 1250 g. RA, right atrium; RV, right ventricle; LA, left atrium.

ACKNOWLEDGMENT

I thank Filippina Giacometti and Carol L. Schurtz for technical assistance and Exa Murray for assistance in preparing the manuscript. The gross photographs were taken by L. Kenzie Edwards and James R. Banks, Jr.

REFERENCES

1. Cooper T, Morrow AG, Roberts WC, Herman LG: Postoperative endocarditis due to *Candida:* Clinical observations and the experimental production of the lesion. Surgery 50:341, 1961
2. Andriole VT, Kravetz HM, Roberts WC, Utz JP: Candida endocarditis. Clinical and pathologic studies. Am J Med 32:251, 1962
3. Roberts WC, Rabson AS: Focal glomerular lesions in fungal endocarditis. Ann Intern Med 56:610, 1962
4. Roberts WC, Braunwald E, Morrow AG: Acute severe mitral regurgitation secondary to ruptured chordae tendineae. Clinical, hemodynamic, and pathologic considerations. Circulation 33:58, 1966
5. Cohn LH, Roberts WC, Rockoff SD, Morrow AG: Bacterial endocarditis following aortic valve replacement. Clinical and pathologic correlations. Circulation 33:209, 1966
6. Archard HO, Roberts WC: Bacterial endocarditis after dental procedures in patients with aortic valve prostheses. J Am Dent Assoc 72:648, 1966
7. Roberts WC, Morrow AG: Bacterial endocarditis involving prosthetic mitral valves. Clinical and pathologic observations. Arch Pathol 82:164, 1966
8. Roberts WC, Ewy GA, Glancy DL, Marcus FI: Valvular stenosis produced by active infective endocarditis. Circulation 36:449, 1967
9. Glancy DL, Marcus FI, Cuadra M, Ewy GA, Roberts WC: Isolated organic tricuspid valvular regurgitation. Causes and consequences. Am J Med 46:989, 1969
10. Buchbinder NA, Roberts WC: Active infective endocarditis confined to mural endocardium. A study of six necropsy patients. Arch Pathol 93:435, 1972
11. Roberts WC, Buchbinder NA: Right-sided valvular infective endocarditis: A clinicopathologic study of twelve necropsy patients. Am J Med 53:7, 1972
12. Buchbinder NA, Roberts WC: Left-sided valvular active infective endocarditis. A study of forty-five necropsy patients. Am J Med 53:20, 1972
13. Buchbinder NA, Roberts WC: Alcoholism, an important but unemphasized factor predisposing to infective endocarditis. Arch Intern Med 132:689, 1973
14. Arnett EN, Roberts WC: Valve ring abscess in active infective endocarditis. Frequency, location and clues to clinical diagnosis from the study of 95 necropsy patients. Circulation 54:140, 1976
15. Arnett EN, Roberts WC: Prosthetic valve endocarditis. Clinico-pathologic analysis of 22 necropsy patients with comparison of observations in 74 necropsy patients with active infective endocarditis involving natural left-sided cardiac valves. Am J Cardiol 38:281, 1976
16. Arnett EN, Roberts WC: Active infective endocarditis: A clinicopathology analysis of 137 necropsy patients. Cur Prob Cardiol 1(7):1, 1976
17. Arnett EN, Roberts WC: Clinicopathology of prosthetic valve endocarditis, in Duma RJ (ed): Infections of Prosthetic Heart Valves and Vascular Grafts. Prevention, Diagnosis, and Treatment. Baltimore, University Park Press, 1977, pp 17–41
18. Andy JJ, Sheikh MU, Ali N, Barnes BO, Fox LM, Curry CL, Roberts WC: Echocardiographic observations in opiate addicts with active infective endocarditis. Frequency of involvement of the various valves and comparison of echocardiographic features of right and left-sided valvular endocarditis. Am J Cardiol 40:, 1977
19. Breyer RH, Arnett EN, Spray TL, Roberts WC: Prosthetic valve endocarditis due to *Listeria monocytogenes*. Am J Clin Pathol (in press)
20. Rokitansky C: Lehrbuch der Pathologischen Anatomie, vol 20 Vienna, Braumuller, 1856

21. Osler W: Malignant endocarditis. Lancet 1:415–418, 459–464, 505–508, 1885
22. Preble HB: Pneumoccus endocarditis. Am J Med Sci 128:782, 1904
23. Clawson BJ: An analysis of two hundred and twenty cases of endocarditis with special reference to the subacute bacterial type. Arch Intern Med 33:157, 1924
24. Thayer WS: Bacterial or infective endocarditis. Edinburgh Med J 38:237–265, 307–334, 1931
25. Goldburgh HL, Baer S, Lieber MM: Acute bacterial endocarditis of the tricuspid valve. Am J Med Sci 204:319, 1942
26. Wilson LM: Pathology of fatal bacterial endocarditis before and since the introduction of antibiotics. Ann Intern Med 58:84, 1963
27. Allen AC: Mechanism of localization of vegetations of bacterial endocarditis. Arch Pathol 27:399, 1939
28. Lepeschkin E: On the relation between the site of valvular involvement in endocarditis and the blood pressure resting on the valve. Am J Med Sci 224:318, 1952
29. Bain RC, Edwards JE, Scheifley CH, Geraci JE: Right-sided bacterial endocarditis and endarteritis. Am J Med 24:98, 1958
30. Luttgens WF: Endocarditis in "main line" opium addicts. Report on eleven cases. Arch Intern Med 83:653, 1949
31. Hussey HH, Katz S: Infections resulting from narcotic addiction. Report of 102 cases. Am J Med 9:186, 1950
32. Louria DB, Hensle T, Rose J: The major medical complications of heroin addiction. Ann Intern Med 67:1, 1967
33. Sapira JD: The narcotic addict as a medical patient. Am J Med 45:555, 1968
34. Reyes MP, Palutke WA, Wylin RF, Lerner AM: Pseudomonas endocarditis in the Detroit Medical Center 1969–1972. Medicine 52:173, 1973
35. Mills J, Drew D: *Serratia marcescens* endocarditis: A regional illness associated with intravenous drug abuse. Ann Intern Med 84:29, 1976
36. Olsson RA, Romansky MJ: Staphylococcal tricuspid endocarditis in heroin addicts. Ann Intern Med 57:755, 1962
37. Cherubin CE, Baden M, Kavaler F, Lerner S, Cline W: Infective endocarditis in narcotic addicts. Ann Intern Med 69:1091, 1968
38. Ramsey RG, Gunnar RM, Tobin JR: Endocarditis in the drug addict. Am J Cardiol 25:608, 1970
39. Menda KB, Gorbach SL: Favorable experience with bacterial endocarditis in heroin addicts. Ann Intern Med 78:25, 1973
40. Dreyer NP, Fields BN: Heroin-associated infective endocarditis. A report of 28 cases. Ann Intern Med 78:699, 1973
41. Banks R, Fletcher R, Ali N: Infective endocarditis in heroin addicts. Am J Med 55:444, 1973
42. Dowling HF, Lepper M, Caldwell ER, Spies HW: Staphylococci-endocarditis: An analysis of 25 cases treated with antibiotics together with a review of the recent literature. Medicine 31:155, 1952
43. Straus AL, Hamburger M: Pneumococcal endocarditis in the penicillin era. Arch Intern Med 118:190,1966
44. Pankey GA: Acute bacterial endocarditis at the University of Minnesota Hospital, 1939–1959. Am Heart J 64: 583, 1962
45. Virmani R, Roberts WC: Aschoff bodies in operatively excised atrial appendages and in papillary muscles. Frequency and clinical significance. Circulation 55:559, 1977
46. Gelfman R, Levine SA: The incidence of acute and subacute bacterial endocarditis in congenital heart disease. Am J Med Sci 204:324, 1942
47. Barker PS: A clinical study of subacute bacterial infection confined to the right side of the heart or the pulmonary artery. Am Heart J 37:1054, 1949

48. Volger WR, Dorney ER: Bacterial endocarditis in congenital heart disease. Am Heart J 64:198, 1962
49. Arnett JH: Splenic and hepatic enlargement in endocarditis: A study of two hundred and eighty-six autopsy findings. Am J Med Sci 163:590, 1922
50. Angrist A, Marquiss J: The changing morphologic picture of endocarditis since the advent of chemotherapy and antibiotic agents. Am J Pathol 30:39, 1954
51. Morgan WL, Bland EF: Bacterial endocarditis in the antibiotic era with special reference to the later complications. Circulation 19:753, 1959
52. Robinson MJ, Ruedy J: Sequelae of bacterial endocarditis. Am J Med 32:922, 1962
53. Roberts WC: The congenitally bicuspid aortic valve. A study of 85 autopsy cases. Am J Cardiol 26:72, 1970
54. Roberts WC: Anatomically isolated aortic valvular disease. The case against its being of rheumatic etiology. Am J Med 49:151, 1970
55. Roberts WC, Perloff JR, Costantino T: Severe aortic stenosis in patients over 65 years of age. A clinicopathologic study. Am J Cardiol 27:497, 1971
56. Traut EF, Carter JB, Gumbiner SH, Hench RN: Bacterial endocarditis in the elderly. A report of 94 autopsied cases. Geriatrics 4:205, 1949
57. Thell R, Martin FH, Edwards JE: Bacterial endocarditis in subjects 60 years of age and older. Circulation 51:174, 1975
58. LeBauer EJ, Perloff JK, Keliher TF: The isolated systolic click with bacterial endocarditis. Am Heart J 73:534, 1967
59. Horder TJ: Infective endocarditis with an analysis of 150 cases and with special reference to the chronic form of the disease. QJ Med 2:289, 1909
60. Morrison H: A study of the incidence of sub-acute bacterial endocarditis at the Massachusetts General Hospital. Boston Med Surg J 197:46, 1927
61. Middleton WS, Burke M: *Streptococcus viridans* endocarditis lenta. A clinico-pathologic analysis of the experience in the Wisconsin General Hospital. Am J Med Sci 198:301, 1939
62. Seabury JH: Subacute bacterial endocarditis. Experiences during the past decade. Arch Intern Med 79:1, 1947
63. Christian HA: The determinative background of subacute bacterial endocarditis. Am J Med Sci 201:34, 1941
64. Kelson SR, White PD: Notes on 250 cases of subacute bacterial (streptococcal) endocarditis studied and treated between 1927 and 1939. Ann Intern Med 22:40, 1945
65. Massell BF, Amezcua F, Pelargonio S: Evolving picture of rheumatic fever. Data from 40 years at the House of the Good Samaritan. JAMA 188:287, 1964
66. Stollerman GH: Rheumatic Fever and Streptococcal Infection. New York, Grune & Stratton, 1975, pp 209–226
67. Lerner PI, Weinstein L: Infective endocarditis in the antibiotic era. N Engl J Med 274:199, 1966
68. Cates JE, Christie RV: Subacute bacterial endocarditis. A review of 442 patients treated in 14 centers appointed by the Penicillin Trials Committee of the Medical Research Council. QJ Med 20:93, 1951
69. Perry EL, Fleming RG, Edwards JE: Myocardial lesions in bacterial endocarditis. Ann Intern Med 36:126, 1952
70. Kalman C, Thomison JB, Shapiro JL: Bacterial endocarditis: Autopsy experience over a thirty year period. South Med J 55:1208, 1962
71. Guze LB, Pearce ML: Hospital-acquired bacterial endocarditis. Arch Intern Med 112:56, 1963
72. Uwaydah MM, Weinberg AN: Bacterial endocarditis—A changing pattern. N Eng J Med 273:1231, 1965

73. Rabinovich S, Evans J, Smith IM, January LE: A long-term view of bacterial endocarditis: 337 cases 1924 to 1963. Ann Intern Med 63:185, 1965
74. Finland M, Barnes MW: Changing etiology of bacterial endocarditis in the antibacterial era. Experiences at Boston City Hospital 1933–1965. Ann Intern Med 72:341, 1970
75. Watanakunakorn C, Tan JS, Phair JP: Some salient features of *Staphylococcus aureus* endocarditis. Am J Med 54:473, 1973
76. Utley JR, Mills J: Annular erosion and pericarditis. Complications of endocarditis of the aortic root. J Thorac Cardiovasc Surg 64:76, 1972
77. Cherubin CE, Neu HC: Infective endocarditis at the Presbyterian Hospital in New York City from 1938–1967. Am J Med 51:83, 1971
78. Steiner I, Patel AK, Huff MSR, Somers K: Pathology of infective endocarditis. A postmortem evaluation. Br Heart J 35:159, 1973
79. Robinson MJ, Ruedy J: Sequelae of bacterial endocarditis. Am J Med 32:922, 1962
80. Cohen L, Freedman LR: Damage to the aortic valve as a cause of death in bacterial endocarditis. Ann Intern Med 55:562, 1961
81. Fowler NO, Hamburger MH, Bove KE: Aortic valve perforation. Am J Med 42:539, 1967
82. Burnside JW, DeSanctis RW: Bacterial endocarditis on calcification of the mitral anulus fibrosus. Ann Intern Med 76:615, 1972
83. Watanakunakorn C: *Staphylococcus aureus* endocarditis on the calcified mitral anulus fibrosus. Am J Med Sci 266:219, 1973
84. Ponfick: Ueber embolische aneurysmen, Nebst bemerkungen Uber das acute herzaneurysma (herzgeschwür). Virchows Arch Pathol Anat 58:528, 1873
85. Beck D: Pericarditis and subacute bacterial endocarditis. J Mt Sinai Hosp 8:364, 1941
86. McColl I: Pericarditis due to a mycotic aneurysm in subacute bacterial endocarditis. Report of a case affecting congenitally stenosed quadricuspid aortic valve. Guys Hosp Rep 107:34, 1958
87. Roberts NK, Somerville J: Pathological significance of electrocardiographic changes in aortic valve endocarditis. Br Heart J 31:395, 1969
88. Buchbinder WC, Saphir O: Heart failure in subacute bacterial endocarditis. Arch Intern Med 64:336, 1939
89. Saphir O: Myocardial lesions in subacute bacterial endocarditis. Am J Pathol 11:143, 1935
90. Correll HL, Lubitz JM, Lindert MCF: Bacterial endocarditis: Clinicopathologic studies of untreated, treated and cured patients. Ann Intern Med 35:45, 1951
91. de Navasquez S: The incidence and pathogenesis of myocardial lesions in subacute bacterial endocarditis. J Pathol Bacteriol 49:33, 1939
92. Roberts WC, Buchbinder NA: Papillary-muscle necrosis in active valvular infective endocarditis. Circulation 33,34 (Suppl 2): II–217, 1971 (abstract)
93. Roberts WC, Buja LM: The frequency and significance of coronary arterial thrombi and other observations in fatal acute myocardial infarction. A study of 107 necropsy patients. Am J Med 52:425, 1972
94. Roberts WC, Cohen LS: Left ventricular papillary muscles. Description of the normal and a survey of conditions causing them to be abnormal. Circulation 46:138, 1972
95. Roberts WC, Perloff JK: Mitral valvular disease. A clinicopathologic survey of the conditions causing the mitral valve to function abnormally. Ann Intern Med 77:939, 1972
96. Roberts WC, Morrow AG: Anatomic studies of hearts containing caged-ball prosthetic valves. Johns Hopkins Med J 121:271, 1967
97. Roberts WC, Morrow AG: Causes of death and other anatomic observations after cardiac valve replacement. Adv Cardiol 7:226, 1972

98. Roberts WC, Bulkley BH, Morrow AG: Pathologic anatomy of cardiac valve replacement: A study of 224 necropsy patients. Prog Cardiovasc Dis 15:539, 1973
99. Fishbein MC, Roberts WC, Golden A, Hufnagel CA: Cardiac pathology after aortic valve replacement using Hufnagel trileaflet prostheses: A study of 20 necropsy patients. Am Heart J 89:443, 1975
100. Fishbein MC, Roberts WC: Late postoperative anatomic observations after insertion of Hufnagel caged-ball prostheses in descending thoracic aorta. Chest 68:6, 1975
101. Roberts WC, Fishbein MC, Golden A: Cardiac pathology after valve replacement by disc prosthesis. A study of 61 necropsy patients. Am J Cardiol 35:740, 1975
102. Roberts WC, Hammer WJ: Cardiac pathology after valve replacement with a tilting disc prosthesis (Bjork-Shiley type). A study of 46 necropsy patients and 49 Bjork-Shiley prostheses. Am J Cardiol 37:1024, 1976
103. Conte JE, Cohen SN, Roe BB, Elashoff RM: Antibiotic prophylaxis and cardiac surgery. A prospective double-blind comparison of single-dose regimens. Ann Intern Med 76:943, 1972
104. Goodman JS, Schaffner W, Collins HA, Battersby EJ, Koenig MG: Infection after cardiovascular surgery: Clinical study including examination of antimicrobial prophylaxis. N Engl J Med 278:117, 1968
105. Nelson RM, Jenson CB, Peterson CA, Sanders BC: Effective use of prophylactic antibiotics in open-heart surgery. Arch Surg 90:731, 1965
106. Stein PD, Harken DE, Dexter L: The nature and prevention of prosthetic valve endocarditis. Am Heart J 71:393, 1966
107. Slaughter L, Morris JE, Starr A: Prosthetic valvular endocarditis. A 12-year review. Circulation 47:1319, 1973
108. Wilson WR, Jaumin PM, Danielson GK, Guilani ER, Washington JA, Gerachi JE: Prosthetic valve endocarditis. Ann Intern Med 82:751, 1975
109. Blakemore WC, McGarrity GJ, Thurer RJ, Wallace HW, MacVaugh H III, Ciriell LL: Infection of air-borne bacteria with cardiopulmonary bypass. Surgery 70:830, 1971
110. Dismukes WE, Karchmer AW, Buckley MJ, Austen WG, Swartz MN: Prosthetic valve endocarditis. Analysis of 38 cases. Circulation 48:365, 1973
111. Chaudhuri MR: Fungal endocarditis after valve replacement. J Thorac Cardiovasc Surg 60:207, 1970
112. Gage AA, Dean DC, Schimert G, Minsley N: Aspergillus infection after cardiac surgery. Arch Surg 101:384, 1970
113. Ostermiller WE Jr, Dye WS, Weinberg M: Fungal endocarditis following cardiovascular surgery. J Thorac Cardiovasc Surg 61:670, 1971
114. Lawrence T, Shockman AT, MacVaugh H III: Aspergillus infection of prosthetic aortic valves. Chest 60:406, 1971
115. Case records of the Massachusetts General Hospital. Weekly clinicopathological exercises. Case 24–1973. N Engl J Med 288:1290, 1973
116. Rubenstein E, Noriega ER, Simberkoff MS, Holzman R, Rahal JJ: Fungal endocarditis: Analysis of 24 cases and review of the literature. Medicine 54:331, 1975
117. Robboy SJ, Kaiser J: Pathogenesis of fungal infection on heart valve prostheses. Hum Pathol 6:711, 1975
118. Kammer RB, Utz JP: *Aspergillus* species endocarditis. The new face of a not so rare disease. Am J Med 56:506, 1974
119. Mann T, McLaurin L, Grossman W, Craige E: Assessing the hemodynamic severity of acute aortic regurgitation due to infective endocarditis. N Engl J Med 293:108, 1975
120. Madison J, Wang K, Gobel FL, Edwards JE: Prosthetic aortic valvular endocarditis. Circulation 51:940, 1975

121. McAllister RG, Samet J, Mazzoleni A, Dillon ML: Endocarditis on prosthetic mitral valves. Fatal obstruction to left ventricular inflow. Chest 66:682, 1974
122. Spray TL, Roberts WC: Structural changes in porcine xenografts used as substitute cardiac valves. Gross and histologic observations in 51 glutaraldehyde-preserved Hancock valves in 41 patients. Am J Cardiol 40:000, 1977
123. Sande MA, Johnson WD JR, Hook EW, Kaye D: Sustained bacteremia in patients with prosthetic cardiac valves. N Engl J Med 286:1067, 1972
124. Weinstein L: Infected prosthetic valves: A diagnostic and therapeutic dilemma. N Engl J Med 286:1108, 1972
125. Koiwai EK, Nahas HC: Subacute bacterial endocarditis following cardiac surgery. Arch Surg 73:272, 1956
126. Denton C, Pappas EG, Uricchio JF, Goldberg H, Likoff W: Bacterial endocarditis following cardiac surgery. Circulation 15:525, 1957
127. Linde LM, Heins HL: Bacterial endocarditis following surgery for congenital heart disease. N Engl J Med 263:65,1960
128. Yeh TJ, Anabtawi IN, Cornett VE, White A, Stern WH, Ellison RG: Bacterial endocarditis following open-heart surgery. Ann Thorac Surg 3:29, 1967
129. Shafer RB, Hall WH: Bacterial endocarditis following open heart surgery. Am J Cardiol 25:602, 1970
130. Dalton JC, Williams B, Atkins L: Staphylococcal endocarditis after mitral valvulotomy. Report of three cases. N Engl J Med 254:205, 1956
131. Morrow AG, Fort L III, Roberts WC, Braunwald E: Discrete subaortic stenosis complicated by aortic valvular regurgitation. Clinical, hemodynamic, and pathologic studies and the results of operative treatment. Circulation 31:163, 1965
132. Roberts WC: Valvular, subvalvular and supravalvular aortic stenosis: Morphologic features. Cardiovasc Clin 5:97, 1973
133. Roberts WC, Dangel JC, Bulkley BH: Non-rheumatic valvular cardiac disease: A clinicopathologic survey of 27 different conditions causing valvular dysfunction. Cardiovasc Clin 5:333, 1973
134. Muna WFT, Ferrans VJ, Pierce JE, Roberts WC: Discrete subaortic stenosis in Newfoundland dogs. Am Heart J (submitted for publication)
135. Johnson DH, Rosenthal A, Nadas AS: A forty-year review of bacterial endocarditis in infancy and childhood. Circulation 51:581, 1975
136. Roberts WC, Buchbinder NA: Healed left-sided infective endocarditis: A clinicopathologic study of 59 patients. Am J Cardiol 40:000, 1977
137. Kelson SR, White PD: Notes on 250 cases of subacute bacterial (streptococcal) endocarditis studied and treated between 1927 and 1939. Ann Intern Med 22:40, 1945
138. Pillsbury PL, Fiese MJ: Subacute bacterial endocarditis. Follow-up study of thirty patients treated with penicillin. Arch Intern Med 85:675, 1950
139. Gorlin R, Favour CB, Emery FJ: Long-term follow-up study of penicillin-treated subacute bacterial endocarditis. N Engl J Med 242:995, 1950
140. Cates JE, Christie RV: Subacute bacterial endocarditis. A review of 442 patients treated in 14 centres appointed by the Penicillin Trials Committee of the Medical Research Council. Q J Med 20:93, 1951
141. Donzelot E, Le Bozec J-M, Kaufmann H, Escalle J-E: Le pronostic de l'endocardite infectieuse subaigua traitee par les antibiotiques. Resultats du traitement de 202 cas. Arch Mal Coeur 46:97, 1953
142. Newman W, Torres JM, Guck JK: Bacterial endocarditis. An analysis of fifty-two cases. Am J Med 16:535, 1954
143. Priest WS, Smith JM, McGee CJ: Penicillin therapy of subacute bacterial endocarditis. A study of the end results in thirty-four cases, with particular reference to dosage,

methods of administration, criteria for judging adequacy of treatment and probable reasons for failures. Arch Intern Med 79:333, 1947

144. Hildebrand E, Priest WS: Cardiac lesions in subacute bacterial endocarditis treated with penicillin. Report of nine cases. Am J Clin Pathol 17:345, 1947
145. Priest WS, Smith JM: The effect of healed subacute bacterial endocarditis on cardiac dynamics. Arch Intern Med 95:646, 1955
146. Henriksen E, Neukirch F: The treatment of subacute bacterial endocarditis. Dan Med Bull 2:208, 1955
147. Mokotoff R, Brams W, Katz LN, Howell KM: The treatment of bacterial endocarditis with penicillin. Results of 17 consecutive unselected cases. Am J Med Sci 211:395, 1946
148. Kaplan SR, Rosenman RH, Katz LN, Brams WA: Healed subacute bacterial endocarditis. A new entity. JAMA 141:114, 1949
149. Mendelson CE, Cahue A, Katz LN, Brams WA: Long-term outlook for healed subacute bacterial endocarditis. JAMA 160:437, 1956
150. Hall B: Long-term follow-up of patients with healed bacterial endocarditis. Ann Intern Med 47:880, 1957
151. Wedgewood J: Prognosis in subacute bacterial endocarditis. Lancet 2:922, 1957
152. Morgan WL, Bland EF: Bacterial endocarditis in the antibiotic era. With special reference to the later complications. Circulation 19:753, 1959
153. Bunn P, Lunn J: Late follow-up of 64 patients with subacute bacterial endocarditis treated with penicillin. Am J Med Sci 279:549, 1962
154. Blount JG: Bacterial endocarditis. Am J Med 38:909, 1965
155. Rabinovich S, Evans J, Smith IM, January LE: A long-term view of bacterial endocarditis. 337 cases 1924 to 1963. Ann Intern Med 63:185, 1965

Prosthetic-valve Endocarditis Due to Listeria monocytogenes

ROBERT H. BREYER, M.D., ERNEST N. ARNETT, M.D., THOMAS L. SPRAY, M.D., AND WILLIAM C. ROBERTS, M.D.

Breyer, Robert H., Arnett, Ernest N., Spray, Thomas L., and Roberts, William C.: Prosthetic-valve endocarditis due to *Listeria monocytogenes*. Am J Clin Pathol 69: 186–187, 1978. Clinical and necropsy observations in the case of a patient with prosthetic-valve endocarditis due to *Listeria monocytogenes* are presented. Although rare cases of *L. monocytogenes* infection of natural cardiac valves have been reported, this represents the first known case of infection of a prosthetic cardiac valve by this organism. (Key words: Prosthetic heart valves; Endocarditis; *Listeria monocytogenes*.)

From the Clinic of Surgery and the Pathology Branch, National Heart, Lung and Blood Institute, National Institutes of Health, Bethesda, Maryland

PROSTHETIC-VALVE ENDOCARDITIS has been caused by a variety of unusual organisms, but, to our knowledge, there has been no report of its being caused by *Listeria monocytogenes*. Such was the case, however, in the patient to be described herein.

Report of a Case

A 64-year-old man who died November 13, 1974, had had his heavily calcified, stenotic, tricuspid aortic valve replaced with a Starr-Edwards prosthesis on January 11, 1973 (22 months before death). His early postoperative course had been complicated by temporary paresis of the right arm. Although the patient had had transient cerebral signs and symptoms 3 months after operation, he had been in functional class II status (New York Heart Association classification) until March 1974 (8 months before death) when he had noticed increasing exertional fatigue.

On September 24, 1974, the patient had had fever and sweats, and two days later he had been hospitalized. Oral temperature at that time was 39.2 C. Examination disclosed the expected prosthetic valve opening and closing sounds and a basal systolic ejection murmur. The leukocyte count was 17,000 cu mm. *Listeria monocytogenes* was grown from each of ten blood cultures of samples drawn serially over a two-day period. The organism was identified and speciated according to growth characteristics standardized by the Center for Disease Control. Minimal inhibitory concentrations (MIC) of antibiotics against this organism were (all in μg/ml): penicillin 0.2, ampicillin 0.2, cephalothin 1.6, erythromycin <0.4, tetracycline <0.4, kanamycin 3.0, gentamicin 1.6, intravenous administration of penicillin, 20 million units daily, was begun, and within 24 hours the fever had subsided. Serum bactericidal titers confirmed the adequacy of the antibiotic therapy (>99.9% bactericidal at 1:8 dilution 30 minutes before the scheduled dose of penicillin; 100% bactericidal at 1:32 dilution 10 minutes after the intravenous penicillin injection).

On October 13, 1974, however, the patient suddenly vomited, and had a severe headache. Two hours later, acute pulmonary edema appeared, followed by shock and finally, cardiac arrest. Although resuscitated, the patient never fully regained consciousness, and he died 30 days later. He had received penicillin intravenously during the entire period, and all further blood cultures were negative.

At necropsy (A74-296), thrombus rimmed the primary orifice of the Starr-Edwards aortic prosthesis (Fig. 1). The site of attachment of the prosthesis was focally necrotic and the prosthesis partially detached (Fig. 1). The necrotic process had burrowed through the wall of the aorta into the space between the aorta and left atrium. Histologic examination of the site of prosthetic attachment disclosed polymorphonuclear leukocytes and fibrin, but no colonies of organisms, and cultures of cardiac blood were negative. Examination of the brain at necropsy revealed subarachnoid hemorrhage over the right cerebellar hemisphere and cavitary lesions in the left frontal and right parietal lobes.

Comments

Although *Listeria monocytogenes* is an infrequent cause of human infection, it is known to cause infection of the meninges and the female pelvic organs. It also may produce infection in newborns and in patients who have lymphoreticular malignancies.[3] This organism is a rare cause of infective endocarditis; only 12 patients with *L. monocytogenes* endocarditis involving native cardiac valves have been reported.[2] Before the infection, five of the 12 patients had had normal cardiac valves, five others were known to have underlying valvular disease, and in two cases the status of the valve before the infection was not mentioned. None had a debilitating disease.

In our patient, the infection was present behind the site of attachment of the prosthesis but colonies of organisms were absent, and postmortem heart blood cultures were negative, presumably because of the intravenous administration of antibiotic therapy for more than 40 days. Organisms may be absent, however, in patients with fatal prosthetic valve endocarditis treated with antibiotics.[1] Although clinical signs of aortic regurgitation were never apparent, partial detachment of the prosthesis occurred. Our patient died, however, not from the effect of prosthetic endocarditis on the heart, but as a result of a central

Received November 29, 1976; received revised manuscript January 25, 1977; accepted for publication January 25, 1977.

Address reprint requests to Dr. Roberts: Chief, Pathology Branch, National Heart, Lung and Blood Institute, National Institutes of Health, Bethesda, Maryland 20014.

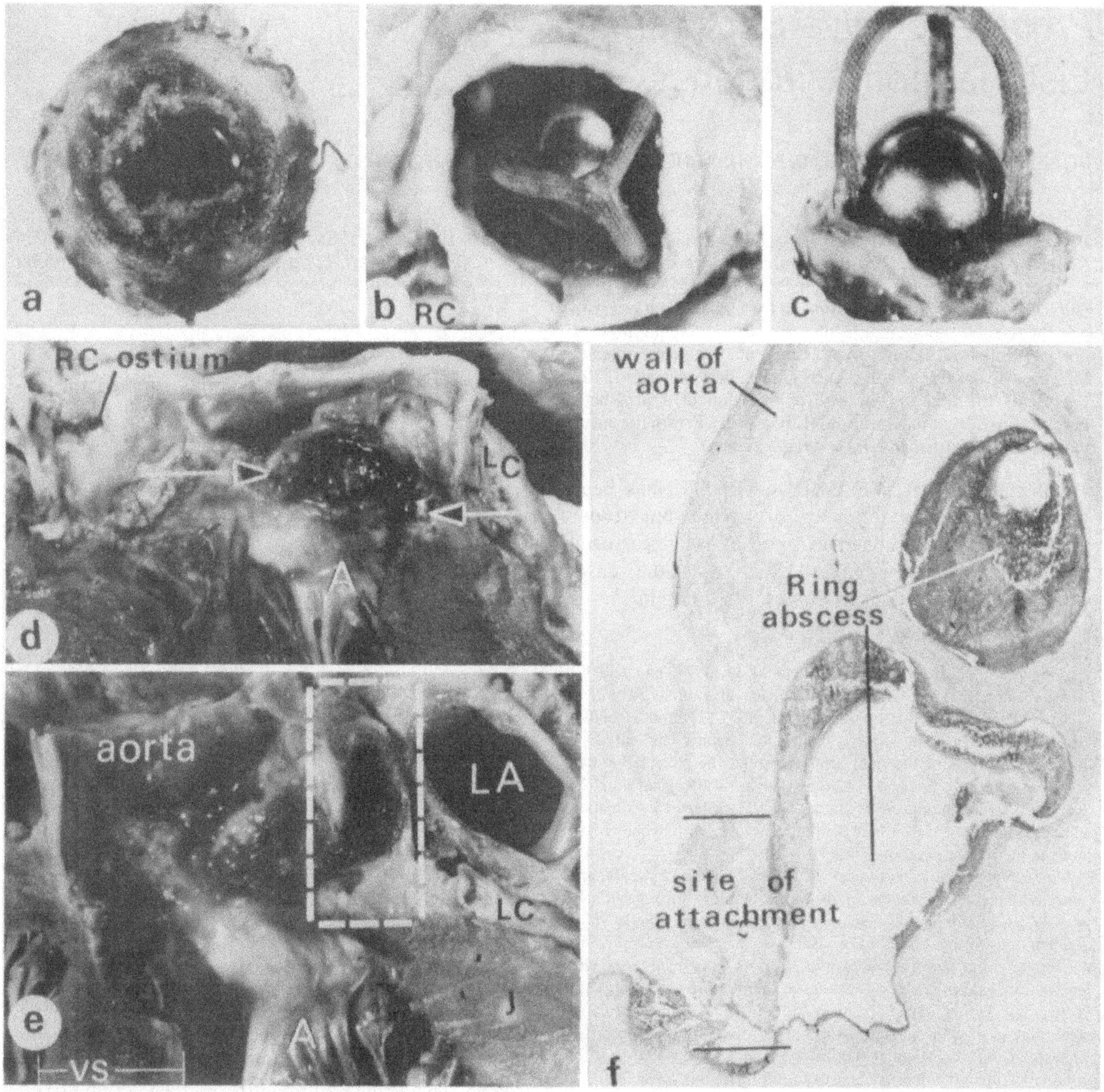

FIG. 1. Infected Starr-Edwards aortic valve prosthesis. *a*, Prosthesis as viewed from left ventricle. Thrombus devoid of organisms and inflammatory cells is present on the margins of the primary orifice. *b*, Prosthesis as viewed from above. RC = right coronary artery. *c*, Prosthesis as viewed laterally. The struts are devoid of thrombus. *d*, Opened aortic valve after removal of the prosthesis. A ring abscess (between the arrows) involves nearly half of the former site of attachment of the prosthesis. A = anterior mitral leaflet; LC = left coronary artery. *e*, Longitudinal cut through the ring abscess, showing extension through the full thickness of the wall of the aorta. Extravasation of blood did not occur because of marked fibrous thickening of the aortic adventitia. LA = left atrium; VS = ventricular septum. *f*, Histologic section through the area enclosed by dashed lines in *e*. Histologic section through the ring abscess, which represents an extension from the site of attachment of the prosthesis. No colonies of organisms were seen in the ring abscess or in the prosthetic anulus. Brown and Brenn stain: ×6.2.

nervous system catastrophe, presumably due to an embolus from the infected prosthetic valve.

References

1. Arnett EN, Roberts WC: Prosthetic valve endocarditis: A clinicopathologic analysis of 22 necropsy patients with comparison of observations to 74 necropsy patients with active infective endocarditis involving natural left-sided cardiac valves. Am J Cardiol 38:281–292, 1976
2. Bassan R: Bacterial endocarditis produced by *Listeria monocytogenes*. Am J Clin Pathol 63:522–527, 1975
3. Buckner LH, Schneierson SS: Clinical and laboratory aspects of *Listeria monocytogenes* infection. Am J Med 45:904–921, 1968

Discrete Subaortic Stenosis in Newfoundland Dogs: Association Of Infective Endocarditis

WALINJOM F. T. MUNA, MD, PhD
VICTOR J. FERRANS, MD, PhD
JOSEPH E. PIERCE, DVM
WILLIAM C. ROBERTS, MD, FACC

Bethesda, Maryland

Necropsy findings are described in eight Newfoundland dogs from the same colony with discrete subaortic stenosis. Infective endocarditis involving the aortic valve occurred in four dogs and in each it proved fatal. Damage to the aortic valve cusps by the jet of blood ejected through the discretely narrowed left ventricular outflow tract predisposes to the development of infective endocarditis in both dogs and human beings with discrete subaortic stenosis. Severe abnormality of the intramural coronary arteries in the ventricular septum, which also occurs in patients with hypertrophic cardiomyopathy, was present in all eight dogs. Myocardial fiber disorganization and asymmetric septal hypertrophy, two other findings observed in patients with hypertrophic cardiomyopathy, were absent in each of the eight Newfoundland dogs with discrete subaortic stenosis.

Discrete subaortic stenosis[1-5] is not unique to man, having been described in the pig,[6] cow[7] and dog.[8] It has been studied extensively in Newfoundland dogs, in which initial breeding experiments suggest that this lesion is inherited as either a polygenic or an autosomal dominant trait with modifiers.[9] Infective endocarditis often complicates discrete subaortic stenosis in man,[5,10,11] but it has not been reported in animals with this anomaly. Recent studies in patients with tunnel subaortic stenosis indicated some similarities to hypertrophic cardiomyopathy, including myocardial fiber disorganization and abnormalities of the intramural coronary arteries.[12,13] Similar abnormalities were sought in eight Newfoundland dogs, four of which experienced infective endocarditis that proved fatal.

Animals Studied

The eight Newfoundland dogs were direct descendants from the original colony of Pyles et al.[9] Certain characteristics in these dogs are summarized in Table I. Each had a precordial systolic murmur compatible with discrete subaortic stenosis. At cardiac catheterization, at age 2 months or older, the peak systolic pressure gradient between the left ventricle and the aorta ranged from 35 to 150 mm Hg; in all but one dog this gradient was more than 60 mm Hg. The animals died at 12 to 36 months of age; three were killed and the other five died naturally, all suddenly. At necropsy, the hearts were weighed and photographed, and histologic sections were prepared. From each animal at least three sections, each measuring at least 2 cm in longest diameter and extending from the endocardium to the epicardium, were prepared for histologic study.

Results

Subaortic stenosis and infective endocarditis: The discrete subaortic narrowing was located 8 to 10 mm below the level of the most caudal extension of the aortic valve cusps (Fig. 1 to 8). The discrete narrowing was circumferential and extended transversely over the ventricular septum and the outflow surface of the anterior mitral leaflet at the level of its attachment to atrial septum. Concentric left ventricular hypertrophy (Fig. 3 to 8) occurred in all eight animals. The ventricular cavities were of normal size except in Dog 3 (Fig. 3 and 4). In-

From the Pathology Branch and the Section on Laboratory Animal Medicine and Surgery, National Heart, Lung, and Blood Institute, National Institutes of Health, Bethesda, Maryland 20014. Manuscript received August 22, 1977; revised manuscript received October 3, 1977, accepted October 5, 1977.

Address for reprints: William C. Roberts, MD, Building 10A, Room 3E30, National Institutes of Health, Bethesda, Maryland 20014.

TABLE I

Clinical and Morphologic Observations in Newfoundland Dogs With Discrete Subaortic Stenosis

Dog no.	Age (mo) & Sex	LV-SA PSG (mm Hg)	Active Infective Endocarditis	Mechanism of Death	Heart Weight (g)	Body Weight (kg)	HW/BW Ratio*
1	12M	35	No	Killed	250	55	0.005
2	12M	150	No	Killed	450	45	0.01
3	15M	>60	No	Killed	700	50	0.01
4	18M	>60	Yes	Sudden	550	50	0.01
5	18F	>60	Yes	Sudden	520	65	0.01
6	24F	145	Yes	Sudden	400	45	0.01
7	28F	130	No	Sudden	400	45	0.01
8	36F	>60	Yes	Sudden	520	60	0.01

* The normal heart weight/body weight ratio in adult Newfoundland dogs without heart disease is not available. This ratio is available in beagles, and it is approximately 0.008. Beagles, however, weigh only up to 15 kg, whereas adult Newfoundland dogs generally weigh between 45 and 70 kg. We therefore believe that the normal heart weight/body weight ratio in adult Newfoundland dogs is somewhat lower than in beagles and is probably about 0.005.

BW = body weight; HW = heart weight; LV = left ventricle; PSG = peak systolic gradient; SA = systemic artery.

fective endocarditis occurred in four of five dogs that died spontaneously (Fig. 5, 7 and 8) but in none of the three killed dogs. In three of the four dogs with infection, vegetations partially obstructed the ostium of the left coronary artery. One or more perforations were present in one or more cusps of the aortic valve in each of the four dogs with infective endocarditis. The infective process also involved the subaortic membrane and the ventricular aspect of the anterior mitral leaflet in two dogs (Fig. 6). Focal necrosis of the left ventricular papillary muscle also occurred in each of the four dogs with infective endocarditis. Large colonies of gram-positive cocci, inflammatory cells (mainly polymorphonuclear leukocytes) and necrotic cell debris were observed histologically in the vegetations in all four dogs. Microabscesses also occurred in the left ventricular myocardium in all four dogs.

Coronary arterial abnormalities: Luminal narrowing, intimal fibrous proliferation, medial hypertrophy and medial smooth muscle disorganization were noted in many intramural coronary arteries in the ventricular septum in all eight dogs (Fig. 2 to 6). In contrast, the extramural branches of the coronary arteries were normal and free of emboli or thrombi. Septic emboli, however, were found in one or more intramural coronary arteries of three dogs with infective endocarditis. Foci of myocardial fiber disorganization, of the kind observed in patients with hypertrophic cardiomyopathy, were not noted in the ventricular septum in any of the eight dogs.

Comments

Mechanism of infective endocarditis: That infective endocarditis develops after damage to the endothelial covering of the aortic valve cusps by blood ejected through the subaortic discrete obstruction under high pressure and velocity is in agreement with the findings in experimental animal models of endocarditis.[14] Endothelial cells can be detached from the vascular surface by mechanical forces generated by a jet of blood.[15,16] Furthermore, denudation of endothelium exposes the subendothelial space, which is covered by a layer of fibrin.[14] Bacteria circulating in the bloodstream adhere to the fibrin deposits. Thus, endothelial damage appears to be an important event in the development of infective endocarditis.

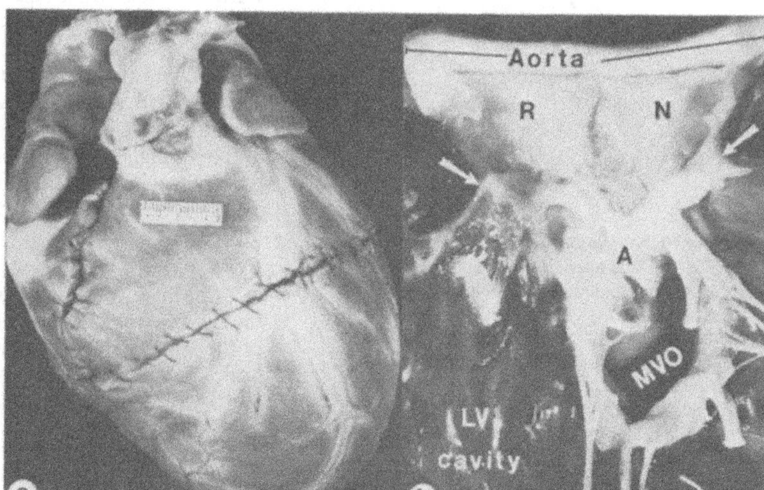

FIGURE 1. Dog 2. **a,** exterior view of heart showing a very large left ventricle. **b,** opened left ventricular (LV) outflow tract showing the discrete "membrane" (between arrows). The peak systolic pressure gradient between the left ventricle and the systemic artery was 150 mm Hg. A = anterior mitral leaflet; MVO = mitral valve orifice; N = noncoronary and R = right aortic valve cusps.

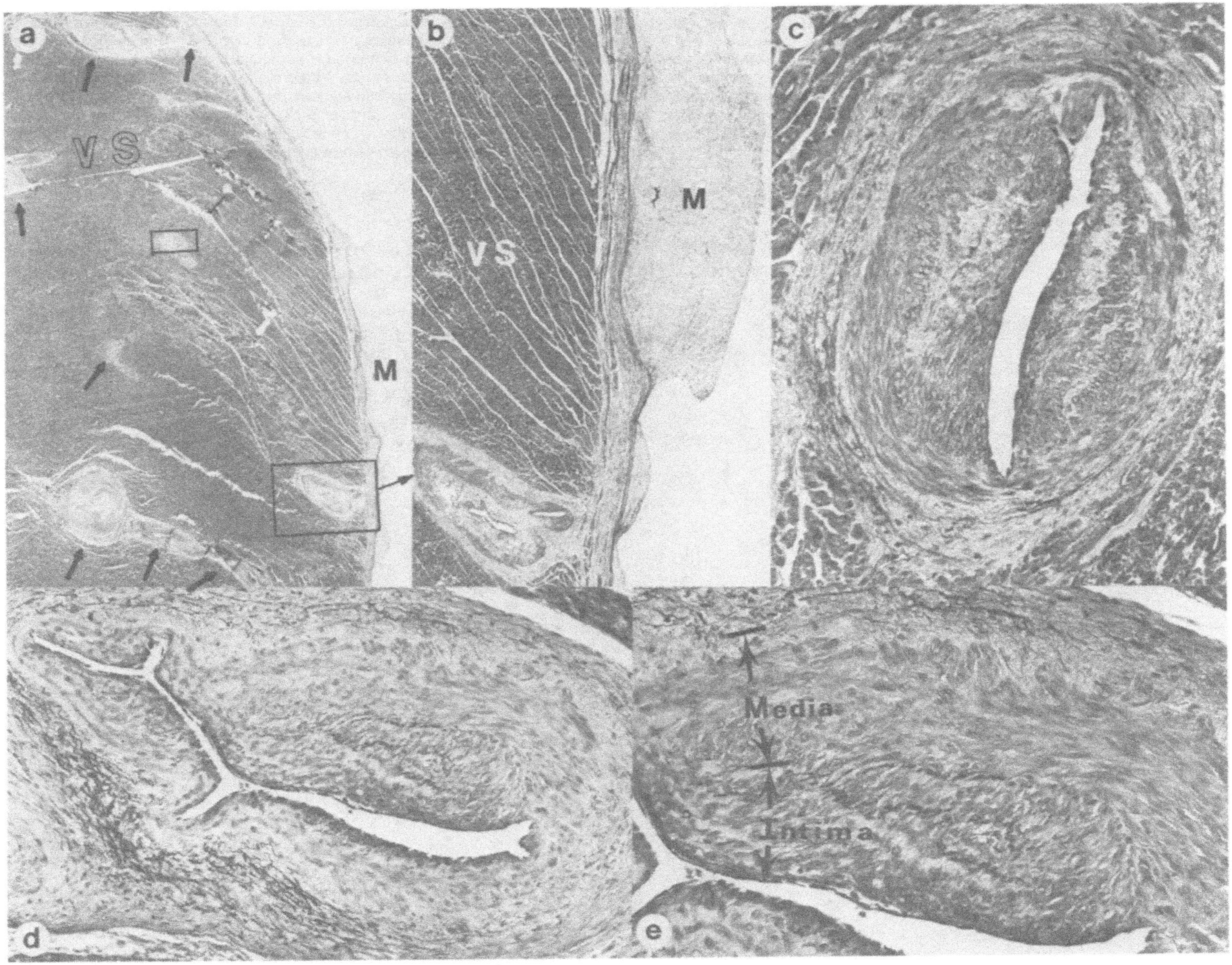

FIGURE 2. Dog 2. Portion of ventricular septum (VS) (**a** and **b**) showing several intramural coronary arteries. **a**, several intramural coronary arteries are designated by either **arrows** or **rectangles.** M = "membrane" of the discrete subaortic stenosis in the left ventricular outflow tract. **b**, a closer view of an area shown in **a**. VS = ventricular septum. **c**, an intramural coronary artery shown in the **rectangle** in **a. d**, another intramural coronary artery, and (**e**) a close-up view of a portion of its wall. (Movat stains ×10 [**a**], ×27 [**b**], ×220 [**c**], ×130 [**d**] and ×250 [**e**], all reduced by 7 percent.)

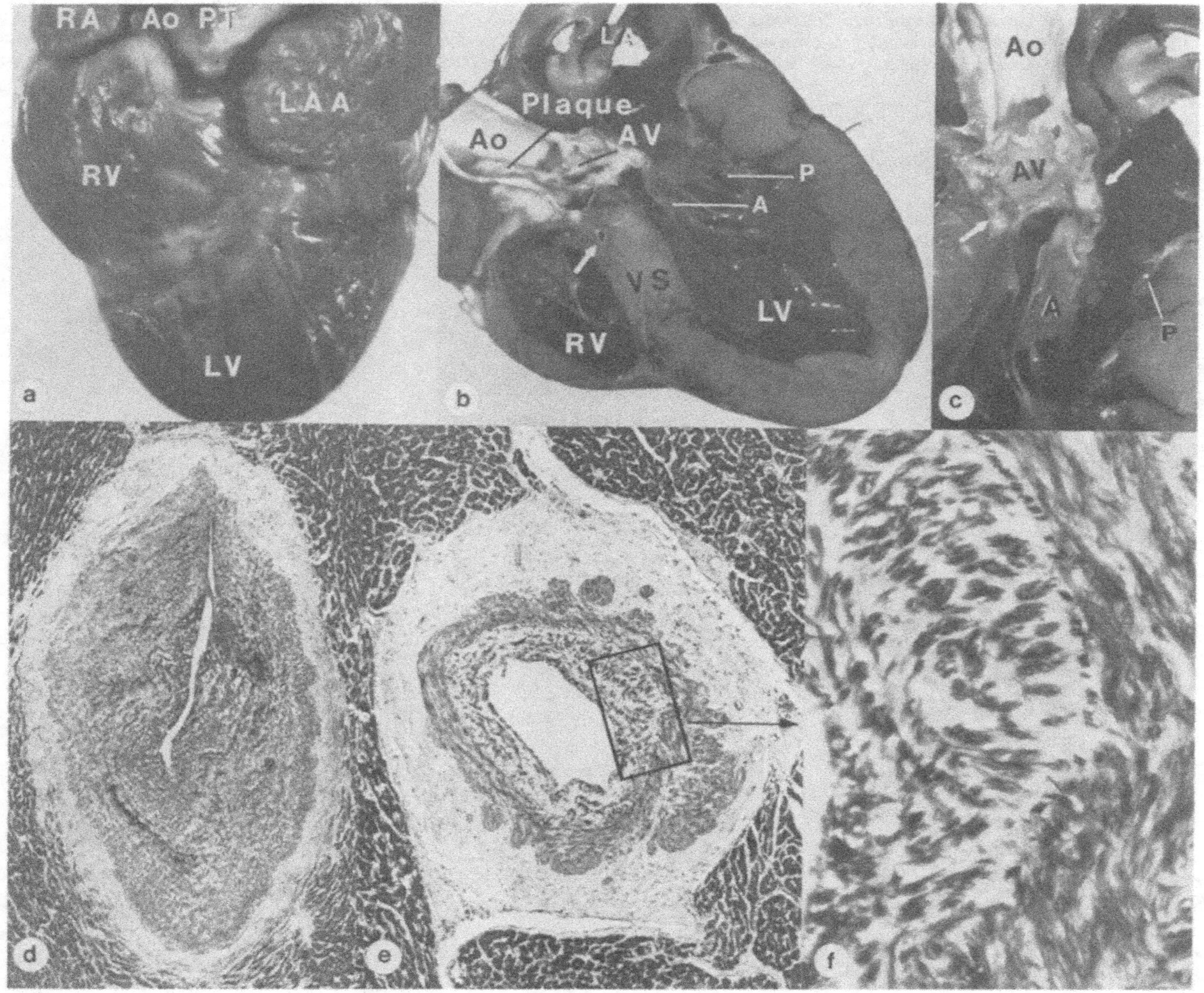

FIGURE 3. Dog 3. Heart **(a, b, c)** and intramural coronary arteries in ventricular septum (VS) **(d, e, f)**. **a,** exterior view showing a very large left ventricle (LV) and left atrial appendage (LAA). Ao = *ascending aorta;* PT = *pulmonary trunk;* RA = *right atrium;* RV = *right ventricle.* **b,** view after removing the anterior half. The left ventricle is dilated. This was the only dog with a dilated left ventricle. The subaortic membrane is located **between the arrows** in the left ventricular outflow tract shown in **c.** The aortic valve (AV) cusps are thickened by fibrous tissue, and the intima in the ascending aorta is focally thickened. A large coronary artery **(white arrow in b)** is present in the cephalad portion of the ventricular septum. A = anterior and P = posterior mitral leaflets; LA = left atrium. **d** and **e,** intramural coronary arteries in ventricular septum. The internal elastic membrane is not discernible in **d,** but it is preserved in **e.** A close-up view of a portion of wall of the artery in **e** is shown in **f.** The cells in the intima are arranged *primarily perpendicular to the lining of the lumen. In contrast,* the cells in the media are arranged more or less parallel to the lining of the lumen. The cells with spindle- or strap-shapes are considered smooth muscle cells. (Movat stains ×54 **[d]**, ×80 **[e]** and ×380 **[f]**, all reduced by 18 percent.)

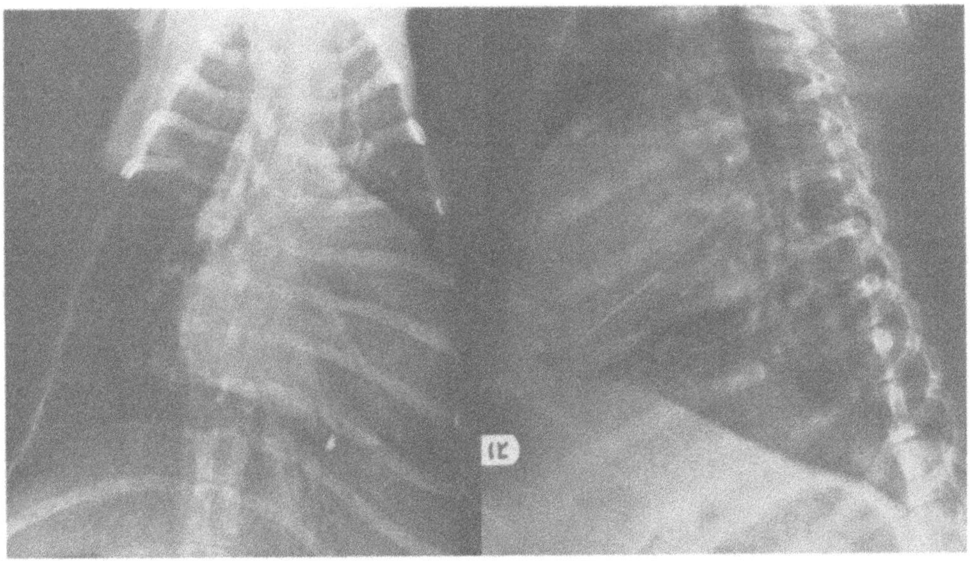

FIGURE 4. Dog 3. Radiographs of heart showing massive cardiomegaly. **Left,** posteroanterior view; **right,** lateral view.

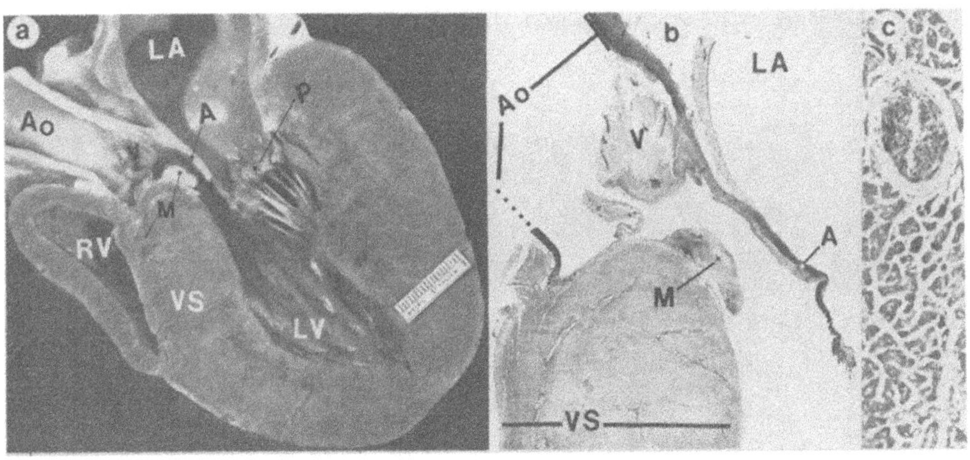

FIGURE 5. Dog 4. **a,** heart in longitudinal view. **b,** photomicrograph of left ventricular outflow tract showing a vegetation (V) occupying much of one sinus of Valsalva. **c,** narrowed intramural coronary artery in ventricular septum. Abbreviations as in previous figures. (Movat stains ×5 [**b**] and ×140 [**c**], both reduced by 34 percent.)

TABLE II

Infective Endocarditis (IE) in Patients with Discrete Subaortic Stenosis (DSS): Summary of Previously Reported Cases

Reference: First Author	Reference: Year	Patients With DSS (no.)	Patients With IE: no.	Patients With IE: %
Nonnecropsy Patients or Clinical Studies				
Brock[17]	1959	16	0	0
Braunwald[1]	1963	20	0	0
Morrow[10]	1965	4	4	100
Campbell[2]	1968	7	0	0
McGoon[3]	1969	30	1*	3
Reis[18]	1971	21	2	10
Shariatzadeh[19]	1972	20	0	0
Kelly[20]	1972	25	0	0
Champsaur[21]	1973	20	0	0
Popp[22]	1974	3	1	33
Mody[23]	1975	6	0	0
Wyman[24]	1976	70	0	0
Newfeld[25]	1976	51	1	2
Chiariello[4]	1976	11	0	0
Necropsy Patients				
Fontana[11]	1962	29	13	45
Roberts[5]	1973	7	4	57

* IE after operation only.

Incidence of infective endocarditis in subaortic stenosis: The frequency of infective endocarditis in animals with discrete subaortic stenosis is not known. Reports of infective endocarditis in patients with discrete subaortic stenosis are summarized in Table II.[1–5,10,17–25] The frequency of infective endocarditis in patients with discrete subaortic stenosis was 45 percent in the 29 necropsy cases collected by Fontana and Edwards from previous reports.[11] This is the highest reported incidence rate of infective endocarditis associated with any congenital or acquired cardiac disorder. Of the seven patients with discrete subaortic stenosis we studied at necropsy (Table I), four had infective endocarditis[5] that was active in two and healed in two. Lower frequencies of infective endocarditis have been reported in other series of patients with discrete subaortic stenosis. The much lower frequency (less than 10 percent) (Table II) of infective endocarditis in the clinical reports of discrete subaortic stenosis may be due in part to early operative treatment (before aortic valve scarring or infection occurred).

Clinical and hemodynamic consequences of infective endocarditis: When infective endocarditis does

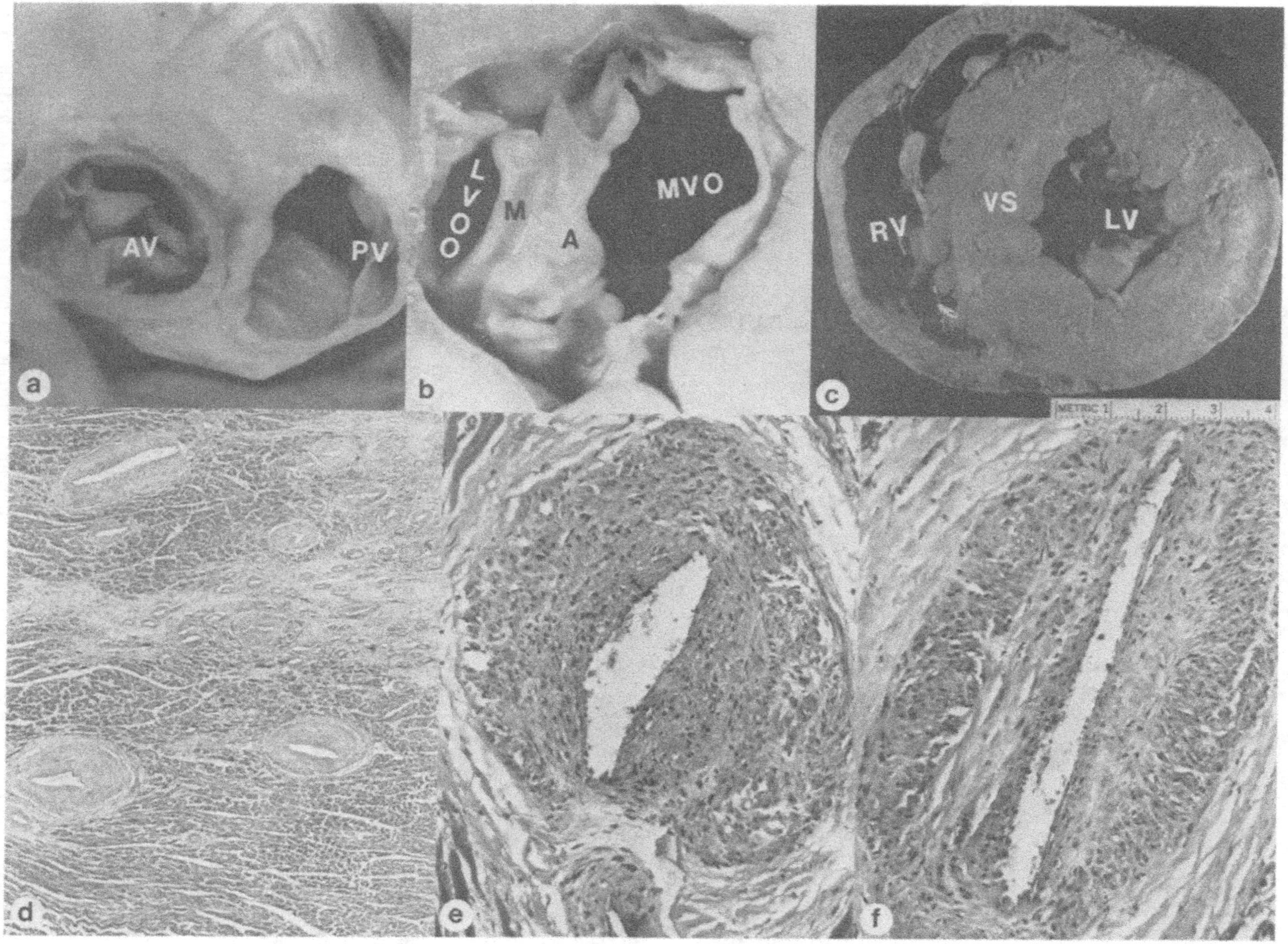

FIGURE 6. Dog 7. Heart **(a, b, c)** and intramural coronary arteries of ventricular septum **(d, e, f)**. **a,** aortic valve (AV) and pulmonary valve (PV) from above. The aortic valve cusps are thick whereas the pulmonary valve cusps are normal. **b,** left ventricular outflow tract as viewed from the left ventricle. The left ventricular outflow obstruction (LVOO) is produced by the subaortic membrane (M), which is attached to the anterior mitral leaflet (A) as well as to the mural endocardium (poorly shown). This dog had a high (130 mm Hg) peak systolic pressure gradient between the left ventricle and the systemic artery. MVO = mitral valve orifice. **c,** transverse section of the ventricles showing symmetric hypertrophy. LV = left ventricle; RV = right ventricle; VS = ventricular septum. **d,** several intramural coronary vessels in the ventricular septum. Most of them have narrowed lumens. The largest diameter of the lumens tends to be similarly oriented in most of the arteries. Replacement myocardial fibrosis also is present. **e** and **f**, close-up views of two arteries. The internal elastic membranes are not distinct. (Movat stains ×40 [**d**], ×330 [**e**] and ×220 [**f**], all reduced by 13 percent.)

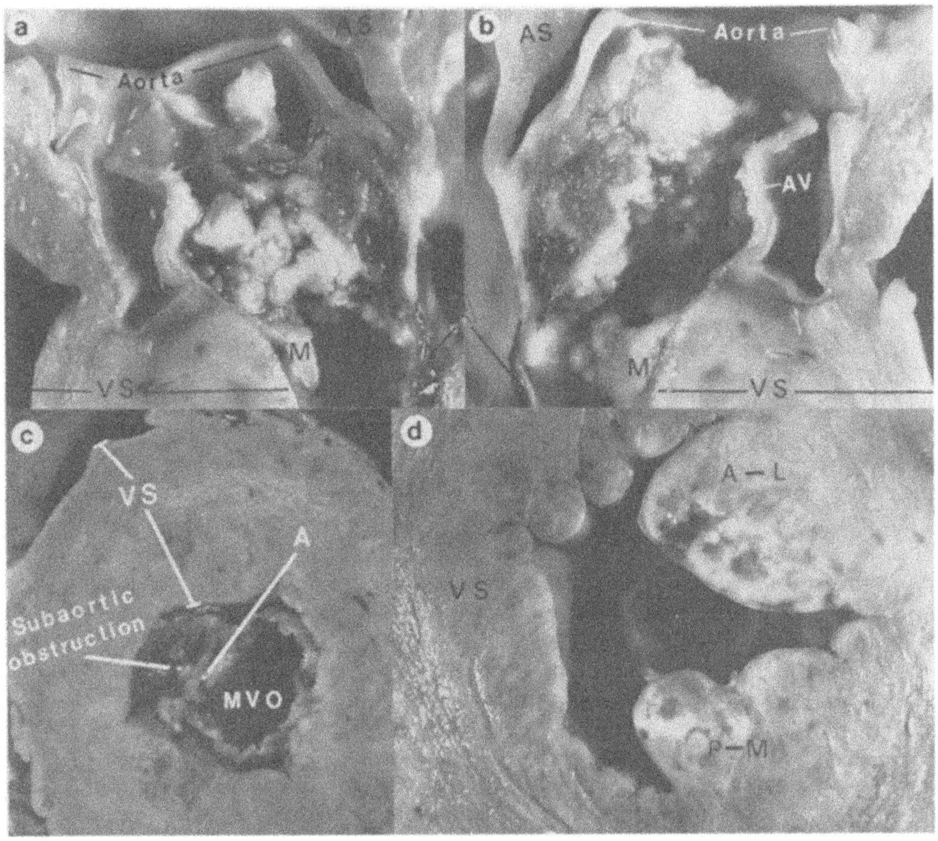

FIGURE 7. Dog 6. Heart with infective endocarditis. A peak systolic pressure gradient between the left ventricle and the systemic artery of 145 mm Hg was measured earlier in life before the cardiac infection occurred. **a**, view of posterior half of the heart as seen anteriorly showing the infected aortic valve. A = anterior mitral leaflet; AS = atrial septum; M = subaortic "membrane"; VS = ventricular septum. **b**, similar anatomy but a view of the anterior half of the aortic valve (AV) as seen posteriorly. The vegetative material has extended to involve the subaortic membrane. A large intramural coronary artery is present in the ventricular septum. **c**, view of subaortic obstruction from below. MVO = mitral valve orifice. **d**, close-up view of the anterolateral (A-L) and posteromedial (P-M) papillary muscles showing extensive necrosis of each.

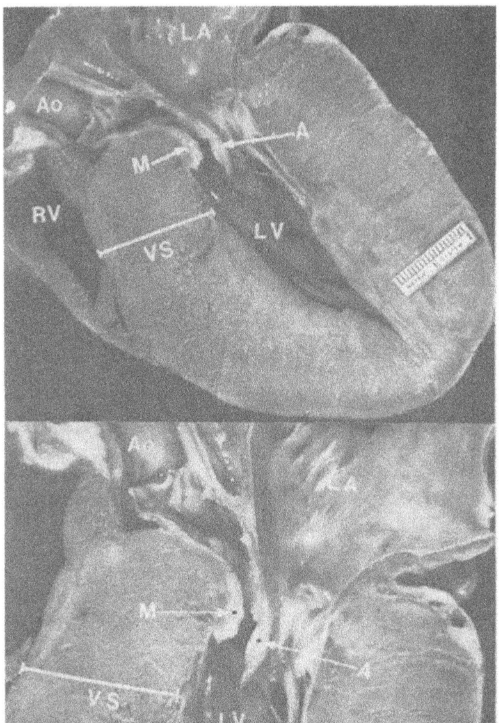

FIGURE 8. Dog 8. Heart with infective endocarditis on the aortic valve. Here, however, the vegetations are not discernible but the aortic valve cusps and subaortic obstruction (due to the close apposition of the "membrane" [M] and the anterior [A] mitral leaflet) are clearly seen. Abbreviations as in previous legends.

complicate discrete subaortic stenosis, clinical manifestations of aortic valve damage may be entirely absent, in contrast to their near universal occurrence in patients with infective endocarditis of the aortic valve and no subaortic obstruction. Damage to the aortic valve from infection in patients without subaortic stenosis generally leads to severe aortic regurgitation, progressive dilatation of the left ventricle and, finally, overt congestive heart failure. In patients with subaortic stenosis, the subaortic obstruction prevents severe aortic regurgitation from occurring because the subvalve chamber above the subaortic obstruction is too small to accommodate much regurgitant volume. As a consequence, diagnosis of infective endocarditis in patients with discrete subaortic stenosis may be unduly delayed. Also, in patients with infective endocarditis of the aortic valve without subaortic stenosis, the hemodynamic consequence is *pure* aortic regurgitation. In contrast, in the person or dog with infective endocarditis of the aortic valve and subaortic stenosis, the vegetations may extend onto the subaortic "membrane" and cause further obstruction to left ventricular outflow. In all four Newfoundland dogs with infective endocarditis, death was sudden and in each the left ventricular outflow obstruction appeared to have been worsened by the vegetations.

Intramural coronary arterial abnormalities: Severe abnormality of the intramural coronary arteries of the ventricular septum occurred in each of the eight dogs. These abnormalities consisted of considerable increase in vessel size, intimal smooth muscle proliferation, medial hypertrophy, disorganization of the media with loss or absence of the internal elastic membrane and luminal narrowing. In addition, the number of intramural coronary arteries in the septum appeared to be increased. These abnormalities were minimal or absent in the left and right ventricular free walls. Similar changes in intramural coronary arteries of dogs with discrete subaortic stenosis were described by Flickinger and Patterson.[26] These changes in intramural coronary arteries are identical to those observed in about half of patients with hypertrophic cardiomyopathy studied at necropsy.[12] The cause of the changes in the intramural coronary arteries is uncertain, but these changes, together with those in patients with hypertrophic cardiomyopathy,[12] are the most impressive changes we have observed in the intramural coronary arteries in any condition. The changes appeared just as extreme in the 12 month old animal as in the 36 month old animal; however, study of eight newborn Newfoundland puppies from the same colony as the eight dogs described here disclosed no abnormalities of the intramural coronary arteries. Similar abnormalities of the intramural coronary arteries in the ventricular septum were also observed in four patients with discrete subaortic stenosis whom we studied at necropsy with histologic examination of the ventricular septum (Roberts WC, unpublished observations).

Coronary blood flow: Although the cause or causes of the alterations in the intramural coronary arteries in our Newfoundland dogs are uncertain, abnormalities in coronary blood flow may be important. Pyle et al.[27] showed in both German shepherd and Newfoundland dogs with discrete subaortic stenosis that flow of blood in the left coronary arteries is diminished and that it is reversed during most of ventricular systole both at rest and during exercise. Significant retrograde flow during any portion of systole has never been observed in the normal dog.[28]

Whether coronary blood flow is abnormal in patients with left ventricular outflow obstruction and morphologically abnormal intramural coronary arteries is uncertain. In human beings, abnormal intramural coronary arteries, particularly those in the ventricular system, were observed in hypertrophic cardiomyopathy,[12] in discrete subaortic stenosis (Roberts WC, unpublished observations) and in tunnel subaortic stenosis,[13] but not in aortic valve stenosis.[12] In the latter condition, the obstruction is usually acquired later in life, whereas in the other three conditions it is present from birth or at least in early life. Early onset of obstruction may be essential for development of the abnormalities in the intramural coronary arteries.

Discrete subaortic stenosis versus hypertrophic cardiomyopathy: Although the alterations we described in the intramural coronary arteries in the ventricular septum suggest a similarity between discrete subaortic stenosis and hypertrophic cardiomyopathy, both dogs and human beings with discrete subaortic stenosis have concentric left ventricular hypertrophy rather than asymmetric septal hypertrophy; and myocardial fiber disorientation in the ventricular septum, as observed in patients with hypertrophic cardiomyopathy,[29] is absent in both dogs and patients with discrete subaortic stenosis. Thus, discrete subaortic stenosis and hypertrophic cardiomyopathy are distinctly separate entities.

References

1. **Braunwald E, Goldblatt A, Aygen MM, et al:** Congenital aortic stenosis. I. Clinical and hemodynamic findings in 100 patients. Circulation 27:426–462, 1963
2. **Campbell M:** The natural history of congenital aortic stenosis. Br Heart J 30:514–526, 1968
3. **McGoon DC, Geha AS, Scofield EL, et al:** Surgical treatment of congenital aortic stenosis. Chest 55:388–394, 1969
4. **Chiariello L, Agosti J, Vlad P, et al:** Congenital aortic stenosis. Experience with 43 patients. J Thorac Cardiovasc Surg 63: 258–262, 1976
5. **Roberts WC, Dangel JC, Bulkley BH:** Nonrheumatic valvular cardiac disease: a clinicopathologic survey of 27 different conditions causing valvular dysfunction. Cardiovasc Clin 5:334–446, 1973
6. **Emsbo P:** Subaortal Stenose; Komparative Studier over Medfodt Subvalvulaer Aortastenose (Venstreisidig Konusstenose) Has Suin og Menneske. Copenhagen, Denmark, Dansk Videnskabs Forlag, 1955, p 1–30
7. **Jubb KVF, Kennedy PC:** Pathology of Domestic Animals, Vol 1. New York, Academic Press, 1970, p 71–88
8. **Patterson DF:** Congenital heart disease in the dog. Ann NY Acad Sci 127:541–569, 1965
9. **Pyle RL, Patterson DF, Chacko S:** The genetics and pathology of discrete subaortic stenosis in the Newfoundland dog. Am Heart J 92: 324–334, 1976
10. **Morrow AG, Fort III L, Roberts WC, et al:** Discrete subaortic stenosis complicated by aortic valvular regurgitation. Clinical, hemodynamic and pathologic studies and the results of operative treatment. Circulation 31:163–171, 1965
11. **Fontana RS, Edwards JE:** Congenital Cardiac Disease: A Review of 357 Cases Studied Pathologically. Philadelphia, London, WB Saunders, 1962, p 291
12. **McReynolds RA, Roberts WC:** The intramural coronary arteries in hypertrophic cardiomyopathy (abstr). Am J Cardiol 35:154, 1975
13. **Maron BJ, Redwood DR, Roberts WC, et al:** Tunnel subaortic stenosis. Left ventricular outflow tract obstruction produced by fibromuscular tubular narrowing. Circulation 54:404–416, 1976
14. **Durack DT:** Experimental bacterial endocarditis. IV. Structure and evolution of very early lesions. J Pathol 115:81–89, 1975
15. **Fry DL:** Acute vascular endothelial changes associated with increased blood velocity gradients. Circ Res 22:165–197, 1968
16. **Fry DL:** Certain histological and chemical responses of the vascular interface to acutely induced mechanical stress in the aorta of the dog. Circ Res 24:93–108, 1969
17. **Brock R:** Aortic subvalvular stenosis. Surgical treatment. Guys Hosp Rep 108:144–158, 1959
18. **Reis RL, Peterson LM, Mason DT, et al:** Congenital fixed aortic stenosis. An anatomical classification and correlations with operative results. Circulation 43, 44:Suppl I:I-11–I-18, 1971
19. **Shariatzadeh AN, King H, Girod D, et al:** Discrete subaortic stenosis. A report of 20 cases. J Thorac Cardiovasc Surg 63:258–262, 1972
20. **Kelly DT, Wulfsberg BA, Rowe RD:** Discrete subaortic stenosis.

Circulation 46:309–322, 1972
21. **Champsaur G, Trusler GA, Mustard WT:** Congenital discrete subvalvular aortic stenosis. Surgical experience and long-term follow-up in 20 pediatric patients. Br Heart J 35:443–446, 1973
22. **Popp RL, Silverman JF, French JW, et al:** Echocardiographic findings in discrete subvalvular aortic stenosis. Circulation 49: 226–231, 1974
23. **Mody MR, Mody GT:** Serial hemodynamic observations in congenital valvular and subvalvular aortic stenosis. Am Heart J 89: 137–143, 1975
24. **Wyman AE, Feigenbaum H, Hurwitz RA, et al:** Localization of left ventricular outflow obstruction by cross-sectional echocardiography. Am J Med 60:33–38, 1976
25. **Newfeld EA, Muster AJ, Paul MH, et al:** Discrete subvalvular aortic stenosis in childhood. Study of 51 patients. Am J Cardiol 38:53–61, 1976
26. **Flickinger GL, Patterson DF:** Coronary lesions associated with congenital subaortic stenosis in the dog. J Pathol Bacteriol 93: 133–140, 1967
27. **Pyle RL, Lowensohn HS, Khouri EM, et al:** Left circumflex coronary artery hemodynamics in conscious dogs with congenital subaortic stenosis. Circ Res 33:34–38, 1973
28. **Gregg DE, Khouri EM, Rayford CR:** Systemic and coronary energetics in the resting unanesthetized dog. Circ Res 16:102–113, 1965
29. **Epstein SE, Henry WL, Clark CE, et al:** Asymmetric septal hypertrophy. Ann Intern Med 81:650–680, 1974

Disseminated Petriellidium boydii and Pacemaker Endocarditis

WILLIAM A. DAVIS, M.D.
Washington, D.C.
JEFFREY M. ISNER, M.D.*
Bethesda, Maryland
ARTHUR W. BRACEY, M.D.
Washington, D.C.
WILLIAM C. ROBERTS, M.D.
Bethesda, Maryland
VINCENT F. GARAGUSI, M.D.
Washington, D.C.

Clinical and morphologic findings are described in a 62 year old woman with "mixed connective tissue disease" who received corticosteroid therapy, and in whom disseminated and fatal Petriellidium boydii infection with right-sided endocarditis developed. The patient was a gardener. The organism is ubiquitous in soil in many parts of the United States; therefore, it is likely that the infection was introduced by this means. Endocarditis due to P. boydii has not been reported previously. In the patient described, massive vegetations nearly obliterated the tricuspid valve orifice, encasing a pacemaker catheter which had been inserted eight years earlier. Although never previously isolated from blood cultures, P. boydii was isolated from 11 consecutive blood cultures. P. boydii is a true fungus and has only recently been appreciated as an opportunistic pathogen in a compromised host.

Infection is one of the major factors limiting survival of a compromised host. Many microorganisms previously considered benign have been recognized more recently to be pathogens in patients whose immunologic status has been compromised. P. boydii (previously Allescheria boydii), a true fungus found in soil, for years was believed to have its pathogenicity primarily limited to maduromycosis of the foot [1]. Recently, this organism has gained increasing recognition as an opportunistic pathogen [2,3]. This report describes previously unreported findings in a patient with widely disseminated, fatal P. boydii infection.

CASE REPORT

A 62 year old black woman, who died August 19, 1977, was first seen at Georgetown University Hospital when she was 41 years old (21 years before death) because of arthralgias, proximal muscle weakness and dermal "tightness," especially of the skin over the face. Upper gastrointestinal tract films at that time suggested changes of scleroderma, and a deltoid muscle biopsy specimen was consistent with polymyositis. The patient was considered to have a mixed collagen vascular syndrome, with elements of both scleroderma and polymyositis. Therapy with prednisone (20 mg per day) resulted in symptomatic improvement.

Subsequent medical problems included chronic anemia (hemoglobin 7.0 g/dl), intermittent mild renal insufficiency (creatinine 1.2–2.0 mg/dl), and congestive heart failure requiring therapy with digoxin and diuretics. Raynaud's phenomenon began at age 46, and the dose of prednisone was increased to 30 mg/day and continued as such until one year before death (age 61) when the dose was reduced to 20 mg/day. In addition, therapy with chloroquine, 500 mg/day was begun and continued for the patient's remaining 16 years. At age 54, syncope occurred, complete heart block was found, and a permanent

From the Infectious Disease Division, Department of Medicine, and the Department of Pathology, Georgetown University Hospital, Washington, D.C., and the Pathology Branch, National Heart, Lung, and Blood Institute, National Institutes of Health, Bethesda, Maryland. Requests for reprints should be addressed to Dr. William A. Davis, Georgetown University Hospital, 3800 Reservoir Road, Washington, D.C. 20007. Manuscript accepted February 4, 1980.

*Present address: Department of Medicine, Tufts University Medical Center, Boston, MA 02111.

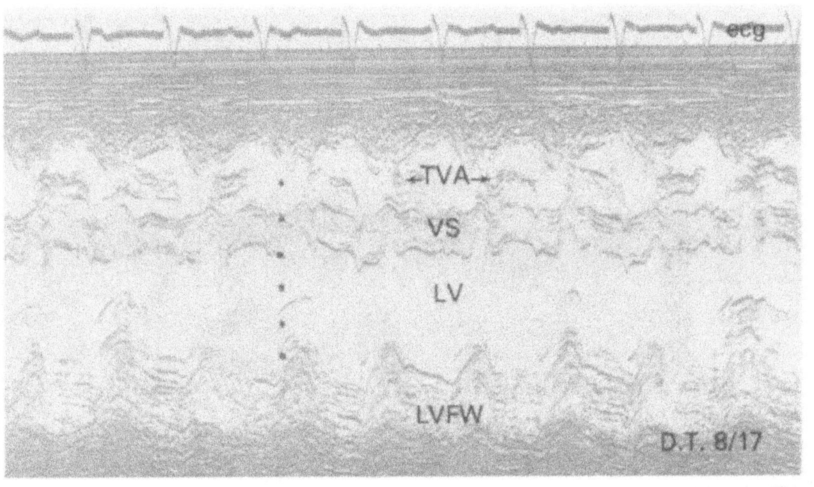

Figure 1. Echocardiogram recorded one day before death. Adventitious echoes are seen in the right ventricular cavity due to the pacemaker and associated tricuspid valve vegetation (TVA). VS = ventricular septum; LV = left ventricle; LVFW = left ventricular free wall; ECG = electrocardiogram.

pacemaker was implanted. The patient encountered no additional problems until age 62 at which time she planted a garden for the first time in several years. After working daily in the garden for one month, she noted the onset of dyspnea, right pleuritic chest pain and right upper quadrant pain; she was hospitalized two months before death. A chest film demonstrated an infiltrate in the lower lobe of the right lung and a bloody effusion in the right pleural cavity. Smears and cultures of sputum, blood, pleural fluid and fluid aspirated from the pacemaker generator site showed no abnormalities. An etiology was never established and the pulmonary process resolved incompletely after therapy with cefazolin and tobramycin. The patient was discharged after two weeks at the family's request. During the next seven weeks, she complained of anorexia and lost 9 kg in weight. Because of increasing lethargy, somnolence and left eye pain, associated with decreased visual acuity of one day's duration, she was rehospitalized seven days before death. On admission, she was cachectic and somnolent. The rectal temperature was 38.6°C. The skin over the face and hands was taut, and there were contractures around the mouth. The left periorbital tissues were swollen, the left eyeball was tender, and the left eye visual acuity was reduced to light perception. A panuveitis was diagnosed. The subcutaneous pacemaker pocket was in the right infraclavicular area. A grade 3/6 holosystolic murmur without respiratory variation was heard at the lower left sternal border. The hemoglobin level was 5.4 g/dl; white blood cell count, 17,000/mm^3 (69 polymorphonuclear cells, 18 band forms, 10 lymphocytes, 3 monocytes); platelet count 16,000/mm^3 and reticulocyte count 8 percent. The erythrocyte sedimentation rate was 45 mm in one hour. Coagulation studies were consistent with disseminated intravascular coagulation. Chest film disclosed an enlarged cardiac silhouette and patchy interstitial infiltrates in the lower lobe of the right lung. Electrocardiogram showed sinus tachycardia at a rate of 120 beats/min. In each QRS complex there was pacemaker artifact from an R-wave triggered pacemaker. An echocardiogram (**Figure 1**) showed abnormal echoes around the expected echoes from a transvenous pacemaker in the right ventricle. The cerebrospinal fluid pressure was 18 cm of water and the fluid contained glucose 19 mg/dl (serum 82 mg/dl), protein 95 mg/dl, erythrocytes 24/mm^3 and leukocytes 130/mm^3 (80 lymphocytes, 20 polymorphonuclear leukocytes). Smears and culture specimens of the cerebrospinal fluid, blood and urine were negative for growth at 36 hours. Sputum cultures grew "normal flora." On the day of death, the heart and respiratory rates increased, chest pain was apparent, and an electrocardiogram showed that the pacemaker was failing to sense and capture. Cardiopulmonary arrest ensued.

The day following the patient's death, growth was observed on the surface of the broth* of several (antemortem) blood cultures. Within one week, all 11 antemortem cultures (both aerobic and anaerobic) had a whitish, floating mass of growth on the surface of the broth, but no growth in the media or at the bottom of the culture bottles. Fluid aspirated from the pacemaker generator pocket eventually was positive on fungal media as were postmortem cultures of the vitreous fluid from the left eye. Studies of the organism on subculture revealed a rapidly growing, cotton-like mass which later became darker in color. Positive identification of the fungus as P. boydii was established by the Center for Disease Control in Atlanta.

At necropsy (GT #77A-130), the patient had a taut face and hands. The pacemaker pocket in the right side of the chest contained a tan-white exudate. The pericardial sac contained 370 ml of serosanguineous fluid, but neither the parietal nor visceral pericardium was scarred or thickened. The heart weighed 410 g. A pacemaker wire was fixed in the right atrium to the atrial septum by fibrous tissue; at the level of the tricuspid valve orifice, it was encased by a vegetation (**Figure 2**), measuring about 4 by 3 by 2 cm, which occupied most of the valve orifice, and pressed the anterior and posterior leaflets against the right ventricular mural endocardium. Distally, the pacemaker wire was encased by collagen; the pacemaker tip made firm contact with the right ventricular apical endocardium. The generator function of the pacemaker was intact with an output of 2.2 milliampere and a postmortem film showed the pace-

* Columbia Broth (Pfizer Diagnostic Division).

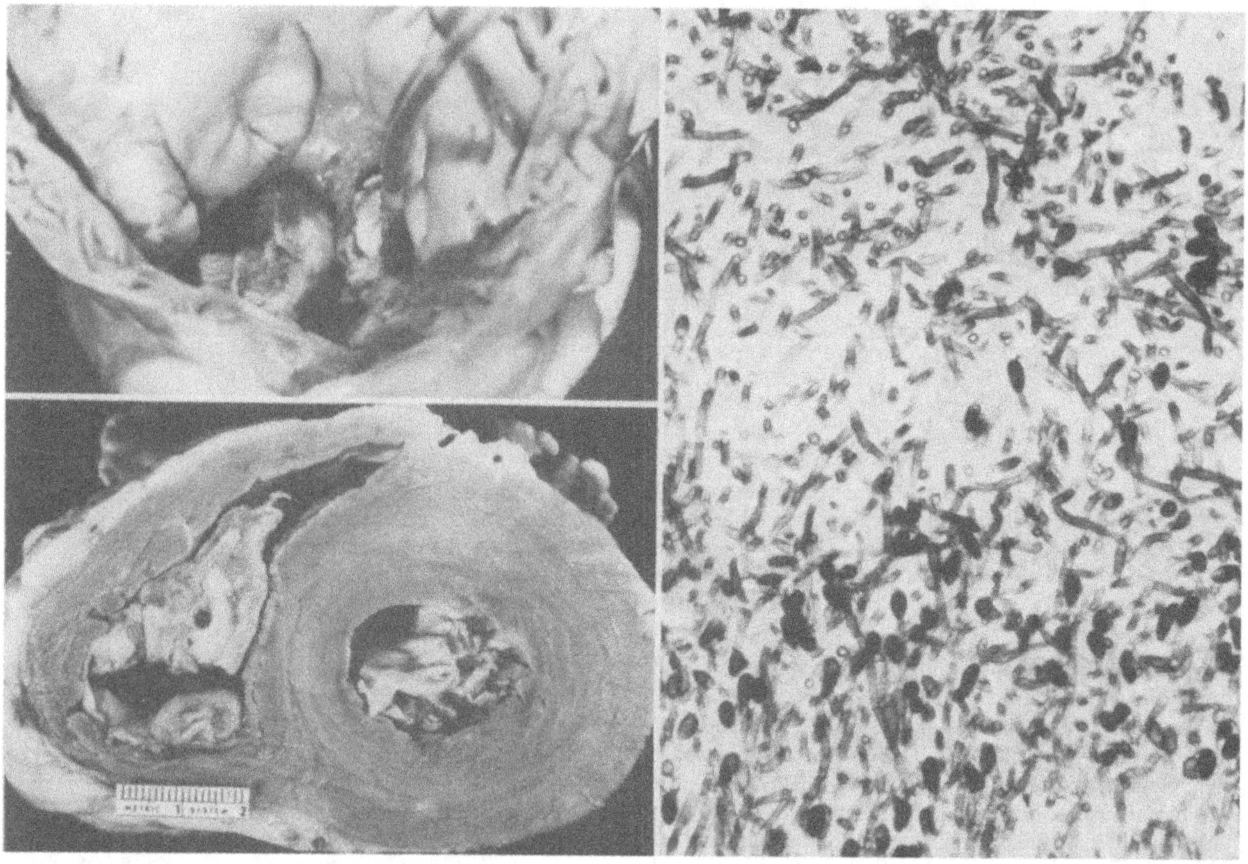

Figure 2. Tricuspid valve vegetation. **Top left,** view of the vegetation and pacemaker wire from the right atrium. **Bottom left,** vegetation in the tricuspid valve orifice and right ventricle as viewed from the ventricular aspect. The hole in the center of the anterior portion of the vegetation was formerly occupied by the pacemaker electrode. **Right,** photomicrograph of histologic section of a portion of the vegetation showing septated hyphal fungi with single terminal conidia, consistent with P. boydii. Gomori methenamine silver stain; magnification × 350, reduced by 65 percent.

maker electrode to be intact. Sections of the vegetation (Figure 2) disclosed septated hyphal fungi with single terminal conidia, consistent with P. boydii, with extensive fibrin deposits and inflammatory cells. There was a 2 by 3 cm transmural scar in the posterior wall of the left ventricle, but all portions of the right, left main, left anterior descending and left circumflex coronary arteries were narrowed less than 75 percent in cross-sectional area by atherosclerotic plaque. There were multiple fresh and organizing pulmonary emboli with a recent infarct in the lower lobe of the right lung but histologically no microorganisms were present. The distal third of the esophagus was fibrotic and ulcerated. The liver (weight 1,000 g) had a nutmeg appearance. The adrenal glands together weighed 5.1 g and their cortices was atrophic. The kidneys weighed 145 and 130 g, respectively, and were within normal limits. The meninges and brain showed no abnormalities; histologically, no microorganisms were found. Postmortem serum for extractable nuclear antigen was positive at a dilution of 1:1,000 and ribonuclease sensitive, consistent with the diagnosis of "mixed connective tissue disease."

COMMENTS

The patient described is most unusual for several reasons. (1) Fatal P. boydii endocarditis with massive vegetations in the tricuspid valve orifice occurred; (2) fungemia was present (11 positive blood cultures); (3) fungal infection of any type of a permanent pacemaker is rare, and P. boydii infection of a permanent pacemaker has not been reported previously. As in several previously described patients with disseminated P. boydii infections, our patient incurred infection of the eye and probably also of the central nervous system. Fewer than 10 patients with disseminated P. boydii infection have been described previously [3].

P. boydii exists in asexual (Monosporium apispermum) or sexual forms (A. boydii); it is similar morphologically to Aspergillus species; grows rapidly in culture and changes in color as it ages; is ubiquitous in soil in many parts of the United States, and causes infection by direct innoculation or by inhalation of ascospores, which are aerosolized when soil, containing the organism, is disturbed [4,5]. Our patient planted and regularly maintained a garden for several weeks before evidence of infection developed.

P. boydii infections may be external or internal or both. Noninvasive localized mycetomas occur on the conjunctivas, lacrimal glands and eyelids, and excisional biopsy is usually required for diagnosis and cure. Pulmonary mycetomas occur in patients with previously normal or abnormal lungs [6], and signs and symptoms of infection may be minimal, or cough and hemoptysis may occur. The mycetomas might require excision. P. boydii was cultured in drainage from purulent sphenoidal sinusitis in a recently reported, presumably normal host [7]. Therapy with intravenous miconazole (41 g) resulted in clearing of the purulent drainage.

Invasive P. boydii infections may be localized, disseminated or both. Local infections may result from direct tissue inoculation and produce a chronic destructive process with abcess and granuloma formation. Maduromycosis of the foot is the most notable of such infections and in the United States is most commonly caused by P. boydii. Both normal and compromised hosts may be infected. Corneal ulceration, endophthalmitis, necrotizing pneumonia, pulmonary abscess, meningoencephalitis and prostatitis have been reported [2,3,5]. Disseminated infection is rare [3], but when present the central nervous system usually is involved [3,8–10], and occasionally the thyroid gland, bone and soft tissues.

Treatment of invasive P. boydii infections is often unsuccessful, especially when it is disseminated. When feasible, surgical resection is preferred for localized disease. Chemotherapy with amphotericin B, and 2-hydroxy-stibamidine, griseofulvin and chloramphenicol has been attempted, but success has been limited [11]. Miconazole is a more recently used agent.

The pacemaker-related vegetation that essentially obstructed the tricuspid valve orifice in our patient is remarkable for several reasons. First, infections involving permanently implanted endocardial pacemakers are uncommon; the reported frequency is less than 6 percent of all units implanted [12–20]. When such infections do occur, they most often are limited to the subcutaneous pocket housing the pacemaker pulse generator. Nearly all of these infections occur soon after implantation and are due to contamination of the operative wound. Local signs of sepsis at the site of the pulse-generator pocket allow early diagnosis and initiation of antibiotic therapy. Such conservative management generally prevents extension of the infective process. As a result, pacemaker infections involving the pacing electrode and tricuspid valve, such as occurred in our patient, account for few pacemaker infections. Second, the etiologic agent of the vast majority of pacemaker infections is Staphylococcus species. Pacemaker-related endocarditis of the tricuspid valve due to a fungus is decidedly rare [21] and, to our knowledge, has never resulted from P. boydii. Third, although the vegetations in patients with fungal endocarditis are generally larger than bacterial endocarditis [22], transorifice vegetations, as occurred in our patient, are unusual. The presence of a foreign body (pacing wire) in the tricuspid valve orifice likely contributed to the size of the vegetations in our patient. The size of the vegetations was almost certainly the factor that allowed echocardiographic identification of the pacemaker-related valvular endocarditis.

REFERENCES

1. Conant NF, Smith DT, Baker RD, et al.: Manual of clinical mycology, 3rd ed. Philadelphia: W.B. Saunders Co., 1971: 458.
2. Lutwick LI, Galgiani JN, Johnson RH, et al.: Visceral fungal infections due to Petrillidium boydii. Am J Med 1976; 61: 632.
3. Winston DJ, Jordan MC, Rhodes J: Allescheria boydii infections in the immunosuppressed host. Am J Med 1977; 63: 830.
4. Emmons CW, Binford CH, Utz JP: Medical mycology, 3rd ed. Philadelphia: Lea & Febiger, 1977: 389–418.
5. Arnett JC, Hatch HB: Pulmonary allescheriasis. Arch Intern Med 1975; 135: 1250.
6. Hainer JW, Ostrow JH, Mackenzie DW: Pulmonary monosporosis: report of a case with precipitating antibody. Chest 1974; 66: 601.
7. Mader JT, Ream SR, Heath PW: Petriellidium boydii (Allescheria boydii) sphenoidal sinusitis. JAMA 1978; 239: 2368.
8. Forno LS, Billingham ME: Allescheria boydii infection of the brain. J Pathol 1972; 106: 195.
9. Rosen F, Deck JH, Remeastle NB: Allescheria boydii unique systemic dissemination to thyroid and brain. Can Med Assoc J 1965; 93: 1125.
10. Selby R: Pachymeningitis secondary to allescheria boydii. J Neurosurg 1972; 36: 225.
11. Utz JP: Mycetoma In: Hoeprich PD, ed. Infectious diseases. New York: Harper & Row, 1978.
12. Imparato AM, Kim GE: Electrode complications in patients with permanent cardiac pacemakers. Ten years' experience. Arch Surg 1972; 105: 705.
13. Linschoten H, Meijne NG, Mellink HM, et al.: Pacemaker implantation and infection. J Cardiovasc Surg 1973; 14: 126.
14. Yarnoz MD, Attai LA, Furman S: Infection of pacemaker electrode and removal with cardiopulmonary bypass. J Thorac Cardiovasc Surg 1974; 86: 43.
15. Kennelly BM, Piller LW: Management of infected transvenous permanent pacemakers. Br Heart J 1974; 36: 1133.
16. Conklin EF, Giannelli S Jr, Nealon TF Jr: Four hundred consecutive patients with permanent transvenous pacemakers. J Thorac Cardiovasc Surg 1975; 69: 1.
17. Grögler FM, Frank G, Greven G, et al.: Complications of permanent transvenous cardiac pacing. J Thorac Cardiovasc Surg 1975; 69: 895.
18. Chavcez CM, Conn JH: Septicemia secondary to impacted infected pacemaker wire. Successful treatment by removal with cardiopulmonary bypass. J Thorac Cardiovasc Surg 1977; 73: 796.
19. Morgan G, Ginks W, Siddons H, et al.: Septicemia in patients with an endocardial pacemaker. Am J Cardiol 1979; 44: 221.
20. Jara FM, Toledo-Pereyra L, Lewis JW, et al.: The infected pacemaker pocket. J Thorac Cardiovasc Surg 1979; 78: 298.
21. Davis JM, Moss AF, Schenk EA: Tricuspid Candida endocarditis complicating a permanently implanted transvenous pacemaker. Am Heart J 1969; 77: 818.
22. Andriole VT, Kravetz HM, Roberts WC, et al.: Candida endocarditis. Clinical and pathologic studies. Am J Med 1962; 32: 251.

M-mode echocardiographic observations in active bacterial endocarditis limited to the aortic valve

Analysis of 37 M-mode echocardiograms recorded during the period of active bacterial endocarditis (ABE) involving the aortic valve (AV) in 17 patients disclosed one or more echocardiographic abnormalities involving the aortic valve cusps or their immediate vicinity in 15 (88%), including "shaggy" echoes indicative of vegetations in 12 (71%). Of the 12 patients with echocardiographic evidence of AV vegetation, 11 developed overt congestive heart failure (CHF) and either died or had AV replacement, and seven had clinical events compatible with systemic emboli; of the five patients without echo-demonstrated vegetations, only one had CHF, none had AV replacement, two died, and one had a systemic embolus. In comparison to our previously reported echocardiographic observations in patients with ABE involving either the mitral (29 patients) or tricuspid valve (23 patients), infection involving the AV was far more liable to produce overt CHF and systemic emboli, to necessitate valve replacement, and to cause death during the period of active infection. (Am Heart J 102:66, 1981.)

Mazhar U. Sheikh, M.D., Edgar A. Covarrubias, M.D. Nayab Ali, M.D., Nasreen M. Sheikh, M.D., Won R. Lee, M.D., and William C. Roberts, M.D.
Washington, D.C., and Bethesda, Md.

Since 1972, a number of reports have described echocardiographic findings in patients with active infective endocarditis involving one or more cardiac valves.[1-9] With few exceptions,[5-7] previous reports have grouped together patients with active infective endocarditis irrespective of which cardiac valve was involved by the infectious process. As a consequence, varying results were obtained by different investigations.[8-13] Previously, we reported M-mode echocardiographic findings in 10 patients with active bacterial endocarditis (ABE) limited to a right-sided cardiac valve[14] and, most recently M-mode echocardiographic findings in 27 patients with ABE limited to the mitral valve.[7] In this report, we describe M-mode echocardiographic finding in 17 patients with ABE involving the aortic valve and compare the observations in this group of patients to those made earlier in patients with infection involving the tricuspid or mitral valve.

From the Section of Cardiology, Georgetown and Howard University Medical Divisions, and Department of Pathology, District of Columbia General Hospital; and the Pathology Branch, National Heart, Lung and Blood Institute, National Institutes of Health.

Received for publication Feb. 27, 1981; accepted March 6, 1981.

Reprint requests: Mazhar U. Sheikh, M.D., Georgetown University Medical Division, District of Columbia General Hospital, Washington, DC 20003.

METHODS

Patients. Satisfactory echocardiograms were performed in 81 patients hospitalized at D.C. General Hospital from 1975 through 1980 with ABE: 16 (20%) had evidence of bacterial endocarditis involving only the aortic valve. In addition, another patient (No. 17, Table I) with ABE was studied at another hospital by one of us and is included. Certain clinical findings in the 17 patients are summarized in Table I. All 17 patients had a single episode of ABE. During ABE, each patient had a precordial murmur characteristic of aortic regurgitation (AR) and fever (greater than 100° F rectally). All had positive blood cultures: Alpha streptococcus in 10; *Staphylococcus aureus* in six; and *Haemophilus parainfluenzae* in one. Of the 17 patients, four (Nos. 4, 10, 16, and 17; Table I) were known to have preexisting heart disease before ABE onset: rheumatic heart disease in two (patients Nos. 4 and 10) and congenitally bicuspid stenotic aortic valves in two (patients Nos. 16 and 17). Eleven of the 17 patients were known users of heroin intravenously.

Sequence of echograms. The initial M-mode echocardiogram in all 17 patients was performed before institution of appropriate antibiotic therapy and during ABE. A total of 37 satisfactory echocardiograms were recorded during the period of ABE in the 17 patients: seven patients had a single echocardiogram and 10 had more than one echocardiogram (range two to five). A Unirad 100 series echograph using a 2.25 MHz transducer was employed. Of the 37 satisfactory echocardiograms performed, 29 were done by the same physician (M.U.S.). The interval from the onset

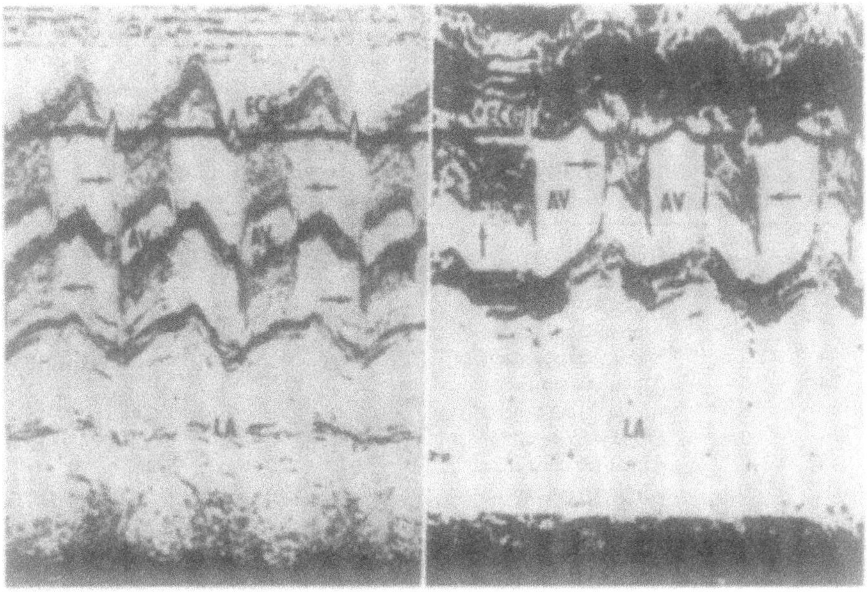

Fig. 1. Echocardiograms showing aortic valve vegetations *(arrows)* in systole *(left)* (Patient No. 16, Table I) and diastole *(right)* (Patient No. 7). *AV* = aortic valve; *ECG* = electrocardiogram; *LA* = left atrium.

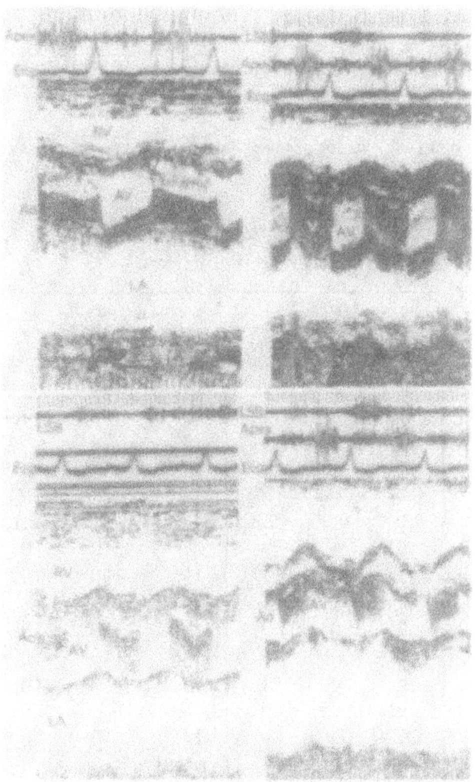

Fig. 2. Patient No. 9. Echocardiogram with phonocardiogram of the aortic valve recorded at different angulations and gain settings showing variable findings 5 days before death. *Top left:* Vegetation on and diastolic fluttering of the aortic valve *(AV)* cusps. *Ao* = aorta; *LA* = left atrium; *RV* = right ventricle. *Top right:* The aortic valve orifice is filled with vegetations *(V)* during diastole. *LSB* = left sternal border. *Bottom left:* Aortic valve vegetation is present in diastole. *Bottom right:* Vegetations fill the aortic valve orifice during systole.

Table I. Clinical and echocardiographic observations in patients with ABE limited to the aortic valve

Pt. no.	Pt	Age (yrs)	Sex	OA	AS before ABE	Infecting bacterium	Interval (days) onset symptoms ABE to E	Interval (days) onset symptoms ABE to death or AVR	CHF	PE	No. echoes recorded
1	RA	26	M	+	0	*Haemophilus parainfluenzae*	10	16	+	0	1
2	RJ	27	M	+	0	*Staphylococcus aureus*	5	24	+	+	1
3	RP	29	M	+	0	Alpha streptococcus	14	56	+	+	2*
4	DB	30	F	0	0	Alpha streptococcus	15	16	+	0	1
5	BT	30	M	+	0	Alpha streptococcus	6	–	0	+	2
6	DA	32	M	+	0	Alpha streptococcus	21	128	+	+	4*
7	LM	34	F	+	0	Alpha streptococcus	21	45	+	0	1
8	GW	35	M	+	0	*Staphylococcus aureus*	18	112	+	0	2
9	DC	36	M	+	0	Alpha streptococcus	12	330	+	+	5*
10	BW	39	M	+	0	Alpha streptococcus	12	–	0	+	3
11	LR	42	M	0	0	*Staphylococcus aureus*	4	–	0‡	0	4
12	JO	44	M	+	0	*Staphylococcus aureus*	7	11	0	0	1
13	LC	45	M	0	0	Alpha streptococcus	20	–	0	0	3
14	GM	54	M	+	0	*Staphylococcus aureus*	15	–	0	+	1
15	OW	69	M	0	0	Alpha streptococcus	28	350	+	0	2
16	RS	24	M	0	+	Alpha streptococcus	20	28	+	0	1
17	PS	30	M	0	+	*Staphylococcus aureus*	14	19	+	+	3*

Abbreviations: ABE = active bacterial endocarditis; AS = aortic valve stenosis; AVC = aortic valve (AV) cusps; AVR = AV replacement; CHF = congestive heart failure; D = death; DE = double echoes; DF = diastolic fluttering; E = first echogram recorded; LV = left ventricle; LVOT = left ventricular outflow tract; No. = number; OA = opiate addiction; PE = peripheral systemic emboli; PMC = premature mitral valve closure; Pt = patient; SA = systemic artery; s/d = systole/diastole; SE = shaggy echoes.

*Changes noted in echocardiograms recorded during period of active infection.

†Autopsy performed.

‡Patient had CHF from atherosclerotic coronary heart disease before ABE.

§AV commissurotomy performed at age 12 years when peak systolic gradient between LV and aorta was 252 mm Hg.

Table II. Comparison of clinical features in ABE of aortic valve (17 patients) to ABE of tricuspid (23 patients) or mitral valves (29 patients) in patients studied by the present authors

Clinical features	Aortic valve +	Aortic valve 0	Aortic valve ±	Mitral valve +	Mitral valve 0	Mitral valve ±	Tricuspid valve +	Tricuspid valve 0	Tricuspid valve ±	Subtotals +	Subtotals 0	Subtotals ±	Totals	
No. patients	12	5	0	22	2	5	14	6	3	48	13	8	69	
Age (years) Range (mean)	26-54 (33)	39-69 (48)	–	18-55 (33)	23-28 (25)	23-69 (49)	15-59 (29)	25-45 (29)	21-35 (27)	15-59	23-69	21-69	15-69	
Female:Male	2:10	0:5	0	6:16	0:2	2:3	3:11	1:5	2:1	11:36	1:12	4:4	16:52	
Previous VHD	3	0	0	5	1	4	3*	0	0	10	1	4	16	(23%)
OA	9	2	0	11	2	1	11	6	3	31	10	4	45	(65%)
Bacterium														
A. *Staph*	4	2	0	7	2	3	11	6	3	22	10	6	38	(55%)
B. α strept	7	3	0	10	0	1	3	0	0	20	3	1	24	(35%)
C. Other	1	0	0	4	0	1	0	0	0	5	0	1	6	(9%)
CHF	10	1	0	9	0	3	1	0	0	20	1	3	24	(35%)
Emboli	7	1	0	6	0	0	14	6	3	26	7	3	37	(54%)
VR [death]	6[1]	0	0	3	0	1	1[1]	0	0	10[2]	0	1	11[2]	(16%)
Death without VR	5	2	0	7	0	2	3	0	0	15	2	2	19	(28%)†
Survival without VR	1	3	0	12	2	2	10	6	3	22	11	5	39	(57%)‡

Valve vegetation by M-mode echogram = + (present); 0 (absent); ± (equivocal).

*Two had ventricular septal defect and one had preexisting right heart Swan-Ganz catheter.

†Total mortality (30%; 21 of 69 patients).

‡Total survival (70%; 48 of 69 patients).

Abbreviations: CHF = congestive heart failure; No. = number; OA = opiate addiction; *Staph* = *Staphylococcus aureus;* strept = streptococcus; VHD = valvular heart disease; VR = valve replacement.

Echocardiogram					Pressures (mm Mg)				
SE AVC	DF AVC	PMC	Echos LVOT	DE AVC	LV (s/d)	SA (s/d)	AVR	D	No. AVC
+	+	0	+	0	125/45	110/54	+	0	3
+	0	0	0	0	–	120/50	0	+	–
+	+	+	0	0	160/21	160/40	+	0	3
+	0	+	0	0	–	120/50	+	0	?
+	+	0	+	0	–	140/40	0	0	–
+	+	±	+	+	140/45	140/65	+	0	
+	0	0	0	0	–	130/40	+	+	3
+	0	+	0	0	110/33	110/45	0	+	–
+	+	+	+	+	–	140/50	0	+†	3
+	0	0	0	0	–	120/68	0	0	–
0	0	0	0	0	110/26	110/70	0	0	–
0	+	0	0	+	–	130/70	0	+†	3
0	+	0	0	+	–	128/64	0	0	–
0	0	0	0	0	–	150/60	0	0	3
0	+	0	0	0	–	130/60	0	+†	3
+	0	0	+	0	–	110/56	0§	+	2
+	0	0	0	+	–	120/80	0	+†	2

of symptoms suggestive or characteristic of ABE to the first echocardiographic recording ranged from 4 to 28 days (mean 17). The interval from the onset of symptoms suggestive or characteristic of ABE to death (seven patients) or aortic valve replacement (four patients) or both (one patient) ranged from 11 to 350 days; in eight patients this interval was less than 60 days (mean 27) and in the other four patients it ranged from 112 to 350 days (mean 230). The indication for aortic valve replacement (six patients) was evidence of overt congestive heart failure (CHF).

Characterization of vegetations and valve rupture. The echocardiographic diagnosis of vegetation on one or more aortic valve cusps was based on the presence of thick, irregular bordered ("shaggy") echoes involving one or more aortic valve cusps in either ventricular systole or diastole or both without significant impairment to cuspal movement. Evidence of significant AR by echocardiogram was premature closure of the mitral orifice due to rapid posterior displacement of the anterior mitral leaflet. Fluttering of one or more aortic valve cusps during ventricular diastole combined with echoes in the left ventricular outflow tract (between mural endocardium of ventricular septum and anterior mitral leaflet) was interpreted as evidence of rupture or perforation of one of more aortic valve cusps. The presence of double echoes in one or more aortic valve sinuses of Valsalva was suggestive evidence of the presence of ring abscess.[6, 15]

RESULTS

Vegetations. Of the 17 patients with ABE limited to the aortic valve, one or more echocardiograms recorded during the period of active infection disclosed the presence of shaggy echoes on the aortic valve cusps (indicative of the presence of one or more vegetations) in 12 (Table I) (Figs. 1 to 8). Of the five patients without shaggy echoes on the aortic valve cusps, three had fluttering of one or more aortic valve cusps during ventricular diastole (Fig. 9). Thus, only 2 of the 17 patients had no echocardiographic abnormalities involving the aortic valve cusps or their immediate vicinity. Following the presence of shaggy aortic valve cusps echoes, the next most frequent echocardiographic abnormality was diastolic fluttering of one or more aortic valve cusps (eight patients); next, double echoes in the aortic valve sinuses of Valsalva (five patients) (Fig. 7); and each of four patients had premature mitral closure (Figs. 3, 5, and 6) or echoes in the left ventricular outflow tract (Figs. 3 and 6). One patient (No. 17; Table I) had a ring abscess which burrowed through the ventricular septum and an echo-clear space was observed by echo in the septum (Fig. 8).

Valve replacements or deaths. The patients who underwent aortic valve replacement or died during the period of ABE had a much higher frequency of echocardiographic evidence of the presence of aortic valve vegetations than did patients who survived without requiring aortic valve replacement during the period of infection. Vegetation by echocardiogram was present in all six patients who underwent aortic valve replacement (one subsequently died), and in five of the seven patients who died without

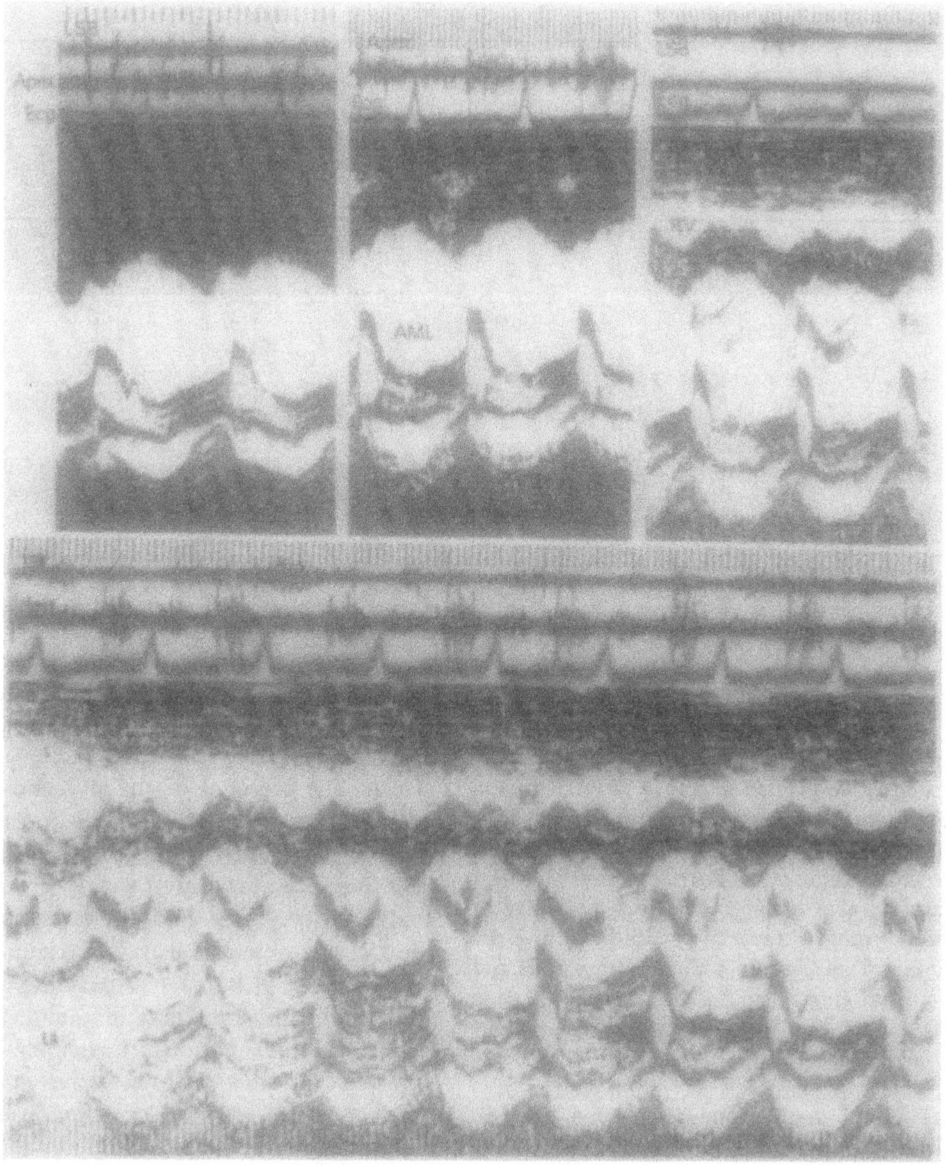

Fig. 3. Patient No. 9. Serial echocardiograms recorded from left ventricle and mitral valve areas showing normal closure of the mitral valve on admission *(top left)*, premature closure of the mitral valve 4 weeks before death *(top middle)*, and abnormal echoes in the left ventricular outflow tract *(arrows)* along with premature closure of mitral valve *(top right)* 5 days before death. Also, the left ventricular cavity gradually increased in size. *AML* = anterior mitral leaflet; *LSB* = left sternal border; *LVW* = left ventricular posterior wall; *PML* = posterior mitral leaflet; *RV* = right ventricle; *VS* = ventricular septum. *Bottom:* Echocardiogram recorded 5 days before death showing abnormal echoes in the left ventricular outflow tract with diastolic fluttering of the prolapsed leaflet *(thick arrows)* and premature closure of the mitral valve *(thin arrows)*. At necropsy, the aortic valve *(AV)* cusps had ruptured.

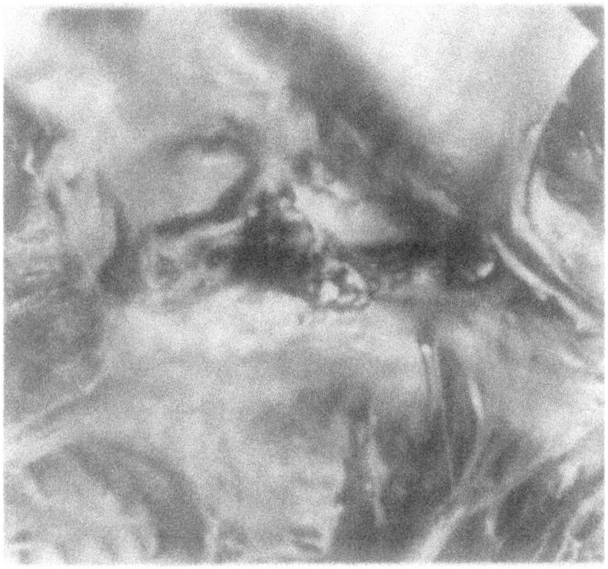

Fig. 4. Patient No. 9. Opened aortic valve showing a large vegetation attached to the noncoronary cusp of the aortic valve which is, for the most part, destroyed. The vegetation pressed against the right anterior cusp during ventricular diastole. The mitral valve is normal.

aortic valve replacement. In contrast, none of the three patients who survived without aortic valve replacement had echocardiographic evidence of vegetation.

CHF and systemic emboli. The frequency of CHF and of systemic emboli was higher in the patients with echocardiographic evidence of aortic valve vegetation compared to those without. Of the 12 patients with echocardiographic evidence of aortic valve vegetation, all 11 had clinical evidence of CHF appearing for the first time during the period of active infection and six had clinical evidence of systemic emboli; of the five patients without echocardiographic evidence of vegetation, only one had CHF and two had systemic emboli.

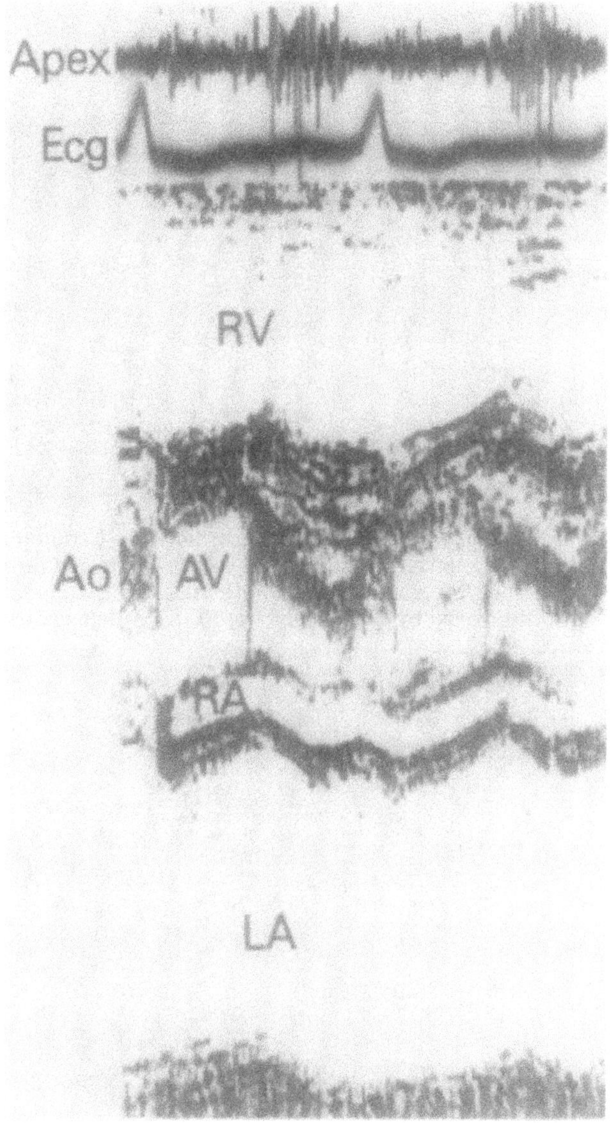

Fig. 5. Patient No. 9. Echocardiogram showing two parallel aortic wall densities separated by an echo-free space suggesting ring abscess *(RA)* which was confirmed at necropsy. *Ao* = aorta; *AV* = aortic valve; *LA* = left atrium; *RV* = right ventricle.

DISCUSSION

Frequency of vegetations. Analysis of 37 M-mode echocardiograms in our 17 patients with ABE limited to the aortic valve disclosed one or more echocardiographic abnormalities involving the aortic valve cusps or their immediate vicinity in 15 (88%), including "shaggy" echoes indicative of vegetations in 12 (71%). Echocardiographic evidence of aortic valve vegetation was found in 10 of 15 patients with ABE of the aortic valve reported by Roy et al,[2] in 10 of 17 patients reported by Wann et al.,[8] in 13 (41%) of 32 patients reported by Pratt et al.,[9] and in 13 (41%) of 32 patients reported by Mintz et al.[6] Thus combining these 96 previously reported patients with ABE of the aortic valve, 46 (48%) had echocardiographic evidence of vegetation on one or more aortic valve cusps.

Relation of vegetations to CHF. Among patients with ABE of the aortic valve, the frequency of development of CHF is much higher in the patients in whom the echocardiogram identifies vegetation on this valve compared to the patients in whom no vegetation is identified by echocardiogram. Of our 12 patients with echocardiographic demonstration of vegetation, 11 had overt CHF appearing for the first time during the period of active infection; of our five patients without echocardiographic evidence of vegetation, only one had CHF. Of the 13 patients with echocardiographic evidence of aortic valve

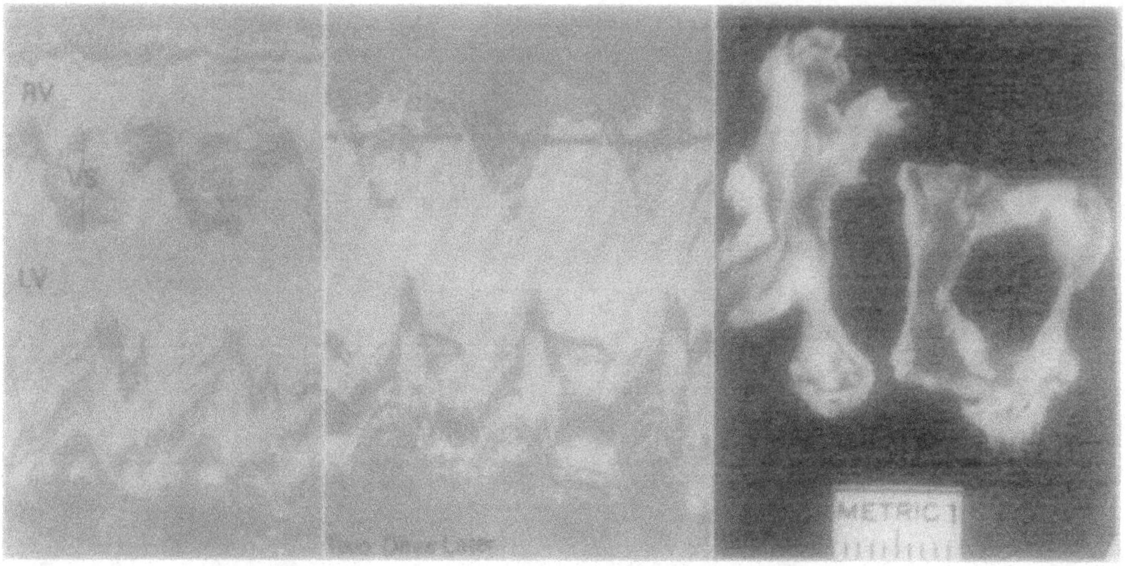

Fig. 6. Patient No. 3. Echocardiograms (*left* and *middle*) recorded from mitral valve areas on admission *(left)* showing normal mitral valve closure and premature closure of the mitral valve *(middle)* 2 days later when congestive heart failure appeared. At operation, both right and left coronary cusps were partially destroyed by vegetations *(right)*. *LV* = left ventricle; *RV* = right ventricle; *VS* = ventricular septum.

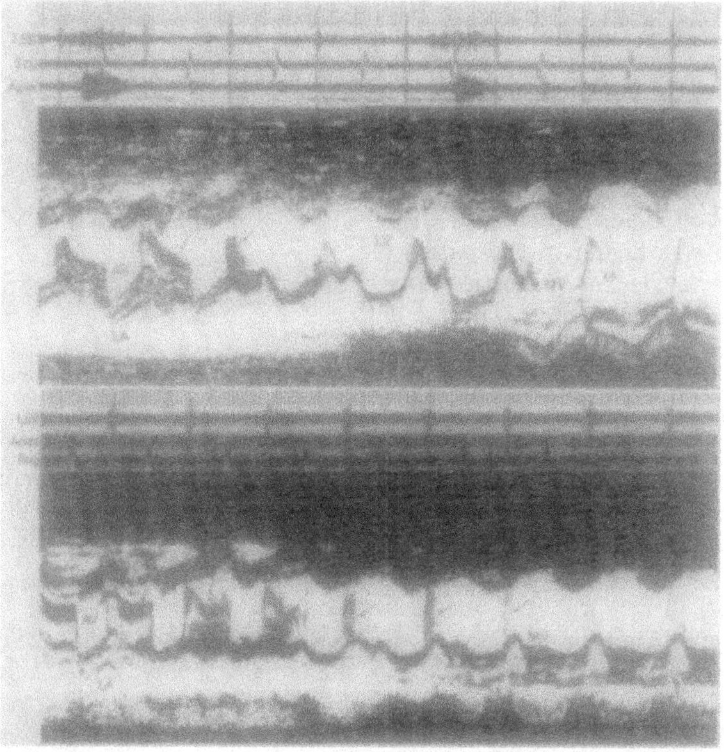

Fig. 7. Patient No. 6. *Top:* Initial echocardiogram showing vegetation *(arrows)* on the aortic valve *(AV)* cusps. Otherwise, the echocardiogram is unremarkable. *LA* = left atrium; *LSB* = left sternal border; *LV* = left ventricle; *MV* = mitral valve. *Bottom:* Follow-up echocardiogram record 91 days after the onset of symptoms, i.e., 45 days after bacteriologic cure, showing diastolic fluttering of the aortic valve cusps *(vertical arrows)*, abnormal echoes in left ventricular outflow tract *(oblique arrows)*, and premature closure of the mitral valve. These findings suggest damage to the aortic valve cusps. Thick echoes suggestive of vegetation are still present. At operation the aortic valve was bicuspid and both cusps were perforated. *VS* = ventricular septum.

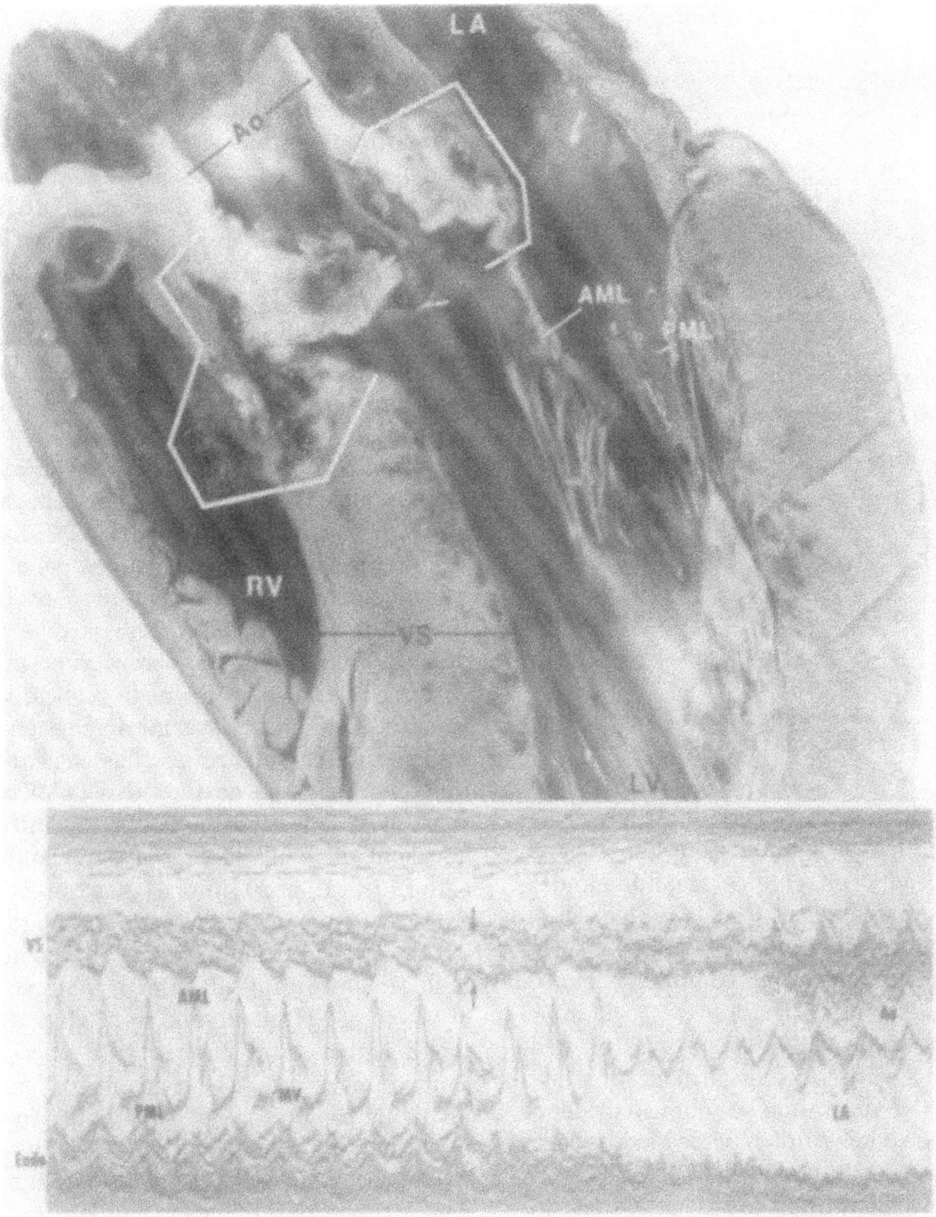

Fig. 8. Patient No. 17. Congenitally bicuspid stenotic aortic valve with superimposed *Staphylococcus aureus* endocarditis in a 30-year-old man. Before the onset of the bacterial endocarditis, the patient was asymptomatic but before the infection the valve was already mildly stenotic and mildly calcified. Nail biting to the point of bleeding apparently was the source of the infection. At necropsy, the heart weighed 560 gm. The infection of the aortic valve burrowed into the adjacent soft tissues *(brackets)* producing large "ring abscesses." Ring abscess caused complete right bundle branch block. There was extensive subendocardial and papillary muscle necrosis of the left ventricle, presumably the result of severely diminished cardiac output. The echocardiogram was recorded several days before death. The *arrows* in the ventricular septum of the echocardiogram designate the probable ring abscess. *Ao* = aorta; *LA* = left atrium; *RV* = right ventricle; *LV* = left ventricle; *AML* and *PML* = anterior and posterior mitral leaflets; *VS* = ventricular septum; *MV* = mitral valve; *Endo* = endocardium.

vegetation reported by Pratt et al.,[9] all had overt CHF, and of the 19 without vegetations, only two had CHF. Of the 13 patients with aortic valve vegetations by echocardiograms reported by Mintz et al.,[6] at least eight had overt CHF.

Relation of vegetations to valve replacement or death. Among patients with ABE of the aortic valve, aortic valve replacement or death or both is much higher in the patients in whom the echocardiogram identifies vegetation on this valve compared to patients in whom no vegetation is identified. Of our 12 patients with aortic valve vegetations by echocardiogram, 11 either underwent aortic valve replacement (five patients; one subsequently died) or died without

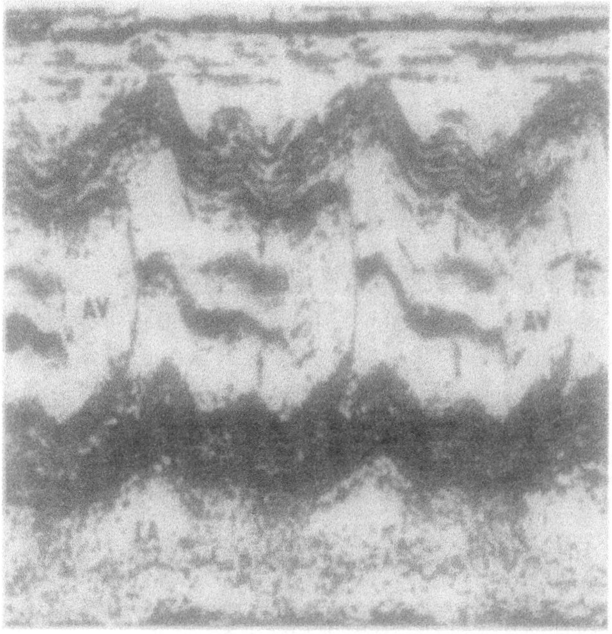

Fig. 9. Patient No. 13. Echocardiogram showing diastolic fluttering *(arrows)* of the aortic valve *(AV)* cusps. *LA* = left atrium.

valve replacement (six patients); of our five patients without vegetation by echocardiogram, none underwent aortic valve replacement but two died. Of 46 patients with echocardiographic evidence of aortic valve vegetations reported by combining figures from four groups of investigators,[2, 6, 8, 9] 40 (87%) either underwent aortic valve replacement or died; of the 34 patients without echocardiographic evidence of aortic valve vegetation but clinical evidence of active infective endocarditis reported in the same combined studies,[6, 8, 9] only four (12%) underwent aortic valve replacement or died. Thus, the presence of vegetation on the aortic valve during the period of ABE is of bad prognostic significance and usually indicates that CHF is present or will occur quickly and that death will follow if aortic valve replacement is not carried out. Nevertheless, we would not recommend at this time aortic valve replacement purely on the basis of echocardiographic demonstration of vegetation in the absence of evidence of CHF or repeated emboli or unresponsive septicemia.

Relation of vegetations to systemic embolism. Echocardiographic identification of aortic valve vegetation is of less but nevertheless of some use in predicting the occurrence of a clinical event compatible with systemic embolism. Of our 12 patients with echocardiographic evidence of vegetation, seven had clinical events compatible with systemic emboli; of our five patients without echocardiographic vegetation, one had a systemic embolus. Of the 10 patients with echocardiographic evidence of aortic valve vegetation reported by Roy et al.,[2] seven had clinical evidence of systemic emboli; of the 13 patients with vegetation reported by Mintz et al.,[6] 10 had evidence of systemic emboli and of the eight without vegetation, none had emboli. In contrast to our results and to those reported by Roy et al.[2] and by Mintz et al.,[6] Pratt et al.[9] found no evidence of systemic embolus in either their 13 with or in their 19 patients without echocardiographic demonstration of aortic valve vegetation.

Comparison of clinical events in ABE of AV to MV or TV. Because most reports on echocardiographic observations in patients with ABE have grouped together the observations irrespective of which valve was involved by the infection, the reported results of these studies as a consequence are variable.[8-13] We delineate in Table II our observations in all patients with ABE studied by M-mode echocardiography by us in the past 5 years, summarizing each subgroup as well as totalling all groups. The patients with infection involving the aortic valve (AV) compared to those with infection on either the mitral (MV) or tricuspid valve (TV) had a higher frequency of CHF (11 of 17 vs 12 of 29 [mitral] and 1 of 23 [tricuspid]), a higher frequency of systemic emboli (8 of 17 vs 6 of 29 [mitral]), a much higher frequency of valve replacement during the period of active infection (6 of 17 vs 4 of 29 [mitral] and 1 of 23 [tricuspid]), and a much higher total mortality (8 of 17 vs 9 of 29 [mitral] and 4 of 23 [tricuspid]). Thus, infection involving the aortic valve compared to that involving either the mitral or tricuspid valve is far more liable to produce CHF and systemic emboli, to necessitate valve replacement, and to cause death during the ABE period.

REFERENCES

1. Dillon JC, Feigenbaum H, Konecke LL, Davis RH, Chang S: Echocardiographic manifestations of valvular vegetations. AM HEART J **86**:698, 1973.
2. Roy P, Tajik AJ, Giuliani ER, Schattenberg TT, Gau GT, Frye RL: Spectrum of echocardiographic findings in bacterial endocarditis. Circulation **53**:474, 1976.
3. Andy JJ, Sheikh MU, Ali N, Barnes BO, Fox LM, Curry CL, Roberts WC: Echocardiographic observations in opiate addicts with active infective endocarditis. Frequency of involvement of the various valves and comparison of echocardiographic features of right- and left-sided cardiac valve endocarditis. Am J Cardiol **40**:17, 1977.
4. Sutton R, Petch M, Parker J: Echocardiography in infective endocarditis. Br Heart J **38**:312, 1976.
5. Wray TM: The variable echocardiographic features in aortic valve endocarditis. Circulation **52**:658, 1975.
6. Mintz GS, Kotler MN, Segal BL, Parry WR: Survival of patients with aortic valve endocarditis. The prognostic

implications of the echocardiogram. Arch Intern Med **139**:862, 1979.
7. Sheikh MU, Covarrubias EA, Ali N, Lee WR, Sheikh NM, Roberts WC: M-mode echocardiographic observations during and after healing of active bacterial endocarditis limited to the mitral valve. AM HEART J **101**:37, 1981.
8. Wann LS, Dillon JC, Weyman AE, Feigenbaum H: Echocardiography in bacterial endocarditis. N Engl J Med **295**:135, 1976.
9. Pratt C, Whitcomb C, Neumann A, Mason DT, Amsterdam EA, DeMaria AN: Relationship of vegetations on echogram to the clinical course and systemic emboli in bacterial endocarditis. Am J Cardiol **41**:384, 1978.
10. Young JB, Walton D, Quinones MA, Ishimozi T, Alexander JK, Miller RR: Prognostic significance of valvular vegetations identified by M-mode echocardiography in infective endocarditis. Circulation **5**:41, 1978.
11. Gura GM, Tajik AJ, Seward JB: Correlation of initial echocardiographic findings with outcome in patients with bacterial endocarditis. Circulation **58**:232, 1978.
12. Stewart JA, Silimperi D, Harris P, Wise NK, Fraker TD, Kisslo JA: Echocardiographic documentation of vegetative lesions in infective endocarditis. Clinical implications. Circulation **61**:374, 1980.
13. Davis RS, Strom JA, Frishman W, Becker R, Matsumoto M, LeJemtel TH, Sonnenblick EH, Frater RWM: The demonstration of vegetations by echocardiography in bacterial endocarditis. An indication for early surgical intervention. Am J Med **69**:57, 1980.
14. Sheikh MU, Ali N, Covarrubias E, Fox LM, Morjaria M, Dejo J: Right-sided infective endocarditis. An echocardiographic study. Am J Med **66**:283, 1979.
15. Hirschfeld DS, Rodriguez HJ, Schiller NB: Duplication of aortic wall seen by echocardiography. Br Heart J **38**:943, 1976.

Congenitally Bicuspid Aortic Valve Causing Severe, Pure Aortic Regurgitation Without Superimposed Infective Endocarditis

Analysis of 13 Patients Requiring Aortic Valve Replacement

WILLIAM C. ROBERTS, MD, FACC
ANDREW G. MORROW, MD, FACC
CHARLES L. McINTOSH, MD
MICHAEL JONES, MD
STEPHEN E. EPSTEIN, MD, FACC

Bethesda, Maryland

Although stenosis and infective endocarditis are commonly appreciated complications of the congenitally bicuspid aortic valve, pure *severe* aortic regurgitation complicating this congenital malformation, unassociated with either stenosis or infection, is not well recognized. Among 189 patients who had aortic valve replacement at the National Heart, Lung, and Blood Institute because of isolated pure aortic regurgitation, the congenitally bicuspid aortic valve, never the site of infective endocarditis, was responsible for the aortic regurgitation in 13 (7 percent). This report describes certain clinical and morphologic findings in 13 men, aged 26 to 65 years (mean 43), who required aortic valve replacement because of severe aortic regurgitation secondary to a noninfected, nonstenotic congenitally bicuspid aortic valve. Although not generally recognized, the noninfected congenitally bicuspid aortic valve is an important cause of pure aortic regurgitation severe enough to warrant aortic valve replacement.

The congenitally bicuspid aortic valve frequently becomes stenotic, and because most stenotic valves are also regurgitant, the most frequent circumstance in which aortic regurgitation is found with this congenital anomaly is in association with aortic valve stenosis.[1] In this situation the aortic regurgitation is usually of only mild or moderate degree. Also, the congenitally bicuspid aortic valve is often the site of infective endocarditis.[1] Although it may be superimposed on a stenotic congenitally bicuspid aortic valve, infective endocarditis far more commonly involves the previously normally functioning bicuspid valve or the one previously only slightly regurgitant.[1,2] The usual consequence of the infection in this circumstance is severe pure aortic regurgitation. Mild degrees of pure aortic regurgitation also are commonly observed in patients with a congenitally bicuspid aortic valve and elevated pressure in the ascending aorta from associated aortic isthmic coarctation. However, *severe* aortic regurgitation due to a nonstenotic and noninfected congenitally bicuspid aortic valve is believed to be decidedly infrequent and, indeed, no reports, to our knowledge, have focused specifically on this complication of the bicuspid valve condition. In this report, we describe observations in 13 men who underwent aortic valve replacement because of severe pure aortic regurgitation unassociated with aortic valve stenosis or infective endocarditis.

From the Pathology, Surgery and Cardiology Branches, National Heart, Lung, and Blood Institute, National Institutes of Health, Bethesda, Maryland. Manuscript received August 4, 1980; revised manuscript received September 16, 1980; accepted September 18, 1980.
Address for reprints: William C. Roberts, MD, Building 10A, Room 3E-30, National Institutes of Health, Bethesda, Maryland 20205.

Clinical Features of Patients

Clinical findings (Table I): At the time of aortic valve replacement, the ages of the 13 men studied ranged from 26 to 65 years (mean 43). Preoperatively, one patient had been in functional class I (New York Heart Association classification[3]), three patients in class II, eight in class III and one in class IV. The one patient who was asymptomatic preop-

TABLE I

Clinical and Operative Observations in 13 Men With Aortic Valve Replacement for Pure Severe Aortic Regurgitation and Noninfected Congenitally Bicuspid Aortic Valve

Case	Age (yr) at AVR	Age (yr) M First Heard	Age (yr) Onset of Cardiac Symptoms	Pressures (s/d) (mm Hg) LV	SA	Site of AV Cusps	AV Raphe	AV Ca^{++}	AV Wt (g)
1	26	17	20	125/25	125/54	R-L	+	0	
2	26	13	21	150/24	150/60	A-P	+	0	1.2
3	28	6	27	200/32	235/70	?		0	1.0
4	30	16	29	135/11	160/55	A-P	0	0	0.9
5	30	27	27	118/6	118/52	R-L	+	0	0.7
6	40	11	35	200/32	200/80	A-P	+	+	2.9
7	46	20	44	125/7	130/50	A-P	+	0	?
8	48	13	40	170/12	170/60	?	+	+	2.2
9	49	20	?	118/5	120/58	R-L	0	0	1.5
10	56	27	27	165/17	165/72	A-P	+	0	1.4
11	57	22	44	160/14	170/75	R-L	+	+	1.8
12	63	45	60	155/7	155/55	?	+	+	2.3
13	65	60	65	138/36	160/53	R-L	+	+	1.7

A = anterior; AV = aortic valve; AVR = aortic valve replacement; Ca^{++} = calcium; L = left; LV = left ventricle; M = murmur; P = posterior; R = right; SA = systemic artery; s/d = peak systole/end-diastole; Wt = weight; ? = not known; + = present or positive; 0 = absent or negative.

eratively underwent aortic valve replacement because of severe aortic regurgitation associated with a dilated left ventricular cavity[4] (left ventricular end-systolic cavity dimension on echocardiogram = 56 mm). None of the 13 patients at any time had had clinical evidence of either active infective endocarditis or acute rheumatic fever.

A precordial murmur had been heard for the first time initially as early as age 6 years to as late as age 60 years (mean 23). By auscultation, all 13 patients had grade 3-5/6 murmurs typical of aortic regurgitation, and by aortic root angiograms the degree of aortic regurgitation was graded in each as either 3+/4+ or 4+/4+. The direct aortic diastolic pressures preoperatively ranged from 45 to 80 mm Hg (mean 61). All 13 patients also had basal precordial systolic murmurs, but at catheterization none had a peak systolic pressure gradient between the left ventricle and a major systemic artery or on pullback from the left ventricle to the aorta. Precordial ejection sounds were absent in all 13 patients. Aortic root angiograms were obtained in all patients, but the bicuspid condition of the aortic valve could not be established by this method. Also, the bicuspid nature of the valve was not recognized in any of the seven patients who had echocardiograms.

Three patients (Cases 3, 4 and 6) had aortic isthmic coarctation, with a peak systolic pressure gradient across the coarctation of 70, 50 and 70 mm Hg, respectively. One (Patient 1) had a right aortic arch. No patient had evidence of mitral regurgitation. The father of Patient 2 had had aortic valve replacement because of a stenotic (60 mm Hg peak systolic pressure gradient) congenitally bicuspid aortic valve.

Surgical and morphologic findings: At aortic valve replacement, only two aortic valve cusps were identified in each of the 13 patients (Fig. 1 to 4). In 10 valves, a

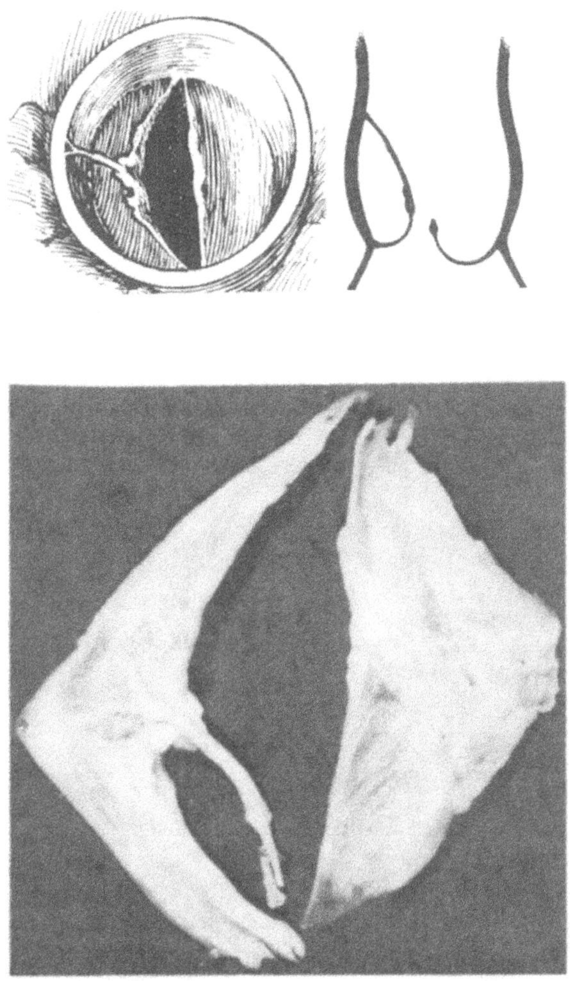

FIGURE 1. Aortic valve in Case 1. The fibrous band on the right cusp (**below**) was attached to the wall of the ascending aorta as shown in the diagram (**above**).

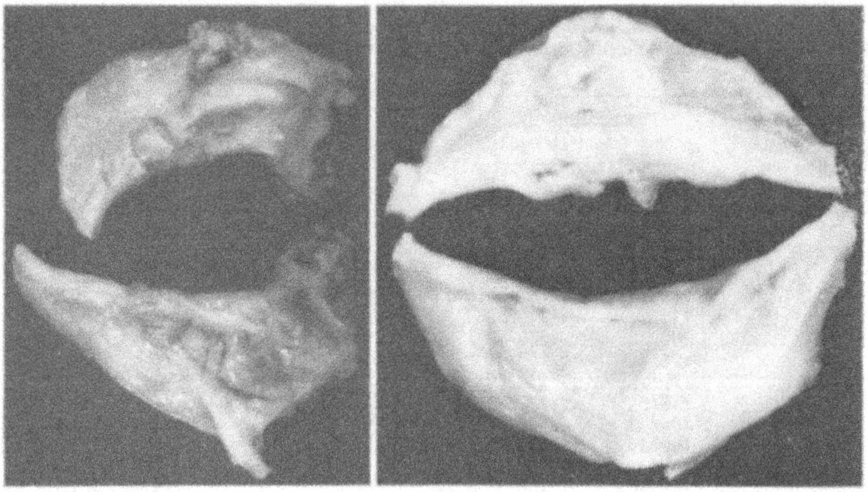

FIGURE 2. Aortic valve in Case 6 (**left**) and Case 7 (**right**). In each valve, the larger cusp is the anterior one. Calcium deposits are present in the valve on the **left**, but not in the one on the **right**.

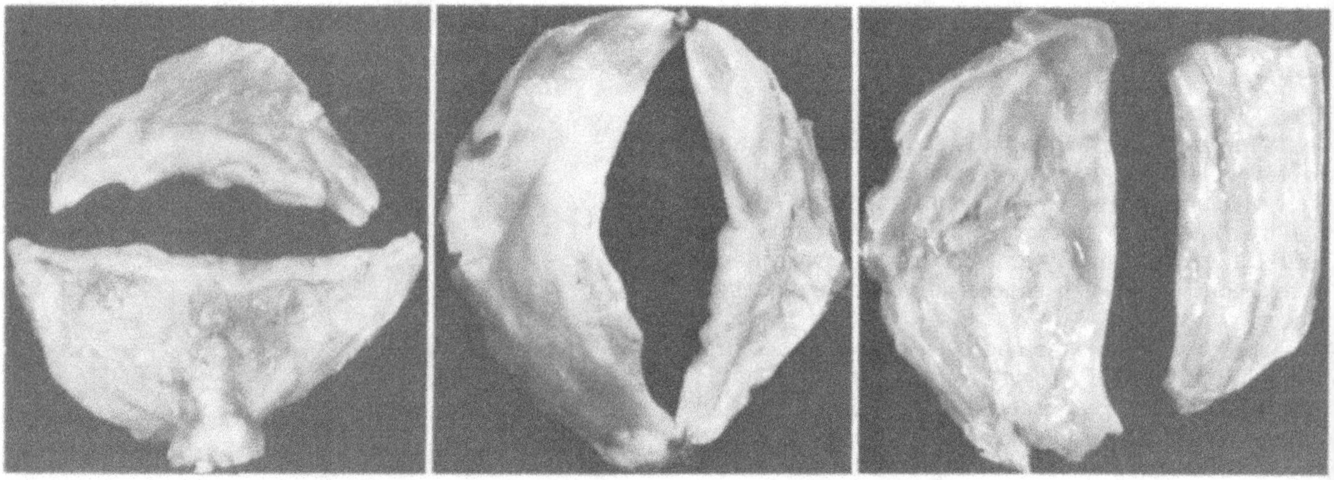

FIGURE 3. Aortic valve in Case 8 (**left**), Case 9 (**middle**) and Case 13 (**right**). The orientation of the cusps is uncertain in Case 8; calcium is present in the raphe in the larger cusp. In both Case 9 and Case 13, the larger cusp is the right one, and the smaller cusp, the left one.

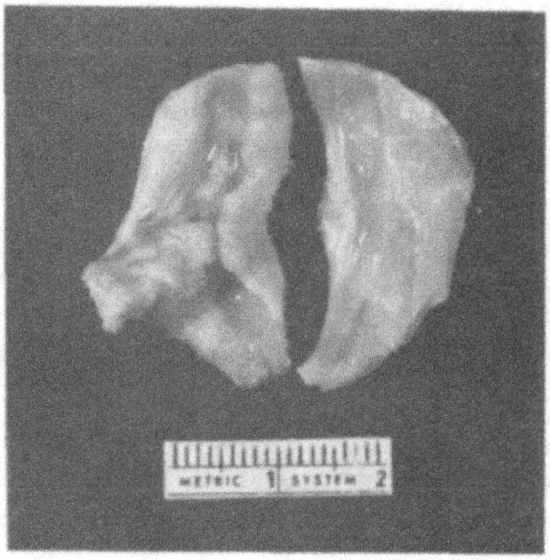

FIGURE 4. Aortic valve in Case 12. The orientation of the two cusps in this patient is not known. The raphe is calcified.

congenital raphe (false commissure) was identified. Each cusp of all 13 aortic valves was thickened by fibrous tissue; no cusp contained vegetations or perforations, indentations, or other evidences of healed infective endocarditis.[5] Calcific deposits, all small, were present in 5 of the 13 excised aortic valves; the deposits in 3 were limited to the raphes.

Comments

Frequency at necropsy of pure regurgitation in bicuspid aortic valve: Each of the 13 patients had aortic regurgitation severe enough to require aortic valve replacement, and at operation each was found to have a congenitally bicuspid aortic valve that neither was stenotic nor had evidence of past infective endocarditis. Furthermore, no patient had had a past clinical illness compatible with active infective endocarditis. Among the complications of a congenitally bicuspid aortic valve, pure severe aortic regurgitation unrelated to infective endocarditis is the least common. Among 200 patients over age 15 years with a congenitally bicuspid aortic valve studied by one of us (W.C.R.) at *necropsy*, only 3 had pure severe aortic regurgitation unassociated with infective endocarditis.[1] Of the 200 necropsy patients, however, 179 had some degree of aortic regurgitation, but it was associated with aortic valve stenosis in 157 and was the result of infective endocarditis in 19; in the remaining 21 patients the bicuspid valve functioned normally. Of 152 necropsy patients with a congenitally bicuspid aortic valve reported on by Fenoglio et al.,[6] 4 apparently had pure aortic regurgitation without evidence of infective endocarditis; however, the severity of the aortic regurgitation in their patients was not stated.

Frequency of congenitally bicuspid valve in pure aortic regurgitation (operative experience): Although the two studies cited provide some information on the frequency of pure aortic regurgitation unassociated with infective endocarditis among *necropsy* patients with a congenitally bicuspid aortic valve, no information is available concerning the frequency of the congenitally bicuspid aortic valve unassociated with infective endocarditis among patients with pure *severe* aortic regurgitation. Accordingly, we reviewed the clinical and operative records and the excised aortic valves in 189 patients aged 18 to 70 years who had aortic valve replacement at the National Heart, Lung, and Blood Institute from 1963 to 1979 because of *isolated* (unassociated with dysfunction of another cardiac valve) *pure* (no element of valve stenosis) aortic regurgitation (Table II). In 13 (7 percent) of the 189 patients the aortic regurgitation was the result of a congenitally bicuspid aortic valve that was not and had not been the site of infective endocarditis. In contrast to the 13 patients that form the basis of this report, only 7 patients (among the 189) had pure aortic regurgitation because of infective endocarditis involving a congenitally bicuspid aortic valve. Thus, the congenitally bicuspid aortic valve unaffected by infective endocarditis is an important cause of pure aortic regurgitation severe enough to warrant aortic valve replacement.

TABLE II

Etiology of Isolated Pure Aortic Regurgitation in 189 Patients Aged 18 to 70 Years Having Aortic Valve Replacement

Cause	Patients n	Patients %
1.* Rheumatic	94	49
2.* Infective endocarditis	41	22
Bicuspid (n = 7)		
Tricuspid (n = 34)		
3. Marfan and Marfan-type	15	8
4.* Congenital (bicuspid valve)	13	7
5.* Prolapse from ventricular septal defect	10	5
6. Syphilis	9	5
7. Aortic dissection	2 }	7 } 4
8. Ankylosing spondylitis	2 }	
9.* With subaortic stenosis	2 }	
Discrete subaortic stenosis (n = 1)		
Hypertrophic cardiomyopathy (n = 1)		
10. Trauma	1 }	
Total	189	100

* Aortic regurgitation resulted from abnormality of the aortic valve only and not from abnormality of the aorta.

References

1. **Roberts WC.** The congenitally bicuspid aortic valve. A study of 85 autopsy cases. Am J Cardiol 1960;23:72–83.
2. **Roberts WC.** Characteristics and consequences of infective endocarditis (active or healed or both) learned from morphologic studies. In: Rahimtoola SH, ed. Infective Endocarditis. New York; Grune & Stratton, 1978;55–123.
3. Criteria Committee of the New York Heart Association. Nomenclature and Criteria for Diseases of the Heart and Great Vessels. 8th ed. Boston; Little, Brown, 1979:349.
4. **Henry WL, Bonow RO, Rosing DR, Epstein SE.** Observations on the optimum time for operative intervention for aortic regurgitation. II. Serial echocardiographic evaluation of asymptomatic patients. Circulation 1980;61:484–92.
5. **Roberts WC, Buchbinder NA.** Healed left-sided infective endocarditis: a clinicopathologic study of 59 patients. Am J Cardiol 1977; 40:876–88.
6. **Fenoglio JJ, McAllister HA, DeCastro CM.** The congenital bicuspid aortic valve after age 20. Am J Cardiol 1977;39:164–9.

Acquired cor triatriatum (left ventricular false aneurysm): Complication of active infective endocarditis of the aortic valve with ring abscess treated by valve replacement

Bruce M. McManus, M.D., Ph.D.,* Nevin M. Katz, M.D., Brian D. Blackbourne, M.D., John S. Gottdiener, M.D., Robert B. Wallace, M.D., and William C. Roberts, M. D.
Bethesda, Md., and Washington, D.C.

Cor triatriatum is a congenital anomaly in which the left atrium (LA) is essentially partitioned into two chambers with a small orifice between them. The cephalad chamber receives the pulmonary veins and the caudal chamber is connected to the mitral valve. The concept of "cor triatriatum" as an *acquired* condition is new. Recently, however, we studied the heart of a 31-year-old opiate addict who had three chambers at the atrial level rather than two. He had developed *Staphylococcus aureus* endocarditis of the aortic valve resulting in severe aortic regurgitation (AR), causing severe congestive heart failure and associated with hemorrhagic pericardial tamponade. At operation, each of the three aortic valve cusps was virtually destroyed by the active infection. A ring abscess was found at operation and the mouth into it was just caudal to the junction of the left and posterior cusps. The cusps were excised and the mouth into the ring abscess was débrided. A porcine

From the Pathology Branch, National Heart, Lung and Blood Institute, National Institutes of Health; the Departments of Surgery and Medicine, Georgetown University; and the Medical Examiner's Office, Washington, D.C.

Received for publication March 29, 1982; accepted Apr. 20, 1982.

Reprint requests: William C. Roberts, M.D., Pathology Branch, NIH-NHLBI, Bldg. 10A, Room 3E-30, Bethesda, MD 20205.

*Present address: Department of Pathology, University of Nebraska Medical Center, Omaha, NE 68105.

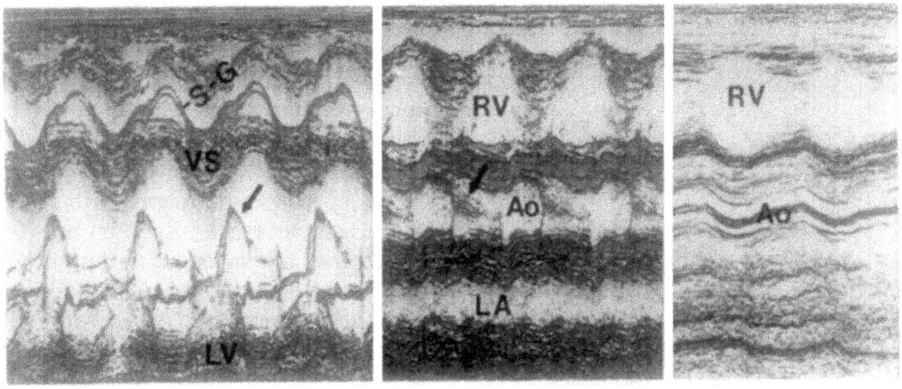

Fig. 1. M-mode echocardiograms. *Left,* Preoperative view showing a Swan-Ganz *(S-G)* catheter in the right ventricular outflow tract, a hyperdynamic ventricular septum *(VS)* and left ventricular free wall *(LV)*, and vibratory movement *(arrow)* of the anterior mitral leaflet and ventricular septum, *Middle,* Preoperative view at the level of aortic valve and left atrium revealing "shaggy" thickenings *(arrow)* of the aortic valve cusps and echo-dense zones between right ventricular outflow tract *(RV)* and aorta *(Ao)*, and between Ao and left atrium *(LA)* that are believed to represent aortic valve ring abscess. *Right,* Postoperative view at the level of aortic valve and left atrium showing the bioprosthesis in aorta and increased echo densities behind the aorta. The latter may represent a portion of the false aneurysm.

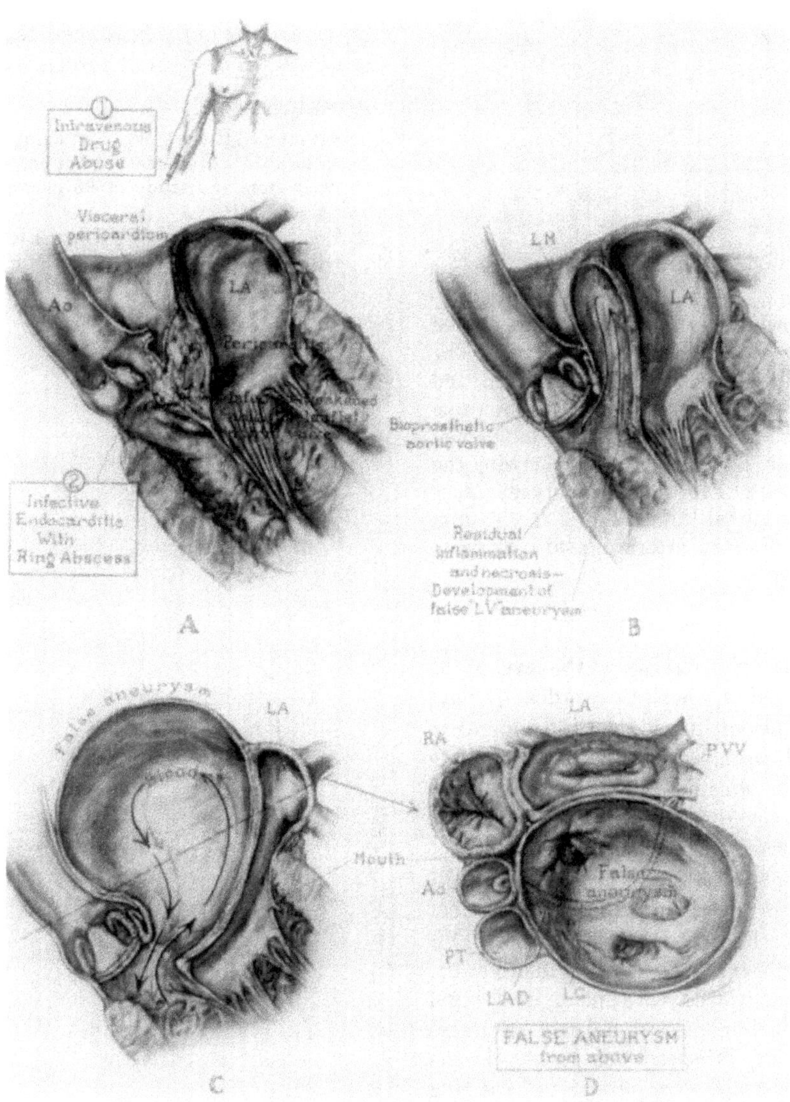

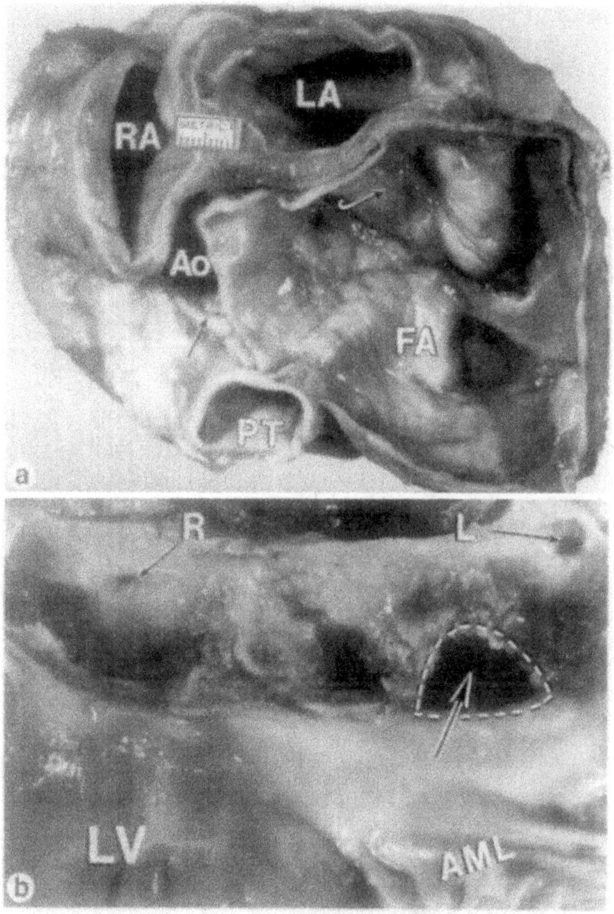

Fig. 3. False aneurysm. *a*, Opened false aneurysm *(FA)* viewed from above showing its fibrous wall and site of communication with the left ventricle *(curved arrow)*. The false aneurysm is much larger than either atrium and overlays the aortic root *(Ao)* where a strut of the bioprosthesis is seen *(arrow)*. *PT* = pulmonary trunk. *b*, Opened aorta and left ventricular *(LV)* outflow tract showing the entry site *(broken-lined area)* into false aneurysm *(large arrow)*. *AML* = anterior mitral leaflet; *L* and *R* = ostium of the left and right coronary arteries *(small arrows)*. (Photos by M.M.M. Moore.)

bioprosthesis (23 mm size) was inserted at the level of the "anulus." The patient died of a narcotic overdose 75 days after an otherwise uneventful clinical postoperative course. A murmur of AR was never present postoperatively and he had received antibiotics for 6 weeks after operation. Echocardiograms recorded 2 days before and 18 days after operation are shown in Fig. 1.

At necropsy, an opening was found just caudal to the ring of the bioprosthesis that led into a large chamber situated adjacent to both atria (Figs. 2 and 3). This accessory chamber, which was much larger than either the right atrium or the compressed LA, ended in a blind pouch, the wall of which consisted entirely of dense fibrous tissue. No residual infection was present in the heart. The bioprosthetic cusps were normal and the ring was securely in place.

Thus, the above described patient had active infective endocarditis on a previously anatomically normal aortic valve and an adjacent ring abscess.[1] The mouth into the abscess was incompletely closed at the time of aortic valve replacement. In retrospect, however, it may have been advisable to have obliterated completely the mouth of the abscess by sutures buttressed with prosthetic material or by a prosthetic patch.[2] Residual infection just caudal to the bioprosthetic valve ring at the aorto-LA angle plus the likely occurrence of a small gradient postoperatively between left ventricle (LV) and aorta are circumstances allowing entrance of blood into the ring abscess. The resulting accessory chamber, which was not present at operation, presumably progressively enlarged postoperatively due to its receiving blood under LV systolic pressure. The aneurysm of the ring abscess represents a false LV aneurysm, although situated at the atrial level, because its wall was not previously myocardium.

The development of a false aneurysm of LV after aortic valve replacement at the site of a ring abscess secondary to infective endocarditis of the aortic valve has not been described previously to our knowledge. Despite the impressive size of the false aneurysm, it apparently caused no symptoms or signs of cardiac dysfunction.

REFERENCES

1. Arnett EN, Roberts WC: Valve ring abscess in active infective endocarditis: Frequency, location, and clues to clinical diagnosis from the study of 95 necropsy patients. Circulation **54**:140, 1976.
2. Frantz PT, Murray GF, Wilcox BR: Surgical management of left ventricular–aortic discontinuity complicating bacterial endocarditis. Ann Thorac Surg **29**:1, 1980.

Mitral Valve Stenosis Produced by or Worsened by Active Bacterial Endocarditis*

Bruce F. Waller, M.D., F.C.C.P.; Bruce M. McManus, M.D.; and William C. Roberts, M.D., F.C.C.P.

Regurgitation is the usual complication of active infective endocarditis involving a cardiac valve. The *development* of valve stenosis entirely from infective endocarditis, of course, is extremely rare and *worsening* of previously existing valve stenosis by infective endocarditis rarely has been documented. In this report we describe one patient who appeared to have mitral stenosis purely on the basis of a large vegetation filling much of the previously normal mitral orifice and another

*From the Pathology Branch, National Heart, Lung, and Blood Institute, National Institutes of Health, Bethesda.
Reprint requests: Dr. Roberts, Bldg 10A, Rm 3E30, National Heart, Lung and Blood Institute, Bethesda 20205

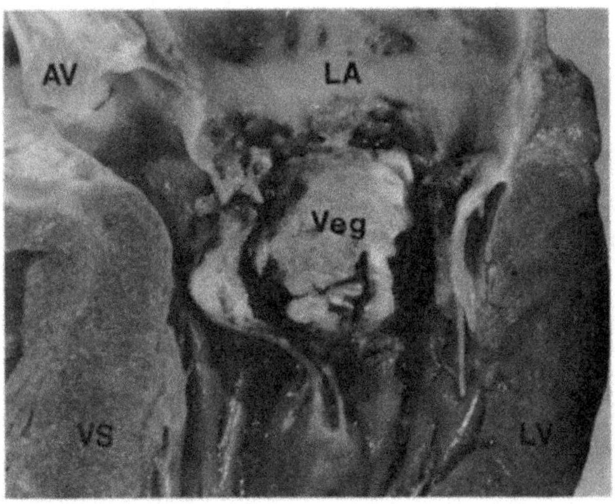

FIGURE 1 (Patient 1). Long axis view of heart showing a large vegetation (veg) in the mitral valve orifice of an otherwise normal mitral valve. AV = aortic valve, LA = left atrium, LV = left ventricle, VS = ventricular septum. *(Photograph by M.M.M. Moore.)*

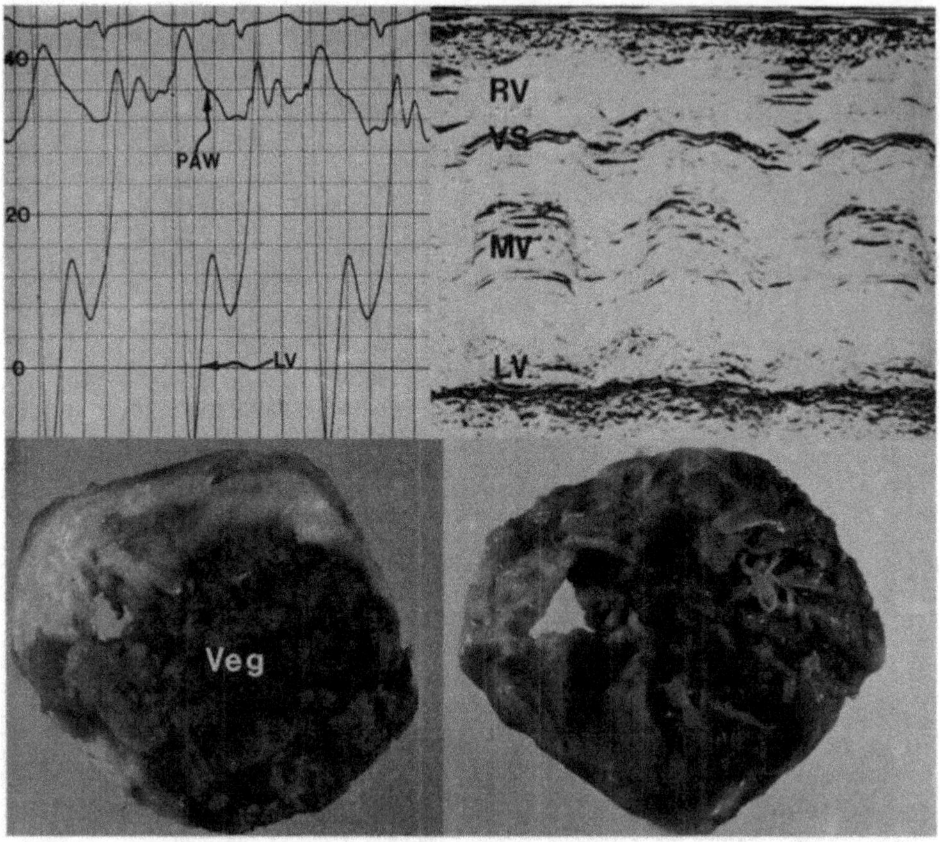

FIGURE 2 (Patient 2). *(Upper left):* Pressure tracing between pulmonary arterial wedge (PAW) position and left ventricle (LV) obtained one week before valve replacement showing a large diastolic gradient. *(Upper right):* M-mode echocardiogram typical of mitral stenosis. Excised mitral valve as seen from left atrium *(lower left)* and from left ventricle *(lower right)*. Veg = vegetation. *(Photograph by M.M.M. Moore.)*

patient in whom active infection clearly worsened preexisting mitral stenosis.

Case Reports

The infecting bacterium in both patients was *Staphylococcus aureus.* Patient 1, a 71-year-old man, initially developed a murmur (grade 3/6) consistent with mitral regurgitation during his last two months of life while febrile (Fig 1). He died from intracerebral bleeding. Patient 2, a 37-year-old man who had had acute rheumatic fever as a child and a grade 1/6 apical diastolic rumble with a loud opening snap for at least three years, increased the intensity of the rumble to grade 3/6 and lost the opening snap when evidence of active infective endocarditis appeared. Cardiac catheterization during the infection disclosed a mean diastolic gradient of 26 mm Hg between pulmonary artery wedge position and left ventricle. The mitral valve was successfully replaced (Fig 2).

Comments

Although hemodynamic confirmation is lacking, the finding of a large vegetation filling the mitral orifice of an otherwise normal valve in patient 1 strongly suggests that mitral stenosis can be produced by active infective endocarditis alone. Roberts and associates[1] previously reported the occurrence of mitral stenosis from infective endocarditis alone due to group B hemolytic Streptococcus in a 21-year-old woman at necropsy, and Davies and associates[2] later described a 38-year-old man in whom both the mitral and aortic orifices at operation appeared to have been obstructed by vegetations alone (group C hemolytic Streptococcus).

The occurrence of active infective endocarditis on a previously stenotic mitral valve, of course, may worsen the degree of stenosis although the degree of worsening has never been documented hemodynamically. In our patient 2 and in three previously reported patients,[3-5] the preexisting mitral stenosis was clearly worsened by the presence of vegetations. Of these four patients, the infecting bacterium in three was *Staphylococcus aureus,* and in one,[5] the blood cultures and cultures of the operatively-excised vegetations were negative. The excised mitral valves in the three previously reported patients were similar in appearance to that in our patient 2.

Thus, active infective endocarditis can by itself *produce* mitral stenosis, and active infective endocarditis may *worsen* preexisting mitral stenosis.

References

1 Roberts WC, Evy GA, Glancy DL, Marcus FI. Valvular stenosis produced by active infective endocarditis. Circulation 1967; 36:449-51

2 Davies MK, Ireland MA, Clarke DB. Infective endocarditis from group C streptococci causing stenosis of both the aortic and mitral valves. Thorax 1981; 36:69-71

3 Reeve R, Reeve FJS, Matula G, Lawson W. Mitral obstruction by vegetations of staphylococcal endocarditis. JAMA 1974; 228:75

4 Matula G, Karpman LS, Frank S, Stinson EB. Mitral obstruction from Staphylococcal endocarditis, corrected surgically. JAMA 1975; 233:58-59

5 Copeland JG, Salomon NW, Stinson EB, Popp RL, Shumway NE. Acute mitral valvular obstruction from infective endocarditis. Echocardiographic diagnosis and report of the second successfully treated case. J Thorac Cardiovasc Surg 1979; 78:128-30

Pathology of Active Infective Endocarditis: A Necropsy Analysis of 192 Patients

E.N. Arnett, and W.C. Roberts

Pathology Branch, National Heart, Lung and Blood Institutes, National Institutes of Health, Bethesda, Maryland, USA

Summary

Successful treatment of infective endocarditis often requires cardiac valve replacement during the active infection. This is especially the case with aortic valve infection, and with infection of valve prostheses in either the aortic or mitral position. Valve excision with or without replacement, however, is also sometimes required for tricuspid valve infection (1). This discussion will focus on the morphologic aspects of active infective endocarditis involving both right and left-sided native cardiac valves. It will also examine certain morphologic aspects of mechanical and bioprosthetic valve substitutes. The information is derived from necropsy examination by the authors of 192 patients with active infective valvular endocarditis (Table 1). Of the 192 patients, 129 were described in an earlier publication (2). Patients with infective endocarditis complicating congenital heart disease with a shunt (6 patients), and those with infective endocarditis following valvulotomy (4 patients) are omitted from this analysis.

Key-Words: Infective endocarditis – Successful treatment – Aortic valve infection

Table 1 Classification of 192 necropsy patients with active infective valvular endocarditis (I.E.)

Group	Patients No.	%
I. I.E. involving right-sided valves	40	(21)
A. Isolated = 22		
B. Combined with left-sided I.E. = 18		
II. I.E. limited to left-sided valve(s)	112	(58)
A. Aortic valve (AV) = 55		
B. Mitral valve (MV) = 35		
C. AV + MV = 22		
III. I.E. involving prosthetic valves	30	(16)
A. Aortic valve = 20		
B. Mitral valve = 10		
IV. I.E. after valvulotomy or valvuloplasty	4	(2)
A. Aortic valve = 1		
B. Mitral valve = 3		
V. I.E. complicating congenital cardiac disease with a shunt	6	(3)
Total	192	(100)

Active infective endocarditis involving right-sided cardiac valves with or without involvement of left-sided cardiac valves

Of the 192 necropsy patients with active infective endocarditis, 40 (20%) had vegetations on right-sided cardiac valves. In 20 patients infection was limited to one or both right-sided cardiac valves, and in 18 patients the infection involved one right-sided cardiac valve and one or both left-sided cardiac valves. The infecting organisms and principle causes of death are shown in Tables 2 and 3. Certain morphologic features of right-sided infective endocarditis are shown in Fig. 1.

Staphylococcus aureus was the most frequent infecting organism causing the infection in 11 (61%) of the 18 patients with isolated right-sided endocarditis in whom the infecting organism was identified. Pneumococcus caused the infection in 7 patients, 5 of whom had vegetations on right and left-sided cardiac valves. In 5 patients fungi caused the infection, and in 6 patients the infecting organism was not identified.

Among the 40 patients, 11 died from generalized sepsis, 5 from meningitis and 3 from pneumonia. Eight patients died from congestive heart failure, but 7 also had left-sided valvular vegetations and in each of them the congestive failure resulted from damage to a left-sided cardiac valve. Eleven patients died from miscellaneous causes not directly related to the infective endocarditis.

Table 2 Active infective endocarditis infecting organisms

Organism	Site of vegetations: Right only or right/left-sided	Left-sided: Normal valve	Left-sided: Abnormal valve	Total
Staphylococcus aureus	18	15	15	48
Staphylococcus epidermis	0	2	2	4
Streptococcus – group D	0	8	6	14
Streptococcus viridans	1	2	10	13
Other streptococci	0	2	5	7
Streptococcus pneumoniae	7	5	4	16
Other bacteria	3	5	1	9
Fungi	5	3	1	9
Unknown or negative	6	16	10	32
	40	58	54	152

In 20 patients infection was limited to the tricuspid valve and in 2 patients infection involved the tricuspid and pulmonic valves. In 16 additional patients the tricuspid valve was infected along with the pulmonic one (2 patients),

Read at the 11th Meeting of the German Society for Thoracic and Cardiovascular Surgery, Bad Nauheim, 1982

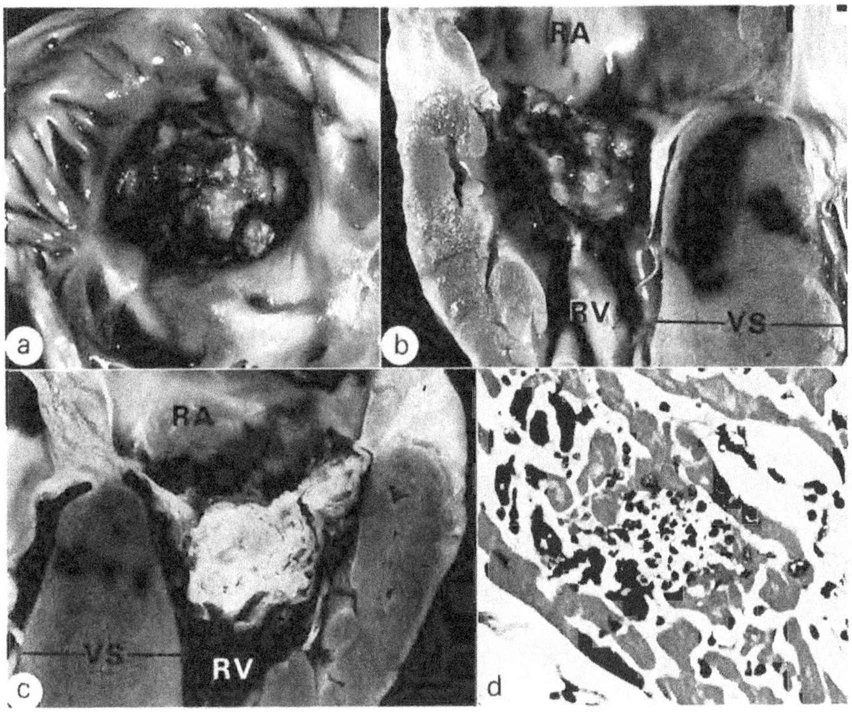

Fig. 1 Tricuspid valve endocarditis in a 26-year-old male heroin addict (A75-84), (a) tricuspid valve viewed from right atrium, (b) posterior portion and (c) anterior portion of a longitudinal cut through right atrium (RA), tricuspid valve and right ventricle (RV). A huge vegetation virtually fills the tricuspid valve orifice. A hemorrhagic abscess is present in the cephalad portion of the ventricular septum (VS), (d) microscopic-sized abscess in left ventricular myocardium (hematoxylin and eosin stain; x450)

Table 3 Active infective endocarditis (AIE)

Principle causes of death				
Cause of death	Site of vegetations			
	Right	Right/left	Left	Total
I. Cardiovascular				
Congestive failure	1	7	57	65
Coronary artery embolism	0	0	2	2
Arrhythmia	0	0	4	4
Tamponade	0	0	1	1
II. Central nervous system				
Embolism	0	0	15	15
Meningitis	2	3	5	10
Diffuse cerebritis	0	0	3	3
III. Generalized sepsis	9	2	12	23
Pneumonia	3	0	0	3
IV. Miscellaneous				
Related to AIE	1[a]	1[b]	4[c]	6
Not related to AIE	6	5	8	19

and one or both left-sided cardiac valves (aortic = 4, mitral = 5, aortic plus mitral = 6). One patient had infection of the pulmonic and mitral valves, and one had infection of the pulmonic and aortic valves.

None of the 40 patients had a history of heart disease before the infective endocarditis. In each of the 40 patients the infected right-sided cardiac valve was normal before infection. Among the 18 patients with infection of right- and left-sided cardiac valves, 15 had normal left-sided cardiac valves before infection. Two patients had normally functioning bicuspid aortic valves (only one of which was infected), and one patient had rheumatic mitral valve disease.

Infective endocarditis appeared to have caused tricuspid regurgitation in 14 of the 38 patients (37%) with tricuspid valve vegetations. Each of these 14 patients had tears or defects in the tricuspid valve or ruptured chordae tendineae. Infective endocarditis caused aortic regurgitation in 8 of the 12 patients with aortic valve vegetations, and mitral regurgitation in 2 of the 13 patients with mitral valve vegetations. Large vegetations appeared to obstruct the tricuspid valve orifice in 2 patients.

Valve ring abscesses were present in 6 of the 38 patients (16%) with tricuspid valve vegetations. Four of these 6 patients also had aortic valve ring abscesses, and in 2 of them the tricuspid valve ring infection had extended through the ventricular septum to involve the aortic valve (and ring). In the other 2 patients, the aortic valve infection was primary, and had extended through the ventricular septum to involve the tricuspid valve.

Comments on right-sided infective endocarditis

Right-sided infective endocarditis is rare compared to left-sided infection. When it occurs it is usually due to a highly virulent organism such as Staphylococcus aureus or Streptococcus pneumoniae. Circumstances associated with an increased risk of infection are almost always present. Intravenous drug addiction and habitual alcoholism are the most frequent predisposing conditions. Signs of pneumonia usually dominate the clinical picture.

Patients with right-sided infective endocarditis almost always have vegetations of the tricuspid valve, and the in-

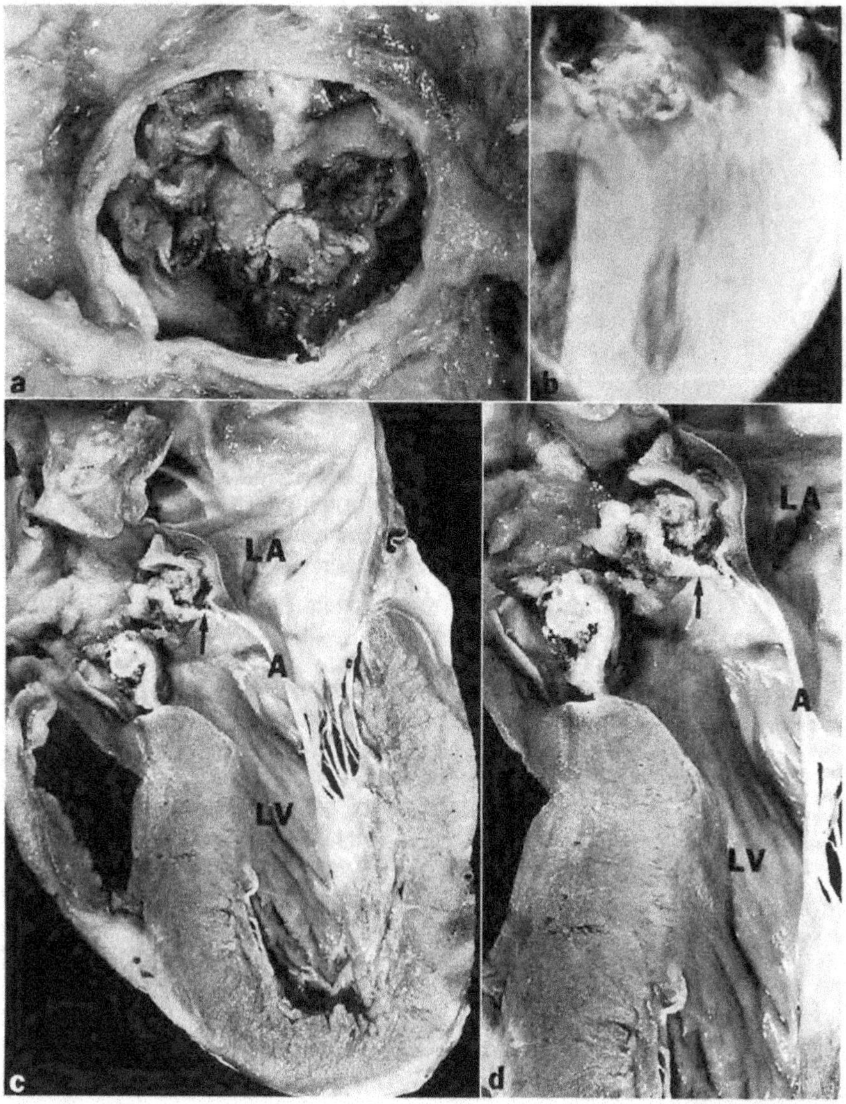

Fig. 2 Streptococcus bovis endocarditis of a calcified stenotic congenitally bicuspid aortic valve in a 65-year-old man (FSH A39 65), (a) aortic valve from above showing extensive vegetations, (b) postmortem roentgenogram of the heavily calcified valve, (c, d) longitudinal cut through the aortic and mitral valves. The aortic valve infection has extended into the wall of the aorta producing ring abscess (arrows). (A = anterior mitral leaflet; L.A. = left atrium; LV = left ventricle)

volved valve, with rare exception, is anatomically and functionally normal before the onset of infective endocarditis. Infection of the tricuspid valve results in tricuspid regurgitation in less than half the patients. Infection of the tricuspid valve ring in isolated tricuspid valve infection is uncommon. Patients with right-sided valvular vegetations often also have vegetations on left-sided cardiac valves. When infection involves both the tricuspid and aortic valves, infection of one or both valve rings is common. Signs of left-sided dysfunction usually dominate when one or both left-sided cardiac valves are infected in combination with a right-sided cardiac valve.

Infective endocarditis limited to one or both left-sided cardiac valves

Among the 192 necropsy patients, 112 (58 %) had vegetations limited to one or both left-sided cardiac valves. The infecting organisms and the causes of death are shown in Tables 1 and 2. Certain morphologic features of left-sided infective endocarditis are shown in Fig. 2 to 5.

Staphylococcus aureus was the most frequent infecting organism (30 patients), and in half the patients with staphylococcal endocarditis the involved valve was normal before infection. Group D streptococcus was the second most frequent infecting organism and also often infected previously normal cardiac valves. Alpha streptococcus, the third most frequent infecting organism, rarely infected previously normal valves. In 9 patients the infection was due to pneumococcus and in 5 of them the involved valve (s) was normal before the infection.

Congestive heart failure from acute valvular regurgitation was, by far, the most common cause of death (57 patients) in patients with left-sided infective endocarditis; central nervous system complications were responsible in 23; generalized sepsis in 12; 7 died from cardiac complications other than valve destruction, and 4 from non-cardiac complications of infective endocarditis.

In the 112 patients with vegetations limited to left-sided cardiac valves, '134 valves were infected; mitral only in 35

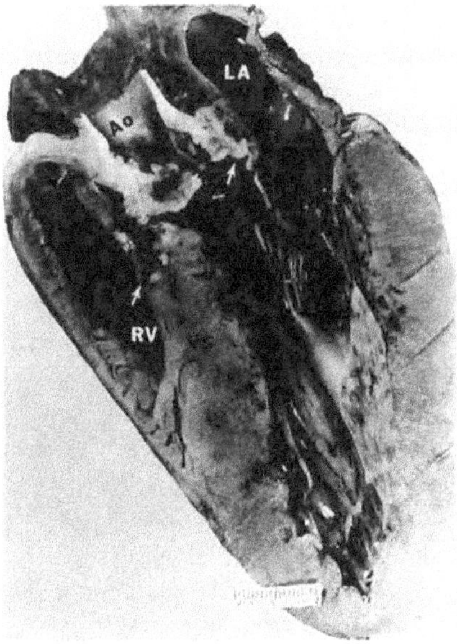

Fig. 3 Congenitally bicuspid aortic valve with superimposed Staphylococcus aureus endocarditis in a 30-year-old mean (GT76A-220). Before the onset of the infective endocarditis the patient was asymptomatic, but the valve was already mildly stenotic and calcified. The infection of the aortic valve burrowed into the adjacent soft tissue (arrows) producing large "ring abscesses". Ring abscess caused complete right bundle branch block. There is extensive subendocardial and papillary muscle necrosis presumably the result of diminished cardiac output. (A = anterior mitral leaflet; Ao = aorta; LA = left atrium; RV = right ventricle; LV = left ventricle; VS = ventricular septum)

patients, aortic only in 55 patients and both the aortic and mitral valves in 22 patients. In at least 15 of the latter 22 patients the mitral valve infection appeared to be secondary to the aortic valve infection.

Among the 77 patients with aortic valve endocarditis, 38 had anatomically normal valves and 39 had anatomically abnormal valves before the onset of infective endocarditis. Of the latter 39 patients, 31 had functionally abnormal valves (stenosis = 18 and pure regurgitation = 13) before the onset of infective endocarditis. The most frequent cause of underlying aortic valve disease was a congenital malformation; bicuspid valve in 18 patients, unicommissural valve in one and discrete subaortic stenosis in 2. Degenerative aortic valve disease was the second most common cause, and was present in 6 patients. Five patients had rheumatic disease of both the aortic and mitral valves, 2 had aortic valve disease of uncertain etiology, and one patient each had syphilis and hypertrophic cardiomyopathy. Four patients had aortic valve disease from a previous episode of infective endocarditis, and in each of them the valve appeared to have been normal before the initial episode of infective endocarditis.

The infective endocarditis caused severe valve damage in 53 (69%) of the 77 patients with aortic valve vegetations. The infective endocarditis caused aortic regurgitation in 50 patients and aortic stenosis in one patient. At necropsy, the aortic valve appeared to have functioned abnormally in 61 patients: from infective endocarditis alone in 30 patients, from infective endocarditis plus the underlying valve deformity in 24 patients, and from the underlying valve deformity alone in 7 patients.

Valve ring abscesses were present in 34 (44%) of the 77 patients. The infective endocarditis had caused severe valvular regurgitation in all but 3 patients with aortic ring abscess, 2 of whom had severe calcific aortic stenosis. The other had a previously normal aortic valve and although extensive vegetations were present, the valve did not appear to have leaked. In 17 of the 34 patients with aortic ring abscess, the infection had burrowed into the pericardial sac causing pericarditis. Ten patients had major conduction defects from extension of the abscess into the ventricular septum, and in 8 patients the infection extended through the left atrial wall into the mitral ring.

Of the 77 patients with aortic valve vegetations, 22 also had vegetations on the mitral valve: in 11 the infective endocarditis caused mitral regurgitation and 8 of them also had aortic regurgitation.

Thirty-five patients had vegetations confined to the mitral valve. In 20 of them the mitral valve appeared to have been anatomically normal, and in 15, anatomically abnormal before the infective endocarditis. Of the 15 anatomically abnormal valves, 11 were functionally abnormal (stenosis in 6 and pure regurgitation in 5). One patient with normal mitral leaflets had mitral regurgitation from an old myocardial infarct. Of the 15 patients with anatomically abnormal mitral valves, 9 had rheumatic disease, 2 had floppy mitral valves and 4 had mitral annular calcium.

Of the 35 patients with isolated mitral valve vegetations, 22 had valve dysfunction from the infective endocarditis. In 21, the infective endocarditis had caused or worsened mitral regurgitation and in one patient, massive vegetations obstructed the mitral orifice. Valve ring abscess was present in 6 patients with isolated mitral valve vegetations and in 3 of them the abscess involved a calcified mitral valve annulus.

Pericarditis was present in 30 of the 112 patients with infective endocarditis involving only left-sided cardiac valves. Of these 30 patients, 27 had vegetations on the aortic valve and only 3 had vegetations limited to the mitral valve. Among the 30 patients, pericarditis resulted from rupture of an aortic valve ring abscess in 17. In 2 patients each the pericarditis resulted from rupture of a myocardial abscess, renal failure, and acute transmural myocardial infarction. Four patients had pericarditis following urgent cardiac valve replacement and 3 patients had pericarditis of uncertain cause.

Comments on left-sided infective endocarditis

A declining incidence rate of acute rheumatic fever and rheumatic heart disease, and the introduction of antibiotic therapy have resulted in important changes in infective endocarditis. Aortic valve infection has become considerably more frequent than mitral valve infection and congenital aortic valve defects account for most of the underlying valve disease. Patients with previously normal cardiac valves constitute a greater proportion of patients with infective endocarditis, and congestive heart failure

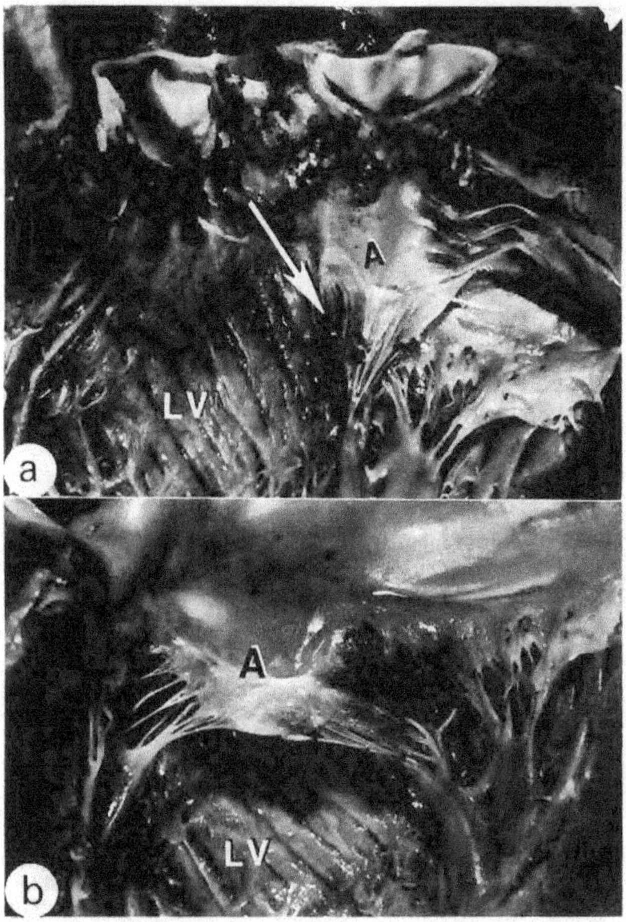

Fig. 4 Streptococcus faecalis endocarditis involving both aortic and mitral valves (A71-120). Both aortic and mitral valves probably were normal before they became sites of infection, (a) opened left ventricle (LV) and aortic valve. The vegetations have partially destroyed each cusp, causing severe aortic regurgitation. Vegetations, on the left ventricular outflow endocardium, mitral leaflet and chordae tendineae almost certainly resulted from retrograde spread of the aortic vegetations by the aortic regurgitation stream (arrow). (A = anterior mitral leaflet), (b) opened mitral valve showing vegetations at the posteriomedial commissure. A number of chordae tendineae are ruptured

from valve damage has become the most frequent cause of death in patients with fatal infective endocarditis.

Among our 112 patients with active infective endocarditis involving native cardiac valves, 77 (69%) had vegetations on the aortic valve and only 35 (31%) had vegetations limited to the mitral valve; 22 patients had vegetations on both left-sided cardiac valves, but in at least 15 of them the mitral valve infection was secondary to the aortic valve infection. Several studies, including one by *Cherubin* and *Neu* (10) involving 656 patients with infective endocarditis seen at Columbia-Presbyterian Medical Center between 1938 and 1967, found a progressive increase in aortic valve infection over the 3 decades, and a decline in mitral valve infection.

Congenitally bicuspid aortic valve is now the single most frequent underlying valve disease. Of our 77 patients with aortic valve vegetations, 38 had underlying valve disease and in 18 of them the aortic valve was congenitally bicuspid. In contrast, only 14 (13%) of the 112 patients, including 35 with vegetations limited to the mitral valve, had underlying rheumatic heart disease. Of 399 necropsy patients with infective endocarditis summarized from several studies, (12, 17, 23, 25, 32) in the preantibiotic era, 258 (65%) had underlying rheumatic valvular disease. Among 424 patients with infective endocarditis studied clinically by *Christian* (11) and by *Kelson* and *White* (19), 381 (90%) had underlying rheumatic valvular disease. The declining frequency of rheumatic heart disease, the lowered frequency of infective endocarditis in patients with rheumatic valvular disease and the increasing age of patients with infective endocarditis appear to account for these changes.

Infective endocarditis on previously normal valves has been considered unusual. Of 1056 necropsy patients with infective endocarditis summarized from several studies, 26% previously had had normal valves (9, 12, 16, 17, 18, 21, 24, 27, 33, 34, 38). Among our 112 patients with active left-sided valvular endocarditis, however, 55 (49%) had anatomically normal valves before the onset of infective endocarditis and 11 of the 57 with anatomically abnormal valves had functionally normal valves before the onset of infective endocarditis. Thus, 59 of our 112 patients had functionally normal valves before the onset of infective endocarditis. *Morgan* and *Bland* (24), *Wilson* (38), *Uwaydah* and *Weinberg* (36), *Lerner* and *Weinstein* (21), and others (7, 37) have noted an increasing number of patients with infective endocarditis involving previously functionally normal valves. In addition, the mortality from infective endocarditis is considerably higher among patients with previously normal valves than among patients with previously abnormal valves. *Rabinovich* and co-workers (28) found infective endocarditis to be fatal in 10 of 12 patients with infective endocarditis involving previously normal valves whereas it was fatal in 61 (48%) of 129 patients with infective endocarditis involving previously abnormal valves. Of 54 patients with active bacterial endocarditis reported by *Pankey* (26), 51 (94%) died and 63% had previously had normal valves.

Congestive heart failure has replaced infection as the leading cause of death among patients with infective endocarditis, and damage to the aortic valve is the most common cause of the failure in patients with infective endocarditis. Of our 112 patients, 57 died from congestive heart failure, and in each of them the infective endocarditis had caused severe valve destruction. In a study by *Robinson* and *Ruedy* (29), congestive heart failure was the cause of death in only 6% of patients with infective endocarditis in the preantibiotic era but caused death in 61% of those with fatal infective endocarditis after the introduction of antibiotic therapy. The increased frequency of congestive heart failure resulted from the increased frequency of valve destruction by the vegetation: 16% of patients with fatal infective endocarditis in the preantibiotic era and 45% in the antibiotic era had cuspal perforations. In nearly all patients in both eras, the perforations involved the aortic valve. Among 33 patients with infective endocarditis stud-

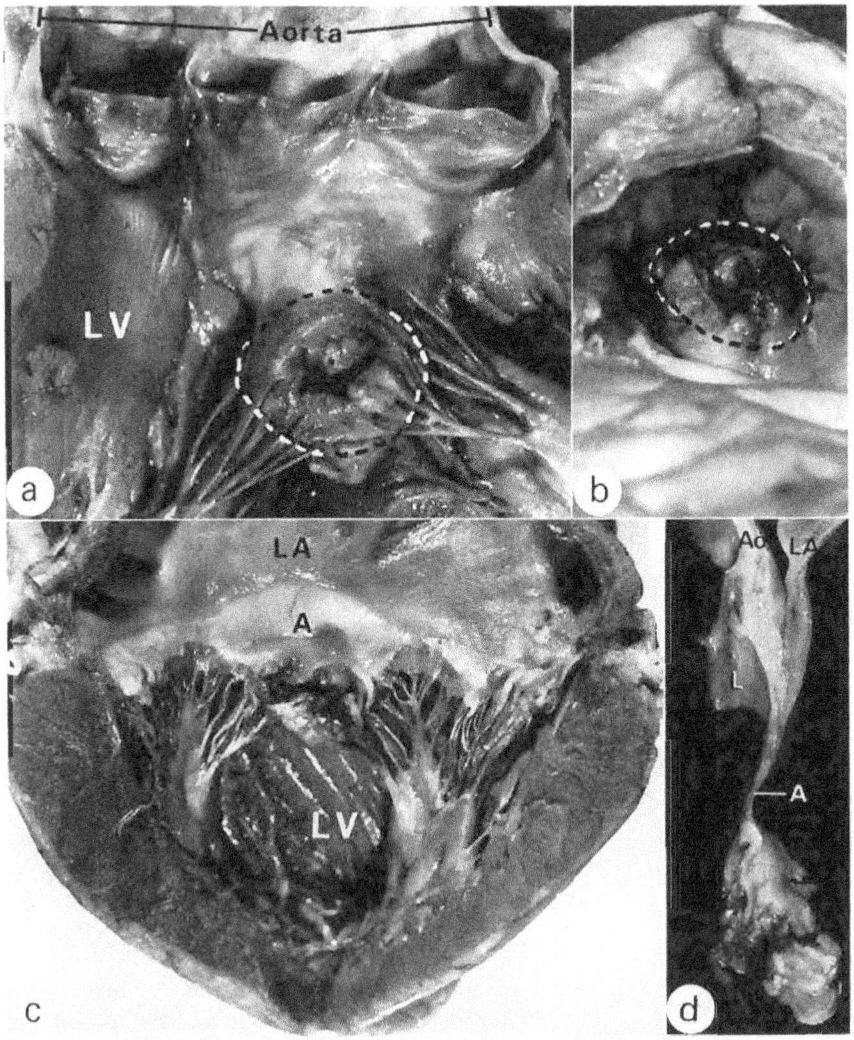

Fig. 5 Serratia marcescens mitral valve endocarditis (A75–123), (a) opened aorta, aortic valve and left ventricle (LV). A large perforation (circle) is present in the anterior mitral leaflet, (b) mitral valve with vegetation (circle) viewed from the left atrium, (c) opened left atrium (LA), mitral valve and left ventricle (LV). The large vegetation on the anterior mitral leaflet (A) is apparent, (d) longitudinal section through aorta (Ao), left atrial wall (LA), left coronary cusp (L) of aortic valve and anterior mitral leaflet (A), showing the large mitral valve vegetation

ied by *Cohen* and *Freedman* (13), damage to the aortic valve was the most common cause of death. Of 14 patients with acute aortic regurgitation from infective endocarditis reported by *Fowler* and co-workers (15), 10 developed severe congestive heart failure within 4 months of the onset of infective endocarditis, and 9 of them died.

The hemodynamic consequence of infective endocarditis is almost always regurgitation. Infective endocarditis caused aortic regurgitation in 50 (65 %) of the 77 patients with aortic valve vegetations and it caused mitral regurgitation in 21 (60 %) of the 35 patients with isolated mitral vegetations. It also caused mitral regurgitation in 11 of the 77 patients with aortic valve vegetations.

Valve ring abscess is frequent in patients with infective endocarditis involving the aortic valve and rare in patients with infective endocarditis of the mitral valve (3). Valve ring abscesses were present in 34 of the 77 patients with aortic valve vegetations and in only 6 of the 35 patients with isolated mitral valve vegetations. In 3 of the latter 6 patients, the infection involved a calcified mitral annulus (8). In 17 of the 34 patients with aortic valve ring abscess, the infection burrowed into the pericardial sac.

Pericarditis in patients with infective endocarditis most often results from ring abscess, and thus usually is a complication of aortic valve infection (3). Pericarditis was present in 30 of our 112 patients and in 27 of them vegetations were present on the aortic valve. In 17 of the 30 patients, the pericarditis resulted from rupture of an aortic valve ring abscess into the pericardial space. Of 43 consecutive necropsy patients with infective endocarditis studied by *Beck* (5), 8 (16 %) had pericarditis and 5 of them had an aortic valve abscess with perforation into the pericardial space. Among 38 patients with aortic valve infective endocarditis reported by *Utley* and *Mills* (35), 15 had ring abscess and 5 of them had pericarditis. Thus, the occurrence of a pericardial friction rub or pericardial effusion during the course of infective endocarditis is highly suggestive of ring abscess.

Active infective endocarditis involving mechanical and bioprosthetic cardiac valve substitutes

Among over 500 patients with one or more substitute cardiac valves studied by us at necropsy, 30 had infection involving a prosthetic valve. In 26 patients the infection in-

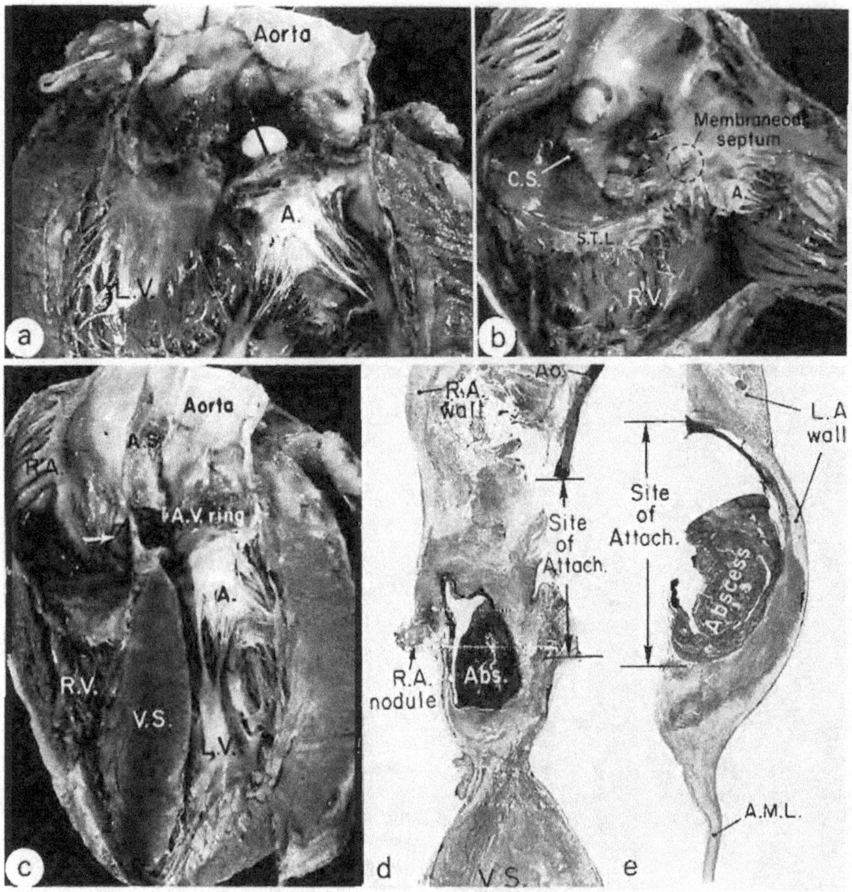

Fig. 6 Staphylococcus epidermidis prosthetic valve endocarditis in a 49-year-old man (A67–22) who died 3 months after aortic replacement, (a) opened aorta, aortic valve and left ventricle (LV) showing a necrotic annulus to which the prosthesis is only partially attached. (A = anterior mitral leaflet), (b) opened right atrium, tricuspid valve and right ventricle (RV) showing vegetative material (arrows) that had burrowed through the atrial septum from the necrotic aortic valve ring (C.S. = ostium of coronary sinus; S.T.L. = septal tricuspid leaflet; A. = anterior tricuspid leaflet), (c) longitudinal section of the heart with the anterior portion removed. The necrotic aortic valve (AV) ring again is seen and the penetration of the infective process through the atrial septum (AS) is apparent. An arrow again designates the vegetation in the right atrium (RA), (V.S. = ventricular septum, (d) and 3, histologic sections through the ring abscess. The site of attachment of the prosthesis, which has been removed, is indicated. The infected nodule, an extension of the ring abscess (Abs.) is showing in the right atrium (RA), (Ao = aortic wall; LA = left atrium; AML = anterior mitral leaflet)

volved a rigid-framed prosthetic valve and in 4 a porcine bioprosthesis. These 30 patients represent 16 % of the 192 patients with active valvular infective endocarditis studied by us. Patients with active infective endocarditis at the time of valve replacement were excluded. Certain morphologic features of the infection in these 30 patients are illustrated in Fig. 6 and 7.

Among the 30 patients, 35 valves had been replaced: 25 patients had one prosthetic valve and 5 patients had 2. Of the 35 prosthetic valves, 30 were infected: aortic in 20 and mitral in 10. Clinical evidence of infective endocarditis was present within 2 months after operation in 11 patients and from 3 months to 17 years after valve replacement in 19. In 10 of the latter 19 patients, evidence of infection did not appear until more than one year after the valve replacement.

Infecting organisms were identified by positive blood cultures in 26 patients and in 19 of them the infection was due to staphylococcus. Listeria species caused the infection in 2 patients, and a different organism in each of the 7 other patients. In 3 patients with negative blood cultures fungi were identified on the prosthetic valve at necropsy.

Five patients underwent valve replacement for prosthetic valve endocarditis. The principle causes of death in the 30 patients were congestive heart failure from prosthetic dysfunction (22 patients), central nervous system emboli (4 patients), generalized infection (2 patients), embolic myocardial infarction (one patient) and small bowel infarction (one patient).

Fourteen of the 17 infected rigid-framed aortic prostheses and 3 of the 9 rigid-framed mitral prostheses were partially or completely detached. In contrast, 5 of the 9 infected mitral prostheses and only one of the 17 infected aortic prostheses were obstructed by vegetative material.

Ring abscesses were present in 25 of the 26 infected rigid-framed prostheses. The abscess involved the entire annulus in 16 patients and only portions of the annulus in the other 10 patients. In 12 of the 17 patients with rigid-framed aortic prosthesis infection, ring infection burrowed into adjacent structures.

Four patients had infected porcine bioprostheses, aortic in 3 and mitral in one patient. In 3 of the 4 patients, the infection was limited to the valve cusps: in one patient it also involved the valve ring. In this patient the aortic porcine bioprosthesis was partially detached. In another patient with an infected aortic porcine graft, vegetations on the ventricular aspect of the cusps appeared to obstruct the valve orifice. All 4 patients with infected porcine valves died from systemic emboli. In no patient did the valve appear to leak as a consequence of the infection.

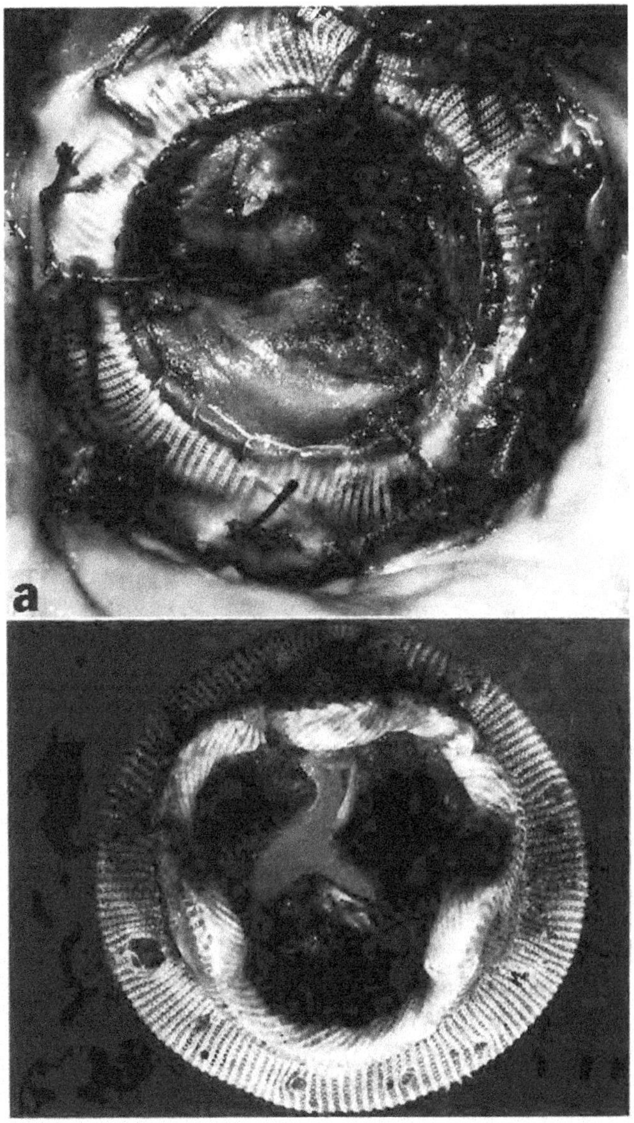

Fig. 7 Staphylococcus aureus infection of a mitral procine bioprosthesis in a 66-year-old woman (A80-51) who died 4 months after mitral valve replacement, (a) bioprosthesis viewed from left atrium. Vegetations are present on all 3 cusps, but not on the sewing ring, (b) ventricular side of the bioprosthesis. All 3 cusps are intact and the valve appeared to have functioned normally

Comments on prosthetic valve endocarditis

Prosthetic valve endocarditis is an infrequent complication of cardiac valve replacement. In most patients with prosthetic valve endocarditis, the infection develops late after valve replacement, but the risk of late prosthetic infection is clearly less than 1% per year (20, 22). Although it has been speculated that porcine valves less often become infected than mechanical valves, *Rutledge* and co-workers' (31) findings did not support this contention. Prosthetic infection occurred in 9 (2.3%) of 397 patients with porcine bioprostheses and in 30 (2.8%) of 1072 patients with mechanical valve prostheses. Similarly, 35 of 1347 Starr-Edwards valves and 16 of 837 bioprostheses described by *Rossiter* and co-workers (30) became infected.

The most consistent morphologic feature of infection involving a rigid-framed prosthesis is infection behind the site of attachment of the valve prosthesis (4). Ring abscesses were present in 25 of the 26 patients with infected rigid-framed prostheses. In over half of them, the entire annulus was necrotic and in 17 the prosthesis was at least partially detached. In 12 patients with infected aortic prostheses, the infection had burrowed extensively into adjacent structures, often causing major conduction defects.

Ring abscess may not be so frequent with infection involving tissue valves. Only one of our 4 patients with infection involving a porcine bioprosthesis had infection behind the sewing ring. In the other 3 patients, infection was limited to the valve cusps. Among 9 necropsy patients with 10 infected porcine valves reported by *Bortolotti* and co-workers (6) one had a ring abscess and only 3 of 43 reported patients with porcine valve infection reviewed by *Ferrans* and co-workers (14) had one.

When a porcine valve becomes infected, the infection appears to involve the valve cusps initially, and only occasionally spreads to involve the valve annulus (14, 30). Consequently, antibiotic cure of infection involving a porcine bioprosthesis may be more frequent than antibiotic cure of infection involving a rigid-framed prosthesis.

The glutaraldehyde-treated porcine valves may be more resistent to destruction by infection than native cardiac valves. Thus, infection of a porcine valve less often results in regurgitation than does infection of a native cardiac valve. Although infection of a native aortic valve resulted in aortic regurgitation in 50 of our 77 patients, none of the 3 with porcine aortic valve infection had regurgitation from the infection.

Large friable vegetations on the porcine valve cusps not infrequently obstruct the valve orifice, and systemic emboli are common. All 4 patients with infected porcine valves died from systemic emboli arising from the infected valve. Five of 9 patients reported by *Bortolotti* and co-workers (6) died from systemic emboli; in 2 of their 9 patients, large vegetations obstructed the porcine valve orifice.

References

1 *Arbulu, A., N.W. Thomas,* and *R.F. Wilson:* Valvulectomy without Prosthetic Replacement. A Lifesaving Operation for Tricuspid Pseudomonas Endocarditis. J. Thorac. Cardiovasc. Surg. 64: 103–107 (1972)
2 *Arnett, E.N.,* and *W.C. Roberts:* Active Infective Endocarditis: A Clinicopathologic Analysis of 137 Necropsy Patients. Curr. Probl. Cardiol. 1: 1–76 (1976)
3 *Arnett, E.N.,* and *W.C. Roberts:* Valve Ring Abscess in Active Infective Endocarditis. Frequency, Location, and Clues to Clinical Diagnosis from Study of 95 Necropsy Patients. Circulation 54: 140–145 (1976)
4 *Arnett, E.N.,* and *W.C. Roberts:* Prosthetic Valve Endocarditis. A Clinicopathologic Analysis of 22 Necropsy Patients with Comparison of Observations in 74 Necropsy Patients with Active Infective Endocarditis Involving Natural Left-sided Cardiac Valves. Am. J. Cardiol. 38: 281–292 (1976)
5 *Beck, D.:* Pericarditis and Subacute Bacterial Endocarditis. J. Mt. Sinai Hosp. 8: 364–375 (1941)
6 *Bortolotti, U., G. Thiene, A. Milano, G. Panizzan, M. Valente,* and *V. Gallucci:* Pathologic Study of Infective Endocarditis on Hancock Porcine Bioprostheses. J. Thorac. Cardiovasc. Surg. 81: 934–942 (1981)

7 *Buchbinder, N.A.*, and *W.C. Roberts:* Left-sided Valvular Active Infective Endocarditis. A Study of Forty-five Necropsy Patients. Am. J. Med. 53: 20–35 (1972)
8 *Burnside, J.W.*, and *R.W. DeSanctis:* Bacterial Endocarditis on Calcification of the Mitral Annulus Fibrosus. Ann. Intern. Med. 76: 615–618 (1972)
9 *Cates, J.E.*, and *R.V. Christie:* Subacute Bacterial Endocarditis. A Review of 442 Patients Treated in 14 Centers Appointed by the Penicillin Trials Committee of the Medical Research Council. Quart. J. Med. 20: 93–130 (1951)
10 *Cherubin, C.E.*, and *H.C. Neu:* Infective Endocarditis at the Presbyterian Hospital in New York City from 1938 to 1967. Am. J. Med. 51: 83–95 (1971)
11 *Christian, H.A.:* The Determinative Background of Subacute Bacterial Endocarditis. Am. J. Med. Sci. 201: 34–40 (1941)
12 *Clawson, B.J.:* An Analysis of Two Hundred and Twenty Cases of Endocarditis with Special Reference to the Subacute Bacterial Type. Arch. Intern. Med. 33: 157–184 (1924)
13 *Cohen, L.*, and *L.R. Freedman:* Damage to the Aortic Valve as a Cause of Death in Bacterial Endocarditis. Ann. Intern. Med. 55: 563–564 (1961)
14 *Ferrans, V.J., S.W. Boyce, M.E. Billingham, T.L. Spray*, and *W.C. Roberts:* Infection of Glutaraldehyde-preserved Porcine Valve Heterografts. Am. J. Cardiol. 43: 1123–1136 (1979)
15 *Fowler, N.O., M.H. Hamburger*, and *K.E. Bove:* Aortic Valve Perforation. Am. J. Med. 42: 539–546 (1967)
16 *Guze, L.B., and M.L. Pearce:* Hospital-acquired Bacterial Endocarditis. Arch. Intern. Med. 112: 56–62 (1963)
17 *Horder, T.J.:* Infective Endocarditis with an Analysis of 150 Cases and with Special Reference to the Chronic Form of the Disease. Q. J. Med. 2: 289–334 (1909)
18 *Kalmar, C., J.B. Thomison*, and *J.L. Shapiro:* Bacterial Endocarditis: Autopsy Experience over a Thirty Year Period. South Med. J. 55: 1208–1211 (1962)
19 *Kelson, S.R.*, and *P.D. White:* Notes on 250 Cases of Subacute Bacterial (Streptococcal) Endocarditis Studied and Treated between 1927 and 1939. Ann. Intern. Med. 22: 40–60 (1945)
20 *Kloster, F.E.:* Diagnosis and Management of Complications of Prothetic Heart Valves. Am. J. Cardiol. 35: 872–885 (1975)
21 *Lerner, P.I.*, and *L. Weinstein:* Infective Endocarditis in the Antibiotic Era. N. Engl. J. Med. 274: 199–206 and 259–266 and 323–331 and 388–393 (1966)
22 *Mayer, K.H.*, and *S.C. Schoenbaum:* Evaluation and Management of Prosthetic Valve Endocarditis. Prog. Cardiovasc. Dis. 25: 43–54 (1982)
23 *Middleton, W.S.*, and *M. Burke:* Streptococcus Viridans Endocarditis Lenta. A Clinicopathologic Analysis of the Experience in the Wisconsin General Hospital. Am. J. Med. Sci .198: 301–323 (1939)
24 *Morgan, W.L.*, and *E.F. Bland:* Bacterial Endocarditis in the Antibiotic Era with Special Reference to the Later Complications. Circulation 19: 753–765 (1959)
25 *Morrison, H.:* A Study of the Incidence of Sub-acute Bacterial Endocarditis at the Massachusetts General Hospital. Boston Med. Surg. J. 197: 46–49 (1927)
26 *Pankey, G.A.:* Acute Bacterial Endocarditis at the University of Minnesota Hospital, 1939 to 1959. Am. Heart J. 64: 583–591 (1962)
27 *Perry, E.L., R.G. Fleming*, and *J.E. Edwards:* Myocardial Lesion in Bacterial Endocarditis. Ann. Intern. Med. 36: 126–137 (1952)
28 *Rabinovich, S., J. Evans, I.M. Smith*, and *L.E. January:* A Long-term View of Bacterial Endocarditis: 337 Cases 1924 to 1963. Ann. Intern. Med. 63: 185–197 (1965)
29 *Robinson, M.J.*, and *J. Ruedy:* Sequelae of Bacterial Endocarditis. Am. J. Med. 32: 922–928 (1962)
30 *Rossiter, S.J., E.B. Stinson, P.E. Oyer, D.C. Miller, J.N. Shapiro, R.P. Martin*, and *N.E. Shumway:* Prosthetic Valve Endocarditis. Comparison of Heterograft Tissue Valves and Mechanical Valves. J. Thorac. Cardiovasc. Surg. 75: 795–803 (1978)
31 *Rutledge, R., J. Kim, R. Applebaum, C.L. McIntosh, A.G. Morrow*, and *W.C. Roberts:* Prosthetic Valve Endocarditis: A Review of 41 Cases. (In press)
32 *Seaburg, J.H.:* Subacute Bacterial Endocarditis. Experiences during the Past Decade. Arch. Intern. Med. 79: 1–21 (1947)
33 *Thayer, W.S.:* Bacterial or Infective Endocarditis. Edinburgh Med. J. 38: 237–265 and 307–334 (1931)
34 *Traut, E.E., J.B. Carter, S.H. Gumbiner*, and *R.N. Hench:* Bacterial Endocarditis in the Elderly. A Report of 94 Autopsied Cases. Geriatrics 4: 205–210 (1949)
35 *Utley, J.R.*, and *J. Mills:* Annular Erosion and Pericarditis. Complications of Endocarditis of the Aortic Root. J. Thorac. Cardiovasc. Surg. 64: 76–81 (1972)
36 *Uwaydah, M.M., and A.N. Weinberg:* Bacterial Endocarditis – A Changing Pattern. N. Engl. J. Med. 273: 1231–1235 (1965)
37 *Weinstein, L.*, and *R.H. Rubin:* Infective Endocarditis – 1973. Prog. Cardiovasc. Dis. 16: 239–274 (1973)
38 *Wilson, L.M.:* Pathology of Fatal Bacterial Endocarditis before and since the Introduction of Antibiotics. Ann. Intern. Med. 58: 84–92 (1963)

Active Infective Endocarditis Complicating Idiopathic Dilated Cardiomyopathy

MARC A. SILVER, MD
WILLIAM C. ROBERTS, MD

The occurrence of infective endocarditis in patients with habitual alcoholism is fairly frequent.[1] A high percentage of patients with idiopathic dilated cardiomyopathy are habitual alcoholics. Yet, the occurrence of infective endocarditis in patients with idiopathic dilated cardiomyopathy is extremely rare. Such was the case, however, in the patient described here.

AW, a 60-year-old man, had been a habitual alcoholic for many years and had the onset of chronic congestive heart failure (CHF) at age 53 years. About 1 year before death, periodic ventricular tachycardia with syncope occurred and he had 2 episodes of ventricular fibrillation with successful resuscitation. The ejection fraction was 19%. His final hospitalization was precipitated by worsening CHF. The blood pressure was 100/80 mm Hg and the temperature 37°C. A grade 3/6 systolic blowing murmur was heard over the cardiac apex. Four of 4 blood cultures grew Staphylococcus aureus *and a chest radiograph showed an infiltrate consistent with acute pneumonia in each lung. Death was attributed to progressive CHF and pneumonia.*

At necropsy, the heart weighed 595 g. The coronary arteries were virtually devoid of atherosclerotic plaques. A thrombus was present in the right atrial appendage. All 4 cardiac chambers were dilated, particularly the ventricles. Several mural endocardial white plaques were present in the left ventricle. A vegetation that measured about 1 cm in maximal diameter and consisted of colonies of Gram-positive organisms, pus and fibrin was present on the atrial aspect of the posterior mitral leaflet (Fig. 1 and 2). The underlying leaflets and chordae tendineae were normal.

Of 165 patients with idiopathic dilated cardiomyopathy studied at necropsy in the Pathology Branch of the National Heart, Lung, and Blood Institute, the patient described in this report is the only 1 with evidence of either active or healed infective endocarditis; we are not aware of any published reports that mention infective endocarditis complicating idiopathic dilated cardiomyopathy. The endocarditis in our patient was probably a consequence of the acute pneumonia, since similar colonies of organisms were present in both the lung and the mitral vegetation.

It has been recognized for decades that active infective endocarditis is a rare occurrence in patients with chronic CHF. Our patient is an exception and illustrates that on rare occasion, a patient with extremely diminished cardiac output can still develop infective endocarditis, even on a previously anatomically normal valve. The endocarditis in our patient was probably secondary to the acute pneumonia. Had the pneumonia not been present, the infective endocarditis likely would not have occurred.

From the Pathology Branch, National Heart, Lung, and Blood Institute, National Institutes of Health, Bethesda, Maryland. Manuscript received and accepted June 3, 1983.

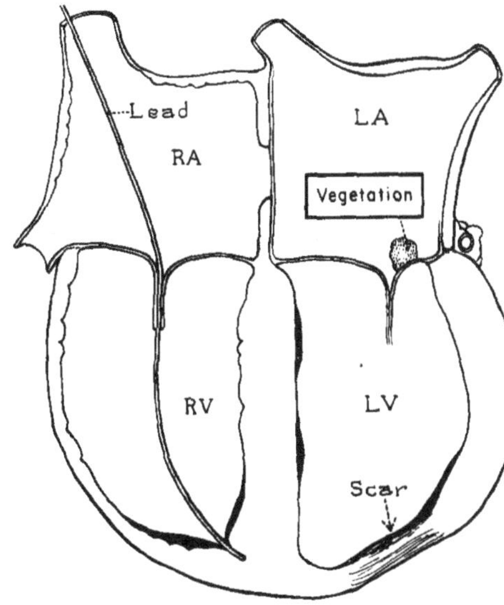

FIGURE 1. Drawing of vegetation on the atrial side of the posterior mitral leaflet. LA = left atrium; LV = left ventricle; RA = right atrium; RV = right ventricle.

Reference

1. **Buchbinder NA, Roberts WC.** Alcoholism. An important but unemphasized factor predisposing to infective endocarditis. Arch Intern Med 1973;132: 689–692.

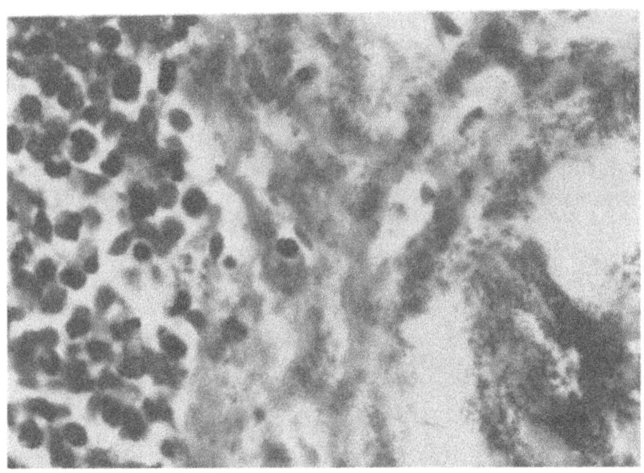

FIGURE 2. Photomicrograph of a section of a portion of the mitral valve vegetation showing colonies of Gram-positive organisms and a collection of polymorphonuclear leukocytes. Hematoxylin-eosin stain; magnification ×860, reduced 13%.

Valve Excision Only Versus *Valve Excision Plus Replacement* for Active Infective Endocarditis Involving the Tricuspid Valve

DEBORAH J. BARBOUR, MD, and WILLIAM C. ROBERTS, MD

M.B., a 28-year-old intravenous (i.v.) drug user, had Group D alpha Streptococcus *endocarditis and underwent tricuspid valve excision without replacement. Late postoperatively, he was asymptomatic, but died from a heroin overdose 11 months after operation (Fig. 1).*

Y.W., a 30-year-old i.v. drug user, had Staphylococcus aureus *endocarditis with severe right-sided congestive heart failure (CHF) and underwent tricuspid valve excision and replacement with a porcine bioprosthesis. Nearly 5 months later the bioprosthesis became infected and it was excised without being replaced (Fig. 2). Shortly thereafter, however, severe right-sided CHF reappeared and, as a consequence, a porcine bioprosthesis was reinserted into the tricuspid valve position. Six weeks after this third operation she was asymptomatic.*

Infective endocarditis involving the tricuspid valve is fairly common in i.v. drug users. The infection on this valve, when bacterial in nature, can usually be eradicated by antibiotic therapy. In an occasional patient, however, persistence of positive blood cultures, repeated pulmonary emboli or development of intractable CHF despite appropriate antibiotic therapy without associated left-sided cardiac valve involvement necessitates operative intervention. But what type of operative intervention should be performed? Excision of the tricuspid valve only or excision plus concurrent replacement (Fig. 3)? This article will examine the arguments for each of these 2 therapeutic options.

Review of previous published reports yielded at least 15 patients who had isolated excision of their infected native tricuspid valves with concurrent placement of either a mechanical prosthesis or a bioprosthesis in the tricuspid valve position.[1-5] Of the 5 patients

From the Pathology Branch, National Heart, Lung, and Blood Institute, National Institutes of Health, Bethesda, Maryland 20205. Manuscript received May 31, 1985, accepted August 13, 1985.

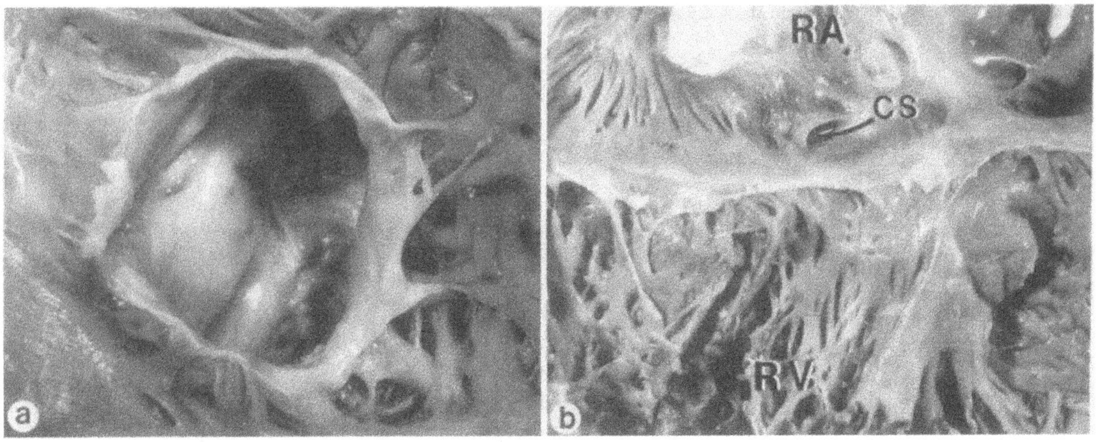

FIGURE 1. Patient M.B. *a*, **intact tricuspid valve anulus viewed from the ventricular side 11 months after excision of most of the leaflets and chordae tendineae.** *b*, **opened tricuspid valve anulus, right atrium (RA) and right ventricle (RV). The tricuspid valve anulus measured 16.5 cm in circumference (normal <12.0 cm). (His mitral valve anulus measured 11.0 cm in circumference [normal <11.0 cm]).**

with mechanical prostheses,[1–4] 2 died in the early postoperative period; 1 patient, who underwent excision of the prosthesis 6 weeks after the initial operation because of prosthetic valve endocarditis, had moderate CHF but no sign of infection 9 months later; and 2 were asymptomatic 12 and 21 months, respectively, after operation. Each of the other 10 patients had tricuspid valve replacement with a porcine bioprosthesis, all since 1980; none died early and 3 died late (1 at 6 months postoperatively from a perforated ulcer and sepsis, and 2 after prosthetic valve endocarditis developed).

In 1971, Arbulu et al[3] reported excision of infected tricuspid valves without replacement in 4 i.v. drug abusers: 1 died of infection 7 weeks later and the other 3 were alive at 1 month, 8 months and 11 years, respectively. In 1981, Arbulu and Asfaw[6] described results of tricuspid valve excision without replacement for tricuspid valve endocarditis (2 patients also concurrently had their infected pulmonic valves excised without replacement) in 61 patients, 29 of whom were operated on by the authors and the other 32 by other surgeons. Of the 61 patients, 6 died within 60 days of operation and 5 died later (2 from "recurrent endocarditis"). Of the remaining 50 patients, 11 subsequently had a prosthesis or bioprosthesis inserted into the tricuspid valve position. Of the 61 patients described by Arbulu and Asfaw,[6] 45 patients between 1970 and 1981 had tricuspid valve excision without replacement, 37 of whom (61%) were reported to have "good" results ("eradication of the infection and absence of hemodynamic problems") and 4 (7%), "fair" results ("eradication of the endocarditis but presence of hemodynamic problems such as tachycardia, mild symptoms and signs of right or left ventricular failure, or biventricular failure"). Actuarial analysis of these patients who underwent tricuspid valve excision without replacement predicted 86% survival at 10 years.

No postoperative hemodynamic data is available in the 13 patients who survived the early postoperative period after isolated replacement of the tricuspid valve for active infective endocarditis.[1,2,4,5] Robin et al[7]

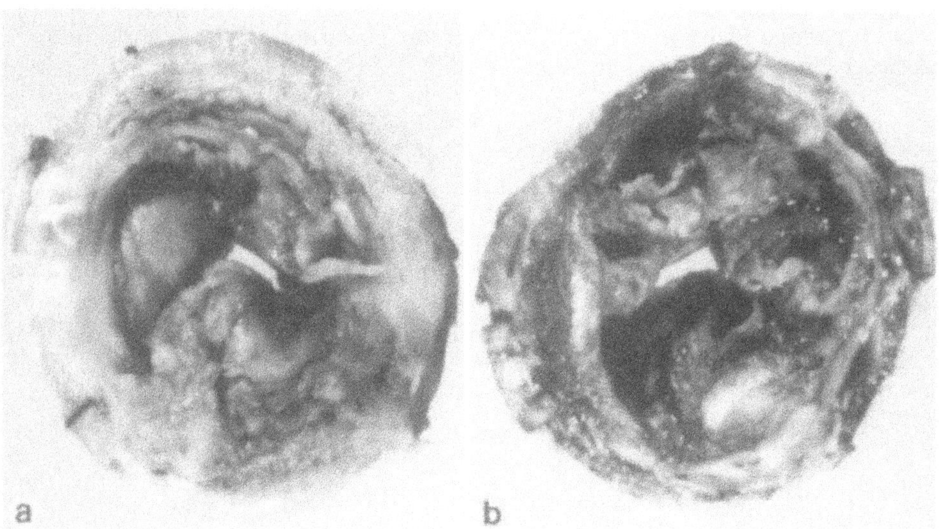

FIGURE 2. Patient Y.W. Operatively excised porcine bioprosthesis from the tricuspid valve position. The bioprosthesis was excised nearly 5 months after its implantation because it became infected. *a*, **right atrial aspect.** *b*, **right ventricular aspect. Infected thrombus (vegetation) is present on both aspects of the cusps.**

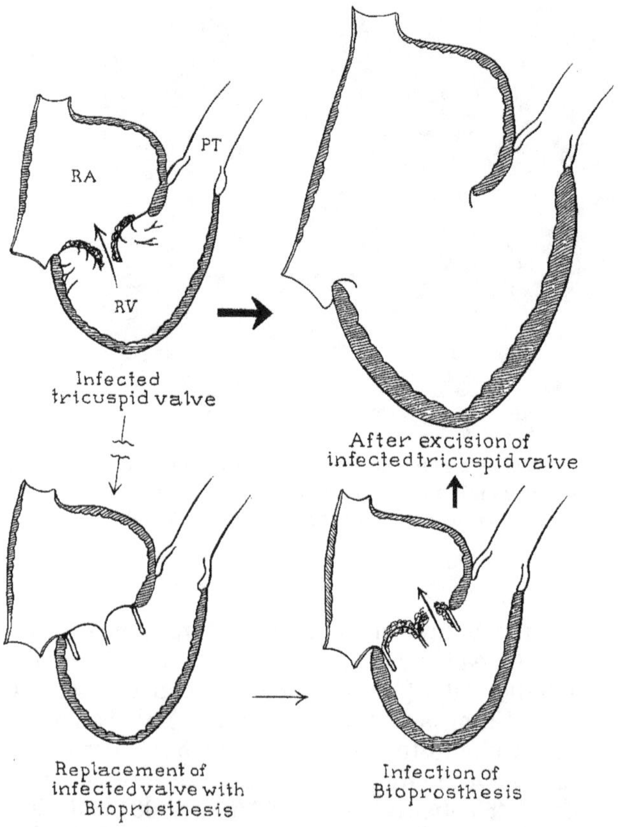

FIGURE 3. Diagram showing the possible operative interventions for resistant infective endocarditis involving the tricuspid valve. *Top panel* shows the expected late consequences of tricuspid valve excision without replacement as occurred in our patient M.B. *Lower panel* shows what happened in our patient Y.W. who initially had replacement of the infected native tricuspid valve with a bioprosthesis, which in turn became infected, necessitating its excision without concurrent replacement.

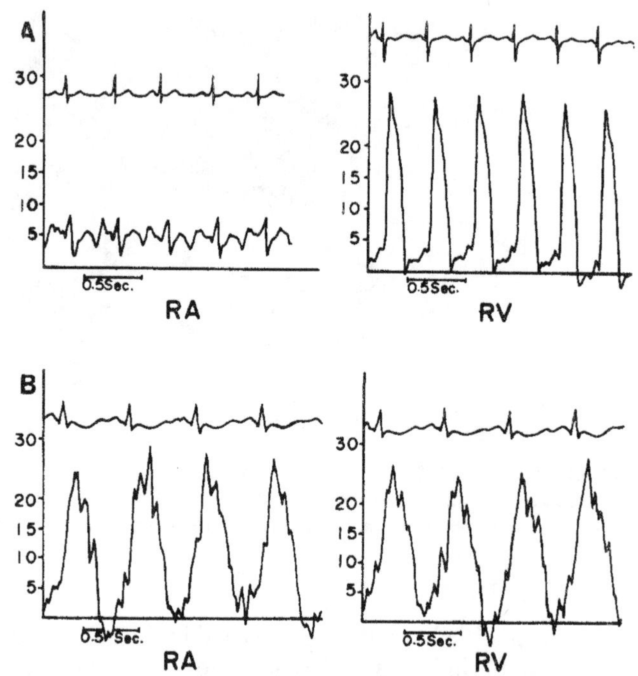

FIGURE 4. Preoperative (*upper panel*) and postoperative (*lower panel*) pressure tracings from right atrium (RA) and right ventricle (RV) in a patient with active tricuspid valve endocarditis reported in 1975 by Robin et al.[7] Postoperatively, the pressure tracing of the right atrium and right ventricle are identical. The numbers in the *vertical columns* in all 4 diagrams are mm Hg. (Reproduced with permission of Robin et al and *The American Journal of Cardiology*.)

described both pre- and postoperative hemodynamic data in 10 patients who had tricuspid valve excision without replacement for active infective endocarditis. Postoperatively, the right atrial and right ventricular pressure tracings were similar, indeed virtually identical (Fig. 4). In their 10 patients, the mean right atrial pressure preoperatively was 4.4 mm Hg (range 3 to 6) and postoperatively it was 13.3 mm Hg (range 10 to 17). The average values of the right and left ventricular systolic and diastolic pressures, pulmonary arterial systolic and diastolic pressures, and the mean aortic pressures were normal and similar preoperatively and postoperatively, whether the patients were free of evidence of right-sided cardiac failure (7 patients) or had right-sided cardiac failure (3 patients). The precise interval between tricuspid valve excision without replacement and postoperative cardiac catheterization was not stated by Robin et al, but the maximal interval was only 48 months, and probably much less.

It is clear that tricuspid valve excision for active infective endocarditis involving this valve removes the source of pulmonary emboli, which occur in virtually all such patients and is the major cause of symptoms. Furthermore, from the aforementioned data, an asymptomatic state can be achieved for varying periods in most patients, in the absence of a tricuspid valve, as long as the right ventricular systolic pressure is normal or near normal. Because most patients with infective endocarditis involving the tricuspid valve are i.v. drug users and their habit usually is not discontinued following a tricuspid valve operation, it appears most reasonable to perform tricuspid valve excision without accompanying valve replacement to prevent the introduction of a "foreign body" which, of course, would be exquisitely sensitive to infection. The insertion of a bioprosthesis or prosthesis provides a nidus more prone to infection than the native tricuspid valve. Furthermore, insertion of the bioprosthesis or prosthesis usually leads to some degree of obstruction between the right atrium and right ventricle during ventricular diastole. Additionally, if the substitute cardiac valve is a bioprosthesis, replacement of it will be indicated some years later because of expected degeneration with long-term wear.[8,9] For these reasons, tricuspid valve excision without replacement appears, in our view, preferable to tricuspid valve excision with concurrent replacement for life-threatening active infective endocarditis involving this valve. It is likely, however, that most patients having tricuspid valve excision without replacement will eventually require the insertion of a prosthesis or a bioprosthesis into the tricuspid valve position, but the interval between operations may be many years and this time may be sufficient to allow cessation of i.v. drug use.

References

1. Kennedy JH, Sabga GA, Fisk AA, Sancetta SM. *Isolated tricuspid valvular insufficiency due to subacute bacterial endocarditis. J Thorac Cardiovasc Surg 1966;51:498–506.*
2. Jimenez-Martinez M, Lopez-Cuellar M, Quinones-Morales R. *Isolated tricuspid endocarditis with ventricular septal defect. J Thorac Cardiovasc Surg 1971;61:665–669.*
3. Arbulu A, Thoms NW, Chiscano A, Wilson RF. *Total tricuspid valvulectomy without replacement in the treatment of Pseudomonas endocarditis. Surg Forum 1971;22:162–164.*
4. Michl L, Shumacker HB Jr, Hobbs D. *Tricuspid valvulectomy. Surg Gynecol Obstet 1973;137:590–592.*
5. Stern HJ, Sisto DA, Strom JA, Soeiro R, Jones SR, Frater RWM. *Immediate tricuspid valve replacement for endocarditis: indications and results (abstr). Am Assoc Thorac Surg, Program of Annual Meeting, 1985: 44.*
6. Arbulu A, Asfaw I. *Tricuspid valvulectomy without prosthetic replacement. Ten years of clinical experience. J Thorac Cardiovasc Surg 1981; 82:684–691.*
7. Robin E, Thoms NW, Arbulu A, Ganguly SN, Magnisalis K. *Hemodynamic consequences of total removal of the tricuspid valve without prosthetic replacement. Am J Cardiol 1975;35:481–486.*
8. Cohen SR, Silver MA, McIntosh CL, Roberts WC. *Comparison of late (62 to 140 months) degenerative changes in simultaneously implanted and explanted porcine (Hancock) bioprostheses in the tricuspid and mitral valve positions in six patients. Am J Cardiol 1984;53:1599–1602.*
9. Silver MA, Cohen SR, McIntosh CL, Cannon RO III, Roberts WC. *Late (5 to 132 months) clinical and hemodynamic results after either tricuspid valve replacement or anuloplasty for Ebstein's anomaly of the tricuspid valve. Am J Cardiol 1984;54:627–632.*

Aortic Valve Perforation With Calcific Aortic Valve Stenosis and Without Infective Endocarditis or Significant Aortic Regurgitation

WILLIAM C. ROBERTS, MD
CHARLES L. McINTOSH, MD
ROBERT B. WALLACE, MD

Small lucunae adjacent to commissures are often observed in the aortic valve cusps of older persons, and they have no functional consequences. Larger perforations in the more central portions of 1 or more aortic valve cusps, in contrast, are uncommon, nearly always the consequence of infective endocarditis; they usually produce severe aortic regurgitation, and rarely involve valves that are either calcified or stenotic.[1,2] Recently, we encountered 3 patients with large perforations in an aortic valve cusp associated with cuspal calcific deposits, large enough in 2 patients to cause aortic valve stenosis and warrant valve replacement; only 1 had associated aortic regurgitation, and none had a clinical event compatible with infective endocarditis. Such cases have not been reported previously.

From the Pathology and Surgery Branches, National Heart, Lung, and Blood Institute, National Institutes of Health, Bethesda, Maryland, and the Department of Surgery, Georgetown University Medical Center, Washington, D.C. Manuscript received and accepted August 21, 1986.

Pertinent findings in the 3 patients are summarized in Table I and illustrated in Figures 1 through 4. Both men had congenitally bicuspid aortic valves that were stenotic, and each was excised and replaced (Fig. 1 to 3). Patient 3, an 85-year-old woman, died from a noncardiac condition. In each of the 3 patients, a protruding calcific nodule on the ventricular aspect of 1 cusp closed the perforation in the apposing cusp. The portion of the cusp in the vicinity of the perforation was devoid of calcific deposits, whereas the cusp in apposition to the perforation contained prominent calcific deposits.

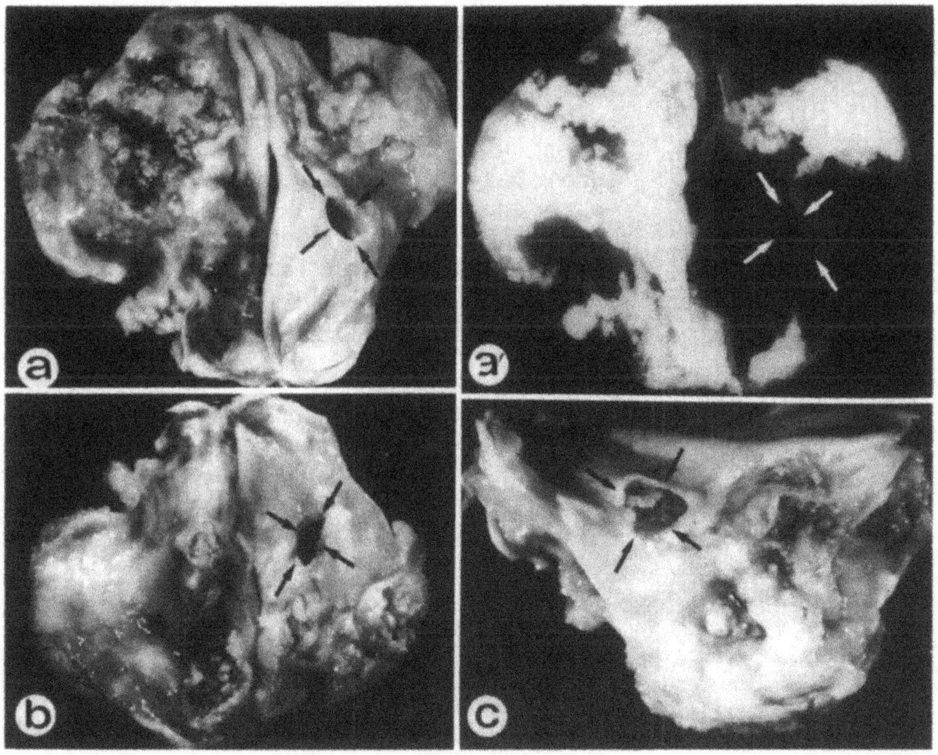

FIGURE 1. Patient 1. Operatively excised congenitally bicuspid aortic valve from the aortic aspect (*a*) and radiograph (*a'*), from the ventricular aspect (*b*), and a view of the aortic aspect of the cusp with calcium protruding into the cusp (*c*). The perforation is designated by the *arrow*.

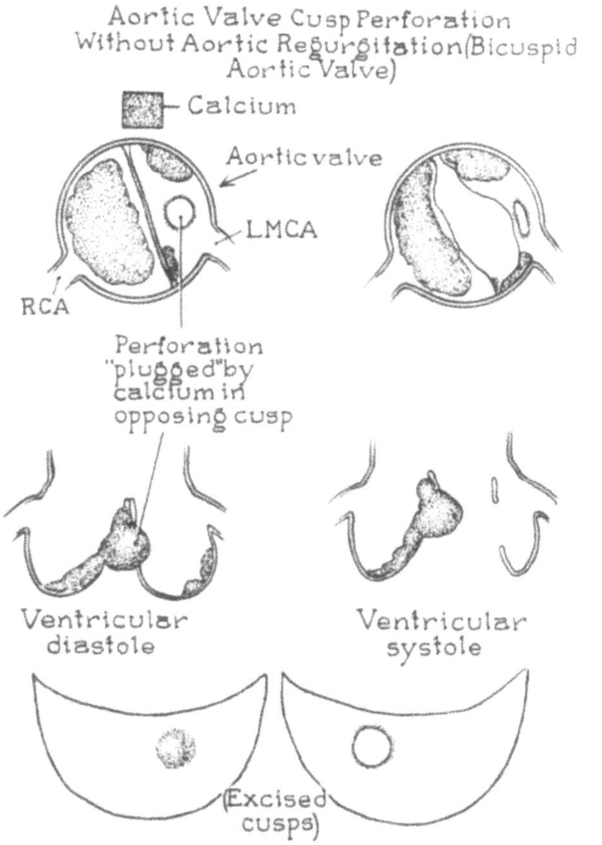

FIGURE 2. Patient 1. Drawing of the aortic valve illustrating the mechanism of the cuspal perforation. LMCA = left main coronary artery; RCA = right coronary artery.

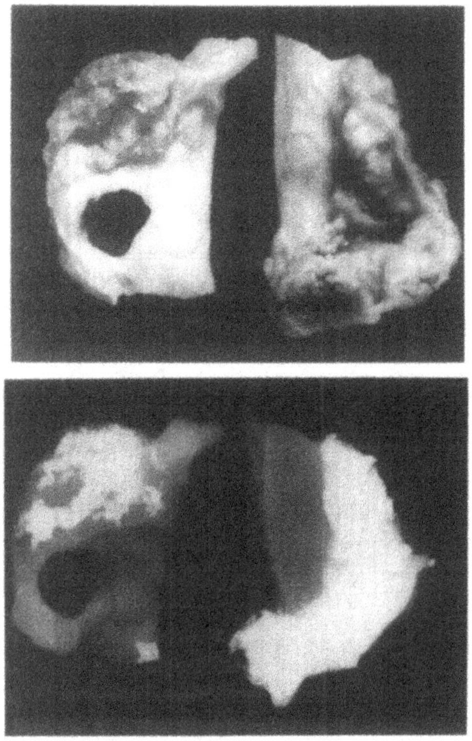

FIGURE 3. Patient 2. Operatively excised congenitally bicuspid aortic valve with radiograph. The perforation is located in the non-calcified portions of the cusp in apposition to heavy calcific deposits in the other cusp.

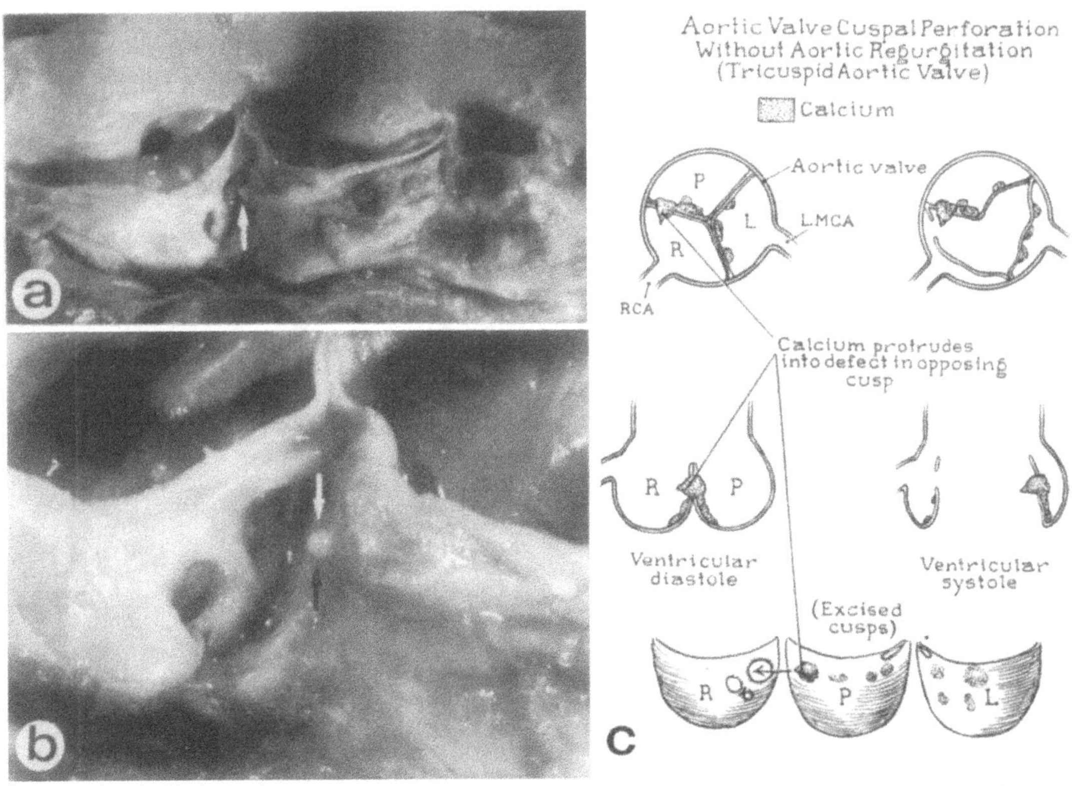

FIGURE 4. Patient 3. *a* and *b*, 2 views of the opened 3-cuspid aortic valve showing 2 large and 1 small perforation in the right cusp and a calcific spur from the posterior cusp protruding into 1 of the perforations in the right cusp. *c*, diagram illustrating the mechanism of cuspal performation. L = left; LMCA = left main coronary artery; P = posterior; R = right; RCA = right coronary artery.

TABLE I Pertinent Observations in the Three Patients

Case	Age (year) at AVR or Death	Sex	Pressures (mm Hg) LV (s/d)	SA (s/d)	LV-SA psg	AR by AA Cine (0-3+)	Murmur of AR	No. AV Cusps	HW (g)
1	62	M	240/20	185/85	55	0	0	2	...
2	64	M	220/9	155/90	65	1+	2/6	2	620
3	85	F	...	160/100	...	...	0	3	440

AA = ascending aorta; AR = aortic regurgitation; AV = aortic valve; AVR = aortic valve replacement; HW = heart weight; LV = left ventricle; psg = peak systolic gradient; SA = systemic artery; s/d = peak systole/end diastole.

Thus, perforation of 1 aortic valve cusp in each of the 3 patients resulted from the trauma engendered by a calcific nodule in 1 cusp, protruding into and finally perforating a noncalcified portion of the apposing cusp. This mechanism of cuspal perforation has not been described previously and neither has aortic valve cuspal perforation without aortic regurgitation.

1. Roberts WC, Buchbinder NA. *Healed left-sided infective endocarditis: a clinicopathologic study of 59 patients. Am J Cardiol 1977;40:876–888.*

2. Roberts WC. *Characteristics and consequences of infective endocarditis (active or healed or both) learned from morphologic studies. In: Rahimtoola SH, ed. Infective Endocarditis. New York: Grune & Stratton, 1978: 55–123.*

Infective Endocarditis in Opiate Addicts: Analysis of 80 Cases Studied at Necropsy

Frederick A. Dressler, MD and William C. Roberts, MD

Eighty opiate addicts were studied at necropsy. Fifty-nine patients had anatomic evidence of active infective endocarditis (IE); 11 had healed IE; and 10 had both. Of the 80 patients, the first episode of IE involved a single right-sided cardiac valve in 24 patients (30%); both a right- and a left-sided valve in 13 patients (16%); a single left-sided valve in 33 patients (41%); and both left-sided valves in 10 patients (13%). Of the 320 cardiac valves in the 80 patients, 103 were sites of vegetations, an average of 1.3 of the 4 valves. Of the 80 patients, the tricuspid valve was infected in 35 (44%), mitral in 34 (43%), aortic in 32 (40%) and pulmonic in 2 (3%). Of the 103 infected cardiac valves, the infection caused sufficient damage to cause dysfunction in 70 (68%): in 28 (88%) of 32 infected aortic valves; in 22 (63%) of 35 infected tricuspid valves; in 19 (56%) of the 34 infected mitral valves; and in 1 of the 2 infected pulmonic valves. Of the 80 patients, 57 (71%) had sufficient valvular damage to cause valvular dysfunction. Of the 80 patients, gross examination of the valves at necropsy indicated that the infected valve almost certainly had been anatomically normal in 65 patients (81%) and abnormal in 15 patients (19%) before the onset of IE. Of the 65 patients with previously anatomically normal valves, 86 (33%) of their 260 cardiac valves were sites of infection (average 1.3 valves/patient); of the 15 patients with infection superimposed on a previously abnormal valve, the infection in each involved previously abnormal valves (21 in the 15 patients) or 17 (28%) of their 60 cardiac valves were sites of infection (average 1.1 valve/patient). Of the 15 patients with abnormal cardiac valves before the infection, 7 had congenitally bicuspid aortic valves and 8 had diffuse fibrous thickening of the mitral valve typical of rheumatic heart disease with (6 patients) or without (2 patients) diffuse fibrous thickening of tricuspid aortic valves. Of the 80 patients, 42 (53%) died during their first episode of active IE, 17 (21%) underwent operative excision with or without valve replacement during the active IE, and in 21 patients (26%) the first episode of active IE healed. In 10 of the latter 21 patients, active IE recurred and was fatal. A total of 19 patients had cardiac valve excision with or without replacement, 17 during active IE and 2 after healing. Of the 19 patients, 5 died within 30 days of operation, 10 (56%) within a year of operation and 16 (80%) within 3 years. Of the 13 patients surviving >30 days after valvular operation, 5 developed prosthetic or bioprosthetic endocarditis, which was fatal in each.

Thus, the first episode of active IE appears to have a high mortality because the infection most often involves previously normal valves that are easily destroyed by vegetations. When the valvular vegetations are operatively excised, with or without replacement, prognosis remains poor because of the danger of prosthetic or bioprosthetic endocarditis. When the active IE is eradicated by antibiotics without operation, recurrence of IE at sites of previously healed IE is common.

(Am J Cardiol 1989;63:1240–1257)

A number of reports have emphasized the propensity of opiate addicts to develop infective endocarditis (IE).[1–12] Several studies have described the distribution of valvular vegetations by echocardiography among opiate addicts,[13,14] and others have focused on echocardiographic features of vegetations involving each of the cardiac valves.[15–18] Although a number of publications have described morphologic features of IE, none describing a large group of patients has focused specifically on characteristics of IE observed at necropsy in opiate addicts. In this report we present clinical and necropsy cardiac findings in 80 opiate addicts who had active or healed IE or both.

METHODS

Cases and sources: Cases accessioned in the Pathology Branch, National Heart, Lung, and Blood Institute, as having *opiate addiction* and *active* and/or *healed IE* were retrieved. The files from 1954 through February 1989 were searched. A total of 168 cases were accessioned as having opiate addiction and of them 80 at necropsy had evidence of either active or healed IE or both. This study is limited to the 80 cases with opiate addiction and either active or healed IE or both. Of the 80 cases, 9 (11%) were studied from 1960 to 1970, 33

From the Pathology Branch, National Heart, Lung, and Blood Institute, National Institutes of Health, Bethesda, Maryland. Manuscript received November 18, 1988; revised manuscript received and accepted February 24, 1989.

Address for reprints: William C. Roberts, MD, Pathology Branch, National Heart, Lung, and Blood Institute, National Institutes of Health, Building 10, Room 2N258, Bethesda, Maryland 20892.

TABLE I Location of Valvular Vegetation During the First Episode of Active Infective Endocarditis in Opiate Addicts (80 Necropsy Cases)

Valve(s) with Vegetations	Pts	Died During First Episode of Active IE Without Operation	Valve Excised With or Without Replacement During Active Infective Endocarditis	First Episode Healed	Causes of Death When First Episode of Active IE Healed: Recurrent Active IE	Other Cardiac	Noncardiac
Single right-sided							
TV	23	14	3	6	2	2	2
PV	1	0	0	1	0	0	1
Single right-sided + Single left-sided							
TV + MV	8	2	1*	5	4	0	1
TV + AV	4	2	1†	1	1	0	0
PV + MV	1	1	0	0	0	0	0
PV + AV	0	0	0	0	0	0	0
Single-left sided							
MV	15	10	2	3	2	0	1
AV	18	8	7	3‡	3§	0	0
Double-left sided							
AV + MV	10	5	3	2	0	0	2
Total	80 (100%)	42 (53%)	17 (21%)	21 (26%)	12/21 (57%)	2/21 (10%)	7/21 (33%)

* Mitral valve excised and replaced; tricuspid valve excised without replacement; † aortic valve excised and replaced; tricuspid valve excised without replacement; ‡ aortic valve replaced after the active IE had healed in 2 of the 3 patients; § site of recurrence was bioprosthetic or prosthetic valve in the aortic valve position in 2 patients.
AV = aortic valve; IE = infective endocarditis; MV = mitral valve; PV = pulmonic valve; TV = tricuspid valve.

TABLE II Infective Endocarditis (IE) in Opiate Addicts: Frequency of Vegetations on Each of the Four Cardiac Valves, of Healing of the Active Infection, of Valve Dysfunction Produced by Valvular Damage By Vegetation, of Underlying Valve Abnormality Before Infection and of Valvular Ring Abscess (80 Necropsy Cases)

Valve	No. Examined	No. (%) with Vegetations	No. (%) in Which Active IE Healed	No. (%) in Which Valvular Infection Caused Sufficient Valve Destruction to Produce Clinical Valve Dysfunction	No. (%) with Underlying Valve Disease Before Active IE	No. (%) with Ring Abscess
Tricuspid	80	35 (44)	12/35 (34)	22 (63)	0/35	2/35 (6)
Pulmonic	80	2 (3)	1/2	1	0/2	0/2
Mitral	80	34 (43)	10/34 (29)	19 (56)	5/34 (15)	3/34 (9)
Aortic	80	32 (40)	6/32 (19)	28 (88)	12/32 (38)	17/31* (55)
Total	320	103/320 (32)	29/103 (28)	70/103 (68)	17/103 (17)	22/102 (21)

* One patient was excluded because it is not known whether a ring abscess was present or absent at the time of aortic valve replacement.

(41%) from 1971 to 1980 and 38 (48%) from 1981 until January 1, 1989. The 80 cases were autopsied in 13 different institutions and subsequently the heart, and often portions of other organs, were submitted to the National Heart, Lung, and Blood Institute for examination. The submitting institutions included the following: District of Columbia Medical Examiner's Office (36 cases); District of Columbia General Hospital (16 cases); Howard University Hospital (Washington, DC) (9 cases); Georgetown University Medical Center (Washington, DC) (6 cases); Veterans Administration Hospital (Washington, DC) (3 cases); Washington Hospital Center (Washington, DC) (3 cases); and 1 case each from 7 hospitals.

At necropsy, 69 (87%) of the 80 patients had cardiac valvular vegetations either at necropsy (52 cases) or at cardiac valve operation (17 cases) for valve excision with or without replacement. Of the remaining 11 patients (14%), 8 had clinical events typical of active IE. They received antibiotics, and the infection disappeared. Three patients, 2 of whom died outside the hospital, had no evidence of a clinical event compatible with active IE: 1 had received antibiotics for an illness: whether or not the other 2 had received antibiotics is unknown. All 11 patients who did not have active vegetations on 1 or more cardiac valves at necropsy or at operation had morphologic evidence of healed IE, i.e., rupture of several chordae tendineae or perforation or indention of a valvular cusp.[19] The active valvular vegetations contained microorganisms, polymorphonuclear leukocytes and fibrin.

Location of valve vegetations during first episode of active infective endocarditis: The cardiac valve(s) containing vegetations during the first episode of active IE is (are) summarized in Tables I and II. In 24 patients (30%) vegetations were limited to a single right-sided cardiac valve (tricuspid in 23) (Figures 1 through 6); in 13 patients (16%), vegetations involved a single right-sided cardiac valve and a single left-sided cardiac valve (Figures 7 through 10); in 33 patients (41%), vegetations were located on a single left-sided cardiac valve (Figures 11 through 14); and in 10 patients (13%), vegetations involved both left-sided cardiac valves (Table I).

Of the 80 patients, the first episode of active IE was fatal in 42 patients (53%) and in another 17 patients (21%) operative valve excision with or without replacement was carried out during the period of active IE (Table I). In the remaining 21 patients (26%), the first episode of active IE healed. Of these 21 patients in whom the vegetations initially healed, 12 had recurrent active IE that was fatal, 2 died from cardiac problems without recurrence of active IE (myocarditis in 1 and congestive heart failure in 1), and 7 died from noncardiac causes (opiate overdose in 3, trauma in 1 and infection [pneumonia and brain abscess] in 3).

The frequency of vegetations on each of the 4 cardiac valves is summarized in Table II. The valve most commonly involved, whether isolated or in association with involvement of another cardiac valve, was the tricuspid one—35 (44%) of the 80 patients. The mitral valve contained vegetations in 34 (43%) patients, the aortic in 32 (40%) patients and the pulmonic valve in 2 patients.

In 70 (68%) of the 103 valves containing vegetations, examination of the valve disclosed so much destruction of leaflet tissue (or associated chordae tendineae) that valvular dysfunction had to be a consequence; in 33

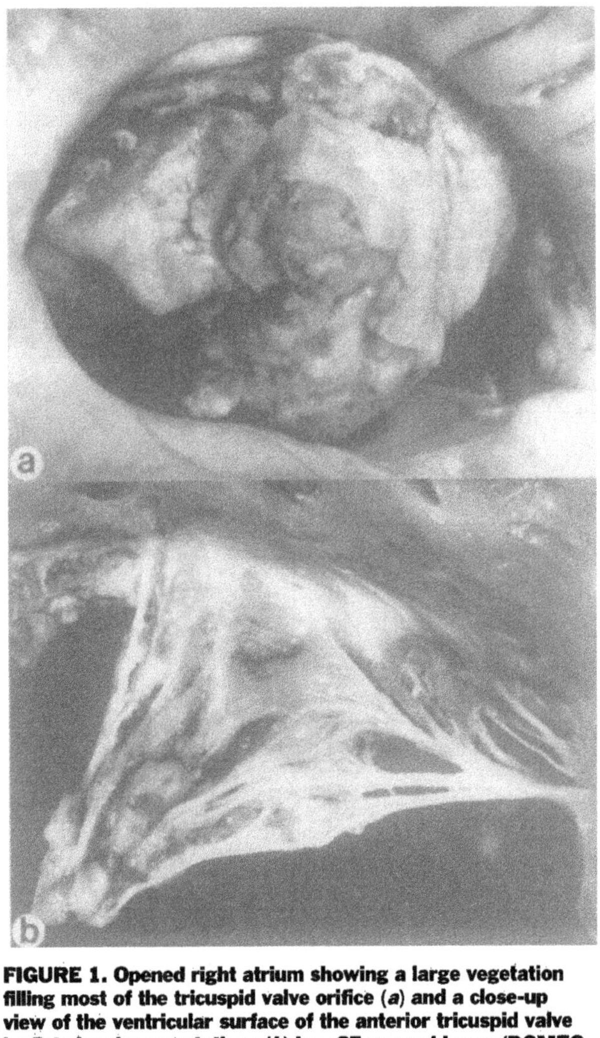

FIGURE 1. Opened right atrium showing a large vegetation filling most of the tricuspid valve orifice (*a*) and a close-up view of the ventricular surface of the anterior tricuspid valve leaflet showing vegetations (*b*) in a 25-year-old man (DCMEO #87-06-549) who had apparently been well until 12 days before death when evidence of pneumonia appeared. He was hospitalized 10 hours before death and blood culture disclosed *Staphylococcus aureus*. The active infective endocarditis, which was limited to the tricuspid valve, was not diagnosed until necropsy.

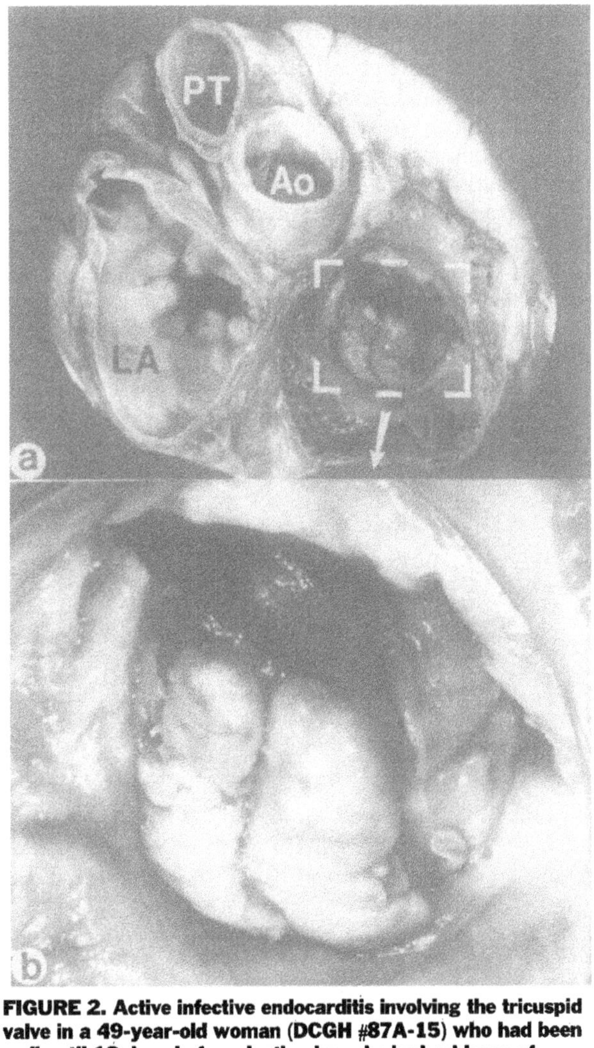

FIGURE 2. Active infective endocarditis involving the tricuspid valve in a 49-year-old woman (DCGH #87A-15) who had been well until 18 days before death when she had evidence of pneumonia. *Staphylococcus aureus* was grown from blood cultures. She developed multiple pulmonary abscesses (from septic emboli) and anasarca. *a*, view of the opened atria from above showing vegetations on the tricuspid valve leaflets (*brackets*). *b*, a close-up of the area in brackets. Ao = aorta; LA = left atrium; PT = pulmonary trunk.

(32%) of the 103 valves containing vegetations leaflet destruction by vegetation was absent or minimal and insufficient to cause valve dysfunction.

Of the 103 cardiac valves containing vegetation, the infective endocarditis healed in 29 (28%).

Of the 37 right-sided cardiac valves that were sites of vegetations, all appeared to have been anatomically normal before the infection. In contrast, of the 66 left-sided cardiac valves that were sites of vegetation, the valve (by morphologic gross examination) appeared to have been previously normal in 49 (74%) and abnormal in 17 (26%).

Valve ring abscess was present in 2 (5%) of the 37 infected right-sided cardiac valves, in 3 (9%) of the 34 infected mitral valves and in 17 (55%) of 31 infected aortic valves.

Analysis of cases in whom the first episode of active infective endocarditis was fatal: Pertinent clinical and necropsy data in the 59 patients who either died or had a cardiac valve operation during the first episode of active IE are summarized in Table III. The 59 patients are divided into 3 categories according to which cardiac valve(s) contained vegetation(s). In 17 patients (29%) the vegetations were limited to a single right-sided cardiac valve, the tricuspid valve in all 17. All of these 17 patients had acute pneumonia as their presenting problem. Of the 13 in whom the information was available, only 6 had a precordial murmur, systolic in each. These 17 patients died primarily as a consequence of the pneumonia. At necropsy, the tricuspid valve in each appeared to have been anatomically normal before the onset of active IE. The pneumonia in each was the consequence of septic emboli, the result of dislodgment of portions of vegetative material from the tricuspid valve.

Of the 59 patients, 7 (12%) had vegetations on 1 right-sided cardiac valve (tricuspid in 6 and pulmonic in 1) and on 1 left-sided cardiac valve (mitral in 4 and aortic in 3). All of these 7 patients had acute pneumonia, presumably secondary to dislodgment of vegetative material from the right-sided cardiac valve. In 3 of the 7 patients there was no clinical evidence of dysfunction of either the right-sided (tricuspid in 2, pulmonic in 1) or the left-sided valve (mitral in 2, aortic in 1); 3 patients had evidence of regurgitation of both tricuspid and aortic valves, the sites of the vegetations; and 1 patient with severe aortic regurgitation had no evidence of tricuspid regurgitation.

Of the 59 patients, 35 (59%) had vegetations limited to 1 or both left-sided cardiac valves: aortic only in 15 patients (43%), mitral only in 12 patients (34%) and both mitral and aortic valves in 8 (23%). In 7 of the latter 8 patients the size of the vegetations on the aortic valve cusps was larger than those on the mitral leaflets and chordae tendineae; all these 8 patients had evidence of severe aortic regurgitation with or without evidence of mitral regurgitation.

Infecting organism during first episode of active infective endocarditis: The microorganism responsible for the first episode of active IE was known in 48 (60%) of the 80 patients. *Staphylococcus aureus* was cultured from the blood in 35 (73%) of the 48 patients, 2 of whom also had other bacteria cultured from the blood: *Pseudomonas aeruginosa* in 1 and *Enterobacter cloacae* in another. The infecting bacterium in 1 patient (2%)

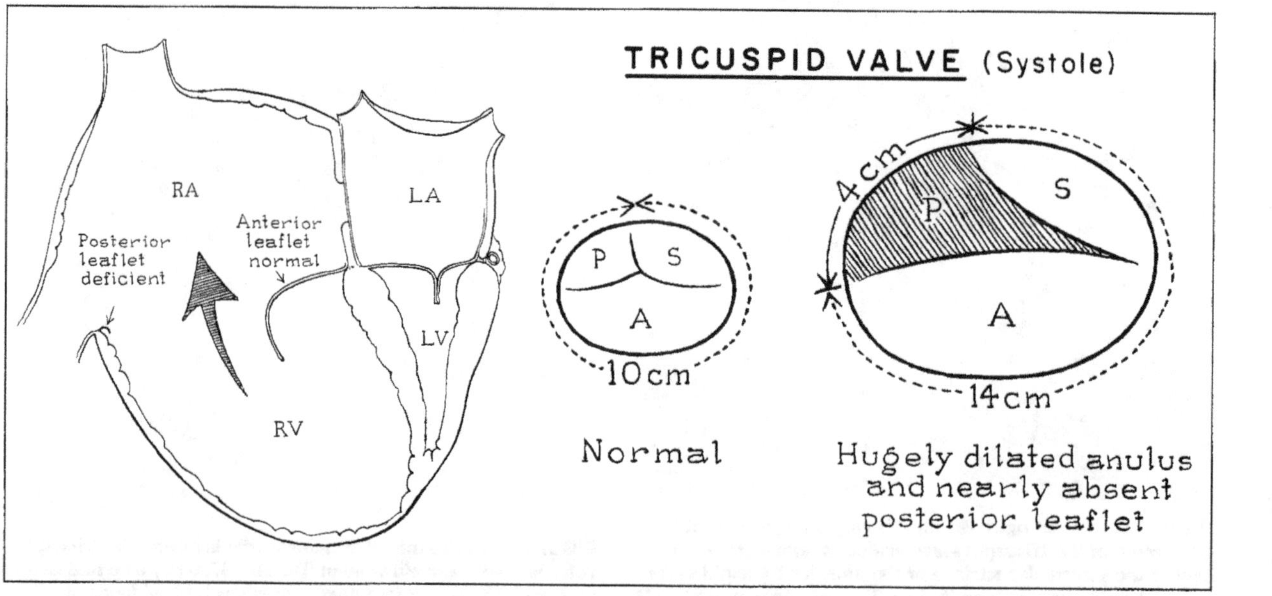

FIGURE 3. Diagram showing a 4-chamber view of the heart in a 32-year-old man (Howard #A83-72) who had active infective endocarditis of the tricuspid valve 10 years before death from chronic congestive heart failure with severe tricuspid valve regurgitation. Necropsy disclosed near total loss of the posterior leaflet by the infective process, which had healed, and a severely dilated tricuspid valve anulus. The tricuspid valve anulus was 18 cm in circumference (normal <11 cm). A = anterior tricuspid leaflet; LA = left atrium; LV = left ventricle; P = posterior tricuspid leaflet; RA = right atrium; RV = right ventricle; S = septal tricuspid leaflet.

TABLE III Infective Endocarditis in Opiate Addicts: Clinical and Necropsy Findings in 59 Patients Who Died or Had a Cardiac Valve Operation During the First Episode of Active Infective Endocarditis (IE)

	Location of Vegetation(s)			
	Right-Sided Valve Only	One Right + One Left-Sided Valve	Left-Sided Valve(s) Only	Total
No. patients (%)	17 (29)	7 (12)	35 (59)	59
Ages (yrs):range [mean]	22–49 [31]	26–55 [37]	20–63 [34]	20–63 [34]
Black:white (%)	16:1	7:0	29:6	52 (88):7 (12)
Men:women (%)	13:4	4:3	27:8	44 (75):15 (25)
Infecting organism (%)				
Bacterium				
Staphylococcus species	9/13	7	15/21	31/41 (76)
Streptococcus species	3/13	0	4/21	7/41 (17)
Mixed	1/13	0	1/21	2/41 (5)
Fungus	0	0	1/21	1/41 (2)
Antibiotic received during active IE (%)	16 (94)	6	30 (86)	52 (88)
Diagnosis of active IE in life (%)	14 (82)	6	28 (80)	48 (81)
Other infections (%)				
Acute pneumonia	17 (100)	7	6/23 (26)	30/47 (64)
Acute meningitis	1 (6)	4	4/21 (20)	9/45 (20)
Valve replacement and/or excision (%)	3* (18)	2‡	12 (34)	17 (29)
Underlying heart disease (%)				
Rheumatic	0	0	6 (17)	6 (10)
Congenital	0	0	6 (17)	6 (10)
Status of valve before IE (%)				
Anatomic status				
Normal	17 (100)	7	23 (66)	47 (80)
Abnormal	0	0	12 (34)	12 (20)
Purely regurgitant	0	0	4 (11)	4 (7)
Stenotic	0	0	1 (3)	1 (2)
Valve function after IE (%)				
Normal	5 (29)	3	8 (23)	16 (27)
Abnormal				
Purely regurgitant	9 (53)	4	25 (71)	38 (64)
Stenotic	3 (18)	0	2 (6)	5 (8)
Death due to IE (%)	15 (88)	7	32 (91)	54 (92)
Congestive heart failure	0	1	3 (9.5)	4 (7)
Prosthetic valve related	1	2	10 (31)	13 (22)
Brain embolus	0	2	10 (31)	12 (20)
Meningitis	0	1	2 (6.5)	3 (5)
Pneumonia	12 (71)	0	1 (3)	13 (22)
Generalized infection	1	1	3 (9.5)	5 (9)
Other	1	0	3 (9.5)	4 (7)
Death due to non-IE cause (%) (narcotic overdose)	2	0	3 (9)	5 (8)
Embolism (gross organ infarcts) (%)				
Brain	0/14†	5	16/25 (64)§	21/46 (46)
Kidney	0/14†	4	19/25 (76)§	23/46 (50)
Spleen	0/14†	3	16/25 (64)§	19/46 (41)
Other systemic	0†	2	9/25 (36)§	11/46 (24)
Lung	14/14†	7	0§	21/46 (46)
Heart weight (g):range [mean]	260–780 [391]	310–600 [425]	210–870 [489]	210–870 [454]
Spleen weight (g):range [mean]	120–1050 [482]	160–840 [407]	70–1000 [384]	70–1050 [410]
>300 g (%)	6/8	1/3	12/21 (57)	19/32 (59)
Liver weight (g):range [mean]	1,390–3,850 [2,480] (n = 8)	1,700–2,750 [2,103] (n = 3)	1,210–3,650 [2,167] (n = 23)	1,210–3,850 [2,235] (n = 34)

* Each of the 3 patients died ≥6 months after operative tricuspid valve excision with or without replacement; † excludes the 3 patients who died late after operative tricuspid valve excision with or without replacement; ‡ the 2 patients died 1 and 5 days, respectively, after replacement of 1 left-sided cardiac valve and tricuspid valve excision without replacement; § excludes the 9 patients who died late after operative mitral (2 patients) or aortic (7 patients) valve excision with replacement.

was *Staphylococcus epidermidis*. The infecting bacterium in 12 patients (26%) was streptococcus species: *faecalis* or *durans* or *liquefaciens* or *zymogenes* in 4 patients; *viridans* in 4 patients; and in 1 patient each *S. pneumoniae* or group A, D or G nutritionally deficient streptococci. *Candida parapsilosis* was the infecting organism in 1 patient.[20]

Valve excision with or without valve replacement during infective endocarditis: Certain clinical and morphologic findings in the 19 patients who had operative valve excision with or without replacement are summarized in Table IV. Of the 19 patients, 17 had the cardiac operation during the period of active IE, and 2 (patients 8 and 17, Table IV) after healing of the IE. Of the 19 patients, 3 had tricuspid valve excision without replacement[21] and 18 patients (2 of whom were among the 3 having tricuspid valve excision) had cardiac valve replacement: tricuspid valve in 2 (11%), mitral valve in 3 (17%) and aortic valve in 13 (72%). Thus, 1 patient (5%) had only tricuspid valve excision, 2 patients (11%) had tricuspid valve excision plus replacement of either the mitral (1 patient) or aortic valve (1 patient), 2 patients (11%) had tricuspid valve replacement alone and 14 patients (74%) had replacement of a single left-sided cardiac valve (mitral in 2 and aortic in 12). The interval from cardiac operation to death was <30 days in 5 pa-

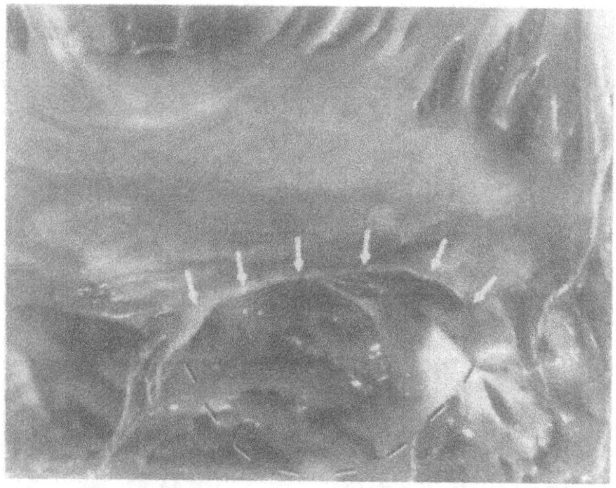

FIGURE 5. Opened right atrium, tricuspid valve and right ventricle showing partial absence of one of the tricuspid valve leaflets in a 33-year-old man (Howard #A83-12) who had active infective endocarditis that healed 5 years before death. He apparently had been well after healing of the endocarditis until 3 months before death when exertional dyspnea appeared. The dyspnea worsened and on the day of death was accompanied by chest pain and shock. Necropsy disclosed a fulminating mononuclear cell myocarditis. *Arrows* show the margins of the partially destroyed leaflet and *dashed line* indicates where the margin of the leaflet, were it normal, would be.

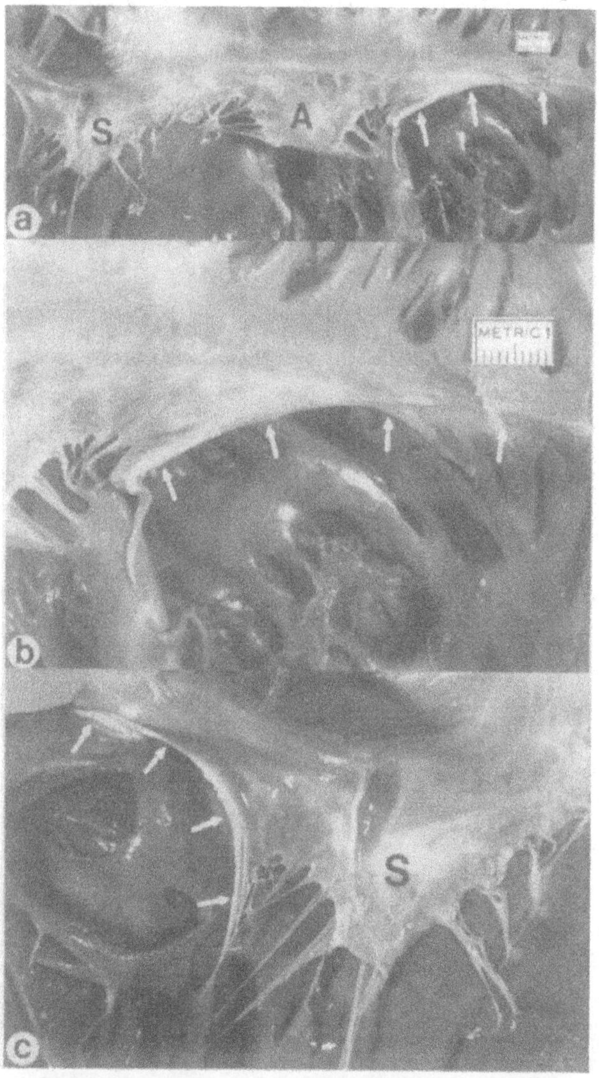

FIGURE 4. Tricuspid valve in the patient described in Figure 3. Opened right atrium, tricuspid valve and right ventricle showing absence of (*arrows*) most of the posterior leaflet (*a*), close-up of the missing leaflet (*b*) near its connection with the anterior leaflet, and near its connection with the septal (S) leaflet (*c*) in a 32-year-old man (Howard #A83-72) who had had active infective endocarditis at age 22, and died of progressive congestive heart failure.

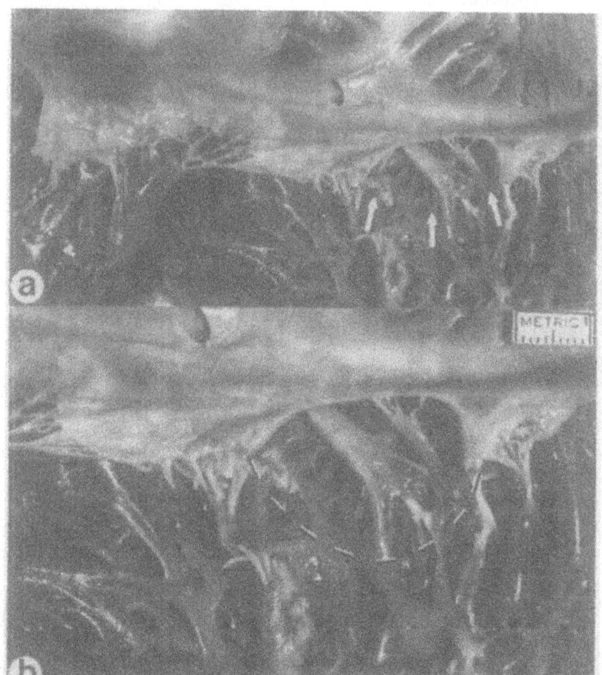

FIGURE 6. Opened right atrium, tricuspid valve and right ventricle showing loss (*arrows*) of a portion of the posterior leaflet from an earlier infection that healed (*a*) and close-up view showing vegetations in the area of the previously damaged leaflet with rupture of several chordae tendineae (*b*) in a 47-year-old man (DCMEO #81-02-128) with *Staphylococcus aureus* tricuspid valve endocarditis. The most recent episode of active infective endocarditis appeared to have started about 60 days before death; it was secondary to massive pulmonary infection with empyema, presumably the consequence of septic emboli.

TABLE IV Infective Endocarditis in Opiate Addicts: Findings in 19 Patients Having Cardiac Valve Excision With or Without Replacement

Pt	Age (yrs), Race, Sex	VR (prosthesis)	TV E Without VR	IE Active at VR or E	Interval VR to Death (days)	Cause of Death
1	26, B, M	AV (BPP)	+	+	1	PO bleeding
2	23, W, M	AV (HD)	0	+	2	Prosthetic misfit
3	47, B, F	AV (BPP)	0	+	4	Operative complication
4	41, B, F	MV (P)	+	+	5	TV active IE
5	53, B, M	AV (P)	0	+	17	PO infection
6	31, B, M	AV (P)	0	+	76	OO
7	33, B, M	TV (P)	0	+	180	PV thrombosis
8	42, B, M	AV (BPP)	0	0	180	PVE
9	50, B, M	AV (S-E)	0	+	240	PV thrombosis
10	36, B, M	MV (SJM)	0	+	300	PVE
11	29, B, M	O	+	+	341	OO
12	34, B, M	AV (P)	0	+	378	OO
13	29, W, M	AV (S-E)	0	+	570	PVE
14	50, B, M	AV (P)	0	+	730	PVE
15	39, B, M	AV (B-S)	0	+	760	PV thrombosis
16	40, B, M	TV (P)	0	+	810	OO
17	34, B, M	AV (SJM)	0	+	1095	PVE
18	39, B, F	AV (S-E)	0	0	2920	PVE
19	38, B, M	MV (P)	0	+	3650	PV thrombosis

AV = aortic valve; B = black; BPP = bovine parietal pericardium; B-S = Bjork-Shiley; E = excision; HD = Hufnagel disc; IE = infective endocarditis; MV = mitral valve; OO = opiate overdose; P = porcine; PO = postoperative; PV = prosthetic or bioprosthetic valve; PVE = prosthetic or bioprosthetic valve endocarditis; SE = Starr-Edwards; SJM = St. Jude Medical; TV = tricuspid valve; VR = valve replacement; W = white; + = present; 0 = absent; – = information not available.

tients (26%), 30 to 180 days in 3 patients (16%) and 8 to 121 months (mean 36) in the remaining 11 patients (58%). Of the 18 patients with a prosthetic or bioprosthetic cardiac valve, 6 (33%) died from consequence of "prosthetic" valve endocarditis (Figures 15 through 18); 5 others (28%) died <30 days from complications of the

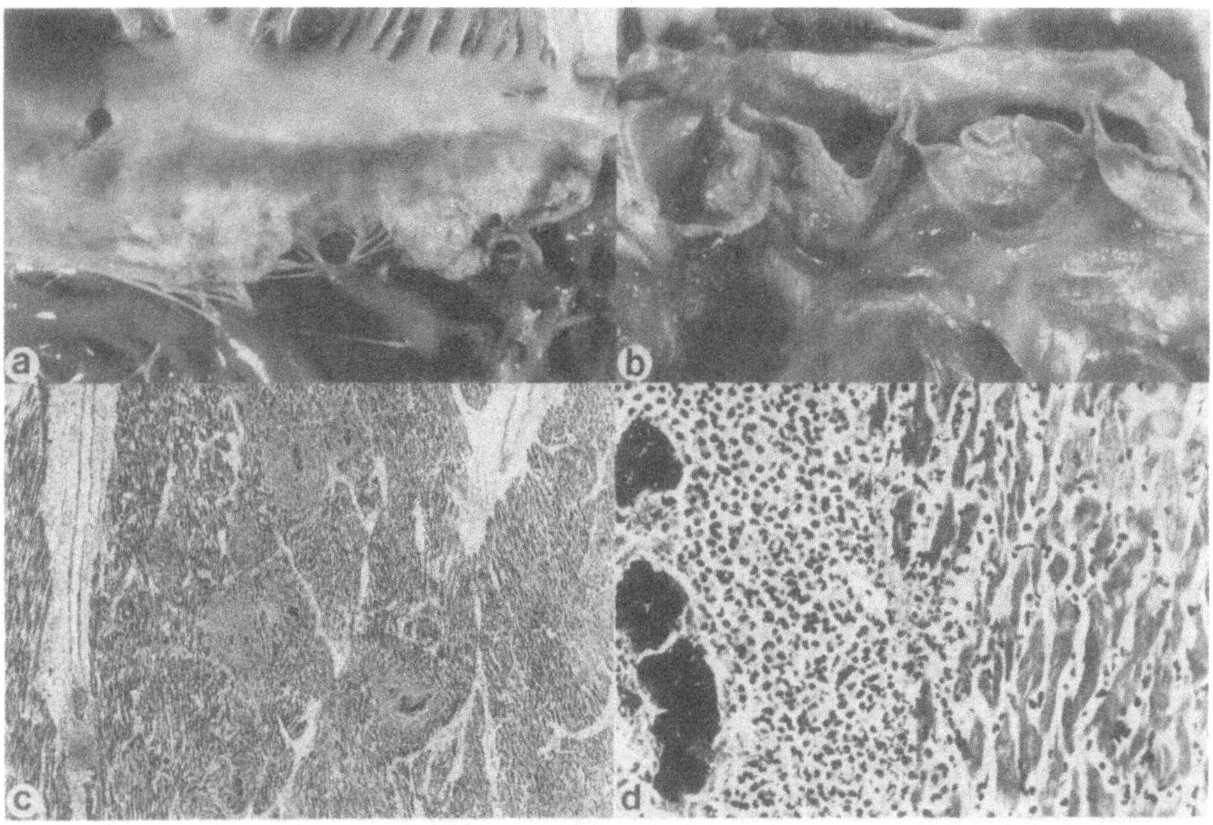

FIGURE 7. Opened right atrium showing vegetations on the tricuspid valve leaflets (*a*), opened aorta and aortic valve showing vegetations on each cusp (*b*) and photomicrographs of abscesses in left ventricular myocardium (*c* and *d*) in a 34-year-old woman (DCMEO #84-03-206) who died suddenly at home. Septic emboli with infarcts were found in the brain and lung. Postmortem blood cultures grew *Staphylococcus aureus*. The active infective endocarditis was not diagnosed until necropsy. The dark material in the photomicrographs in both *c* and *d* are colonies of organisms.

operation; 4 (22%) died from "prosthetic" valve thrombosis without infection; and 3 (17%) died from opiate overdose.

Follow-up in patients in whom the first episode of active infective endocarditis healed: In 21 (26%) of the 80 patients the first episode of active IE healed. Certain findings in these 21 patients are summarized in Table V. Of the 21 patients, the first episode of IE involved the tricuspid valve in 12 patients (isolated in 6 and associated with involvement of either the mitral or aortic valve in 6); the pulmonic valve was involved in 1 patient, the mitral valve in 10 patients (isolated in 3), and the aortic valve in 6 (isolated in 3). Thus, of the 84 cardiac valves in these 21 patients, 29 valves (35%) or an average of 1.4/4.0 valves/patient were sites of active IE that healed. Of the 21 patients in whom the first episode of active IE healed, active IE recurred once in 8 patients and twice in 2 patients and in each of these 10 patients the recurrent infection was fatal. The sites of the valvular vegetations in the recurring and fatal active IE were tricuspid valve in 5 patients (isolated in 3), mitral valve in 5 patients (isolated in 3) and aortic valve in 2 patients (isolated in both). Thus, of the 40 cardiac valves in the 10 patients with recurrent active IE, 12 valves (30%), or an average of 1.2/4.0 valves/patient, were sites of recurrent active IE. Two of the 21 patients had valve replacement after healing of the first episode of active IE and death in both was due to "prosthetic" valve endocarditis. Three other patients died from opiate overdose, 2 from pneumonia and 1 each from trauma, valvular regurgitation, myocarditis and brain abscess.

The infecting microorganism causing a second or third episode of active IE was known in 6 of these 10 patients: *Streptococcus viridans* in 3 patients, *Staphylococcus aureus* in 2 patients and *Streptococcus faecalis*

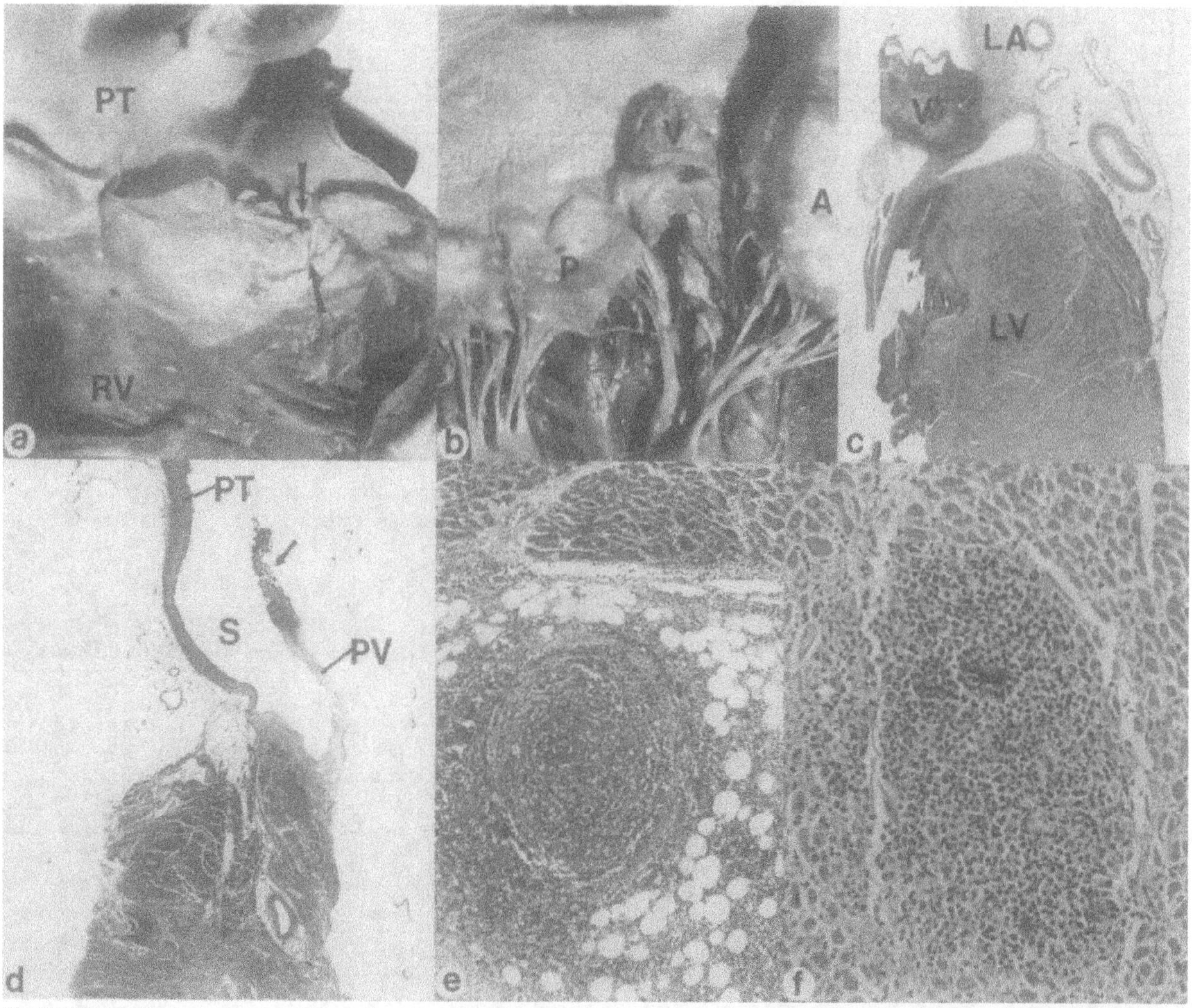

FIGURE 8. Active *Staphylococcus aureus* endocarditis involving the pulmonic and mitral valves in a 55-year-old man (DCGH #70A-171) who had onset of clinical signs and symptoms of infective endocarditis about 70 days before death. *a*, vegetative material (between *arrows*) on 2 cusps. PT = pulmonary trunk; RV = right ventricle. *b*, opened mitral valve with vegetation (V) on the posterior (P) leaflet near the anterior (A) leaflet. *c*, photomicrograph of a section that includes left atrium (LA), vegetation (V) on posterior mitral leaflet and left ventricular wall (LV). Hematoxyin and eosin stain, × 3.5. *d*, photomicrograph of section through the infected pulmonic valve (PV). *Arrow* points to vegetative material on 1 cusp. S = sinus. *e*, photomicrograph of an epicardial coronary artery occluded by vegetative embolic material. Hematoxylin and eosin stain, × 80. *f*, photomicrograph of an abscess in left ventricular wall. Hematoxylin and eosin stain, × 220. Reproduced with permission from Roberts WC and Buchbinder NA.[3]

in 1 patient. Of the 6 patients in whom the responsible bacterium for the recurrent and fatal episode of active IE was known, the responsible organism for the first episode of active IE was known in 4: the organism was the same in both episodes in 3 patients and different organisms were causative in 1 patient.

Comparison of cardiac valve(s) involved by infection in the patients who died or had cardiac operation during the first episode of active infective endocarditis to those in whom the first episode healed: Table VI summarizes the sites of vegetations in these patients. No significant differences were observed in comparison of the 2 groups.

Active infective endocarditis involving previously anatomically abnormal cardiac valves: In 15 (19%) of the 80 patients the cardiac valve(s) that was (were) the site(s) of active IE was (were) anatomically abnormal before the active IE occurred. Certain findings in these 15 patients are summarized in Table VII. Eight patients had anatomic evidence of previous rheumatic heart disease with diffuse fibrous thickening of the mitral valve in each and also of the aortic valve in 6. The other 7 patients had congenitally bicuspid aortic valves: none was stenotic and 3 were mildly regurgitant. Of these 15 patients with previously anatomically abnormal valves, 6 had aortic valve replacement—during the period of active IE in 5 and after healing of the IE in 1.

Myocardial lesions: In 45 patients in whom the active IE was fatal and in whom a cardiac operation had not been performed, 2 to 9 (mean 5) histologic sections of left ventricular wall and ventricular septum extending through the full thickness of the wall were exam-

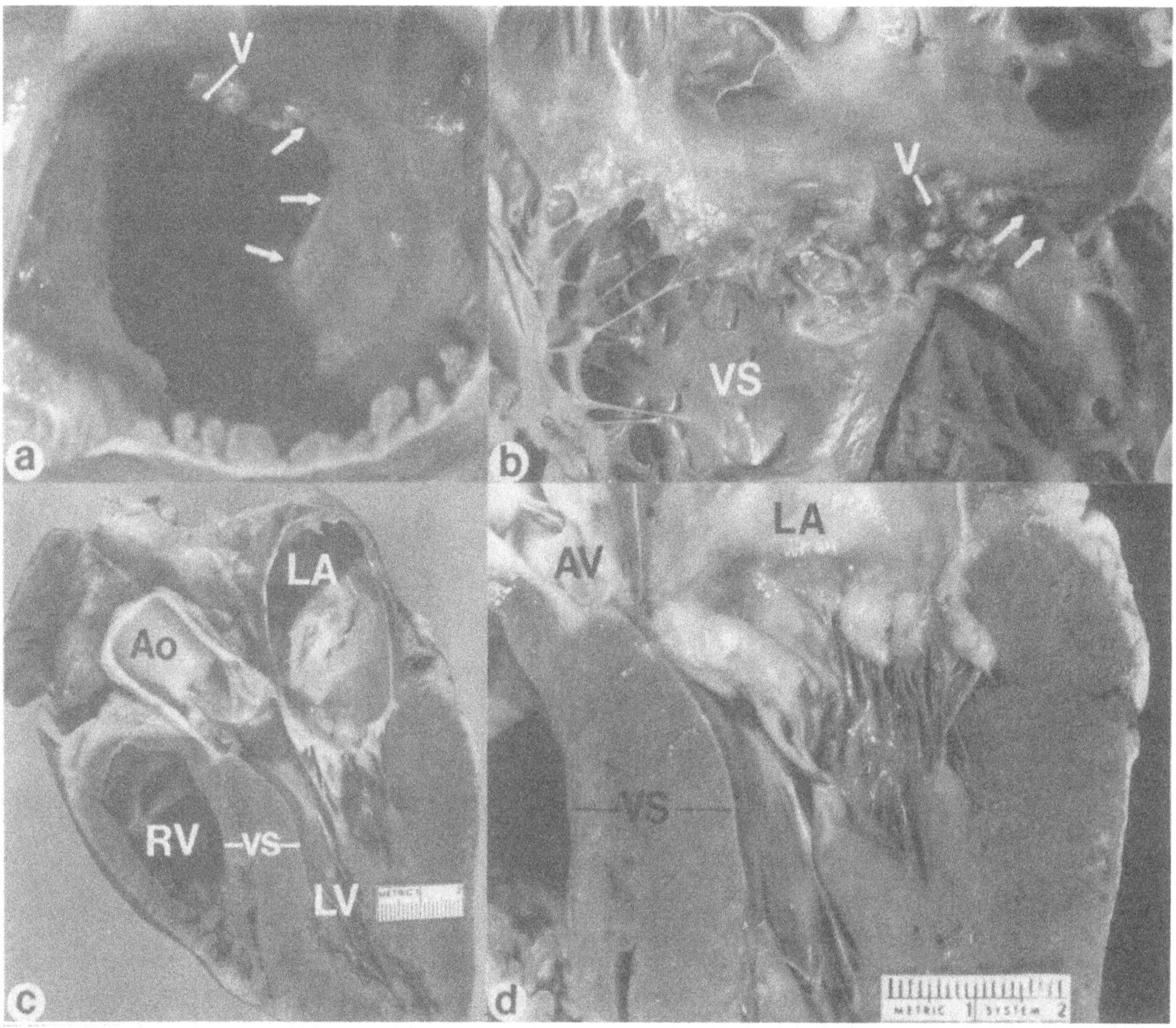

FIGURE 9. Healed infective endocarditis of the tricuspid and mitral valve and recurrent active infection involving the tricuspid valve in a 21-year-old woman (DCGH #79A-101). She had active infection at age 18 and again 3 weeks before death. *a*, opened right atrium showing a partially absent anterior tricuspid valve leaflet (*arrows*). V = vegetation. *b*, opened right atrium, tricuspid valve and right ventricle showing vegetation (V) on septal and anterior tricuspid valve leaflets. *Arrows* point to the anterior leaflet, which is partially absent from the previous infection. *c*, longitudinal view of heart showing both left-sided cardiac valves. Ao = aortic; LA = left atrium; LV = left ventricle; RV = right ventricle; VS = ventricular septum. *d*, close-up of the scarred mitral valve from the previously healed infection. AV = aortic valve.

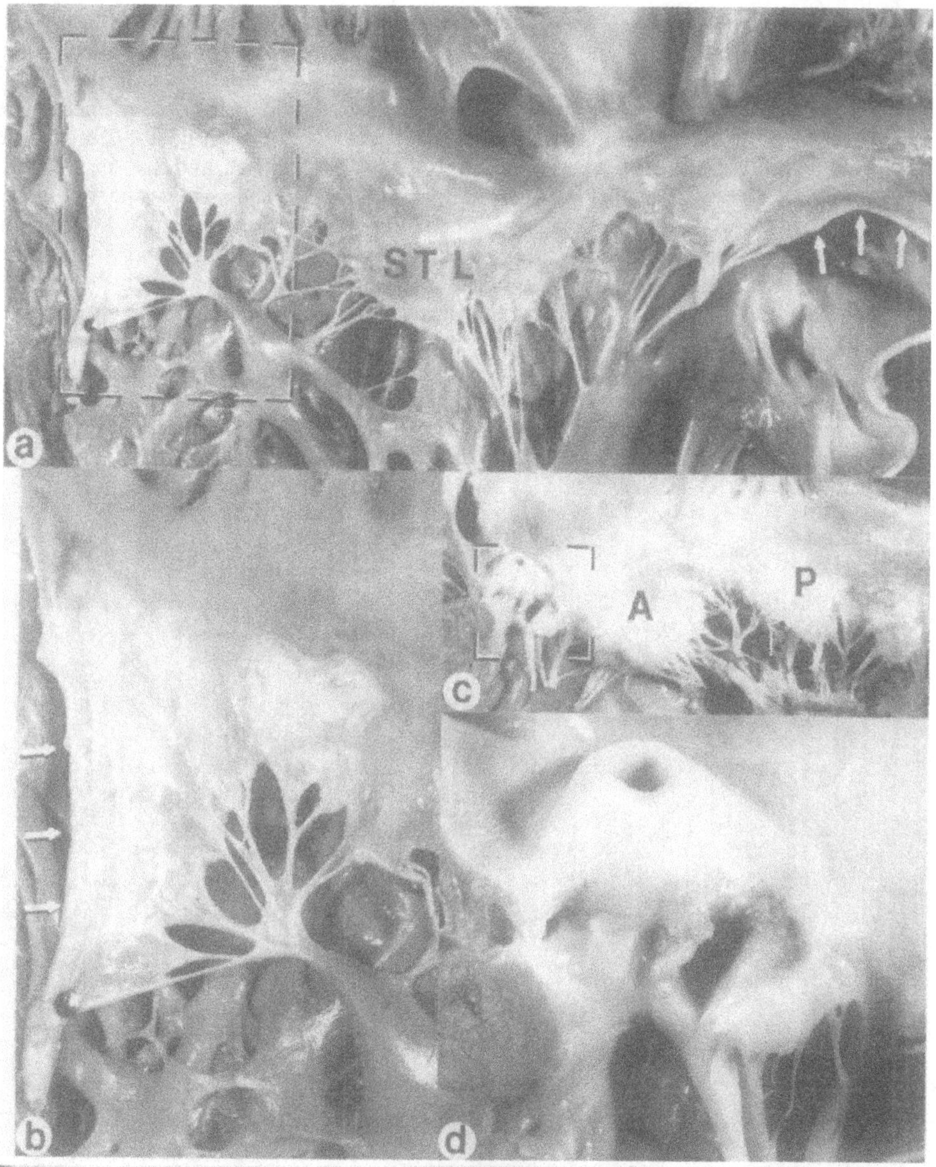

FIGURE 10. Healed and active infective endocarditis involving both tricuspid and mitral valves in a 35-year-old man (DCMEO #87-03-187) who was found comatose at home. He was known to have infective endocarditis, which healed, in the past and he had evidence of chronic congestive heart failure. *a*, opened tricuspid valve showing loss of a large portion of anterior leaflet (*arrows*) from previous infection that healed and a new vegetation (*brackets*). *b*, close-up of area in brackets in *a*, showing loss of leaflet (*arrows*). *c*, opened mitral valve showing a domed lesion with a central opening (*brackets*). *d*, close-up of the domed lesion, presumably the result of infective endocarditis that healed.

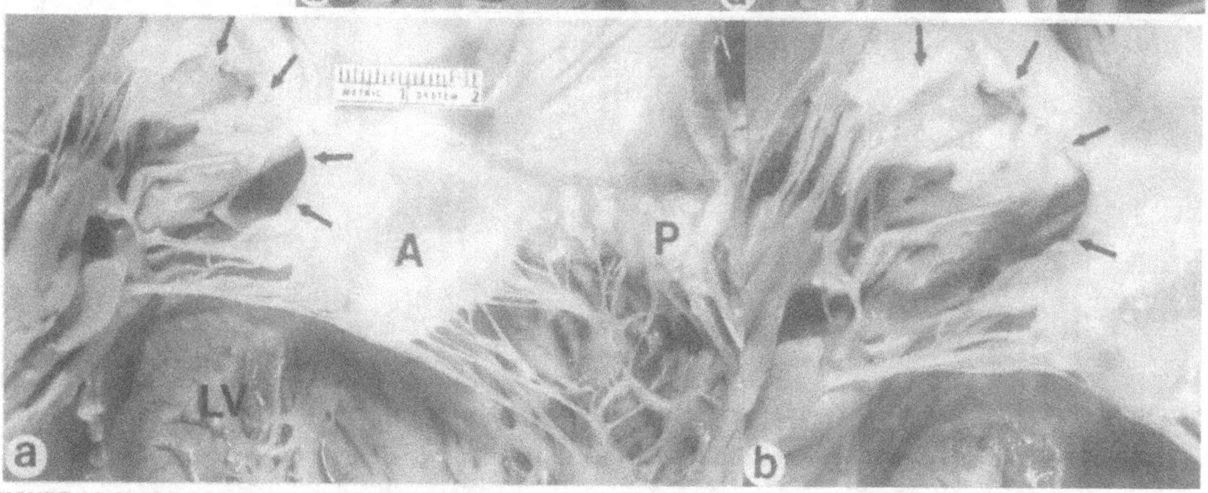

FIGURE 11. Healed infective endocarditis involving the mitral valve in a 29-year-old man (DCMEO #79-01-68) who died of a brain abscess. He had had active infective endocarditis, which healed, on 3 occasions (6, 4 and 1 years before death). *a*, opened mitral valve showing absent (*arrows*) portions of both posterior (P) leaflet and anterior (A) leaflets. *b*, close-up of the area of previous infection (*arrows*) located near the anterolateral commissure.

TABLE V Infective Endocarditis in Opiate Addicts: Findings in 21 Patients in Whom the First Episode of Active Infective Endocarditis Healed

Pt	Age (yrs), Race, Sex	Active IE Diagnosed in Life	Interval Between Active IE That Healed and Death	Valve Anatomically Abnormal Before First Active IE	Organism Grown From Blood During First Episode of IE	Cause of Death	Location of Vegetations That Healed				Organism Grown From Blood During Second Episode of IE	Location of Vegetation in Recurrent Active IE				HW (g)
							TV	PV	MV	AV		TV	PV	MV	AV	
1	24, B, F	+	—	0	—	Recurrent IE	+	0	0	0	—	+	0	0	0	—
2	32, B, M	+	10 yrs	0	—	TR	+	0	0	0	—	—	—	—	—	570
3	33, B, M	+	5yrs	0	—	Myocarditis	+	0	0	0	—	—	—	—	—	875
4	36, B, F	0	—	0	—	Pneumonia	+	0	0	0	—	—	—	—	—	585
5	43, B, M	0	—	0	—	OO	+	0	0	0	—	—	—	—	—	460
6	47, W, M	+	225 days	0	*Straph. aureus*	Recurrent IE	+	0	0	0	—	+	0	0	0	350
7	21, B, F	+	3 yrs	0	—	Recurrent IE	+	0	+	0	—	+	0	0	0	410
8	29, B, F	+	386 days	0	*Staph. aureus*	Recurrent IE	+	0	+	0	*Staph. aureus*	+	0	+	0	440
9	35, B, M	+	—	0	—	Recurrent IE	+	0	+	0	—	+	0	+	0	470
10	37, B, F	0	—	0	—	Pneumonia	+	0	+	0	—	—	—	—	—	320
11	39, B, M	+	8 mos	0	*Group G Strept.*	Recurrent IE	+	0	+	0	*Staph. aureus*	0	0	+	0	485
12	45, B, M	+	3 yrs	0	—	Recurrent IE	+	0	0	+	—	0	0	0	+	840
13	39, B, F	+	6 yrs	0	*Enterococcus*	OO	0	+	0	0	—	—	—	—	—	500
14	28, B, M	+	4 yrs	0	—	Recurrent IE	0	0	+	0	*Strept. viridans*	0	0	+	0	380
15	29, B, M	+	6 yrs	0	—	Brain abscess	0	0	+	0	—	—	—	—	—	400
16	36, B, M	+	10 mos	0	*Enterococcus*	Recurrent IE	0	0	+	0	*Enterococcus*	0	0	+	0	500
17	30, B, M	+	2 yrs	+ (RHD)	—	Trauma	0	0	+	+	—	—	—	—	—	600
18	41, B, M	0	—	0	—	OO	0	0	+	+	—	—	—	—	—	825
19	35, B, M	+	10 mos	+ (BAV)	*Strept. viridans*	Recurrent IE	0	0	0	+	*Strept. viridans*	0	0	0	+	760
20	39, B, F	+	10 yrs	+ (RHD)	*Strept. viridans*	PVE	0	0	0	+	—	—	—	—	—	550
21	42, B, M	+	15 mos	0	—	PVE	0	0	0	+	*Strept. viridans*	—	—	—	—	780

BAV = bicuspid aortic valve; HW = heart weight; IE = infective endocarditis; PV = pulmonic valve; RHD = rheumatic heart disease; Staph. = Staphylococcus; Strept. = Streptococcus; TR = tricuspid regurgitation; W = white; other abbreviations as in Table IV.

ined. In addition, 33 of the hearts were reexamined specifically searching for myocardial lesions.

The most common lesion observed in the left ventricular wall (includes septum) was myocardial abscesses and these were found in 18 patients (40%). In each patient the abscesses were multifocal. The abscesses consisted of collections of polymorphonuclear cells and in 17 (94%) of the 18 patients colonies of bacteria also were observed in the abscesses. In some patients most abscesses contained colonies of organisms (Figure 7) and in other patients only a rare abscess contained colonies of organisms. In all 18 patients, colonies of organisms also were observed in 1 or more intramural coronary arteries in the vicinity of the abscesses. Four of the 18 patients also had embolic material—infected in each case—in an epicardial coronary artery, and in each case the epicardial artery was a branch of a major trunk, not the major trunk itself. Of the 18 patients, 14 had vege-

TABLE VI Infective Endocarditis in Opiate Addicts: Location of Vegetations in Those Who Died or Had Operation Compared to Those Who Healed During the First Episode of Infective Endocarditis

Infected Valve(s)	Died or Had Operation During First Episode	First Episode Healed	p <0.05
Right-sided only (%)	17 (29)	7 (33)	0
TV	17	6	0
PV	0	1	0
Right + left-sided (%)	7 (12)	6 (29)	0
TV-MV	3	5	0
TV-AV	3	1	0
PV-MV	1	0	0
PV-AV	0	0	0
Left-sided only (%)	35 (59)	8 (38)	0
MV	12	3	0
AV	15	3	0
MV + AV	8	2	0
Total	59	21	

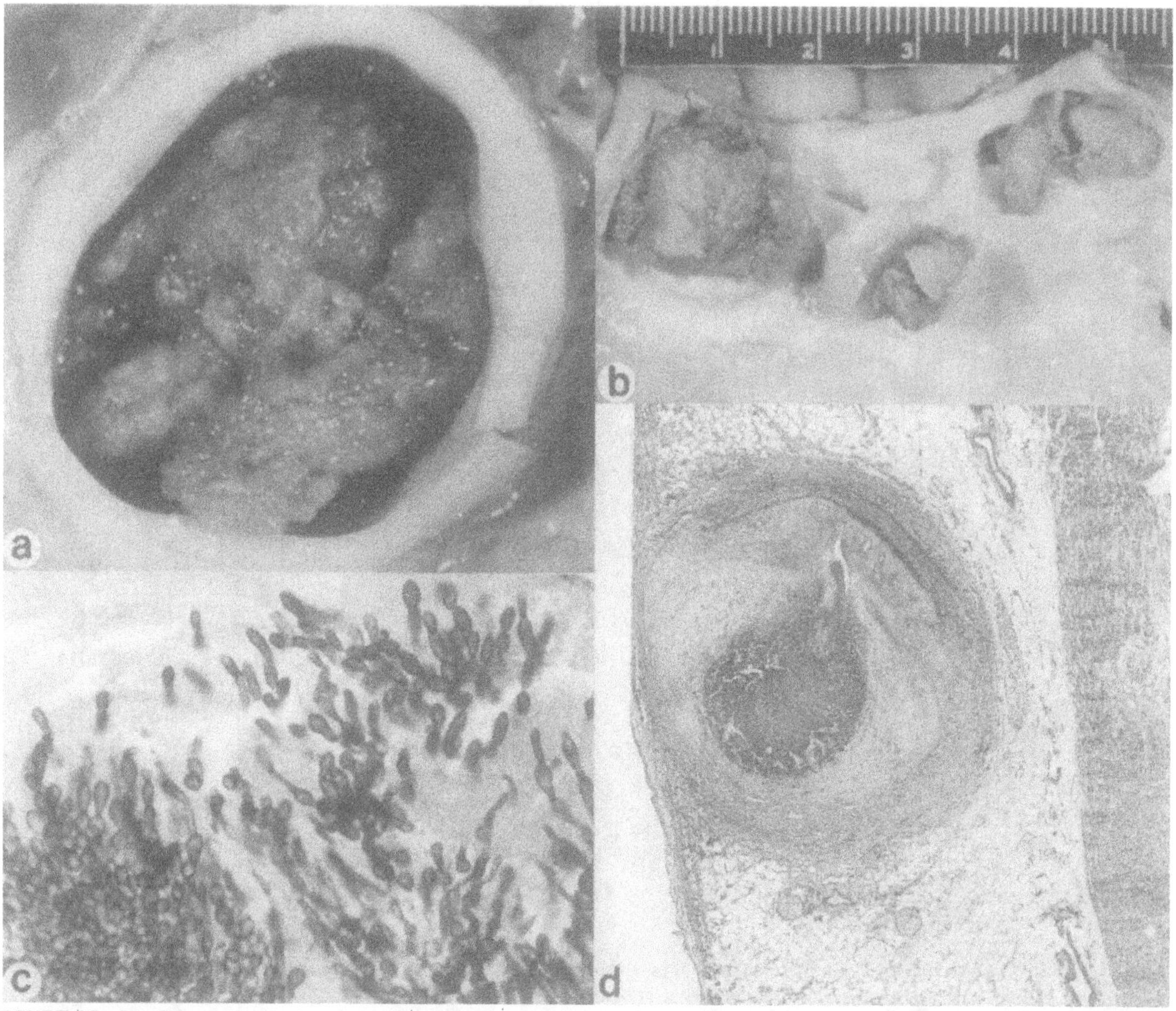

FIGURE 12. ***Candida parapsilosis*** **endocarditis involving the aortic valve of a 26-year-old man (NIH #A60-36). This patient lived for 8 months after initial symptoms and signs of infective endocarditis. He had an embolus to the left anterior descending coronary artery with a huge transmural acute myocardial infarct 2 months before death. *a*, aortic valve viewed from above. The large vegetations appear to obstruct the valve orifice. *b*, opened valve showing vegetations on each cusp. *c*, photomicrograph of vegetation showing pseudomycelia of *C. parapsilosis* (methenamine silver stain; × 775). *d*, photomicrograph of section of left anterior descending coronary artery occluded by vegetative material that is now partially organized into fibrous tissue. Candida organisms were present in the more central portions. Elastic tissue stain, × 21. Reproduced with permission from Andriole VT, Kravetz HM, Roberts WC, and Utz JP.[20]**

tations involving one or both left-sided cardiac valves, and 4 had vegetations limited to a tricuspid valve. Only 1 of the latter 4 patients had a patent foramen ovale.

The second most common lesion observed in the left ventricular wall was myocardial infarction, occurring in 10 patients. None of these 10 patients had intramyocardial collections of polymorphonuclear leukocytes containing colonies of organisms. Of the 10 patients, 3 had unifocal, transmural, huge anterior wall infarcts, and each of them had an embolus in a major coronary trunk—the left anterior descending coronary artery in 2 and right in 1. One of these patients was 26 years old and had *Candida parapsilosis* endocarditis of the aortic valve (Figure 12). The other patients were 43 years old and had bacterial endocarditis of the aortic valve. In each patient, the acute myocardial infarction was diagnosed clinically. The other 7 patients had multiple small left ventricular infarcts, which were mainly subendocardial, and in 3 patients limited to both left ventricular papillary muscles. In all 7 patients, however, portions of 1 or both left ventricular papillary muscles were necrotic. In none of these 7 patients was myocardial infarction diagnosed clinically. Of the 7 patients, the active IE was limited to 1 or both left-sided valves in 4 patients, and

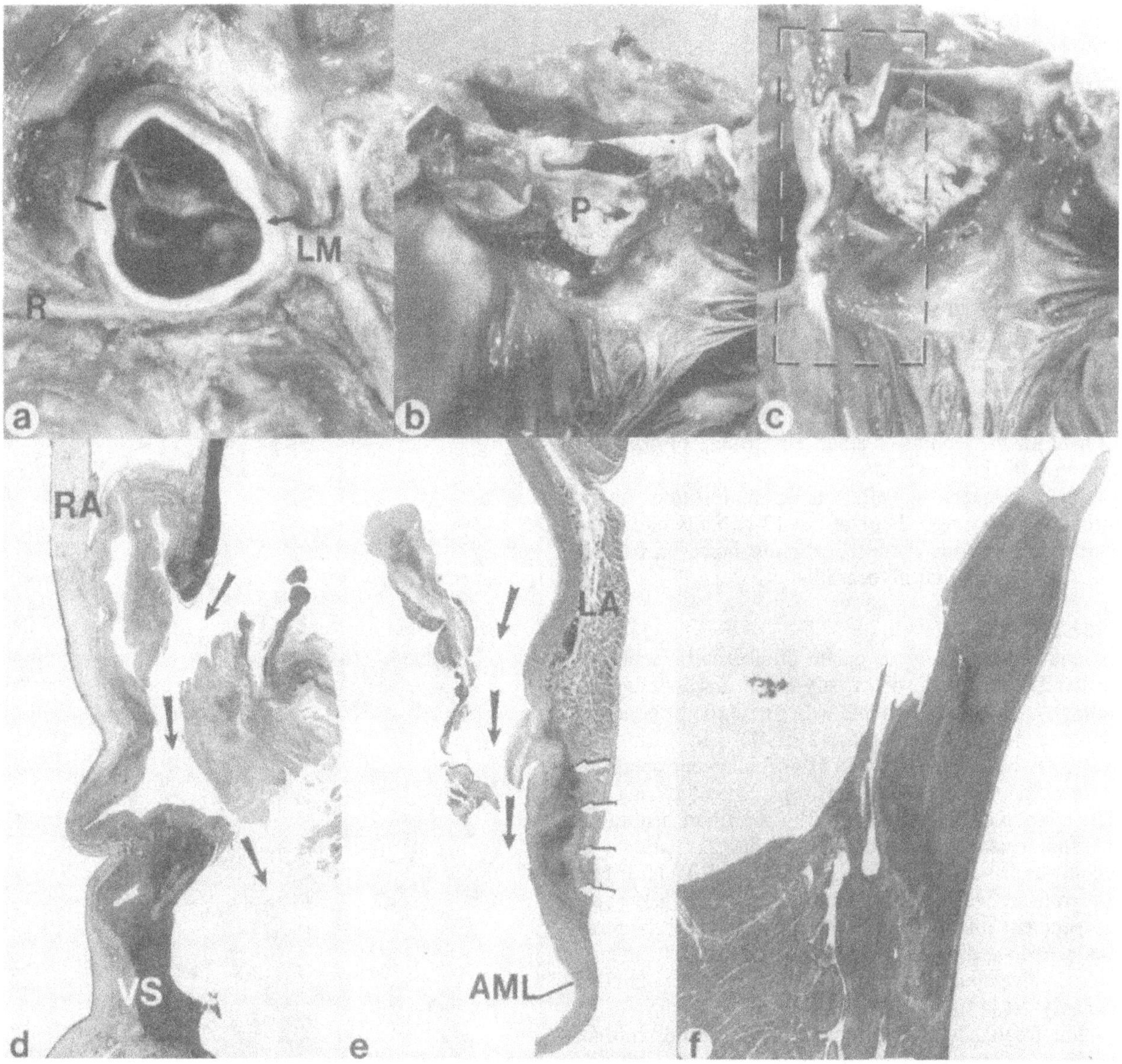

FIGURE 13. ***Staphylococcus epidermidis*** **endocarditis in a 22-year-old man (DCGH #69A-47) superimposed on a congenitally bicuspid aortic valve, which apparently was mildly incompetent before becoming infected. *a*, aortic valve from above showing 2 cusps. The arrows point to the 2 commissures. LM = left main and R = right coronary artery. *b*, opened aortic valve. P = posterior cusp which is perforated. *c*, longitudinal section through posterior cusp showing ring abscess (*arrow*). *d*, photomicrograph of a section of wall of aorta, right atrium (RA) and ventricular septum (VS) showing a large vegetation on the aortic valve cusp, right abscess and perforation of the cusp (*arrows*). *e*, photomicrograph of section that includes perforated aortic cusp (*black arrows*), and ring abscess (*black and white arrows*) in the area between left atrial wall (LA) and anterior mitral leaflet (AML). Elastic tissue stains, × 3.5 (*c*) and 3.0 (*d*). *f*, posteromedial papillary muscle, which is necrotic. Hematoxylin and eosin stain, × 4. The coronary arteries were normal. The necrosis of the papillary muscle was probably related to the severely decreased cardiac output. Reproduced with permission from Buchbinder NA and Roberts WC.[4]**

TABLE VII Infective Endocarditis in Opiate Addicts: Findings in 15 Patients with Abnormal Cardiac Valves Before the First Episode of Active Infective Endocarditis

Pt	Age (yrs), Race, Sex	History of ARF	Etiology of Valvular Anatomic Abnormality	Anatomically Abnormal Valves Before IE		Diffuse Valvular Thickening		No. of AV Cusps	Valvular Function Before Active IE				Location of Vegatation		VR	HW (g)
				MV	AV	MV	AV		MR	MS	AR	AS	MV	AV		
1	20, B, F	0	R	+	0	+	0	3	0	0	0	0	+	0	0	210
2	22, B, M	+	R	+	+	+	+	3	+	0	+	0	+	0	0	540
3	24, B, F	0	R	+	+	+	+	3	+	0	+	0	+	+	0	—
4	30, B, M	+	R	+	+	+	+	3	0	0	0	0	+	+	0	600
5	34, B, M	0	R	+	+	+	+	3	0	0	0	0	0	+	+(AV)	530
6	37, B, M	0	R	+	0	+	0	3	0	+	0	0	+	0	0	350
7	39, B, F	+	R	+	+	+	+	3	+	0	+	0	0	+	+(AV)	550
8	50, B, M	—	R	+	+	+	+	3	0	0	0	0	0	+	+(AV)	—
9	22, B, M	0	C	0	+	0	+	2	0	0	+	0	0	+	0	670
10	23, W, M	0	C	0	+	0	0	2	0	0	0	0	0	+	+(AV)	500
11	28, W, F	0	C	0	+	0	+	2	0	0	0	0	+	+	0	310
12	29, W, M	0	C	0	+	0	0	2	0	0	0	0	0	+	+(AV)	580
13	35, B, M	0	C	0	+	0	0	2	0	0	+	0	0	+	0	760
14	44, B, M	0	C	0	+	0	0	2	0	0	0	0	0	+	0	425
15	53, B, M	0	C	0	+	0	0	2	0	0	+	0	+	+	+(AV)	690

AR = aortic regurgitation; ARF = acute rheumatic fever; AS = aortic stenosis; C = congenital; IE = infective endocarditis; MR = mitral regurgitation; MS = mitral stenosis; MV = mitral valve; R = rheumatic heart disease; VR = valve replacement; other abbreviations as in Table IV.

only the tricuspid valve in 3 patients. Two of the 7 patients also had small multifocal left ventricular scars: one of these patients also had a previous episode of active IE that healed and the second patient had had evidence of active IE for 50 days. Embolic material was seen in an intramural or small epicardial coronary artery in 6 of the 7 patients.

In 17 patients, no left ventricular abscesses or infarcts were observed. Four of the 17 patients had valve ring abscesses. One of the 17 patients, however, had focal, acute interstitial myocarditis.

DISCUSSION

The present study of opiate addicts with active or healed IE or both involves only those cases studied at necropsy. Of the 80 patients with anatomic evidence of active or healed IE or both, 42 (53%) died during the first episode of active IE, 17 (21%) underwent operative valve excision with or without replacement during the first episode of active IE, and 21 (26%) had healing of the first episode of active IE. Of the 21 patients in whom the first episode of active IE healed, 10 later had recurrent active IE that was fatal, 2 others had valve replacement and both later had prosthetic or bioprosthetic endocarditis that was fatal. Of the 17 patients having valve operations during the first episode of active IE, only 7 (44%) survived >1 year.

The frequency of involvement of the various cardiac valves in opiate addicts with fatal IE may be a bit different from that observed in opiate addicts who survive an episode of active IE. Of our 59 patients in whom the cardiac valves were examined anatomically at the time of the first episode of active IE, the vegetations were limited to a right-sided cardiac valve in 17 (29%) patients, they involved both right and left-sided valves in 7 (12%) and they involved only 1 or both left-sided valves in 35 (59%). Among our 21 patients in whom the first

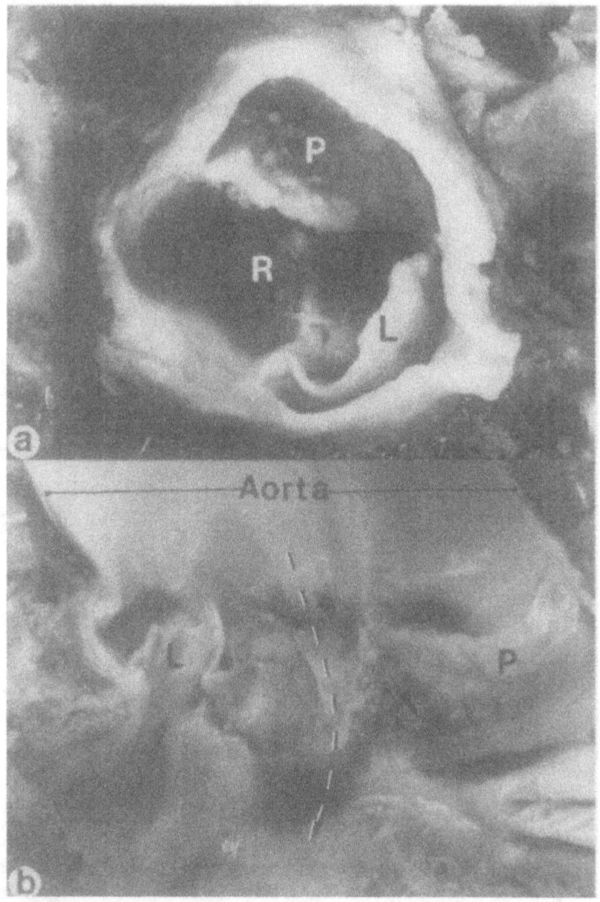

FIGURE 14. Active infective endocarditis involving the aortic valve in a 40-year-old man (DCMEO #80-06-466) who died from an overdose of opiates. Infective endocarditis was never diagnosed clinically. *a*, aortic valve from above showing prolapse of the right (R) cusp and vegetative material on the right and posterior (P) cusps, but not on the left (L) cusp. *b*, opened aortic valve showing a large opening (*arrow*) in the right cusp.

episode of active IE healed, the infection was limited to a right-sided cardiac valve in 7 patients (33%), to both right- and left-sided cardiac valves in 6 patients (29%) and to 1 or both left-sided valves in 8 patients (38%) (difference not significant).

Several previous reports have described, by clinical examination only, the valves involved in active IE in opiate addicts. Of 21 surviving addicts with IE studied by Menda et al,[5] the infection involved a right-sided valve only in 11 patients (52%), both a right- and left-sided cardiac valve in 2 (10%) and 1 or both left-sided valves only in 8 (38%). Banks et al[7] studied 50 opiate addicts with IE clinically; IE was fatal in 12. The infection was limited to a right-sided valve in 38 (76%), to both a right- and left-sided valve in 5 (10%) and to 1 or both left-sided valves in 7 (14%). Hubbell et al[10] described 94 episodes of active IE in 76 patients, 21 of whom died during the infection; the infection was limited to a right-sided cardiac valve in 32 patients (34%), to both right- and left-sided valves in 3 patients (3%) and to 1 or both left-sided valves in 59 patients (63%).

Whether a study yields a high frequency of left-sided infection may be dependent on the frequency of anatomically abnormal cardiac valves before the infection. Of the 94 opiate addicts with IE studied by Hubbell et al,[10] >40% apparently had clinical evidence of heart disease before the infection: 66% of the episodes of active IE in their 94 patients involved a left-sided cardiac valve and only 34% were limited to a right-sided valve. In contrast, only 22% of the 50 patients studied by Banks et al[7] had clinical evidence of cardiac disease before the infection, and only 24% of their patients had clinical evidence of left-sided valve infection.

The frequency of healing of active IE in opiate addicts has received attention previously. Of our 80 patients, the first episode of active IE healed in 21 (26%).

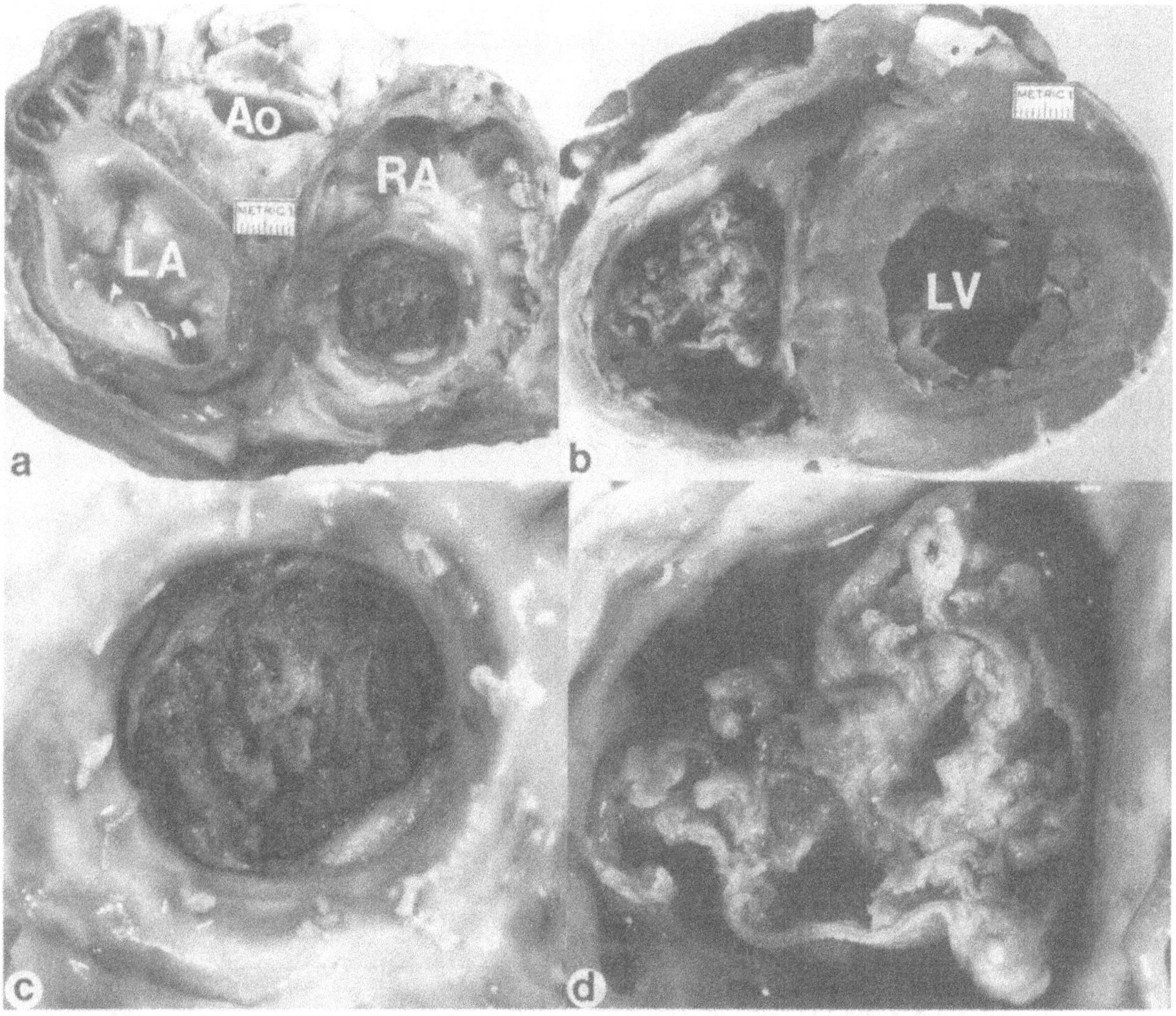

FIGURE 15. Thrombosis of the porcine bioprosthesis in the tricuspid valve position in a 33-year-old man (DCMEO #83-12-862). He had tricuspid valve replacement for infective endocarditis 6 months before death. He had syncope on several occasions after operation and became comatose shortly before death. At necropsy, the orifice of the tricuspid valve bioprosthesis was occluded by thrombus. *a*, view from above with atria removed showing thrombus filling the bioprosthetic orifice. Ao = aorta; LA = left atrium; RA = right atrium. *b*, ventricular aspects of the atrioventricular valves are visible after transverse excision of the walls of the ventricles. LV = left ventricle. *c*, close-up view of the right atrial aspect of the occluded bioprosthetic orifice. *d*, close-up view of ventricular aspect of the bioprosthesis containing thrombus.

Of the 23 patients studied by Menda et al,[5] the infection healed in all 23. Of the 50 cases studied by Banks et al,[7] the infection healed in 38 (76%), and of the 94 patients studied by Hubbell et al,[10] the infection healed in 73 (78%).

The frequency of recurrence of active IE after healing of active IE has received little attention. Among our 21 patients in whom the first episode of active IE healed, the infection recurred in 10 patients (48%) and in each the recurrent IE was fatal. Our study is the first, to our knowledge, to illustrate morphologic features of active IE superimposed on healed IE.

The prognosis in opiate addicts having valve replacement is not good.[22–26] Of our 18 patients having valve replacement (16 during active IE and left-sided in 16), 10 (55%) died within 1 year and 16 (89%) within 3 years of the replacement. Furthermore, of the 13 patients surviving >30 days after valve replacement, 6 (46%) developed prosthetic or bioprosthetic endocarditis, fatal in each. Of 24 opiate addicts with left-sided valve replacement for IE reported by Hubbell et al,[10] 9 had died within 1 year and 4 others within 3 years; of 18 opiate addicts having valve replacement and reported by Mammana et al,[22] 9 died within 1 year; of 14 addicts reported by Silverman et al,[23] 5 died within 1 year of valve replacement, all from prosthetic endocarditis.

Only 1 of our patients had tricuspid valve excision as the only cardiac operation for IE and he died of opiate

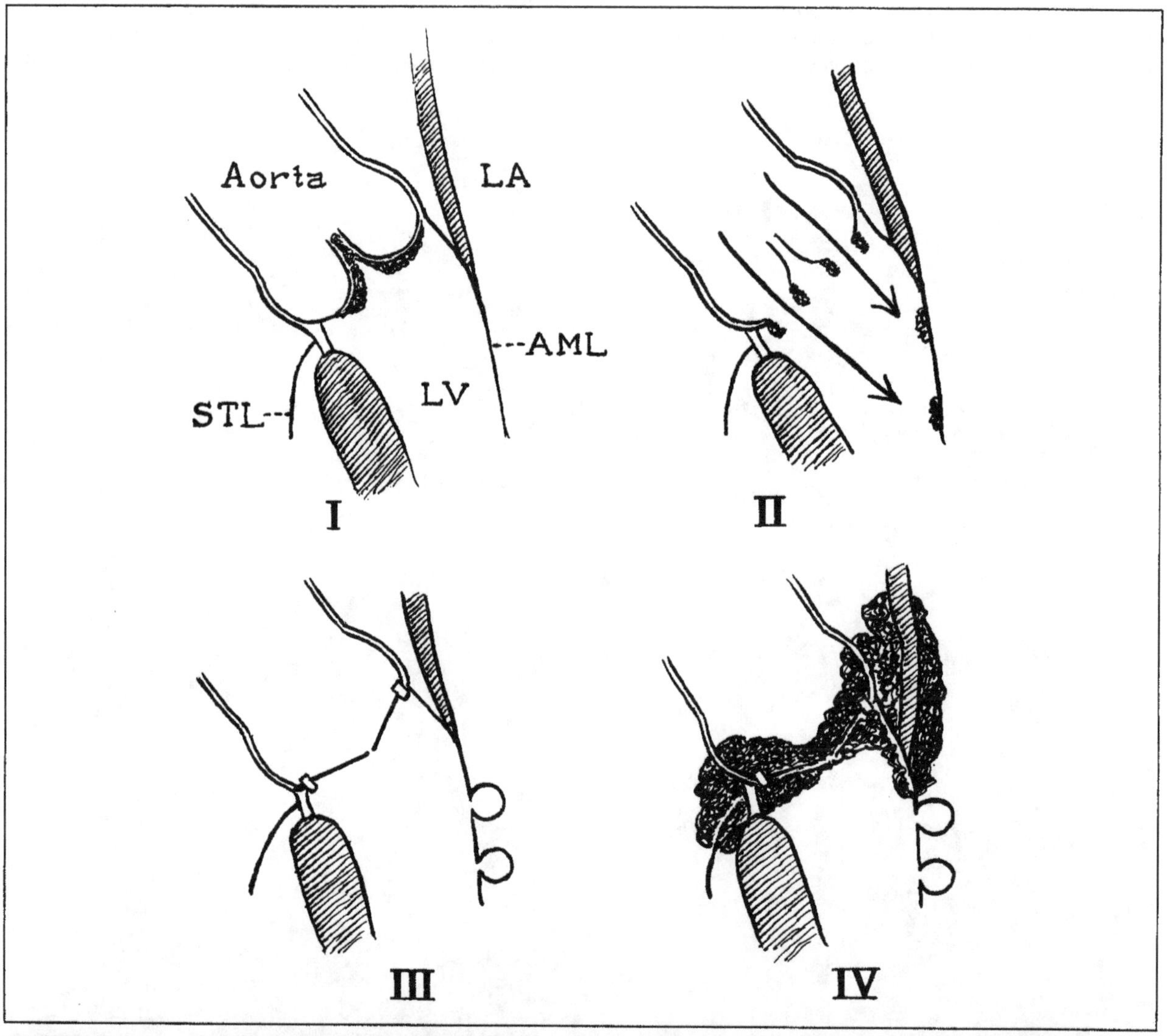

FIGURE 16. Stages of active infective endocarditis, which healed, with perforated aortic valve cusps and 2 aneurysms of the anterior mitral leaflet, and later fatal prosthetic valve endocarditis in a 34-year-old man (DCGH #87A-37). At age 31, three years before death, the patient had *Staphylococcus aureus* endocarditis involving the aortic valve (stage I). AML = anterior mitral leaflet; LA = left atrium; LV = left ventricle; STL = septal tricuspid leaflet. The aortic valve cusps were perforated by the infective process causing regurgitation with seeding of the anterior mitral valve leaflet with organisms (stage II). The regurgitant aortic valve was replaced with a St. Jude Medical prosthesis. Two aneurysms of the anterior mitral leaflet remain (stage III). At age 34, the prosthesis became infected (alpha hemolytic streptococcus), and the infection spread to adjacent tissue (stage IV). The patient continued to use opiates after the valve replacement. In his last month of life he developed aortic regurgitation, complete heart block and episodes of ventricular tachycardia.

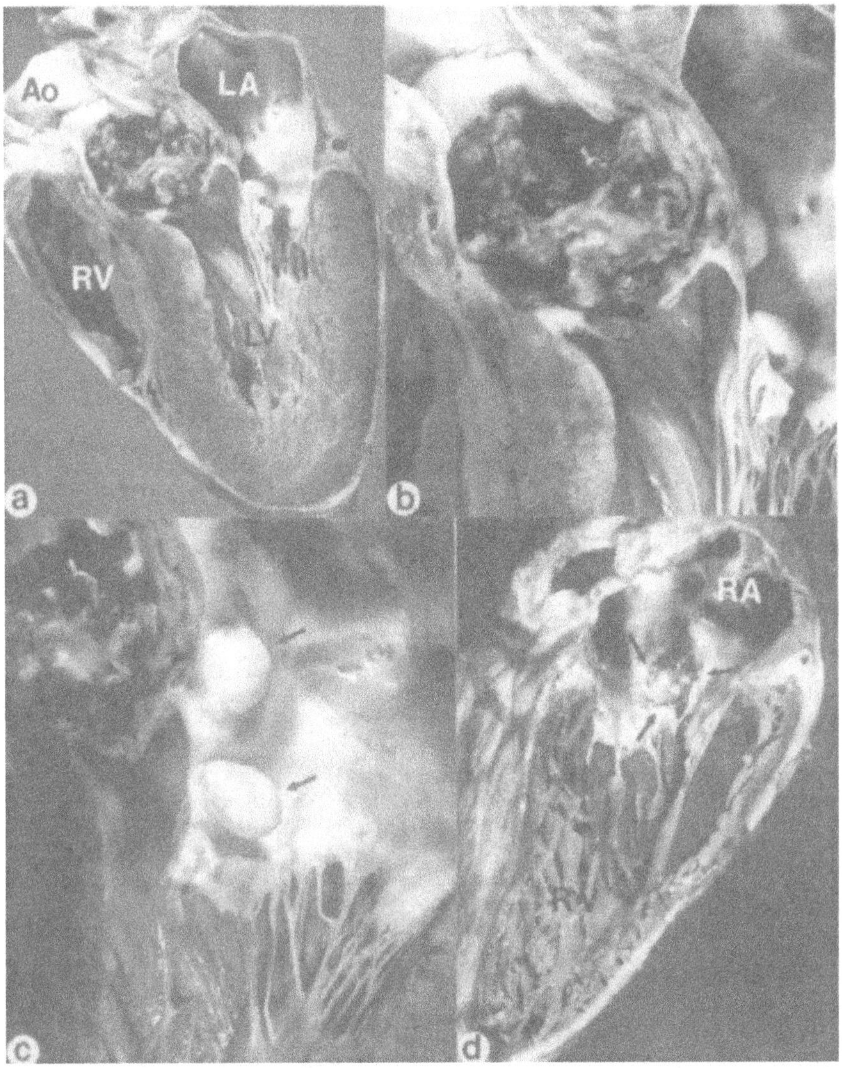

FIGURE 17. The heart in the patient described in Figure 16. *a*, longitudinal view of heart. Ao = aorta; LA = left atrium; LV = left ventricle; RV = right ventricle. *b*, close-up of the infected prosthesis. *c*, close-up showing the 2 aneurysms (*arrows*) in the anterior leaflet (residua from active infection that healed). *d*, Longitudinal view of right side of the heart showing ring abscess (*arrows*) just cephalad to the tricuspid valve. The ring abscess had burrowed through the ventricular septum from the prosthetic infection.

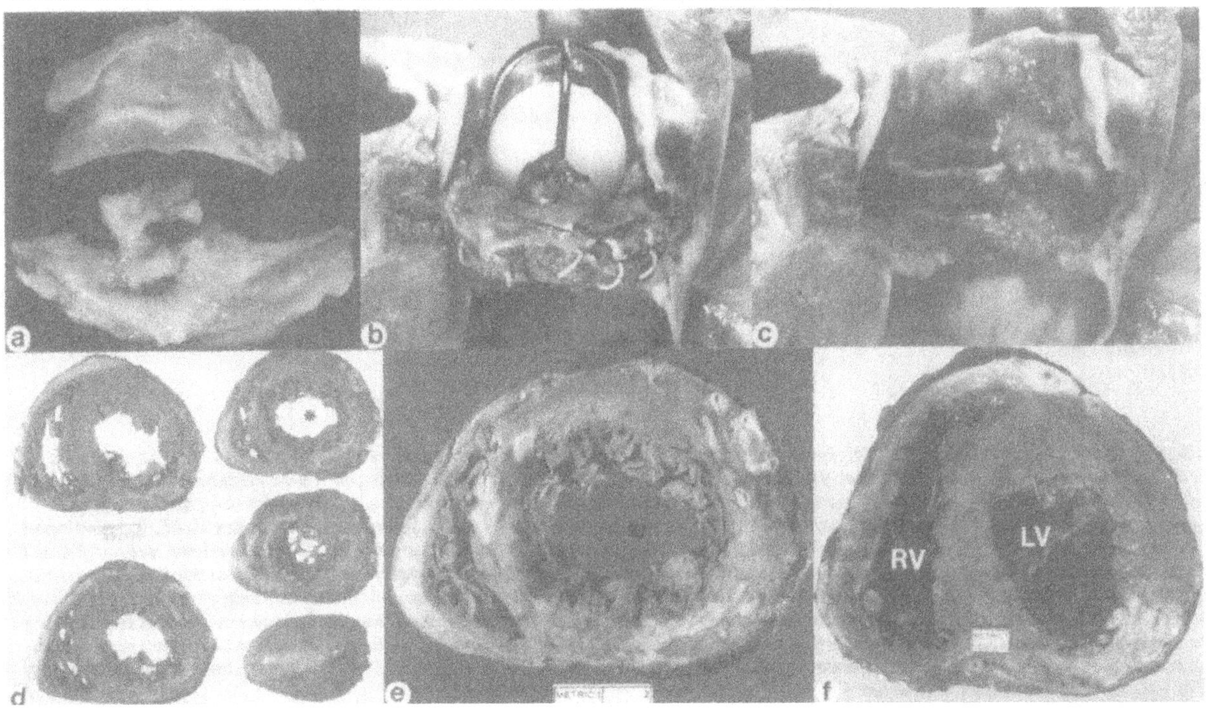

overdose 341 days later. Of the 48 patients having tricuspid valve excision for IE reported by Arbulu and Asfaw,[27] 6 died within 60 days and 10 later (time not specified). Persistent infection was the cause of death in 5 of the 6 patients who died within 60 days and all 10 patients dying after 60 days continued to use opiates. Although the risk of recurrent infection apparently is greater in opiate addicts receiving tricuspid valve replacement compared to those having excision alone, death beyond the immediate postoperative period is related primarily to consequences of continued opiate use.

REFERENCES

1. Luttgens WF. Endocarditis in "main line" opium addicts. Report on eleven cases. *Arch Intern Med 1949;83:653–664.*

2. Ramsey RG, Gunnar RM, Tobin JR Jr. Endocarditis in the drug addict. *Am J Cardiol 1970;25:608–618.*

3. Roberts WC, Buchbinder NA. Right-sided valvular infective endocarditis. A clinicopathologic study of twelve necropsy patients. *Am J Med 1972;53:7–19.*

4. Buchbinder NA, Roberts WC. Left-sided valvular active infective endocarditis. A study of forty-five necropsy patients. *Am J Med 1972;53:20–35.*

5. Menda KB, Gorbach SL. Favorable experience with bacterial endocarditis in heroin addicts. *Ann Intern Med 1973;78:25–32.*

6. Dreyer NP, Fields BN. Heroin-associated infective endocarditis. A report of 28 cases. *Ann Intern Med 1973;78:699–702.*

7. Banks T, Fletcher R, Ali N. Infective endocarditis in heroin addicts. *Am J Med 1973;55:444–451.*

8. Curtis J, Richman BL, Feinstein MA. Infective endocarditis in drug addicts. *South Med J 1974;67:4–9.*

9. Lange M, Salaki JS, Middleton JR, Sen P, Kapila R, Gocke M, Louria DB. Infective endocarditis in heroin addicts: epidemiological observations and some unusual cases. *Am Heart J 1978;96:144–152.*

10. Hubbell G, Cheitlin MD, Rapaport E. Presentation, management, and follow-up evaluation of infective endocarditis in drug addicts. *Am Heart J 1981;102:85–94.*

11. Chambers HG, Korzeniowski OM, Sande MA. The National Collaborative Endocarditis Study Group. Staphylococcus aureus endocarditis: clinical manifestations in addicts and nonaddicts. *Medicine 1983;62:170–177.*

12. Rouveix E, Witchitz S, Bouvet E, Friedlander G, Wolff M, Regnier B, Vachon F. Tricuspid infective endocarditis: 56 cases. *Eur Heart J 1984;5:111–115.*

13. Andy JJ, Sheikh MU, Ali N, Barnes BO, Fox LM, Curry CL, Roberts WC. Echocardiographic observations in opiate addicts with active infective endocarditis. Frequency of involvement of the various valves and comparison of echocardiographic features of right- and left-sided cardiac valve endocarditis. *Am J Cardiol 1977;40:17–23.*

14. Dubois RW, Ginzton LE. Role of echocardiography in suspected infective endocarditis in intravenous drug abusers. *Am J Cardiol 1986;58:649–650.*

15. Berger M, Delfin LA, Jelveh M, Goldberg E. Two-dimensional echocardiographic findings in right-sided infective endocarditis. *Circulation 1980;61:855–861.*

16. Ginzton LE, Siegel RJ, Criley JM. Natural history of tricuspid valve endocarditis: a two-dimensional echocardiographic study. *Am J Cardiol 1982;49:1853–1859.*

17. Sheikh MU, Covarrubias EA, Ali N, Lee WR, Sheikh NM, Roberts WC. M-mode echocardiographic observations during and after healing of active bacterial endocarditis limited to the mitral valve. *Am Heart J 1981;101:37–45.*

18. Sheikh MU, Covarrubias EA, Ali N, Sheikh NM, Lee WR, Roberts WC. M-mode echocardiographic observations in active bacterial endocarditis limited to the aortic valve. *Am Heart J 1981;102:66–75.*

19. Roberts WC, Buchbinder NA. Healed left-sided infective endocarditis: a clinicopathologic study of 59 patients. *Am J Cardiol 1977;40:876–888.*

20. Andriole VT, Kravetz HM, Roberts WC, Utz JP. Candida endocarditis. Clinical and pathologic studies. *Am J Med 1962;32:251–285.*

21. Barbour DJ, Roberts WC. *Valve excision only* versus valve *excision plus replacement* for active infective endocarditis involving the tricuspid valve. *Am J Cardiol 1986;57:475–478.*

22. Mammana RB, Levitsky S, Sernoque D, Beckman CB, Silverman NA. Valve replacement for left-sided endocarditis in drug addicts. *Ann Thorac Surg 1983;35:436–441.*

23. Silverman NA, Levitsky S, Mammana R. Acute endocarditis in drug addicts: surgical treatment for multiple valve infection. *JACC 1984;4:680–684.*

24. Nelson RJ, Harley DP, French WJ, Bayer AS. Favorable ten-year experience with valve procedures for active infective endocarditis. *J Thorac Cardiovasc Surg 1984;87:493–502.*

25. Cukingnan RA Jr, Carey JS, Wittig JH, Cimochowski GE. Early valve replacement in active infective endocarditis. Results and late survival. *J Thorac Cardiovasc Surg 1983;85:163–173.*

26. Stern HJ, Sisto DA, Strom JA, Soeiro R, Jones SR, Frater RWM. Immediate tricuspid valve replacement for endocarditis. Indications and results. *J Thorac Cardiovasc Surg 1986;91:163–167.*

27. Arbulu A, Asfaw I. Management of infective endocarditis: seventeen years' experience. *Ann Thorac Surg 1987;43:144–149.*

FIGURE 18. Opposite, recurrent *Staphylococcus aureus* endocarditis in a 29-year-old man (GT #A85-75). Nineteen months before death he had *Staphylococcus aureus* infection on a congenitally bicuspid aortic valve and it was replaced with a Starr-Edwards prosthesis. He continued his opiate addiction after operation. About a month before death he developed fever, altered mental status, evidence of an acute myocardial infarction and *Staphylococcus aureus* was grown from the blood. He developed cardiogenic shock and died. *a,* operatively excised congenitally biscuspid aortic valve showing infection involving only 1 of the 2 cusps. *b,* longitudinal view of the infected prosthesis in the aortic valve position. *c,* same view after the prosthesis has been excised. *d,* cardiac ventricles after they have been cut transversely at approximately 1 cm intervals. Multiple abscesses are present in the walls. *e,* close-up of the transverse cut containing an asterisk in *d.* The abscesses are more apparent. *f,* most basal view of cardiac ventricles showing a large myocardial abscess in the posterior left ventricular wall. The abscesses contain polymorphonuclear leukocytes and colonies of organisms and the myocardium in the areas of abscess are necrotic. The epicardial coronary arteries were insignificantly narrowed. LV = left ventricle; RV = right ventricle.

Severe Mitral or Aortic Valve Regurgitation, or Both, Requiring Valve Replacement for Infective Endocarditis Complicating Hypertrophic Cardiomyopathy

WILLIAM C. ROBERTS, MD, FACC, JOAN C. KISHEL, MD, CHARLES L. McINTOSH, MD, FACC, RICHARD O. CANNON III, MD, FACC, BARRY J. MARON, MD

Bethesda, Maryland

Certain clinical and morphologic findings are described in 11 patients with hypertrophic cardiomyopathy complicated by infective endocarditis that produced severe mitral or aortic valve regurgitation, or both, necessitating valve replacement. All 11 patients had changes in the operatively excised valve or valves characteristic of healed infective endocarditis. The infection involved only the mitral valve in seven patients, only the aortic valve in three patients and both valves in one patient.

Study of the operatively excised mitral valves indicated that the healed vegetations were located most commonly on the left ventricular aspects of the anterior mitral leaflet, indicating that vegetation had formed at contact points of this leaflet with mural endocardium of the left ventricular outflow tract. In all 11 patients, the infective endocarditis either worsened preexisting valve regurgitation or initiated valve regurgitation and led to worsened signs and symptoms of cardiac dysfunction, necessitating valve replacement. Functional class improved in the nine patients who survived 7 to 101 months after valve replacement.

Hypertrophic cardiomyopathy appears to be a factor predisposing to infective endocarditis. Patients with hypertrophic cardiomyopathy should receive prophylactic antibiotic therapy during procedures that predispose to infective endocarditis.

(J Am Coll Cardiol 1992;19:365–71)

From 1961 through October 1989, 626 patients with hypertrophic cardiomyopathy underwent a cardiac operation at the Surgery Branch of the National Heart, Lung, and Blood Institute: partial septotomy/septectomy alone in 539 patients (86%); septotomy/septectomy followed later by mitral valve replacement in 19 patients (3%) and mitral valve replacement alone in 68 patients (11%). Of the 87 patients undergoing mitral valve replacement with or without septotomy/septectomy, mitral valve replacement was performed because of severe left ventricular outflow obstruction unassociated with severe thickening of the ventricular septum in 65 patients; damage to either the mitral or aortic valve at the time of earlier septotomy/septectomy in 5 patients; inability to wean the patient from cardiopulmonary bypass after septotomy/septectomy in 3 patients; severe regurgitation of uncertain etiology in 3 patients; and valvular regurgitation caused by or worsened by infective endocarditis in 11 patients. This report describes certain clinical and morphologic cardiac findings in the 11 patients with hypertrophic cardiomyopathy with severe mitral or aortic valvular regurgitation, or both, from infective endocarditis.

From the Pathology, Cardiology and Surgery Branches, National Heart, Lung, and Blood Institute, National Institutes of Health, Bethesda, Maryland.
Manuscript received May 8, 1991; revised manuscript received July 15, 1991, accepted July 29, 1991.
Address for reprints: William C. Roberts, MD, Building 10, Room 2N258, NHLBI-NIH, Bethesda, Maryland 20892.

Methods

Clinical characteristics (Tables 1 to 3). All 11 patients had clear clinical evidence of hypertrophic cardiomyopathy: 1) each had evidence of left ventricular hypertrophy on both the electrocardiogram (ECG) and the M-mode echocardiogram; 2) immediately before cardiac valve replacement, only 1 patient had a dilated left ventricular cavity as determined by left ventricular angiography and the dilation was of mild degree; 3) none had a history of systemic hypertension and, with one exception, all had systemic arterial indirect pressure recordings ≤140 mm Hg systolic and ≤90 mm Hg diastolic (Patient 3 had a systemic arterial direct pressure of 160/90 mm Hg recorded immediately before valve replacement, but other pressures recorded were normal); 4) although cardiac index was normal in only four of nine patients in whom it was recorded, the other five had evidence of severe valvular regurgitation (worsened by infective endocarditis) at the time of the recording; 5) the maximal thickness of the ventricular septum was greater than that of the left ventricular free wall in all patients before either valve replacement or partial ventricular septotomy/septectomy; and 6) all patients had hemodynamic documentation of subaortic obstruction at some time.

Characteristics of infective endocarditis. All 11 patients had evidence of active infective endocarditis at some time (Fig. 1 to 7). Ten patients had a typical clinical illness of active infective endocarditis. Of the nine patients with one

Table 1. Clinical and Morphologic Features in 11 Patients Having Valve Replacement for Valvular Regurgitation Due to or Worsened by Infective Endocarditis Complicating Hypertrophic Cardiomyopathy

Pt No.	Age (yr) at VR/ Gender	Diagnosis of HCM		NYHA Functional Class (I–IV)			Septotomy/Septectomy (7 patients)				Follow-Up After Valve Replacement (mo)	NYHA Class at Latest Follow-Up	Interval IE to VR (mo)	Type Valve Prosthesis		Morphology of Operatively Excised Valve				
																MV			AV	
		Before IE	After IE	Just Before IE	After IE	Just Before VR	Before IE	After IE	Before VR	With VR				MV (size)	AV (size)	Calcium	P	RCT	Calcium	P
1	12/M	+	0	II	IV	IV	0	0	0	0	7	I	17	SE	–	+	+	+	–	–
2	25/M	+	0	II	III	III	+	+	0	+	21	I	10	H (27 mm)	–	+	+	+	–	–
3	43/M	+	0	II	III	III	0	0	0	0	10	II	19	H (25 mm)	–	+	+	+	–	–
4	46/M	–	–	–	–	III	0	+	0	+	101	III	–	H (25 mm)	–	0	+	+	–	–
5	63/M	+	0	III	IV	IV	0	0	0	0	90	II	8	H (31 mm)	–	+	+	+	–	–
6	64/M	0	+	II	II	III	0	0	0	0	18	I	156	H (31 mm)	–	+	+	+	–	–
7	71/M	+	0	II	III	IV	0	–	+	0	30 days	Dead	204	H (31 mm)	–	+	+	+	–	–
8	51/M	0	+	I	IV	IV	0	–	0	+	72	I	3	–	SE (9A)	–	–	–	+	+
9	52/F	+	0	II	III	III	0	–	0	+	33	II	7	–	SE (9A)	–	–	–	+	+
10	64/F	0	+	I	III	IV	0	+	0	+	12	I	60	–	H (21 mm)	–	–	–	0	+
11	58/M	+	0	III	IV	IV	0	+	+	0	3 days	Dead	168	H (29 mm)	H (23 mm)	+	+	+	0	+

AV = aortic valve; F = female; H = Hancock; HCM = hypertrophic cardiomyopathy; IE = infective endocarditis; M = male; MV = mitral valve; NYHA = New York Heart Association; P = perforation or indentation (deficiency of leaflet tissue); Pt = patient; RCT = ruptured chordae tendineae; SE = Starr-Edwards; VR = valve replacement; 0 = absent or negative; + = present or positive; – = no information available or not applicable.

clinical episode of active infective endocarditis, the interval between active infective endocarditis and valve replacement ranged from 3 to 204 months (mean 54, median 17). This interval was <1 year in four patients. Patient 11 (Table 1) had two episodes of active infective endocarditis that occurred 168 and 27 months, respectively, before valve replacement (Fig. 7). Only the second episode caused clinical worsening of this patient's cardiac status. Patient 4 apparently never had a clinical illness diagnosed as active infective endocarditis, but examination of the operatively excised mitral valve disclosed a large deficit in the anterior mitral leaflet adjacent to several ruptured chordae tendineae, anatomic findings diagnostic of healed infective endocarditis (1). Of the 11 patients, 9 had active infective endocarditis before they were admitted to the National Institutes of Health; 1 had active infective endocarditis treated at another hospital, but hypertrophic cardiomyopathy had previously been diagnosed at the National Institutes of Health; and 1 patient had active infective endocarditis while hospitalized at the National Institutes of Health. Diagnosis of hypertrophic cardiomyopathy had been established previously in 7 of the 10 patients with a clinical illness diagnosed as active infective endocarditis; it was made in the other 3 patients after active infective endocarditis had healed. In five patients, a factor other than hypertrophic cardiomyopathy predisposing to infective endocarditis was apparent: dental procedures in Patients 4 and 5, cardiac catheterization in Patients 6 and 10 and opiate addiction in Patient 11.

During active infective endocarditis, information regarding the results of blood cultures were known in eight patients: in two, the blood cultures were negative and in six a bacterium was identified (alpha streptococcus in Patients 7, 10 and 11; group D streptococcus in two patients [nonenterococcal in Patient 2 and enterococcus in Patient 6]; and *Cardiobacterium hominis* in Patient 4). All 11 patients, however, had anatomic deficiencies of mitral or aortic valve cusps, and in those with infective endocarditis involving the mitral valve, there were associated ruptured chordae tendineae. The 10 patients with clear clinical evidence of active infective endocarditis received appropriate antibiotic treatment, and by the time of valve replacement, the infection had healed in all 10 patients. The M-mode echocardiogram immediately before valve replacement showed "echo densities" compatible with healed vegetations in four of seven patients in whom healed infective endocarditis involved the mitral valve and two of four in whom it involved the aortic valve.

Valvular regurgitation caused by infective endocarditis. Active infective endocarditis worsened the symptomatic status in nine patients by at least one New York Heart Association functional class. It also increased the intensity of the precordial systolic murmur (mitral regurgitation) in three of three patients in whom this information was known and caused the appearance of a basal diastolic murmur in all four patients with aortic regurgitation. Despite the appearance or worsening of valvular regurgitation, the left ventric-

Table 2. M-Mode Echocardiographic Data Before and After Operation in the 11 Patients With Infective Endocarditis Complicating Hypertrophic Cardiomyopathy and Requiring Valve Replacement

Pt No.	Interval Echo to VR (days)	Wall Thickness (mm)		Cavity (mm)			FS (%)	Echo Density		Flail		SAM
		VSd	LVd	LVd	LVs	LA		MV	AV	MV	AV	
1	9 (MVR)	20	13	41	18	45	56	+	0	+	0	+
	PO	16	10	37	18	35	51	−	0	−	0	−
2												
3	78 (MVR)	17	14	36	16	56	55	0	0	+	0	+
	PO	—	—	—	—	—	—	−	−	−	−	−
4	12 (MVR)	19	15	40	18	40	55	0	0	0	0	−
	PO	15	—*	—*	—*	57	—	−	0	−	0	−
5	65 (MVR)	32	14	46	28	55	39	±	0	0	0	+
	PO	14	—	—	—	57	—	−	0	−	0	−
6	16 (MVR)	26	13	56	38	68	32	+	0	0	0	+
	PO	—	—	—	—	—	—	−	−	−	−	−
7	33 (MVR)	—	—	—	—	72	—	0	0	±	0	−
	PO	—	—	—	—	63	—	−	0	−	0	−
8	8 (AVR)	20	13	40	22	43	45	0	+	0	−	0
	PO	10	10	—*	—*	40	—	0	−	0	−	0
9	37 (AVR)	26	14	44	22	49	50	0	+	0	+	0
	PO†		11	51	29	45	43	0	−	0	−	0
10	41 (AVR)	24	13	53	41	60	23	0	0	0	0	−
	PO	11	11	—*	—*	52	—	0	−	0	−	0
11	10 (MVR, AVR)	—	—	—	—	54	—	0	0	0	0	0
	PO	—	—	—	—	—	—	−	−	−	−	−

*Paradoxical movement; †ventricular septal defect created at operation. AV = aortic valve; AVR = aortic valve replacement; d = end-diastole; Echo = echocardiography; FS = fractional shortening; LA = left atrium; LV = left ventricle; MV = mitral valve; MVR = mitral valve replacement; PO = after operation; s = peak systole; SAM = systolic anterior motion of the anterior mitral leaflet; VS = ventricular septum; − = not applicable; other abbreviations as in Table 1.

Table 3. Hemodynamic and Angiographic Data Immediately Before and ≥6 Months After Valve Replacement in 11 Patients With Infective Endocarditis Complicating Hypertrophic Cardiomyopathy

Pt No.	Time of Cath (mo PO)	PA* (s/d)	RV* (s/d)	RA* (m)	Mean PAW*	LA*		LV* (s/d)	SA* (s/d)	LV-SA psg*	MR by LV Cine (0–4+)	AR by AA Cine (0–4+)	CAD by Cine	CI
						a	v							
1	Pre-VR	66/40	65/16	7	26	36	38	180/25	118/60	62	4+	—	—	3.8
	PO (6)	32/14	32/4	4	9	16	10	130/12	125/65	5	—	—	—	2.1
2	Pre-VR	80/40	80/18	18	45	AF	50	138/24	138/60	0	4+	1+	—	2.1
3	Pre-VR	88/40	88/14	11	32	32	44	140/30	114/65	26	4+	0	0	1.8
	PO (6)	44/20	44/6	4	14	16	12	150/14	158/88	0	0	0	—	3.3
4	Pre-VR	90/40	90/10	8	30	27	40	165/32	120/70	45	3+	—	0	2.0
5	Pre-VR†	50/25	50/10	5	15	—	—	245/40	160/90	85	3+	—	—	3.7
	PO (10)‡	—	120/30	19	35	23	55	130/24	130/65	0	2+	0	—	2.0
	PO (21)	60/25	60/9	11	24	—	32	—	—	—	—	—	—	2.5
6	Pre-VR	45/23	45/8	4	20	28	36	110/10	105/70	5	3+	—	—	2.5
	PO (6)	—	24/5	3	—	—	—	105/6	105/60	0	0	—	—	2.3
7	Pre-VR	50/25	50/5	6	31	AF	50	120/20	130/75	0	4+	—	§	1.5
8	Pre-VR	85/35	85/12	—	38	AF	55	120/14	120/60	0	4+	—	—	—
9	Pre-VR	50/25	50/15	6	27	40	45	164/34	86/40	78	1+	3+	0	—
	PO (12)	24/11	24/7	4	6	13	8	115/16	110/65	5	—	—	—	2.0
10	Pre-VR	60/30	65/15	9	20	10	22	200/28	130/68	70	1+	2+	0	3.1
	PO (8)	—	—	—	16	20	28	105/20	105/55	0	—	—	—	4.4
	PO (58)	30/12	30/5	6	12	—	—	—	120/70	—	—	—	—	—
11	Pre-VR	55/30	55/6	5	17	26	20	240/30	100/30	140	3+	3+	0	1.7
	PO (76)	75/35	75/16	15	31	28	44	150/24	145/85	5	3+	1+	0	2.1

*Pressures in mm Hg. †Cardiac catheterization (Cath) 36 months before valve replacement; ‡peribasilar bioprosthetic communication found by left ventricular cineangiography (Cine) and it was operatively closed after this cardiac catheterization procedure. §This patient was the only one with significant coronary narrowing and he had aortocoronary bypass grafting in addition to valve replacement (VR). a = a wave; AA = ascending aorta; AF = atrial fibrillation; AR = aortic regurgitation; CAD = coronary artery narrowing >50% in diameter of >1 major artery; CI = cardiac index in liters/min per m^2; LA = left atrium; LV = left ventricle; MR = mitral regurgitation; PA = pulmonary artery; PAW = pulmonary artery wedge; PO = after operation (months); Pre = before; psg = peak systolic gradient; Pt = patient; RA = right atrium; RV = right ventricle; SA = systemic artery; s/d = peak systole/end-diastole; v = v wave.

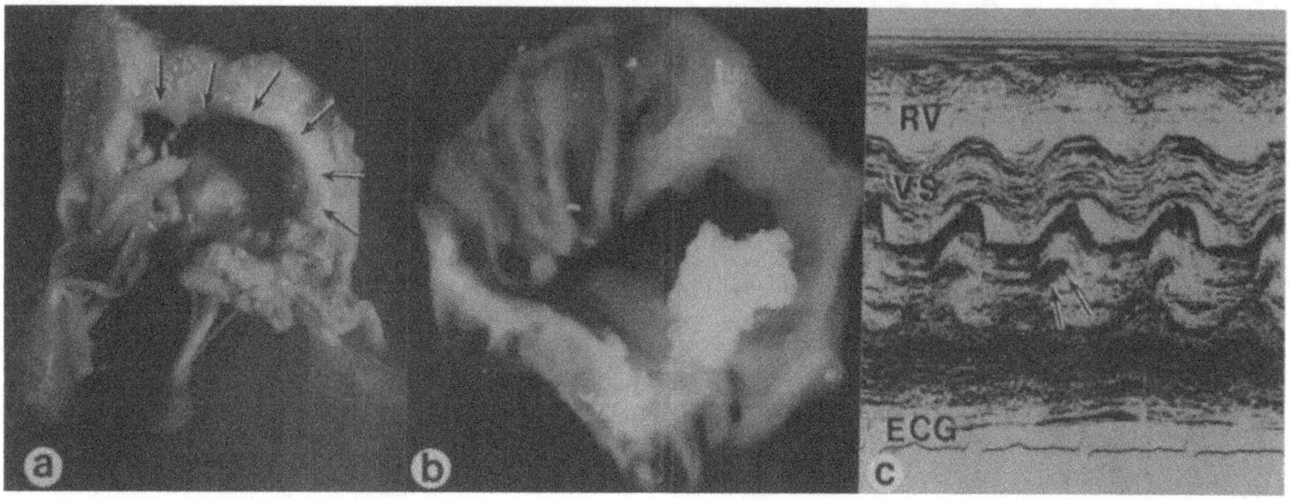

Figure 1 (above). Patient 1. Operatively excised mitral valve. **a,** Leaflets, chordae tendineae and attached papillary muscles showing loss of tissue in the posterior leaflet and absence of chordae tendineae (**arrows**). A large deposit of calcium is present and is better seen in **b,** a radiograph of the excised valve. **c,** M-mode echocardiogram taken shortly before mitral valve replacement, showing thickening and impaired mobility of the anterior mitral leaflet and fluttering (**arrows**) of the posterior leaflet. ECG = electrocardiogram; RV = right ventricular cavity; VS = ventricular septum.

Figure 2 (below). Patient 2. Operatively excised mitral valve (**a, b,** and **c**) and M-mode echocardiogram (**d**). **a,** Radiograph of the opened valve. The **arrows** point to a calcific deposit. **b** and **c,** Close-up views of the atrial aspect of a portion of both leaflets. The anterior leaflet contains two perforations (**solid arrows**) and the posterior leaflet one perforation (**dashed arrow**). **d,** Typical echocardiogram in hypertrophic cardiomyopathy with asymmetric thickening of the anterior ventricular septum (VS). The **arrows** point to dense echoes of the thickened anterior mitral leaflet, which contacts the ventricular septum in diastole. Mild mitral systolic anterior motion is present (*). PW = posterior wall; RV = right ventricular cavity.

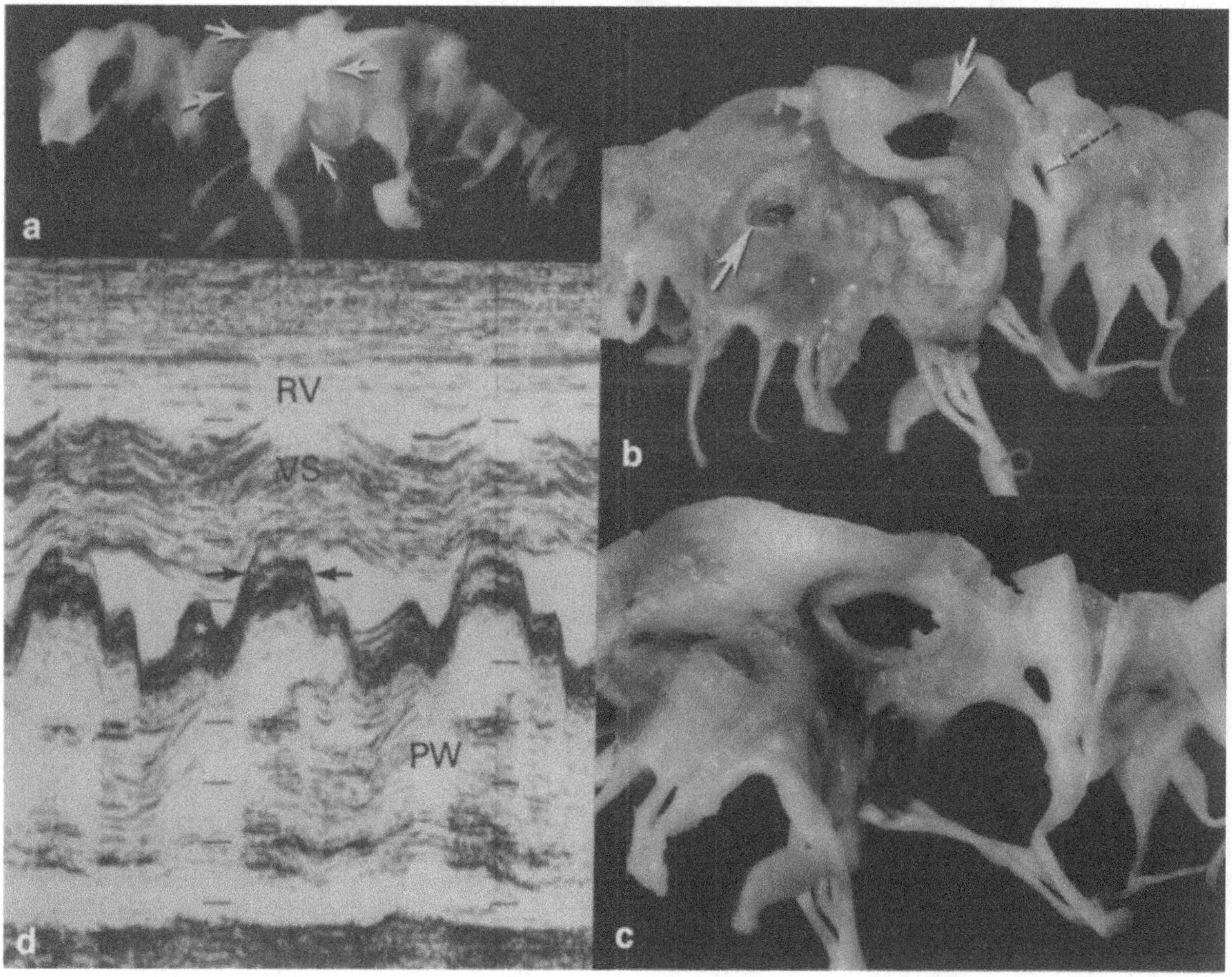

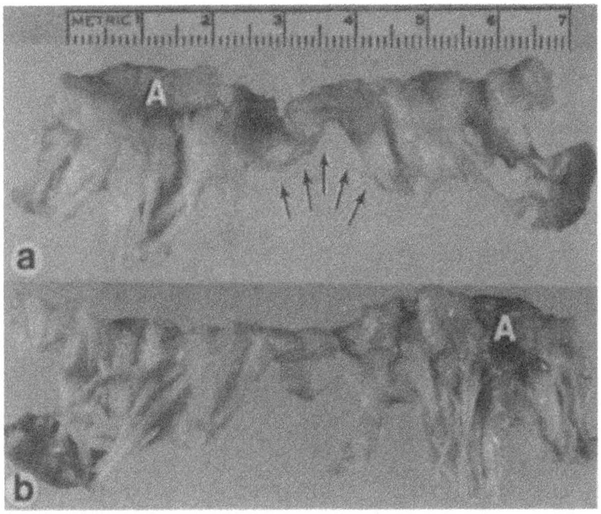

Figure 3. Patient 3. Opened mitral valve. **a,** Atrial surface. **b,** Ventricular surface. The **arrows** designate the area where chordae tendineae are missing (ruptured) and a site where a portion of the leaflet is absent (destroyed by the previous infection). A = anterior mitral leaflet.

ular cavity was of normal size on the echocardiogram immediately before valve replacement in nine of nine patients; left ventricular angiograms in the other two patients disclosed mild left ventricular cavity dilation in one of them. The degree of valvular regurgitation immediately before valve replacement in each of the 11 patients was severe: in the 7 patients with isolated mitral valve replacement, the degree of mitral regurgitation by left ventricular angiography was either 3+/4+ or 4+/4+; in the 3 patients with isolated aortic valve replacement, the degree of aortic regurgitation by aortic root angiography was 3+/4+ in 2 and 2+/4+ in 1; in the single patient with replacement of both left-sided cardiac valves, the degree of mitral regurgitation was 4+/4+ and aortic regurgitation, 1+/4+.

Effect of infective endocarditis on the left ventricular outflow pressure gradient. Active infective endocarditis involving the mitral valve was associated with a decrease in

Figure 4. Patient 5. Opened mitral valve from its atrial aspect, showing a large perforation (**arrow**) in the anterior leaflet (A) with adjacent focal calcific deposits. The perforation represents a site where vegetation had been present.

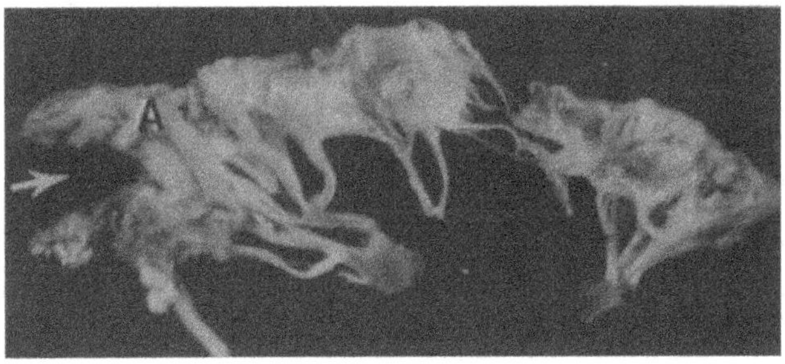

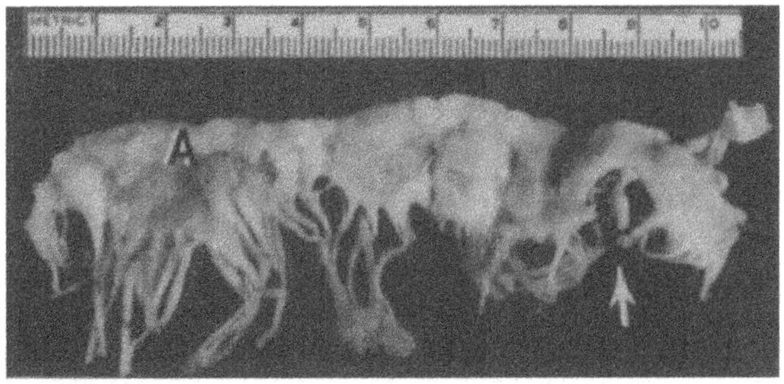

Figure 5. Patient 6. Opened mitral valve from its atrial aspect, showing a large indentation (**arrow**) in the posterior leaflet. Both anterior (A) and posterior leaflets are thickened by fibrous tissue. The indentation represents a site of previous vegetation.

the peak systolic pressure gradient between the left ventricle and a systemic artery. In the three patients who had cardiac catheterization before and after active infective endocarditis, the peak systolic pressure gradient decreased from 90 to 62 mm Hg in Patient 1, from 100 to 5 mm Hg in Patient 4 and from 76 to 55 mm Hg in Patient 6.

Results of cardiac valve replacements. Valve replacement was successful in nine patients. The other two patients (Patients 7 and 11), each of whom died within 30 days of valve replacement, were the only patients who had had partial septectomy and septotomy before cardiac valve replacement. Of the nine hospital survivors after valve replacement (combined with partial septotomy and septectomy in four), eight were in functional class I or II and one was in class III when seen 6 to 21 months after valve replacement, whereas preoperatively three had been in functional class III and five in functional class IV. Cardiac catheterization was performed 6 to 21 months (mean 14) after valve replacement in seven of the nine long-term survivors (Table 3). In three of the seven patients, no left ventricular outflow tract obstruction was present preoperatively and the postoperative study disclosed no pressure gradient between the left ventricle and a systemic artery during peak systole. In the other four patients, the peak systolic pressure gradient before valve replacement (combined with partial septotomy and septectomy in three patients) decreased from an average of 74 mm Hg (range 62 to 85) preoperatively to ≤5 mm Hg postoperatively.

Discussion

Major findings of present study. Although 30 reports describing one or more patients (19 were single case studies) with hypertrophic cardiomyopathy and infective endocarditis have appeared (cases tabulated by Alessandri et al. [2]), the presence of infective endocarditis was confirmed anatomically (2–11) only in 15 of the reported 56 cases and in none was the type of valvular damage illustrated. The present study analyzed 11 patients from the same center with

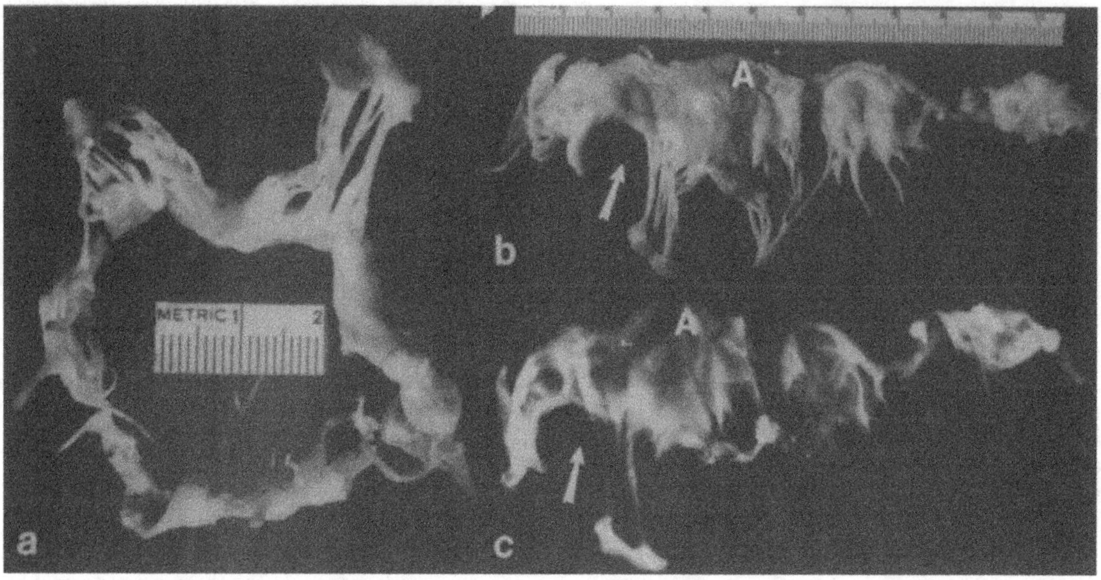

Figure 6. Patient 7. **a,** Unopened mitral valve. **b,** Opened mitral valve showing its atrial aspect. The **arrow** points to an indentation at the junction of the anterior (A) and posterior leaflets. Several chordae tendineae are missing (ruptured) at this site. **c,** Radiograph of the opened mitral valve. Several calcific deposits are present in the annular region of the posterior leaflet.

hypertrophic cardiomyopathy complicated by infective endocarditis necessitating replacement of one or more cardiac valves in each, and in each the operatively excised valve was studied. It is apparent that infective endocarditis should be recognized as a complication of hypertrophic cardiomyopathy and that the latter predisposes to infective endocarditis. The frequency with which the complication occurs is unclear. The present study suggests that among patients with hypertrophic cardiomyopathy with mitral or aortic valve regurgitation, or both, severe enough to warrant valve replacement, infective endocarditis often is responsible for the severe regurgitation. Of the 87 patients with hypertrophic cardiomyopathy who underwent valve replacement at our institution, 11 underwent this procedure because of damage by infective endocarditis. None of the other operatively excised valves had cusp perforations or tears or ruptured chordae tendineae and therefore it is unlikely that any of these other patients had had infective endocarditis at any time.

Location of the vegetations in infective endocarditis complicating hypertrophic cardiomyopathy. The most frequent site of vegetations in patients with hypertrophic cardiomyopathy is the mitral valve and specifically its anterior leaflet. It is this leaflet, of course, which tends to contact the mural endocardium of the ventricular septum during one or both phases of the cardiac cycle and it is likely that vegetations form at these contact sites. Of our 11 patients, 8 had vegetations that left telltale residua of infective endocarditis on the mitral valve (1 also had damage to the aortic valve, but the damage was not diagnostic of healed infective endocarditis [1]) and 3 had both clinical and anatomic evidence of damage to one or more aortic valve cusps by infective endocarditis. The vegetations on the anterior mitral leaflet appear to have been on their ventricular aspects, unlike those in most patients with active infective endocarditis involving the mitral valve. The mechanism of formation of aortic valve vegetations in patients with hypertrophic cardiomyopathy is unclear. In three of our four patients having aortic valve replacement, the left ventricular aortic

Figure 7. Patient 8. Three-cusped aortic valve with severe destruction of one of the three cusps by the infective process.

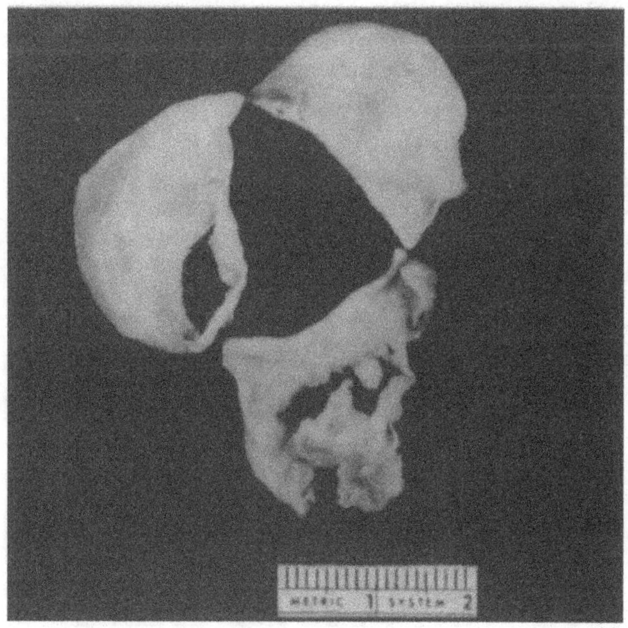

peak systolic pressure gradient was high (70, 78 and 140 mm Hg, respectively), whereas only one of the seven patients with isolated mitral valve replacement had a left ventricular outflow pressure gradient of this magnitude. The vegetations on the aortic valve appear to have been located on the ventricular aspects of these cusps, the usual location of vegetations on this valve.

Valvular regurgitation after infective endocarditis in hypertrophic cardiomyopathy. The present study shows that infective endocarditis complicating hypertrophic cardiomyopathy can result in serious consequences. In all 11 patients, the symptomatic status was unequivocally worsened by active infective endocarditis that healed. Additionally, the intensity of the precordial systolic murmur increased in the patients with infective endocarditis involving the mitral valve, and infective endocarditis involving the aortic valve caused the appearance of a murmur of aortic regurgitation, which was confirmed in each by angiography. The degree of valvular regurgitation was severe in all 11 patients; however, despite the severe degree of regurgitation, the left ventricular cavity immediately before valve replacement was not dilated in any patient on M-mode echocardiography and was only mildly dilated in one of two patients studied by angiography.

Benefit of valve replacement. Despite recognized potential complications of mitral valve replacement in patients with hypertrophic cardiomyopathy (12), the present study indicates that valve replacement for infective endocarditis complicating hypertrophic cardiomyopathy may result in a striking diminution or disappearance of previous symptoms of cardiac dysfunction.

References

1. Roberts WC, Buchbinder NA. Healed left-sided infective endocarditis: a clinicopathologic study of 59 patients. Am J Cardiol 1977;40:876–88.
2. Alessandri N, Pannarale G, del Monte F, Moretti F, Marino B, Reale A. Hypertrophic obstructive cardiomyopathy and infective endocarditis: a report of seven cases and a review of the literature. Eur Heart J 1990;11:1041–8.
3. Nagle JP. Idiopathic hypertrophic subaortic stenosis and bacterial endocarditis. JAMA 1967:200:643–5.
4. Vecht RJ, Oakley CM. Infective endocarditis in three patients with hypertrophic obstructive cardiomyopathy. Br Med J 1968;2:455–9.
5. Caramanian M, Joly F, Fouchard J, Guerinon J. Endocardite infectieuse sur stenose musculaire hypertrophique du ventricule gauche. Arch Mal Coeur 1971;64:1117–31.
6. Chretien EH, Limas C, Garagusi VF. Association of bacterial endocarditis in idiopathic hypertrophic subaortic stenosis. South Med J 1973;66: 269–72.
7. Wang K, Gobel FL, Gleason DF. Bacterial endocarditis in idiopathic hypertrophic subaortic stenosis. Am Heart J 1975;89:359–65.
8. Heret JF, Jandin M, Rigaud M, et al. Endocardite a staphylocoque dore au cours d'une cardiomyopathic obstructive. Arch Mal Coeur 1977;70: 1227–32.
9. Greenland P, Murphy GW. Acute valvular insufficiency complicating hypertrophic obstructive cardiomyopathy. Chest 1979;75:182–3.
10. LeJemtel TH, Factor SM, Koenigsberg M, O'Reilly M, Frater R, Sonnenblick EH. Mural vegetations at the site of endocardial trauma in infective endocarditis complicating idiopathic hypertrophic subaortic stenosis. Am J Cardiol 1979;44:569–74.
11. Pueyo JM, Shahin A, Benazet JM, Camaeno AM, San Miguel JG. Endocarditis infecciosa en estenosis subaortica hipertrofica idiopatica: a proposito de una observacion. Med Clin Barcelona 1981;76:129–31.
12. Roberts WC. Operative treatment of hypertrophic obstructive cardiomyopathy: the case against mitral valve replacement. Am J Cardiol 1973;32: 377–81.

Comparison of Active Infective Endocarditis Involving a Previously Stenotic Versus a Previously Nonstenotic Aortic Valve

William C. Roberts, MD, B. Olusola Oluwole, MB, BS, and Daniel J. Fernicola, MD

No previous studies, either clinical or morphologic, have compared findings in patients with active infective endocarditis (IE) involving a previously stenotic versus a previously nonstenotic aortic valve. Clinical and cardiac necropsy findings were analyzed in 96 patients with active IE involving the aortic valve. Of the 96 patients, 25 (26%) had active IE superimposed on a previously stenotic aortic valve and 71 (74%) on a previously nonstenotic aortic valve. The patients with stenotic aortic valves compared with those with nonstenotic aortic valves had significantly higher mean ages (61 vs 47 years), a higher percentage >60 years of age (52 vs 24%), a higher percentage of men (92 vs 73%), a higher frequency of an absent or unknown predisposing factor to infection (68 vs 38%), a lower frequency of a precordial murmur of aortic regurgitation (44 vs 79%), a lower percent with a long duration (>60 days) of signs and symptoms of active IE (4 vs 23%), a larger mean heart weight (594 vs 514 g), a higher percentage with aortic valve calcific deposits (100 vs 24%), and a higher frequency of associated ring abscess (84 vs 52%). Thus, active IE superimposed on a stenotic aortic valve differs in some features compared with active IE on a nonstenotic aortic valve. Because ring abscess is so common when active IE involves a stenotic aortic valve in adults, operative intervention at an early stage may be warranted.

(Am J Cardiol 1993;71:1082–1088)

From the Pathology Branch, National Heart, Lung, and Blood Institute, National Institutes of Health, Bethesda, Maryland. Manuscript received and accepted December 1, 1992 (see addendum).

Address for reprints: William C. Roberts, MD, Baylor Cardiovascular Institute, Baylor University Medical Center, 3500 Gaston Avenue, Dallas, Texas 75246.

Studies from this laboratory[1–31] and others indicate that the cardiac valve most likely to be involved by active infective endocarditis (IE) is the one which is anatomically abnormal but functionally normal. Next is the valve which is anatomically abnormal and which functions slightly abnormally. The usual functional disturbance in the latter situation is mild valvular regurgitation. IE superimposed on a severely regurgitant cardiac valve is extremely uncommon and indeed has not been encountered by us from a study of >200 cases of active IE involving 1 or more native cardiac valves at necropsy. Infective endocarditis involving a previously stenotic valve is relatively uncommon, and when it occurs the valve involved is most often the aortic one. The degree of valve stenosis may vary from mild to severe. When active IE involves a previously stenotic aortic valve the consequences may be quite different from that which occurs when active IE involves a previously nonstenotic valve, i.e., one that functioned normally or was only slightly regurgitant before the active IE appeared. To better understand these clinical and morphologic differences, we studied at necropsy 25 patients with active IE involving a previously stenotic aortic valve and compared the findings with those in 71 patients in whom active IE involved a previously nonstenotic aortic valve.

METHODS

Method of retrieving cases and exclusion criteria: Records of cases accessioned in the Pathology Branch, National Heart, Lung, and Blood Institute from 1954 until July 1, 1991, under the code "active infective endocarditis" were retrieved and examined. All cases had been classified originally by WCR. Cases in which the native aortic valve was not involved by active IE, i.e., no vegetations were present on the aortic valve, were excluded. The present study was limited to patients studied at necropsy in whom active IE involved the aortic valve. A total of 104 such cases were identified. To make comparisons among cases most meaningful, however, cases of active IE of the aortic valve in which other complicating conditions or circumstances were present were eliminated. Thus, the following cases were eliminated from further analysis: 2 patients with discrete subaortic stenosis, 1 patient with associated ventricular septal defect, 4 patients with associated mitral valve stenosis, and 1 patient who developed active IE shortly after "open" aortic valve commissurotomy. The remaining 96 patients with active IE were included in the present study. Although 21 (22%) of the 96 patients had aortic valve replacement during the period of active IE, all 96 patients had active IE of the native aortic valve.

TABLE I Clinical and Necropsy Observations in Active Infective Endocarditis Superimposed on Preexisting Aortic Valve Stenosis

Pt. No.	Age (year) & Sex	Diagnosis AS in Life	Diagnosis IE in Life	Infecting Organism	Murmur (intensity 1–6) AS	Murmur (intensity 1–6) AR	Duration S & S of IE (days)	HB	PE	AVR	HW (g)	No. AV Cusps	AV Calcium (0–3+)	No. AV Cusps with V	V on MV	Ring Abscess	MAC (0–4+)	CA Embolus	AMI
1	21M	+ (CC)	+	*H. parainfluenzae*	+(−)	+(−)	21	+*	+(300 ml)	+	–	2	0	2	0	+	0	+	0
2	30M	+ (A)	+	*S. aureus*	+(4/6)	0	18	0	0	0	560	2	3+	2	0	+	0	0	0
3	45M	+ (E)	+	*α-Streptococcus*	0	0	12	0	+(150 ml)	0	920	2	2+	2	+	+	0	0	0
4	54M	+ (E)	+	*S. aureus*	+(2/6)	+(2/6)	35	0	0	0	480	2	2+	2	+	+	0	+	+
5	54M	+ (E)	+	*α-Streptococcus*	+(4/6)	+(3/6)	23	0	0	0	850	2	3+	2	+	+	0	0	0
6	55M	+ (A)	0	—	+(−)	0	2	0	—	0	600	2	2+	2	0	0	0	0	0
7	59M	+ (E)	+	—	+(−)	+(−)	—	0	—	+	315	2	2+	2	0	+	0	0	0
8	60M	+ (CC)	+	*Strept. pneumoniae*	+(−)	+(−)	7	+	—	0	540	2	3+	2	0	+	0	0	0
9	63M	+ (A)	+	*α-Streptococcus*	+(3/6)	+(2/6)	90	+	—	0	620	2	3+	2	0	+	0	0	0
10	71M	0	0	*S. epidermidis*	—	—	30	0	0	0	520	2	3+	2	0	+	0	+	+
11	31M	+ (A)	+	*H. parainfluenzae*	+(−)	+(−)	23	0	+(600 ml)	0	425	3	0	2	0	+	0	0	0
12	45F	+ (A)	+	—	+(−)	+(−)	—	–	0	0	490	3	2+	3	0	0	0	–	0
13	49M	+ (A)	+	*S. aureus*	+(4/6)	0	16	+*	0	0	580	3	2+	3	0	+	0	0	0
14	52M	+ (A)	+	*Gram -ve bacilli*	+(−)	+(−)	18	0	—	+	—	3	2+	—	0	+	0	0	0
15	53M	+ (E)	+	*Escherichia coli*	+(3/6)	0	42	0	+(1,000 ml)	0	—	3	3+	3	0	+	0	0	+
16	60M	+ (E)	+	*S. aureus*	+(3/6)	+(−)	60	+	—	0	580	3	2+	3	0	+	0	0	0
17	62M	+ (A)	+	*S. epidermidis*	+(−)	0	—	0	0	0	650	3	2+	3	+	0	2+	0	0
18	65M	+ (A)	+	*α-Streptococcus*	+(2/6)	0	28	0	+(100 ml)	0	610	3	3+	3	0	+	0	0	0
19	67M	+ (A)	+	*S. aureus*	+(2/6)	0	30	0	0	0	700	3	3+	2	0	0	0	+	+
20	70M	+ (A)	+	*β-Streptococcus*	+(3/6)	+(−)	42	0	—	0	560	3	3+	1	+	+	0	0	0
21	72M	0	+	*Strept. pneumoniae*	+(−)	0	7	—	—	0	700	3	3+	3	0	+	0	0	0
22	77F	+ (A)	+	*α-Streptococcus*	+(−)	0	14	0	—	0	450	3	3+	2	+	+	4+	0	0
23	77M	+ (A)	0	—	+(3/6)	0	—	0	—	0	590	3	3+	2	0	0	4+	0	0
24	83M	+ (A)	0	*Strept. pneumoniae*	+(−)	0	1	0	0	0	550	3	2+	3	0	+	2+	0	0
25	86M	+ (A)	0	—	+(−)	0	14	0	+(80 ml)	0	710	3	3+	1	0	+	0	0	0

*Second-degree heart block present.
A = auscultation; AMI = acute myocardial infarction; AR = aortic regurgitation; AS = aortic stenosis; AV = aortic valve; AVR = aortic replacement; CA = coronary artery; CC = cardiac catheterization; E = echocardiogram; HB = heart block; HW = heart weight; IE = infective endocarditis; MAC = mitral annular calcium; MV = mitral valve; PE = pericardial effusion; S and S = signs and symptoms; V = vegetation.

Sources of cases: The 96 patients included in this study had the autopsy performed at 23 different medical institutions: 12 institutions were local and 84 of the 96 cases came from them; the remaining 12 cases were submitted from 12 different nonlocal hospitals. Only 6 of the 96 cases had an autopsy performed at the Clinical Center of the National Institutes of Health. The hearts of all 96 patients were examined initially by WCR and classified by him. Photographs were prepared of the heart in 60 of the 96 cases and all were available for examination. Histologic sections of the heart including aortic valve were examined in 72 of the 96 patients; in the remaining 24 cases the reports of the necropsy findings were examined. The hearts in 32 of the 96 cases were reexamined for this study.

Division of cases: The 96 cases were divided into 2 groups based on whether or not there was evidence that the aortic valve was stenotic before the valve be-

TABLE II Comparison of Patients with Active Infective Endocarditis Involving Stenotic and Nonstenotic Aortic Valves

	Stenotic (n = 25)	Nonstenotic (n = 71)	p Value
1. Age (year): range (mean)	21–86 (61)	17–81 (47)	0.002
≤30	2 (8%)	12 (17%)	0.278
31–60	10 (44%)	42 (59%)	0.098
>60	13 (52%)	17 (24%)	0.009
2. Men: women	23 (92%): 2 (8%)	52 (73%): 19 (27%)	0.051
3. Diagnosis of AS in life	23 (92%)	—	—
4. Diagnosis of IE in life	20 (80%)	48 (68%)	0.241
5. Infecting organism			
Bacterium			
Staphylococcal	7 (28%)	20 (28%)	0.987
Streptococcal	9 (36%)	22 (31%)	0.645
Mixed	4 (16%)	10 (14%)	0.816
Fungus	0	2 (3%)	1.0
Unknown	5 (20%)	17 (24%)	0.687
6. Predisposing factor			
Alcoholism	5 (20%)	20 (28%)	0.424
Opiate addiction	0	11 (15%)	0.06
Dental procedure	2 (8%)	5 (7%)	0.874
Hemodialysis	1 (4%)	4 (6%)	0.752
Previous IE	0	4 (6%)	0.57
Unknown	17 (68%)	27 (38%)	0.010
7. Aortic regurgitation murmur	11 (44%)	56 (79%)	0.001
8. Duration of IE (days)			
≤60	20 (80%)	45 (63%)	0.126
>60	1 (4%)	16 (23%)	0.037
Uncertain	4 (16%)	10 (14%)	0.816
9. Complete heart block	3 (12%)	4 (6%)	0.292
10. Pericardial effusion (>50 ml)	6/15 (40%)	11/43 (26%)	0.446
11. Aortic valve replacement	3 (12%)	18 (26%)	0.165
12. Heart weight (g): range (mean)	315–920 (594)	240–980 (514)	0.013
Men (n = 62)	315–920 (604)	340–980 (549)	0.098
Women (n = 14)	490 and 500	240–570 (389)	—
13. Number of aortic valve cusps			
2	10 (40%)	21 (30%)	0.338
3	15 (60%)	47 (66%)	0.577
Uncertain	0	3 (4%)	0.533
14. Aortic valve calcium			
0–1+	2 (8%)	17 (24%)	0.0001
2+–3+	23 (92%)	0	0.0001
15. No. of cusps with vegetation			
Bicuspid aortic valves	10	21	—
1	0	4 (19%)	0.28
2	10 (100%)	15 (71%)	0.060
Uncertain	0	2 (10%)	0.548
Tricuspid aortic valve	15	47	—
1	2 (13%)	13 (28%)	0.471
2	4 (27%)	12 (26%)	0.930
3	8 (53%)	20 (42%)	0.465
Uncertain	1 (7%)	2 (4%)	—
16. Vegetation on mitral valve	6 (24%)	19 (22%)	0.787
17. Ring abscess	21 (84%)	37 (52%)	0.005
18. Mitral annular calcium	4 (16%)	6 (8%)	0.288
19. Coronary artery embolus	4 (16%)	5 (7%)	0.186
20. Acute myocardial infarct	4 (16%)	4 (6%)	0.107
21. Stroke	2 (8%)	5 (7%)	0.874

AS = aortic stenosis; IE = infective endocarditis.

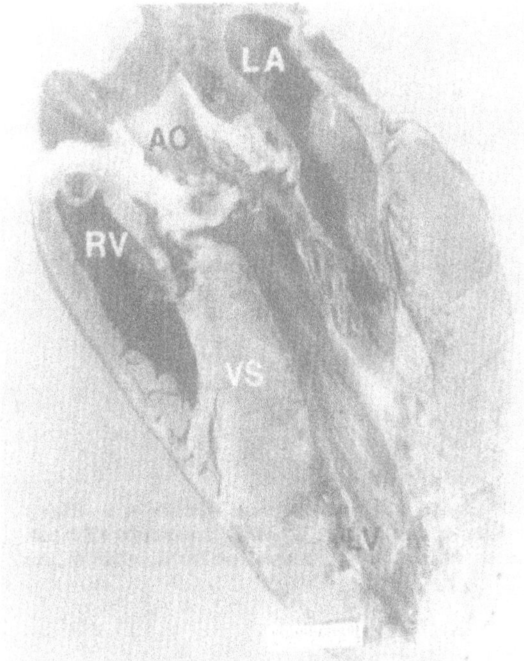

FIGURE 1. Case 1, Table I. Longitudinal view of heart (GT #76A-220) showing active infective endocarditis of a congenitally bicuspid and mildly stenotic aortic valve with extension of the infection into the right ventricular cavity via the ventricular septum (VS) and also with extension into the left atrial wall just cephalad to the anterior mitral leaflet. Left ventricular myocardium of the papillary muscle and of the subendocardial region is focally necrotic. Ao = aorta; LA = left atrium; LV = left ventricle; RV = right ventricle; VS = ventricular septum. (Reproduced with permission from Roberts WC, editor, Congenital Heart Disease in Adults, Philadelphia: FA Davis, 1979:422.)

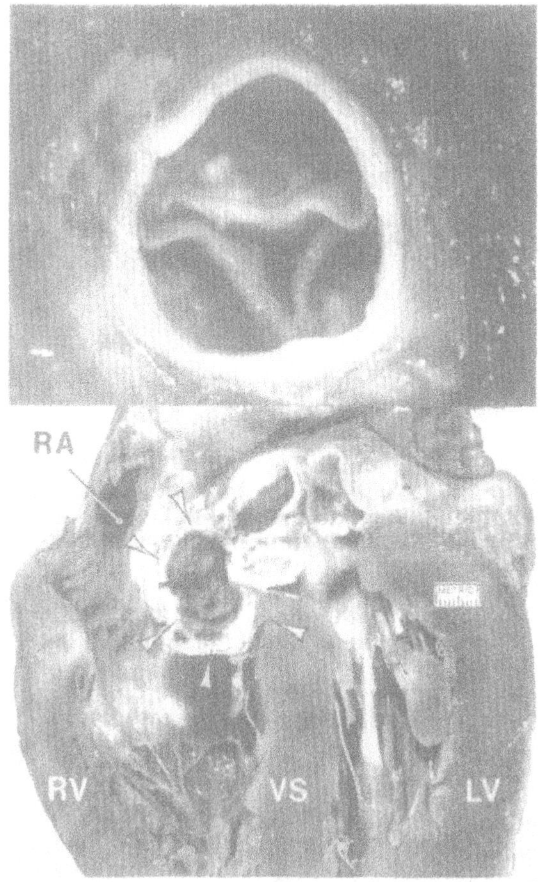

FIGURE 2. Case 6. *Top,* aortic valve seen from above (FSH# 4256). Each cusp is thickened and calcific deposits are present on their aortic surfaces. *Bottom:* longitudinal view of heart showing a large ring abscess *(arrows)* extending from the aortic valve toward the right atrial cavity. LV = left ventricular wall; RA = right atrial cavity; RV = right ventricular wall; VS = ventricular septum.

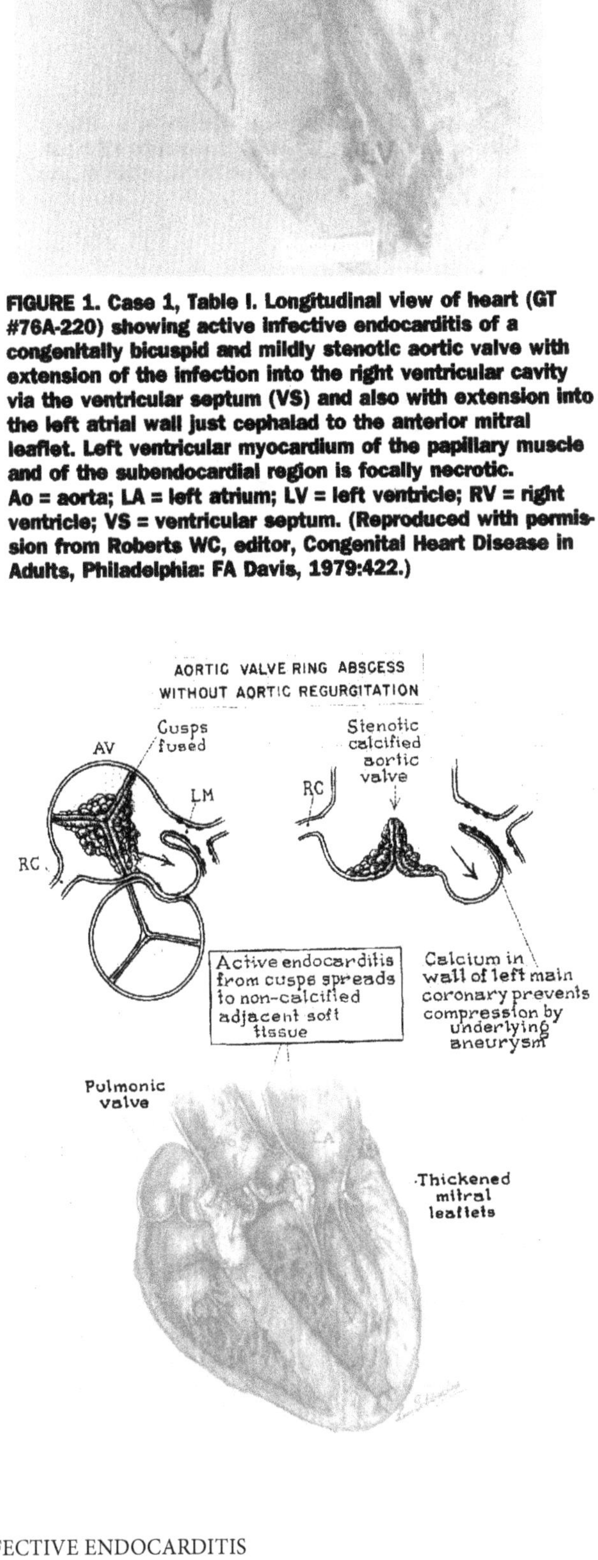

came the site of active IE. Of the 96 cases, 25 had preexisting aortic valve stenosis (Tables I and II) and 71 had nonstenotic aortic valves (Table II). The evidence of preexisting aortic stenosis was based on the finding at necropsy of heavy calcific deposits on the aortic aspects of the cusps resulting in loss of or severe reduction of mobility of the cusps leading to a clearly stenotic orifice. Twenty-three (92%) of the 25 patients had precordial ejection murmurs consistent with aortic valve stenosis, 6 had M-mode echocardiograms consistent with aortic valve stenosis, and 3 had cardiac catheterization with peak systolic pressure gradients recorded between the left ventricle and a systemic artery. Additionally, the presence of significant cardiomegaly without a history of systemic hypertension or the actual recording of an elevated systemic arterial diastolic blood pressure without

FIGURE 3. Case 8, Table I. Diagram of aortic valve (AV) (#33445) as seen from above *(upper left)* showing heavy calcific deposits and ring abscess *(arrow)* and longitudinal view of the valve *(upper right)* showing the ring abscess just beneath the left main (LM) coronary artery. *Lower,* longitudinal view showing large ring abscesses extending from the infection on the aortic valve. Ao = aorta; LA = left atrium; LV = left ventricle; RC = right coronary.

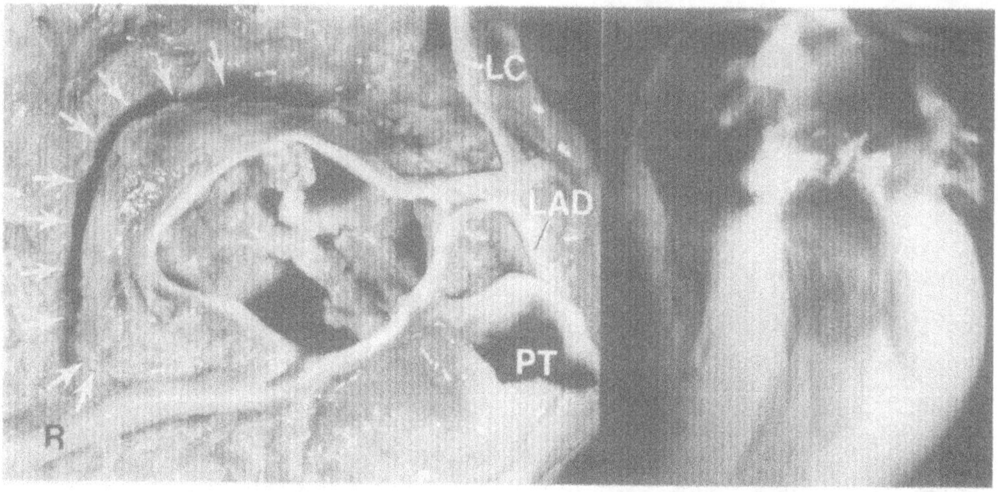

FIGURE 4. Case 9. ***Left,*** **Aortic valve (A75-55) seen from above showing a heavily calcified, severely stenotic valve with a large ring abscess *(arrows)* bulging toward the right atrium. LAD = left anterior descending; LC = left circumflex; PT = pulmonary trunk; R = right coronary arteries.** ***Right,*** **radiograph of the heart specimen showing heavy calcific deposits on the aortic valve.**

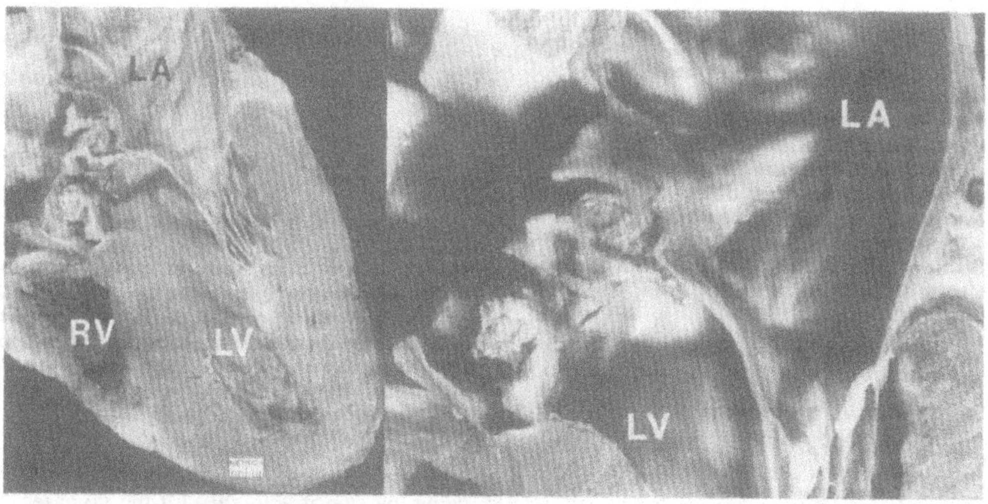

FIGURE 5. Case 15. ***Left,*** **longitudinal view of heart (FSH# A3965) showing active infective endocarditis of the aortic valve.** ***Right,*** **close-up view of the valve which is heavily calcified. Ring abscess is present in the area between aortic wall and wall of left atrium (LA). LV = left ventricle; RV = right ventricle.**

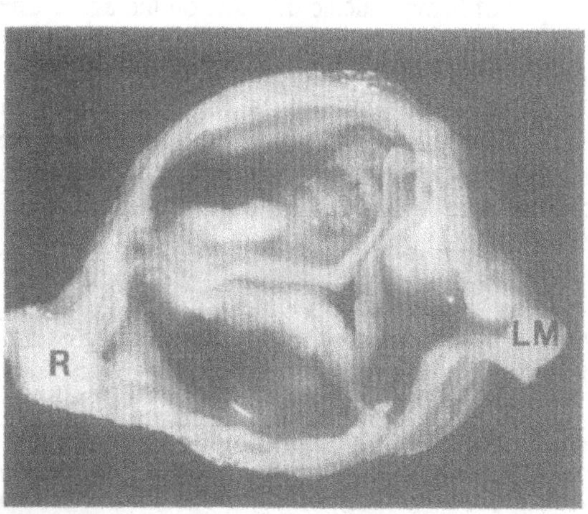

FIGURE 6. Case 20. Aortic valve (SH# A75-27) seen from above showing a small vegetation on the posterior cusp and calcific deposits in all 3 cusps. LM = left main; R = right coronary arteries.

significant aortic regurgitation supported the view of significant preexisting aortic valve stenosis.

Statistical analysis: Data were analyzed using SAS-PC, Stat View 512+, and MRTOD statistical software packages. Categorical comparisons were made with 2-tailed chi-squared analysis or with Fisher's exact test (where appropriate). Numerical comparisons were made using a 2-tailed paired *t* test. Frequency distributions were analyzed using the Stat View software package. Statistical significance was defined as $p < 0.05$.

RESULTS

Pertinent findings in each of the 25 patients with preexisting aortic valve stenosis are presented in Table I, and comparison of the findings in the 25 stenotic cases with those in the 71 nonstenotic cases are summarized in Table II. Some morphologic features of the active IE in the patients with preexisting aortic stenosis are illus-

FIGURE 7. Case 24. *Lower left,* diagram of the aortic and pulmonic valves seen from above *(left)* showing calcific deposits on the ventricular aspects of all 3 aortic valve cusps and the infection in the area between aortic and pulmonic valves causing compression of the wall of the pulmonic trunk. *Right,* longitudinal view (FSH# A4188) showing active infection of the aortic valve with extension of the infection into the most cephalad portion of the ventricular septum (VS) via a perforation of the right coronary cusp. The ring abscess extended also into the wall of the right atrium. LV = left ventricle; PT = pulmonary trunk; RV = right ventricle.

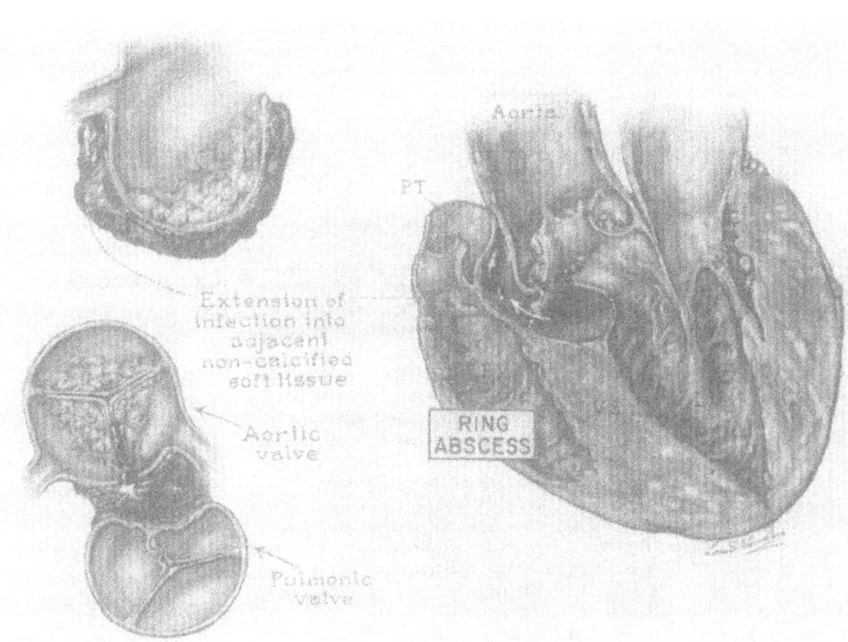

trated in Figures 1 to 7. The patients with stenotic aortic valves compared with those with nonstenotic aortic valves had significantly higher mean ages (61 vs 47 years), a higher percentage >60 years of age (52 vs 24%), a higher percentage of men (92 vs 73%), a higher frequency of an absent or unknown predisposing factor to infection (68 vs 38%), a lower frequency of a precordial murmur of aortic regurgitation (44 vs 79%), a lower percentage with a long duration (>60 days) of infection (4 vs 23%), a larger mean heart weight (594 vs 514 g), a higher percentage with aortic valve calcific deposits (100 vs 24%), and a higher frequency of associated ring abscess (84 vs 52%).

DISCUSSION

The present study indicates that active IE commonly affects previously stenotic aortic valves and that infection on previously stenotic aortic valves, in contrast to that involving previously nonstenotic ones, affects older patients (over 50% >60 years of age), mainly men (>90%), and that ring abscess is a frequent complication (>80%). Despite the presence of a ring abscess, associated aortic regurgitation occurred in less than half the patients with previously stenotic valves, whereas aortic regurgitation occurred in >80% of those with active IE involving a previously nonstenotic aortic valve.

Why is ring abscess significantly more common in patients with active IE superimposed on a previously stenotic valve than on a previously nonstenotic aortic valve? The answer probably is related to the presence of and amount of calcific deposits on the previously stenotic aortic valve. Microorganisms appear to grow poorly in calcific deposits ("rocks"), which were present in all patients with stenotic aortic valves and in <25%, and then of small size, of the patients with nonstenotic aortic valves. Because microorganisms appear to grow poorly in "rocks," the infective process spreads quickly to the adjacent noncalcific soft tissues and extension of the infection outside the aortic valve cusps results in ring abscess.

Because infection superimposed on a calcified aortic valve so often leads to the development of a ring abscess, which then makes valve replacement more difficult and decreases the frequency of a successful outcome, earlier operative intervention may be warranted in these patients compared with patients with active IE on previously nonstenotic aortic valves.

Although other publications have mentioned active IE complicating a previously stenotic aortic valve,[32–36] none have compared either clinical or necropsy findings in patients with previously stenotic to those with previously nonstenotic aortic valves. Indeed, review of 7 books on infective endocarditis disclosed no information on differences observed in patients with active IE superimposed on a previously stenotic valve compared with those on a previously nonstenotic aortic valve.[37–43]

1. Cooper T, Morrow AG, Roberts WC, Herman LG. Postoperative endocarditis due to Candida: clinical observations the experimental production of the lesion. *Surgery* 1961;50:341–346.
2. Andriole VT, Kravetz HM, Roberts WC, Utz JP. Candida endocarditis. Clinical and pathology studies. *Am J Med* 1962;32:251–285.
3. Roberts WC, Rabson AS. Focal glomerular lesions in fungal endocarditis. *Ann Intern Med* 1962;56:610–618.
4. Roberts WC, Braunwald E, Morrow AG. Acute severe mitral regurgitation secondary to ruptured chordae tendineae. Clinical, hemodynamic, and pathologic considerations. *Circulation* 1966;33:58–70.
5. Cohn LH, Roberts WC, Rockoff SD, Morrow AG. Bacterial endocarditis following aortic valve replacement. Clinical and pathologic correlations. *Circulation* 1966;33:209–217.
6. Archard HO, Roberts WC. Bacterial endocarditis after dental procedures in patients with aortic valve prostheses. *J Am Dent Assoc* 1966;72:648–652.
7. Roberts WC, Ewy GA, Glancy DL, Marcus FI. Valvular stenosis produced by active infective endocarditis. *Circulation* 1967;36:449–451.
8. Buchbinder NA, Roberts WC. Active infective endocarditis confined to mural endocardium. A study of six necropsy patients. *Arch Pathol* 1972;45:769–792.
9. Roberts WC, Buchbinder NA. Right-sided valvular infective endocarditis. A clinicopathologic study of twelve necropsy patients. *Am J Med* 1972;53:7–19.
10. Buchbinder NA, Roberts WC. Left-sided valvular active infective endocarditis. A study of forty-five necropsy patients. *Am J Med* 1972;53:20–35.

11. Buchbinder NA, Roberts WC. Alcoholism, an important but unemphasized factor predisposing to infective endocarditis. *Arch Intern Med* 1973;132:689–692.
12. Arnett EN, Roberts WC. Valve ring abscess in active infective endocarditis. Frequency, location, and clues to clinical diagnosis from the study of 95 necropsy patients. *Circulation* 1976;54:140–145.
13. Arnett EA, Roberts WC. Prosthetic valve endocarditis. Clinicopathologic analysis of 22 necropsy patients with comparison of observations in 74 necropsy patients with active infective endocarditis involving natural left-sided cardiac valves. *Am J Cardiol* 1976;38:281–292.
14. Arnett EN, Roberts WC. Active infective endocarditis: a clinicopathology analysis of 137 necropsy patients. *Curr Probl Cardiol* 1976;7:1–76.
15. Arnett EN, Roberts WC. Clinicopathology of prosthetic valve endocarditis. In: Duma RJ, ed. Infections of Prosthetic Heart Valves and Vascular Grafts. Prevention, Diagnosis, and Treatment. Baltimore: University Park Press, 1977:17–41.
16. Arnett EN, Kastl DG, Garvin AJ, Roberts WC. A conversation on prosthetic valve endocarditis. *Am Heart J* 1977;93:510–517.
17. Andy JJ, Shekh MU, Ali N, Barnes BO, Fox LM, Curry CL, Roberts WC. Echocardiographic observations in opiate addicts with active infective endocarditis. Frequency of involvement of the various valves and comparisons of echocardiographic features of right and left-sided cardiac valve endocarditis. *Am J Cardiol* 1977;40:17–23.
18. Roberts WC, Buchbinder NA. Healed left-sided infective endocarditis: a clinicopathologic study of 59 patients. *Am J Cardiol* 1977;40:876–888.
19. Roberts WC. Characteristics and consequences of infective endocarditis (active or healed or both) learned from morphologic studies. In: Rahimtoola SH, ed. Infective Endocarditis. New York: Grune & Stratton, 1978:55–123.
20. Breyer RH, Arnett EN, Spray TL, Roberts WC. Prosthetic valve endocarditis due to *Listeria monocytogenes*. *Am J Clin Pathol* 1978;69:186–187.
21. Ferrans VJ, Boyce SW, Billingham ME, Spray TL, Roberts WC. Infection of glutaraldehyde-preserved porcine valve heterografts. *Am J Cardiol* 1979;43:1123–1136.
22. Billingham ME, Ferrans VJ, Boyce SW, Spray TL, Roberts WC. Bacterial infection in implanted porcine valve heterografts: a histopathologic and ultrastructural study. In: Sebening F, Klovekorn WP, Meisner H, Struck E, eds. Proceedings of the Symposium on Bioprosthetic Cardiac Valves; Munich, April 5–7, 1979. Deutsches Herzzentrum Muncehn, Federal Republic of Germany, 1979:281–294.
23. Davis WA, Isner JM, Bracey AW, Roberts WC, Garagusi VF. Disseminated petriellidium boydiii and pacemaker endocarditis. *Am J Med* 1980;69:929–932.
24. Sheikh MU, Covarrubias EA, Ali N, Lee WR, Sheikh NM, Roberts WC. M-mode echocardiographic observations during and after healing of active bacterial endocarditis limited to the mitral valve. *Am Heart J* 1981;101:37–45.
25. Sheikh MU, Covarrubias EA, Ali N, Sheikh NM, Lee WR, Roberts WC. M-mode echocardiographic observations in active bacterial endocarditis limited to the aortic valve. *Am Heart J* 1981;102:66–75.
26. McManus BM, Katz NM, Blackbourne BD, Gottdiener JS, Wallace RB, Roberts WC. Acquired cor triatriatum (left ventricular false aneurysm): complication of active infective endocarditis of the aortic valve with ring abscess treated by valve replacement. *Am Heart J* 1982;104:312–314.
27. Arnett EN, Roberts WC. Pathology of active infective endocarditis: a necropsy analysis of 192 patients. *Thorac Cardiovasc Surg* 1982;30:327–335.
28. Silver MA, Roberts WC. Active infective endocarditis complicating idiopathic dilated cardiomyopathy. *Am J Cardiol* 1983;52:651–652.
29. Barbour DJ, Roberts WC. Valve excision only versus valve excision plus replacement for active infective endocarditis involving the tricuspid valve. *Am J Cardiol* 1986;57:475–478.
30. Dressler FA, Roberts WC. Infective endocarditis in opiate addicts: Analysis of 80 cases studied at necropsy. *Am J Cardiol* 1989;63:1240–1257.
31. Roberts WC, Kishel JC, McIntosh CL, Cannon RO III, Maron BJ. Severe mitral or aortic valve regurgitation, or both, requiring valve replacement for infective endocarditis complicating hypertrophic cardiomyopathy. *J Am Coll Cardiol* 1992;19:365–371.
32. Bayles TB, Lewis WH Jr. Subacute bacterial endocarditis in older people. *Ann Intern Med* 1940;13:2154–2163.
33. Gouley BA, Sickel E. Aortic regurgitation caused by dilatation of the aortic orifice and associated with a characteristic valvular lesion. *Am Heart J* 1943;26:24–38.
34. Seabury JH. Subacute bacterial endocarditis. Experiences during the past decade. *Arch Intern Med* 1947;79:1–21.
35. Lichtman P, Master AM. The incidence of valvular heart disease in people over fifty and penicillin prophylaxis of bacterial endocarditis. *NY State J Med* 1949;49:1693–1698.
36. Applefeld MM, Hornick RB. Infective endocarditis in patients over age 60. *Am Heart J* 1974;88:90–94.
37. Kerr A Jr. Subacute Bacterial Endocarditis. Springfield, IL: Charles C. Thomas, 1955:343.
38. Kay D, editor. Infective Endocarditis. Baltimore: University Park Press, 1976:272.
39. Kaplan EL, Taranta AV, editors. Infective Endocarditis. An American Heart Association Symposium. Dallas, Texas: The American Heart Association, Inc., 1977:95.
40. Rahimtoola SH, editor. Infective Endocarditis. New York: Grune & Stratton, 1978:386.
41. Freedman LR. Infective Endocarditis and Other Intravascular Infections. New York: Plenum Medical Book Co., 1982:243.
42. Sande MA, Kaye D, Root RK, editors. Endocarditis. New York: Churchill Livingstone, 1984:234.
43. Magilligan DJ Jr, Quinn EL. Endocarditis. Medical and Surgical Management. New York: Marcel Dekker, 1986:269.

ADDENDUM

The manuscript of this article had initially been sent to the *Journal of the American College of Cardiology* (JACC) (their #JAC921143) and it was declined by that journal because ". . . its priority is [was] too low to warrant publication in JACC."

The comments of the 2 JACC reviewers were as follows:

Reviewer #1

"A well conceived and presented paper giving new information regarding infective endocarditis. I have only two suggestions:

1. a reduction in the number of figures (2, 5, 6, 8 and 9) since I believe with the artistic drawings and the remaining specimens [present] the message you wish to transmit is accomplished;

2. with 52% of the non-stenotic valves having ring abscess, this group also warrants careful evaluation and believe paper would be strengthened by some comment about this. Dr. Roberts needs to decide if he is first or last author?"

Reviewer #2

"1. It should be made clear that since the information presented in this paper was derived from a study of necropsy cases, the data cannot necessarily be applied to the treatment of living patients. For example, the authors suggest that those patients with infectious endocarditis and aortic stenosis should be operated earlier because of the propensity of this group to develop ring abscesses. It may be correct, but, on the other hand, it may be that those patients with ring abscesses and aortic stenosis are those who came to autopsy. Unless one knew the denominator, i.e., the entire set of patients with aortic valve disease and infectious endocarditis, one could not justify this conclusion.

2. The observation that older men with large hearts are those with aortic stenosis is in keeping with the well know propensity for this group to have this pathology.

3. The explanation for the formation of ring abscesses in patients with aortic stenosis is extremely speculative and not substantiated by any fact. The suggestion that the micro-organisms do not grow well on 'rocks' and consequently spread out into the peri-aortic tissue is interesting but certainly not substantiated. One could easily speculate in the same way that the hemodynamics of aortic stenosis in some way influence the perivalvular tissue to make it less resistant to infection, but, again, this would be without evidence. The concept of bacteria seeking out a place to grow because one atmosphere is hostile is hard to substantiate.

4. The number of illustrations submitted is excessive. Many of them are redundant and could be eliminated."

Clinicopathologic Features of Active Infective Endocarditis Isolated to the Native Mitral Valve

Daniel J. Fernicola, MD, and William C. Roberts, MD*

Although a number of clinicopathologic studies in patients with active infective endocarditis (IE) have been reported, none have focused on patients studied at necropsy with active IE isolated to the mitral valve. We studied at necropsy 63 patients (aged 12 to 88 years [mean 50], 44 males [70%]) with active IE limited to the native mitral valve: 21 (33%) had preexisting mitral valve disease (rheumatic in 8, prolapse in 3, hypertrophic cardiomyopathy in 1, and mitral annular calcium in 9), and the other 42 patients (67%) had previously normal mitral valves. Of the latter 42 patients, 22 (52%) had recognized predisposing factors to IE: opiate addiction in 14, habitual alcoholism in 6 and/or chronic hemodialysis in 4. *Staphylococcus aureus* or *epidermidis* was the responsible organism in 32 patients (51%), and the active IE was associated with an infection elsewhere in the body in 31 patients (50%). The active IE caused rupture of mitral chordae tendineae in 11 patients (18%), perforation of the anterior mitral leaflet in 7 patients (11%), and mitral ring abscess in 10 patients (16%). Grossly visible systemic emboli were found in 44 patients (70%) and 33 (52%) had infarcts in 1 or more body organs.

Thus, active IE isolated to the mitral valve in necropsied patients appears to be more common in males than females (2 to 1); the infection more commonly than not involves a preexisting anatomically normal valve rather than a preexisting abnormal one (2 to 1); the vegetations often do not cause or worsen valvular dysfunction; a predisposing factor is commonly present (2 of 3 patients), and the IE commonly is part of a generalized or systemic infection (1 of 2 patients).

(Am J Cardiol 1993;71:1186–1197)

From the Pathology Branch, National Heart, Lung, and Blood Institute, National Institutes of Health, Bethesda, Maryland. Manuscript received November 10, 1992; revised manuscript received and accepted December 4, 1992.

*Present address: Baylor Cardiovascular Institute, Baylor University Medical Center, 3701 Junius Street, P.O. Box E010, Dallas, Texas 75246.

Address for reprints: Pathology Branch, National Heart, Lung, and Blood Institute, National Institute of Health, Building 10, Room 2N258, Bethesda, Maryland 20892.

Although numerous reports from this laboratory and elsewhere have described clinical and morphologic features of active infective endocarditis (IE) involving native left-sided cardiac valves,[1–12] surprisingly, few have focused on patients with active IE limited to the mitral valve, and none have described both clinical and morphologic features in patients with active IE limited to the mitral valve. Such is the purpose of the present report.

METHODS

Patients studied: The files of patients in the Pathology Branch, National Heart, Lung, and Blood Institute, were searched for cases coded as active IE on 1 or more native cardiac valves (active infection involving patients with prostheses or bioprostheses and those in patients with congenital cardiovascular shunts were excluded). A total of 217 cases were retrieved. Of this number, 74 (34%) had vegetations limited to the aortic valve,[12] 27 (12.5%) had vegetations on both aortic and mitral valves,[12] 67 (30.5%) had vegetations limited to the mitral valve, and 49 (23%) had vegetations on 1 or both right-sided cardiac valves with or without involvement of 1 or both left-sided cardiac valves. This report is limited to the patients with vegetations limited to the mitral valve. Of the 67 patients, 3 were eliminated from this study because 2 with mitral stenosis had had mitral commissurotomy, and 1 patient, who had hypertrophic cardiomyopathy, had had ventricular septal myotomy and myectomy.

Inclusion criteria: To be included in this study the following criteria were met: (1) age at death >10 years; (2) 1 or more vegetations on the mitral valve at necropsy and no vegetations on any of the other 3 cardiac valves; and (3) never a cardiac operation. Of the 63 patients, 52 (82%) had received 1 or more antibiotics shortly before death, and 11 (17%) had not received antibiotics during the last month of life.

Sources of cases: The 63 patients had necropsies performed at 16 different medical institutions and the hearts were subsequently submitted to the Pathology Branch, National Heart, Lung, and Blood Institute, for examination. The medical records from the submitting medical center subsequently were examined. Of the 63 cases, 12 had the necropsy performed at the Clinical Center of the National Institutes of Health; 9 at Georgetown University Medical Center; 8 at the District of Columbia Medical Examiners' Office; 7 at the District of Columbia General Hospital; 5 at the District of Columbia Veterans' Administration Hospital; 5 at Howard University Hospital; 5 at the Washington Hospital Center; 3 at George Washington University Hospital; 2 at Suburban Hospital (Bethesda, Maryland), and 1 each from 7 different medical centers. The hearts in all 63 patients were

TABLE I Clinical and Morphologic Features of 21 Patients with Anatomically Abnormal Mitral Valves Prior to Infective Endocarditis

Case	Age (years)	Race	Sex	RHD	HC	MVP	MAC	Predisposing Factors: O	HA	H	P	Mn	Infecting Organism	Mode of Death: Sepsis	Embolus	CHF	HW (g)	LV: Fi	N	Ring Abscess	RCT	PAML	SE	Gross Organ Infarcts: Brain	Spleen	Kidney	Heart	Other
1	21	B	F	+	0	0	0	0	0	0	0	0	Beta streptococcus	0	+	0	400	0	0	0	+	0	+	+	+	+	0	0
2	37	B	M	+[1]	0	0	0	+	0	0	+	+	—	+	0	0	350	0	0	0	0	0	+	+	+	+	0	+
3	49	W	M	+[1]	0	0	0	0	+	0	0	0	Alpha streptococcus	0	0	0[2]	530	+	0	0	+	0	+	—	—	—	0	—
4	58	W	M	+	0	0	0	0	0	0	0	0	*Staphylococcus aureus*	+	0	0	450	0	0	0	0	0	+	+	+	+	0	+
5	59	W	M	+[1]	0	0	0	0	0	0	0	0	*Pseudomonas aeruginosa*	0	+	0	350	0	0	0	0	0	+	—	—	—	0	—
6	62	W	M	+	0	0	0	0	—	0	—	—	Beta streptococcus	0	+	0	—	+	0	0	0	0	+	—	—	—	0	—
7	66	W	F	+[1]	0	0	0	0	0	0	0	0	Group D streptococcus	0	0	+	600	0	0	0	0	0	+	0	+	0	0	+
8	72	W	F	+[1]	0	0	0	0	0	0	0	0	*Staphylococcus aureus*	+	0	0	480	0	0	+	0	0	—	—	—	—	0	—
9	49	W	M	0	+	0	0	0	0	0	0	0	*Staphylococcus aureus*	0	0	+	650	0	+	0	0	0	+	0	0	+	+	0
10	52	W	M	0	0	+	0	0	0	0	0	0	*Staphylococcus aureus*	0	+	0	—	0	0	0	0	0	+	+	+	+	0	+
11	54	W	M	0	0	+	0	0	0	0	+	+	*Staphylococcus aureus*	0	+	0	500	0	0	0	0	0	+	+	+	+	0	0
12	64	W	F	0	0	+	0	0	0	0	0	0	Alpha streptococcus	0	+	0	275	0	0	0	0	0	+	+	0	0	0	0
13	45	B	F	0	0	0	+	0	0	+	0	0	*Staphylococcus aureus*	—	—	—	—	0	0	0	0	0	—	—	—	0	0	—
14	50	B	M	0	0	0	+	0	0	+	0	0	*Staphylococcus aureus*	0	0	0[3]	520	0	0	0	0	0	0	0	0	0	0	0
15	55	B	F	0	0	0	+	0	0	+	0	0	*Staphylococcus aureus*	+	0	0	360	0	0	+	0	0	+	0	0	+[4]	0	+
16	58	W	F	0	0	0	+	0	0	+	0	0	*Staphylococcus aureus*	—	—	—	—	0	+[5]	0	0	0	—	—	—	—	0	—
17	63	W	M	0	0	0	+	0	0	+	0	0	*Staphylococcus aureus*	0	+	0	530	0	+[5]	0	0	0	+	0	0	0	0	0
18	79	W	M	0	0	0	+	0	0	0	0	0	*Staphylococcus aureus*	—	—	—	530	+	+	0	0	0	—	—	—	—	+	—
19	83	W	M	0	0	0	+	0	0	0	0	0	Beta streptococcus	0	—	0	535	0	0	0	0	0	—	—	—	0	—	—
20	84	W	M	0	0	0	+	0	0	0	+	0	*Staphylococcus aureus*	0	0	0	505	+	0	0	0	0	0	0	0	0	0	0
21	85	W	M	0	0	0	+	0	0	0	+	0	Beta streptococcus	+	0	0	540	0	+	+	0	0	+	0	+	+	+	+
Total or mean	59			8	1	3	9	1	1	5	4	2		5	7	2	479	4	5	3	2	0	14	6	7	8	3	6

[1]Mitral stenosis present; [2]sudden cardiac death without coronary artery embolus but atherosclerotic coronary artery disease; [3]died from hyperkalemia; [4]abscesses of transplanted kidney; [5]myocardial abscess.
B = black; CHF = congestive heart failure; CT = chordae tendineae; F = female; Fi = fibrosis; H = hemodialysis; HA = habitual alcoholism; HC = hypertrophic cardiomyopathy; HW = heart weight; LV = left ventricular; M = male; MAC = mitral annular calcium; Mn = meningitis; MVP = mitral valve prolapse; N = necrosis; O = opiate addict; P = pneumonia; PAML = perforated anterior mitral leaflet; RCT = ruptured chordae tendineae; RHD = rheumatic heart disease; SE = systemic emboli; W = white.

examined initially by WCR, and in 27 patients the hearts were reexamined by DJF. Photographs of the heart were available in 43 cases (68%).

Year of necropsy: Of the 63 cases, 2 (3%) died in the decade 1951–1960; 8 (13%), from 1961–1970; 22 (35%) from 1971–1980; and 31 (49%) from 1981–1990.

Methods of examining the hearts: After "cleaning" each heart of extraneous tissue, the heart was weighed. All portions of the heart including epicardial coronary arteries, valves, and myocardium were carefully examined for lesions (abnormalities) and those observed were recorded. Histologic sections were prepared of myocardium and valvular vegetations and often of epicardial coronary arteries.

Statistical analysis: Data were analyzed using StatView 512+ statistical software package. Categorical comparisons were made with 2-tailed chi-squared analysis. Numerical comparisons were made using a 2-tailed, unpaired *t* test. Statistical significance was defined as $p < 0.05$.

RESULTS

CLINICAL FINDINGS

Age, sex, race: The 63 patients ranged in age from 12 to 88 years (mean 50); 31 were white, 28 were black, and 1 was Hispanic; 19 (30%) were female and 44 (70%) were male. Two patients (3%) were in their teens and 7 patients (11%) were over 70 years of age.

Underlying heart disease: Of the 63 patients, 21 (33%) had underlying cardiac valve disease before active IE: rheumatic heart disease in 8 patients (13%) (mitral stenosis in 5)[13]; mitral valve prolapse in 3 patients (5%)[14]; hypertrophic cardiomyopathy in 1 (2%)[15]; and mitral annular calcium in 9 patients (15%).[16] Certain clinical and necropsy findings in each of the 21 patients with underlying heart disease are tabulated in Table I and illustrated in Figures 1 to 7, and the findings in each of the 42 patients without underlying structural heart disease are listed in Table II and illustrated in Figures 8 to 16.

Other risk factors to infective endocarditis: In addition to underlying structural heart disease (21 patients), other predisposing factors to IE were present in 29 patients (46%), 7 of whom also had underlying structural valvular heart disease: opiate addiction in 15 patients (24%)[11]; habitual alcoholism in 7 patients (11%),[5] and chronic hemodialysis in 9 patients (14%).[16] Four patients (cases 29, 31, 34 and 33, Table I) had ≥2 episodes of active IE. The initial episode appeared to predispose to a subsequent one. The data recorded in the table concerns only the last episode of active IE. One patient (no.

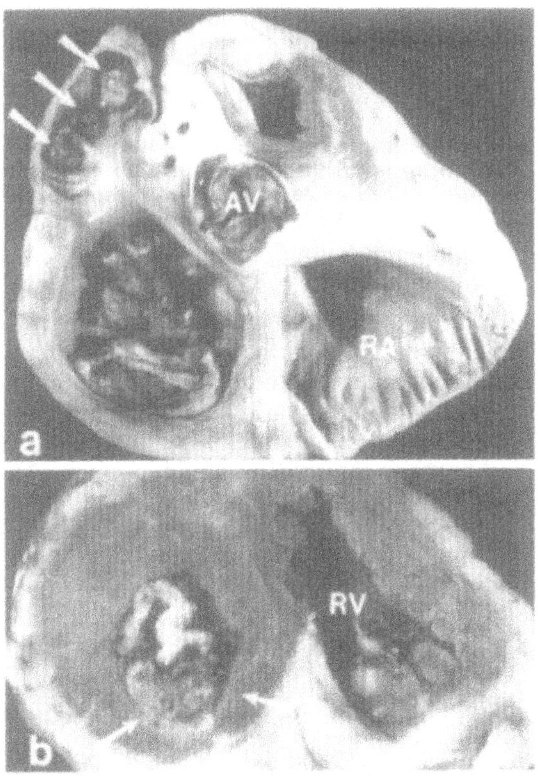

FIGURE 1. (Case 5, Table I.) Views of the base of the heart in a 66-year-old woman with mitral stenosis (NIH# A76-175) who developed infective endocarditis due to group D enterococcus 3 months before death. *a*, the opened left atrial cavity discloses vegetation attached to the atrial aspect of the mitral leaflet and also thrombi *(arrows)* in the left atrial appendage. *b*, vegetation *(arrows)* on the ventricular aspect of the mitral leaflets. The mitral orifice is diminished by the vegetative material and the mitral leaflets are considerably thickened. AV = aortic valve; RA = right atrium; RV = right ventricle.

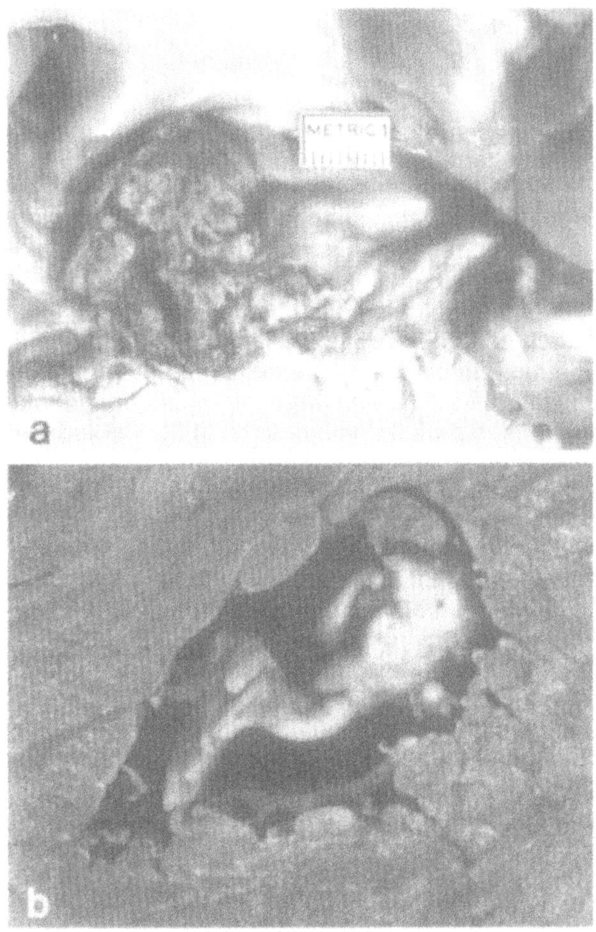

FIGURE 2. (Case 7, Table I.) Mitral valve with superimposed vegetation in a 59-year-old man (NIH# A84-134) with mitral stenosis. *a*, view of vegetation on the opened mitral valve. *b*, stenotic valve from the left ventricular aspect.

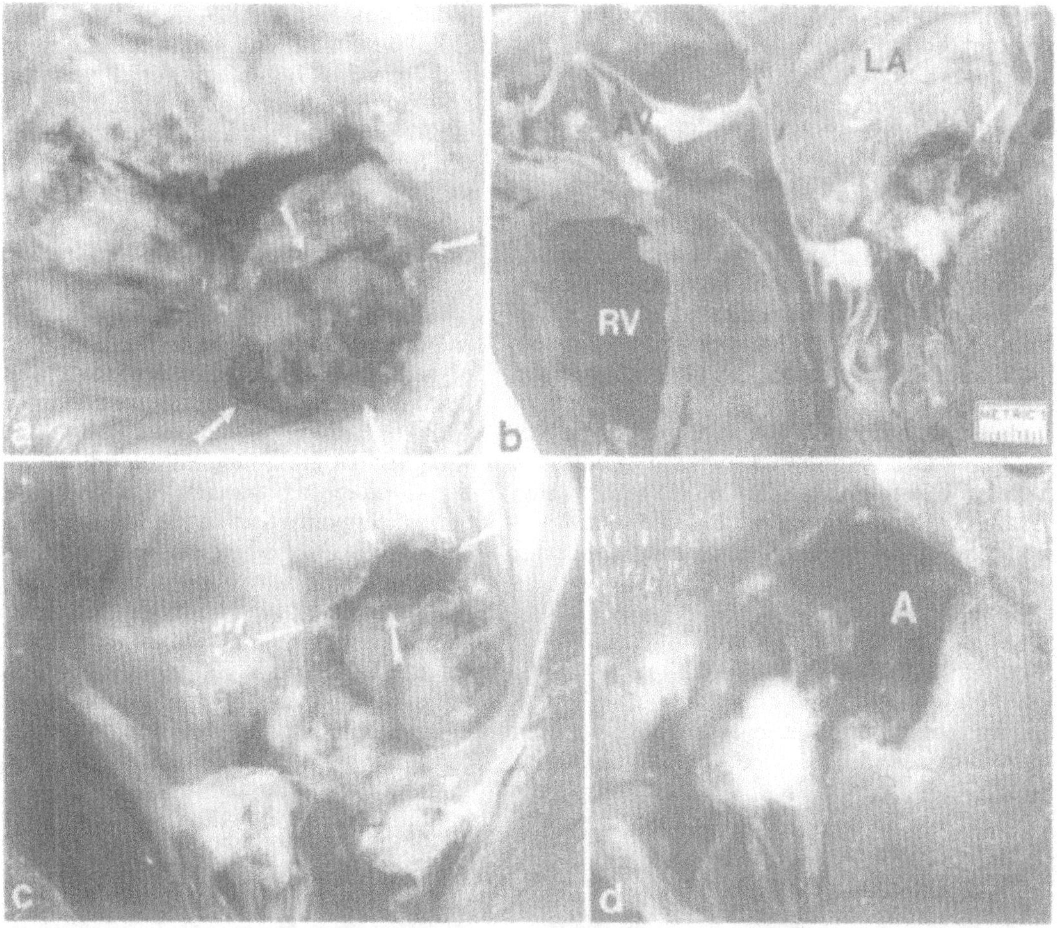

FIGURE 3. (Case 9, Table I.) Mitral valve in a 72-year-old woman with severe mitral stenosis. *a*, view from left atrium showing a vegetation *(arrows)* and the stenotic orifice. *b*, view of valve after longitudinal cut showing the thickened mitral leaflets and the vegetation *(arrow)*. *c*, close-up view of entrance *(arrows)* into a ring abscess. *d*, view of the ring abscess (A). AV = aortic valve; LA = left atrium; RV = right ventricle.

18, Table II), who had structurally normal cardiac valves, had idiopathic dilated cardiomyopathy.[17]

Organisms causing the infective endocarditis: The microorganisms responsible for the active IE are listed in Tables I and II. *Staphylococcus aureus* or *epidermidis* was responsible in 32 patients (51%); streptococcus species in 11 patients (17%); a gram-negative organism in 6 patients (10%); fungal species in 3 patients[1] (5%); and *Streptococcus pneumoniae* in 2 patients (3%). In 7 patients (11%), no information was available regarding the results of blood cultures. In 2 patients (3%) repeated blood cultures were negative but antibiotics were being administered at the time.

Infection in noncardiac organs and tissues: Infection involving organs other than the heart occurred in at least 31 (49%) of the 63 patients. Of the 31 patients, 25 had associated acute pneumonia or meningitis or both, 3 had huge renal abscesses, and 3 had systemic fungal infections involving 1 or more noncardiac organs.[1]

NECROPSY FINDINGS

Heart weight: At necropsy, the hearts in the 63 patients ranged in weight from 195 to 715 g (mean 432). Those in the 19 women ranged from 195 to 600 g (mean 333), and those in the 44 men from 270 to 715 g (mean 471) ($p < 0.05$). The heart weights in the 42 patients without preexisting heart disease ranged from 195 to 715 g (mean 410) (women = 289 g, men = 459 g), and in the 21 with preexisting heart disease from 275 to 650 g (mean 479) (women = 423 g, men = 499 g).

Mitral valve consequences: The active IE caused rupture of mitral chordae tendineae in 11 patients (18%), perforation of the anterior mitral leaflet in 7 patients (11%), and mitral ring abscess in 10 patients (16%).

Systemic emboli and infarcts: Grossly visible systemic emboli were found in 44 patients (70%) and 33

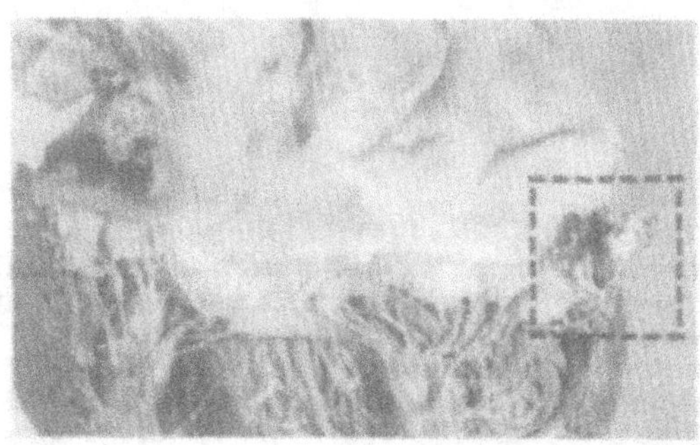

FIGURE 4. (Case 11, Table I.) Opened mitral valve showing a vegetation *(box)* on the posterior leaflet in a 54-year-old man (NIH# A60-27) with preexisting mitral regurgitation from prolapse.

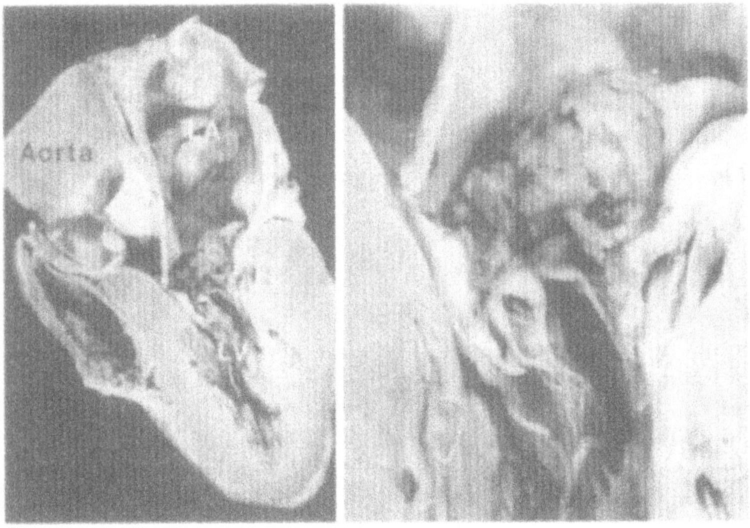

FIGURE 5. (Case 12, Table I.) Mitral valve in a 64-year-old woman (GT# 83A-173) whose first symptom of infective endocarditis was a cerebrovascular accident. *a*, longitudinal view showing a huge vegetation on a "floppy" mitral valve. *b*, close-up view. LA = left atrium; LV = left ventricle.

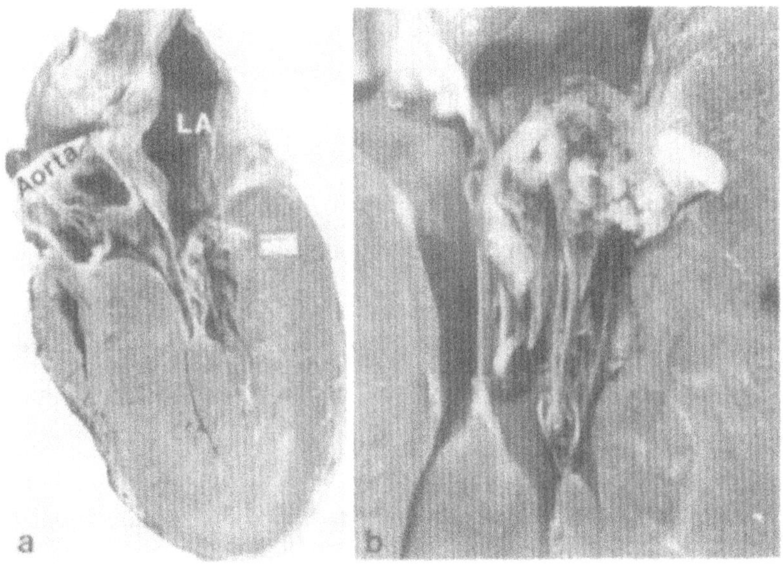

FIGURE 6. (Case 19, Table I.) Infective endocarditis involving a calcified mitral valve annulus in an 83-year-old man (GT# 85A-11) with bullous pemphigoid. *a*, longitudinal cut showing the vegetation on the mitral valve and mitral annular calcium extending into left ventricular myocardium. *b*, close-up view of the mitral valve showing vegetative material and "annular" calcium. At no time before or during the episode of active infective endocarditis were signs or symptoms of heart disease present. The diagnosis of infective endocarditis was not made until autopsy. LA = left atrium.

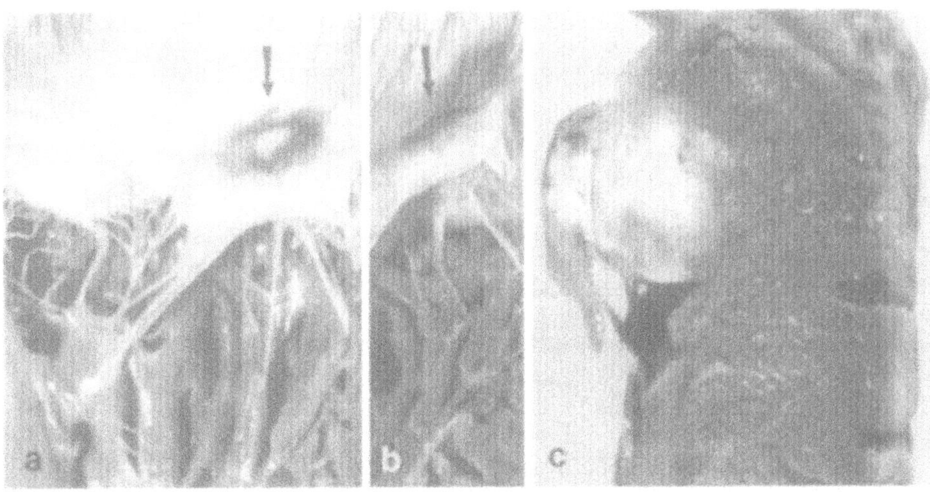

FIGURE 7. (Case 20, Table I.) Mitral valve with infective endocarditis superimposed on mitral annular calcium in an 84-year-old man (DCGH# 82A-34) who presented with pneumonia and was found to have *Staphylococcus aureus* in blood cultures. *a*, view of opened valve showing infection on the atrial aspect of the posterior leaflet. *b*, similar view but underlying annular calcium is now visible. *c*, longitudinal view of calcified mitral "annulus" with superimposed infection.

TABLE II Clinical and Morphologic Features of 42 Patients with Previously Normal Mitral Valves Prior to Active Infective Endocarditis

Case	Age (years)	Race	Sex	Predisposing Factors: O	HA	H	P	Mn	Infecting Organism	MR	Mode of Death: Sepsis	Embolus	CHF	HW (g)	LV: Fi	N	Ring Abscess	RCT	PAML	SE	Gross Organ Infarcts: Brain	Spleen	Kidney	Heart	Other
1	12	W	F	0	0	0	0	0	*Staphylococcus aureus*	0	0	+	0	205	0	+[1]	+	0	0	+	+	—	0	0	—
2	20	B	F	+	0	0	0	+	*Staphylococcus aureus*	0	+	0	+	210	0	0	0	0	0	+	—	—	+	0	—
3	28	W	F	0	0	0	0	+	*Staphylococcus aureus*	0	+	0	0	280	0	0	0	0	0	+	+	+	+	0	+
4	28	B	F	+	0	+	+	0	*Staphylococcus aureus*	0	+	0	0	390	0	+[1]	0	0	0	+	—	+	—	+	+
5	32	B	M	+	0	0	0	0	—	0	0	—	—	335	0	0	0	+	0	0	0	0	0	0	0
6	36	B	M	+	0	+	+	0	Alpha streptococcus	0	+	0	0	715	0	0	0	0	0	0	0	0	0	0	0
7	43	B	M	0	+	0	+	+	*Streptococcus pneumoniae*	0	0	0	0[3]	440	0	+	0	0	+	+	—	—	—	+	—
8	43	His	M	+	0	0	0	0	—	0	0	+	0	535	0	+	0	0	0	+	—	—	—	+	—
9	46	B	M	0	0	0	0	0	*Escherichia coli*[4]	0	0	0	0[5]	620	0	0	+	0	0	+	+	0	0	0	0
10	49	W	M	0	0	0	0	0	*Staphylococcus aureus*[4]	0	0	0	0[3]	280	0	0	0	0	0	0	0	0	0	0	0
11	52	B	M	0	0	+	0	0	*Aspergillus fumigatus*	0	+	0	0	—	0	0	0	0	0	+	+	+	+	0	0
12	54	W	F	0	0	0	+	0	*Pseudomonas aeruginosa*	0	0	+	0	195	0	0	+	0	0	+	0	+	+	0	0
13	54	B	M	0	0	0	0	0	—	0	0	+	0	520	0	0	0	0	0	+	+	—	—	0	—
14	55	—	M	0	0	0	0	0	—	0	—	—	—	—	0	0	0	0	0	+	—	+	+	0	—
15	58	W	M	0	+	0	+	0	*Staphylococcus aureus*	0	+	0	0	420	0	+[1]	0	0	0	+	0	0	+	0	—
16	58	W	M	0	0	0	0	0	*Mucormycosis*	0	0	+	0	340	0	+[1]	0	0	0	+	+	+	+	0	0
17	58	W	M	0	0	0	+	0	*Staphylococcus epidermis*	0	0	+[6]	0	370	0	0	0	0	+	+[2]	0	0	0	0	0
18	60	B	M	0	+	0	0	0	*Staphylococcus aureus*	0	+	0	0	600	0	0	0	0	0	—	—	—	—	0	—
19	62	W	F	0	0	0	0	+	*Staphylococcus aureus*	0	0	—	—	—	0	0	0	0	0	—	—	—	—	0	—
20	63	W	F	0	0	0	0	0	*Escherichia coli*	0	0	0	0[3]	380	0	0	0	0	0	0	—	0	0	0	0
21	64	B	M	0	+	0	+	+	*Streptococcus pneumoniae*	0	+	0	0	—	0	0	0	0	0	—	—	—	—	0	—
22	74	W	M	0	0	0	+	0	*Staphylococcus aureus*	0	+	0	0	390	0	0	0	0	0	+	+	0	0	0	0
23	88	—	F	0	0	0	+	0	Klebsiella species	0	+	0	0	—	0	0	0	0	0	—	—	—	—	0	—
24	15	W	F	0	0	0	+	+	*Staphylococcus aureus*	+	+	0	0	200	0	+[1]	0	0	0	+	—	+	+	0	0
25	15	W	M	0	0	0	0	+	*Staphylococcus aureus*	+	0	+	0	440	0	+[1]	+	0	0	+	+	+	+	0	+
26	22	B	M	+	0	0	0	0	*Staphylococcus aureus*	+	+	0	0	540	0	0	0	0	0	+	+	+	+	0	0
27	27	B	M	+	0	0	0	0	—[7]	+	0	+	0	345	0	+	0	+	0	+	+	+	+	+	0
28	27	B	F	0	0	0	0	0	Negative[8]	+	+	0	0	360	0	+	0	+	0	—	—	—	—	+	—
29	28	B	M	+	0	0	+	0	Alpha streptococcus	+	0	+	0	380	0	0	+	0	0	+[2]	0	0	0	0	+
30	29	B	F	+	0	0	0	0	*Staphylococcus aureus*	+	0	+	0	320	0	+[1]	0	0	0	+	+	+	+	0	—
31	29	B	M	0	0	0	0	0	*Staphylococcus aureus*	+	+	0	0	270	0	0	+	0	0	—	—	—	—	0	—
32	34	B	M	+	0	0	0	0	*Staphylococcus aureus*	+	0	+	0	485	0	0	0	+	0	+	+	+	+	0	0
33	36	B	M	+	0	0	0	0	Group D streptococcus	+	0	0	+	500	0	+	0	+	+	+	0	+	+	0	0
34	39	B	M	+	0	0	—	—	*Staphylococcus aureus*	+	0	+	0	485	0	+[1]	0	0	+	+	+	+	+	+	—
35	41	B	F	+	0	0	+	0	*Staphylococcus aureus*	+	+	0	0	350	0	0	0	+	0	0	0	0	0	0	0
36	42	B	M	—	—	0	0	0	Negative[8]	+	0	0	+	620	+	0	0	+	+	+	+	—	—	+	—
37	43	B	M	+	0	0	0	0	—	+	0	+	0	—	+	0	0	+	0	+[2]	+	0	+	0	+
38	54	W	M	0	+	0	0	0	Group D streptococcus	+	0	0	+	510	0	+[9]	0	0	0	—	—	—	—	0	—
39	59	B	M	0	+	0	0	0	*Serratia marcescens*[4]	+	+	0	0	360	0	0	0	0	+	+	—	+	0	0	0
40	58	—	M	0	0	+	0	0	*Staphylococcus aureus*	+	0	+	0	670	0	+	0	+	+	+	+	0	0	+	0
41	66	W	M	0	0	0	0	0	*Staphylococcus aureus*	+	0	+	0	300	0	0	+	0	0	+	+	0	0	0	0
42	68	W	M	0	0	0	0	0	*Candida parapsilosis*	+	+	0	0	480	+	0	0	0	0	+	0	+	0	0	0
Total or mean	44			14	6	4	12	7		19	17	15	4	412	3	15	7	9	7	30	17	16	16	8	5

[1]Myocardial abscess; [2]pulmonary emboli also; [3]death due to cancer; [4]endocarditis not diagnosed (postmortem blood cultures positive); [5]death due to chronic renal failure 2° to systemic hypertension; [6]pulmonary embolus 2° hypercoagulable state; [7]sudden death before cultures obtained; [8]cultured while on antibiotics; [9]necrosis limited to papillary muscle.

A = alcoholism; B = black; CHF = congestive heart failure; F = female; Fi = fibrosis; H = hemodialysis; His = Hispanic; HW = heart weight; LV = left ventricle; M = male; Mn = meningitis; MR = mitral regurgitation; N = necrosis; O = opiate addict; P = pneumonia; PAML = perforated anterior mitral leaflet; RCT = ruptured chordae tendineae; SE = systemic emboli; + = present; 0 = absent; — = no information available.

(52%) had infarcts in 1 or more body organs (Tables I and II).

Comparison of cases without to those with mitral valve structural abnormalities before the active infective endocarditis: The 42 patients with normal mitral valves before the active IE compared to those with previously structurally abnormal valves were significantly (p <0.05) younger (mean age 44 vs 59 years); were more likely to be opiate addicts (33% vs 5%); were less likely to have beta streptococcus as the infecting organism

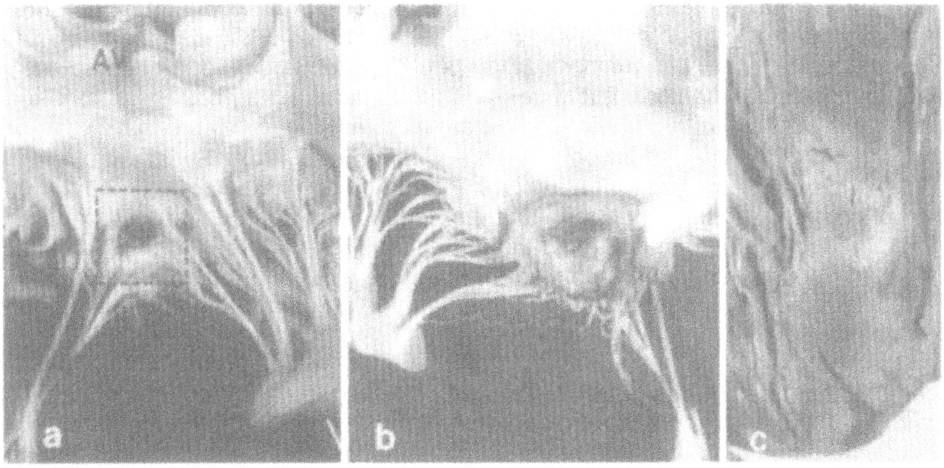

FIGURE 8. (Case 8, Table II.) Active infective endocarditis involving a previously normal valve in 43-year-old man (DCGH# 71A-70). *a*, view of ventricular side of the anterior mitral leaflet showing a perforation *(dashed box)* filled with vegetative material. *b*, view of atrial side of anterior mitral leaflet. The vegetation covers the perforation. *c*, close-up view of left ventricular free wall showing an area of necrosis, the result of a coronary artery embolus. (Reproduced with permission from *The American Journal of Medicine* 1972;53:20–35.[4])

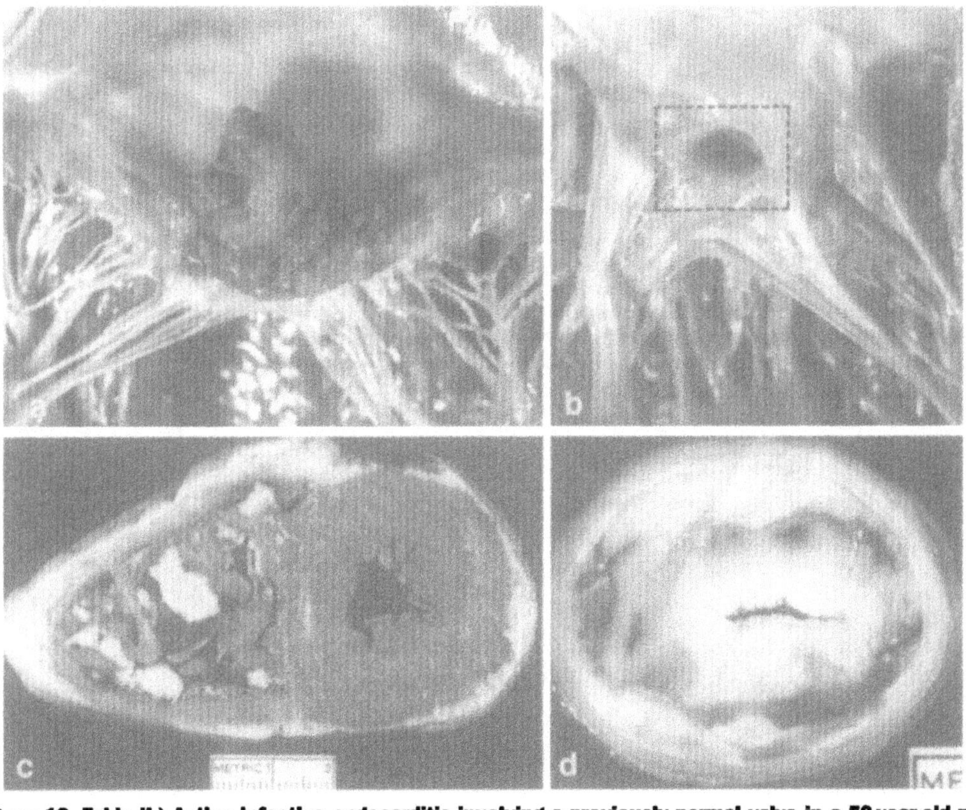

FIGURE 9. (Case 19, Table II.) Active infective endocarditis involving a previously normal valve in a 58-year-old man (NIH# A85-34) who had metastatic colonic carcinoma. *a*, opened mitral valve with a vegetation on the atrial aspect of the anterior mitral leaflet. *b*, view of the ventricular side of the anterior mitral leaflet showing a perforation *(dashed box)* that is filled with vegetative material. *c*, transverse section of the cardiac ventricles showing multiple thrombi in the right ventricular cavity. The patient was in a hypercoagulable state. He died from a pulmonary embolus. *d*, thromboembolic material filling the lumen of a portion of descending thoracic aorta. Apparently no clinical consequences resulted from the near total occlusion of a portion of aorta. The material filling the aorta is different from that of the vegetation on the mitral valve.

(0 of 35 vs 4 of 20 patients), and were more likely to have a perforation of the anterior mitral leaflet (7 of 41 [17%] vs 0 of 21). No significant differences in the 2 groups were observed in sex; the type of infecting organism other than beta streptococcus; or the frequency of habitual alcoholism, hemodialysis, systemic emboli, ring abscess, or ruptured chordae tendineae.

Comparison of patients with and without ruptured chordae tendineae: The 11 patients with compared to the 52 patients without ruptured chordae tendineae were significantly younger ($p < 0.05$) (mean age 37 vs 52 years), and had a higher frequency of opiate addiction (60% vs 15%).

Comparison of patients with and without perforation of the anterior mitral leaflet: The 7 patients with compared to the 56 patients without a perforation in the anterior mitral leaflet had a significantly higher frequency of previously normal mitral leaflets (100% vs 63%), a history of habitual alcoholism (33% vs 9%), and of ruptured chordae tendineae (50% vs 14%).

Comparison of patients with and without ring abscess: Comparison of the 10 patients with to the 53 patients without mitral valve ring abscess disclosed no significant differences in the variables listed in Tables I and II. Complete heart block, however, was present in 3 of the 10 patients with ring abscess and in 1 of the 53 patients without ring abscess. One other patient with ring abscess had right bundle branch block, but the latter patient had clear evidence of digitalis toxicity.

Comparison of patients with to those without mitral annular calcium: The 9 patients with mitral annular calcium compared to the 54 without were significantly (p

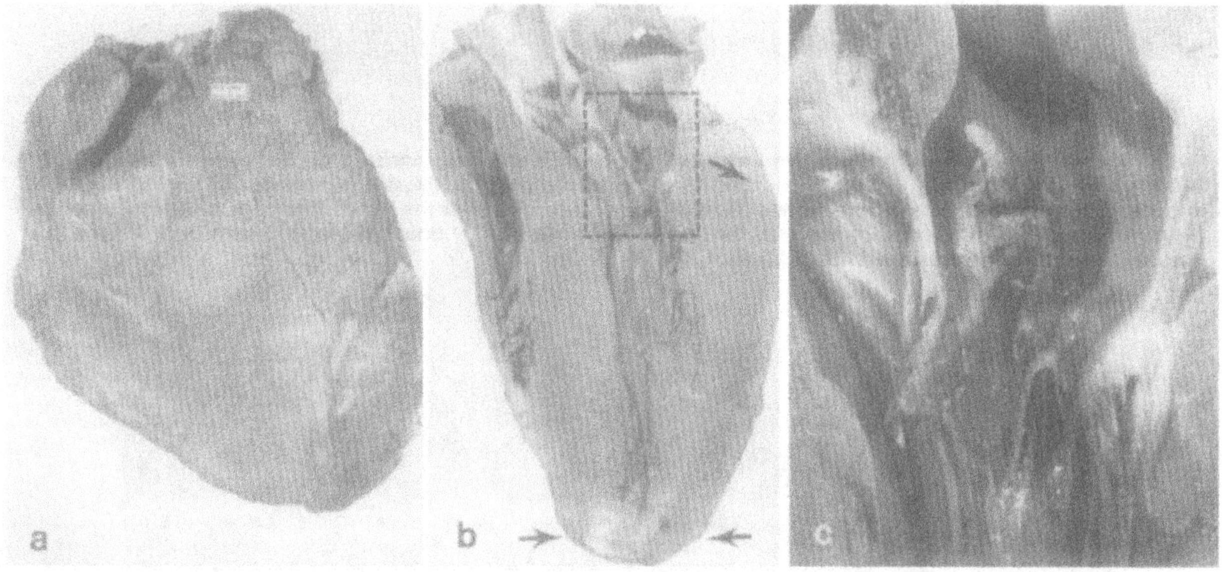

FIGURE 10. (Case 25, Table II.) Active infective endocarditis involving a previously normal valve in a 15-year-old boy (GT# 81A-186). ***a,*** **exterior of the heart showing a diffuse purulent pericarditis but without colonies of microorganisms on histologic study.** ***b,*** **longitudinal view showing a partially destroyed mitral valve by the infection. An abscess** ***(arrows)*** **is present in the ventricular wall at the apex.** ***c,*** **close-up of mitral valve. This boy had been well until he cut his finger while repairing his bicycle 3 weeks before death. The infecting organism was** ***Staphylococcus aureus.***

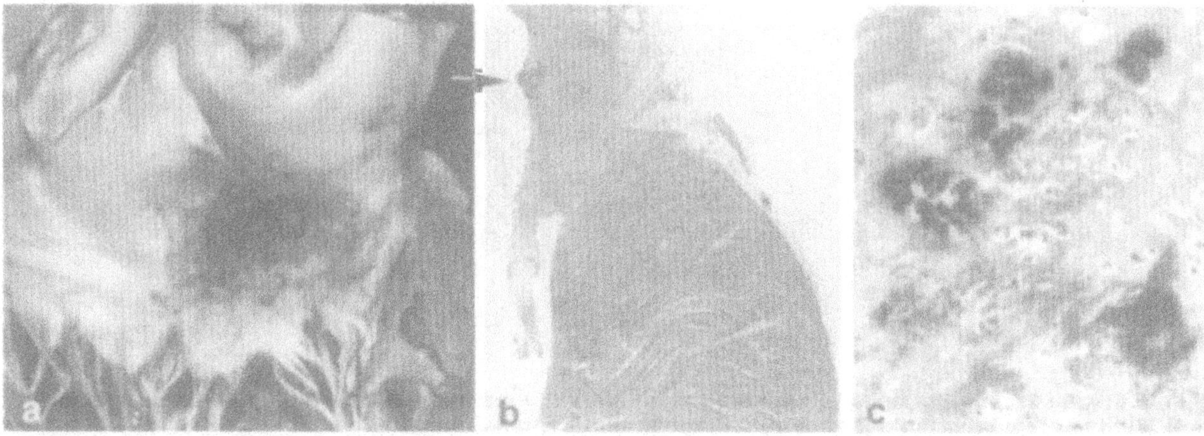

FIGURE 11. (Case 27, Table II.) Active infective endocarditis involving a previously normal valve in a 22-year-old opiate addict (DCGH# 75A-65). ***a,*** **opened mitral valve showing vegetative material on both the posterior leaflet and left atrial endocardium.** ***b,*** **histologic section after longitudinal cut through posterior mitral leaflet. The infection also involves mural endocardium of left atrium** ***(arrow).*** ***c,*** **close-up of colonies of organisms in the vegetation. This man died of a ruptured mycotic aneurysm in the brain. (Hematoxylin-eosin stains × 4** ***(b),*** **and × 530** ***(c);*** **reduced by 25%.)**

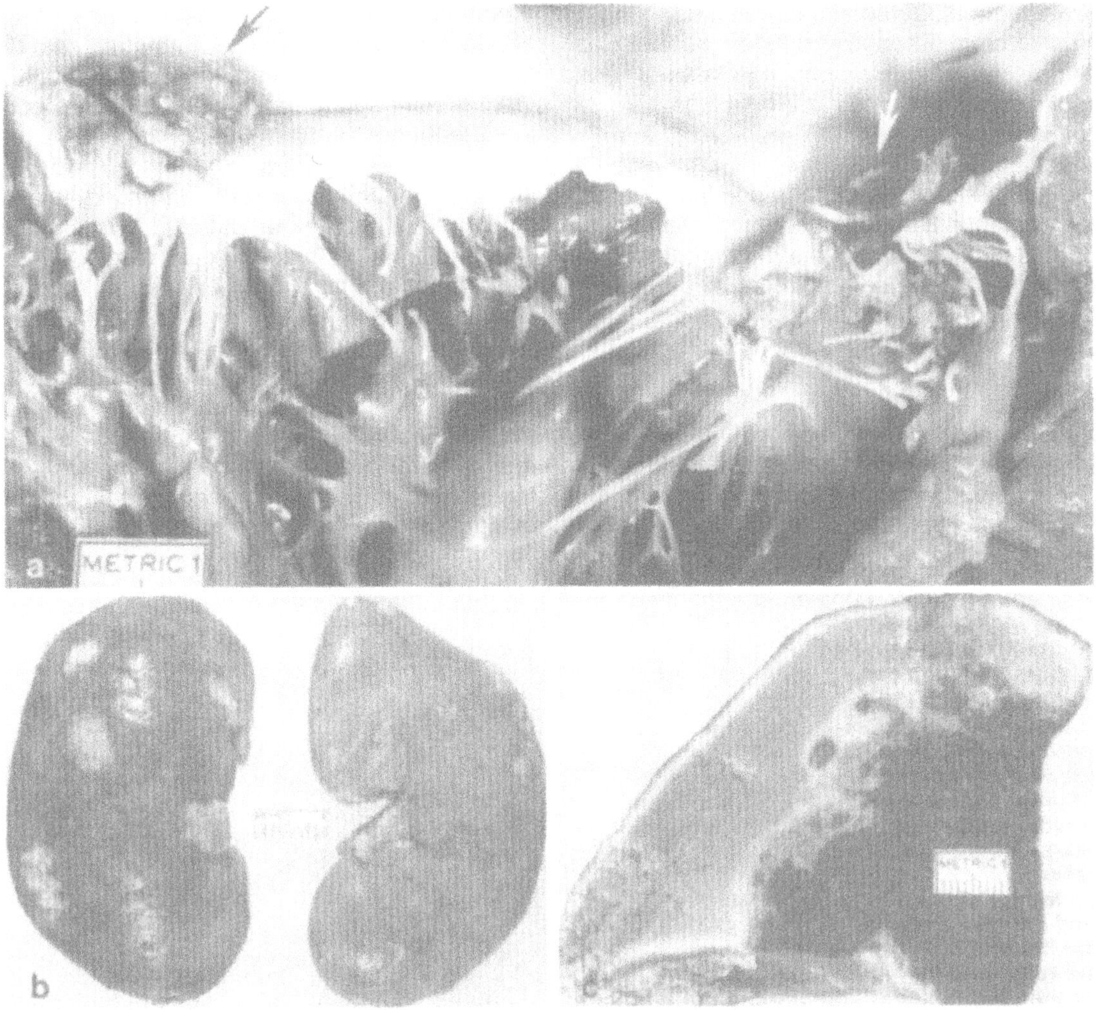

FIGURE 12. (Case 28, Table II.) Opened mitral valve with superimposed vegetations *(arrows) (a)*, exterior of kidneys showing multiple infarcts *(b)*, and cut surface of spleen showing a huge infarct *(c)* in a 27-year-old opiate addict (DCMEO# 83-08-574) who developed signs and symptoms consistent with active infective endocarditis 26 days before death. Despite antibiotic therapy he developed evidence of mitral regurgitation but died from consequences of multiple systemic emboli. The mitral valve was normal before the infection.

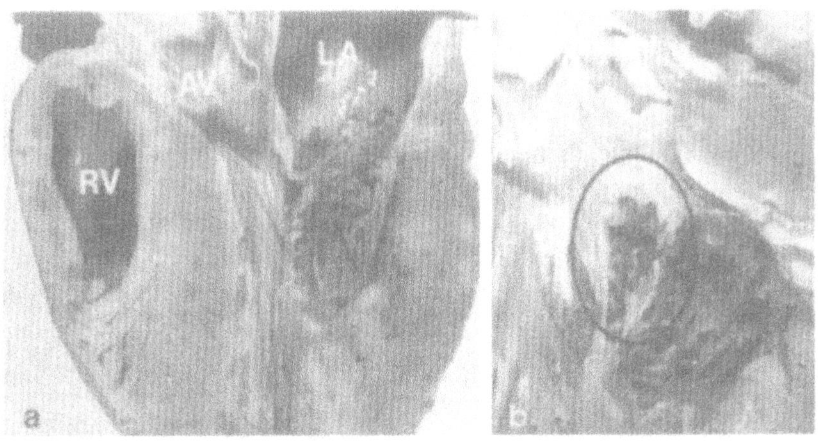

FIGURE 13. (Case 33, Table II.) Infective endocarditis involving a previously normal valve in a 36-year-old opiate addict (DCGH# 75A-159) who died 34 days after onset of congestive heart failure. The infection virtually destroyed the mitral valve which was severely incompetent. *a*, view after a longitudinal cut of the heart. Large vegetations are visible. Multiple abscesses without colonies of organisms were present in the left ventricular wall and the lumens of several intramural coronary arteries contained embolic material. *b*, close-up view showing a perforation in the anterior mitral leaflet *(circle)*.
AV = aortic valve; LA = left atrium; RV = right ventricle.

<0.05) older (mean age 66 vs 46 years); had a higher frequency of chronic hemodialysis (56% vs 18%); and a lower frequency of systemic emboli (60% vs 88%) and cerebral infarcts (0 of 9 vs 21 of 54 [61%]).

Comparison of patients with and without systemic emboli: No significant differences were observed in mean age, sex, infecting organism, and frequency of perforated anterior mitral leaflet, ruptured chordae tendineae, ring abscess, grossly visible organ infarcts, and presence of or type of underlying heart disease in the 44 patients with morphologic evidence of systemic emboli compared to the 7 patients without such evidence.

DISCUSSION

The heretofore described findings in necropsied patients with active IE limited to the mitral valve without operative intervention showed that more patients were males than females (2 to 1); that the infection more commonly involved a previously anatomically normal than a previously anatomically abnormal mitral valve (2 to 1); that vegetations on previously normal mitral valves often did not cause severe valvular dysfunction and that vegetations on previously abnormal valves did not cause or worsen valvular dysfunction; that a predisposing factor to IE (previously abnormal mitral valve, opiate addiction, habitual alcoholism and/or chronic hemodialysis) was common (2 of 3 patients); and that the IE often was simply part of a generalized or systemic infection (1 of 2 patients).

One of the more difficult evaluations in the present study was the determination of the presence or absence of mitral regurgitation as a consequence of vegetations on the mitral valve. When the vegetations are small (≤5 mm in maximal diameter), it is unlikely that mitral regurgitation would result unless chordae tendineae are ruptured and the latter event is infrequent when vegeta-

FIGURE 14. (Case 34, Table II.) Active infective endocarditis involving a mitral valve in a 39-year-old opiate addict (DCMEO# 88-08-887). This man had clinical evidence of active infective endocarditis involving the tricuspid valve 9 months before death. Another episode of infective endocarditis probably occurred 4 months before death when he had a stroke during a febrile period. He again had evidence of cerebral problems including seizures 7 days before death and blood cultures were positive for *Staphylococcus aureus*. At necropsy, a vegetation was present on the mitral valve bordering a leaflet perforation. The perforation probably was produced during an earlier episode of active infective endocarditis.

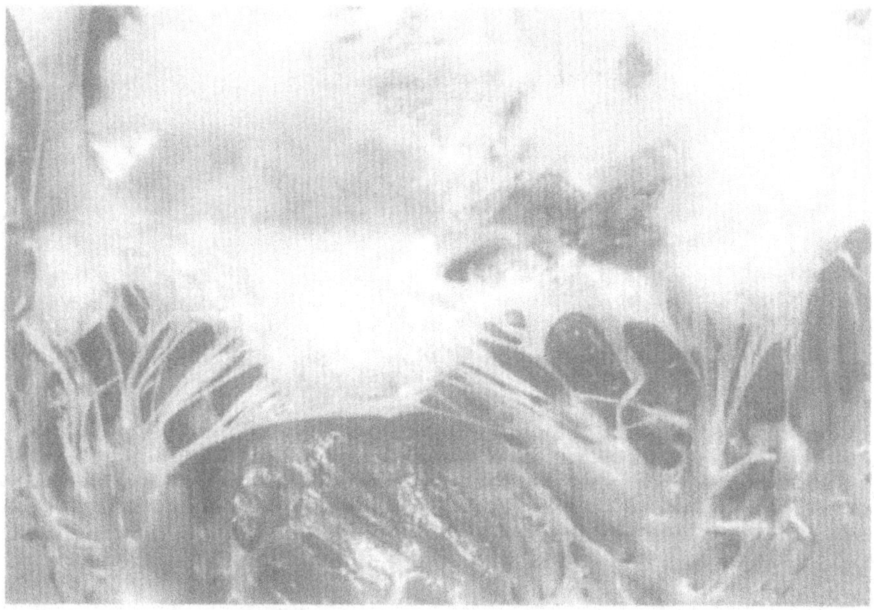

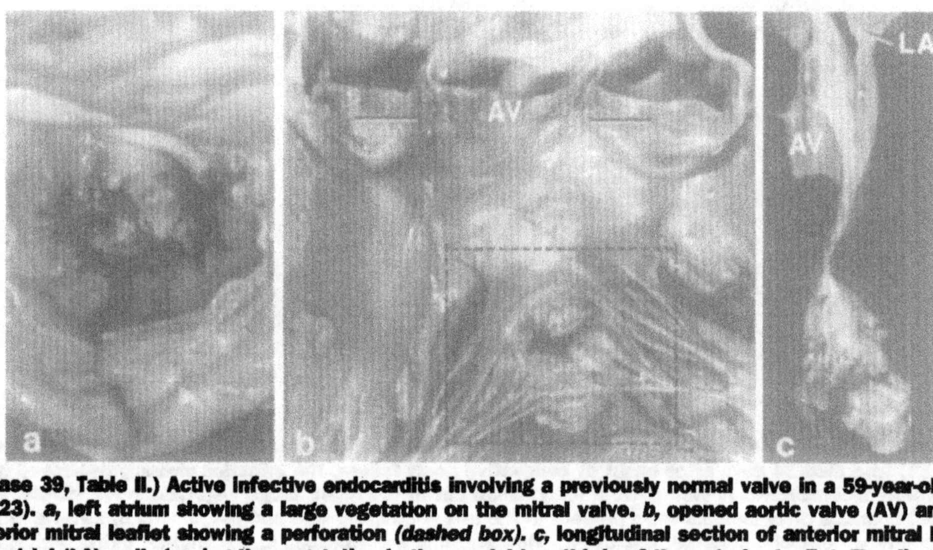

FIGURE 15. (Case 39, Table II.) Active infective endocarditis involving a previously normal valve in a 59-year-old man (DCGH# 75A-123). *a,* left atrium showing a large vegetation on the mitral valve. *b,* opened aortic valve (AV) and ventricular aspect of anterior mitral leaflet showing a perforation *(dashed box)*. *c,* longitudinal section of anterior mitral leaflet, aortic valve and left atrial (LA) wall showing the vegetation in the caudal two thirds of the anterior leaflet. The diagnosis of active infective endocarditis was not suspected in life. The patient presented with pneumonia.

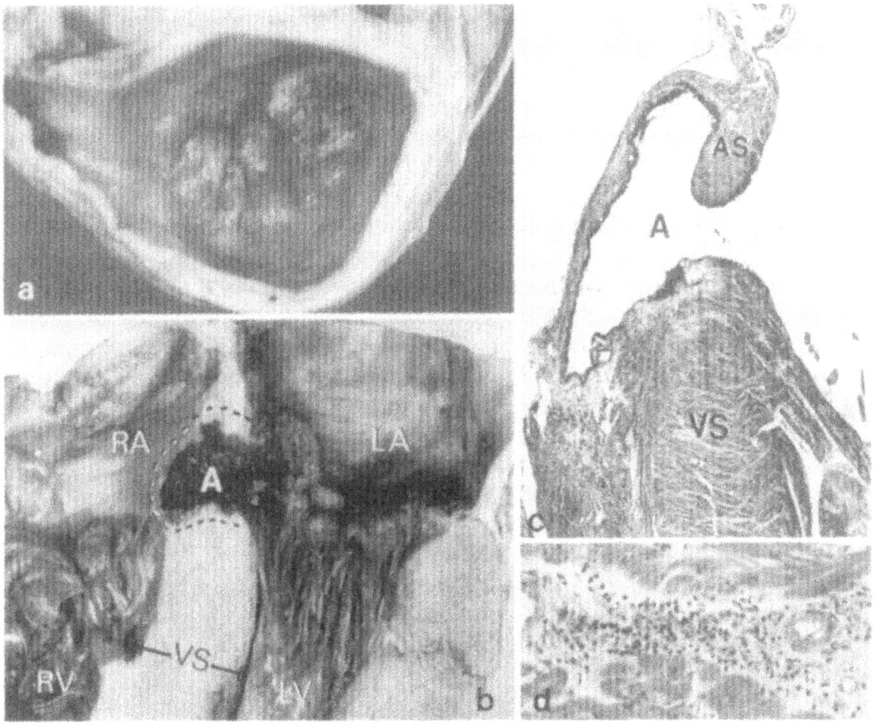

FIGURE 16. (Case 41, Table II.) Active infective endocarditis involving a previously normal mitral valve in a 66-year-old man (MHCMH# A4826) who developed symptoms of active infective endocarditis 20 days before death and complete heart block 14 days before death. *a,* view of left atrium (LA) showing a vegetation at the posteromedial commissure. *b,* 4-chamber view showing a huge ring abscess *(dashed area)* in the caudal half of the atrial septum (AS). *c,* photomicrograph through the area of the ring abscess (A) (Movat stain × 3; reduced by 30%). *d,* foci of acute inflammation were present in the ventricular walls (hematoxylineosin stain × 220; reduced by 30%). LV = left ventricle; RA = right atrium; RV = right ventricle; VS = ventricular septum. (*a* and *b* are reproduced with permission from *Circulation* 1976;54:140–145.[6])

tions are small. Large vegetations, however, even in the absence of ruptured chordae tendineae or perforation of a valvular leaflet probably often cause mitral regurgitation because of their interfering with leaflet coaptation during ventricular systole.

One anatomic finding that usually indicates mitral regurgitation is rupture of chordae tendineae.[2] In the present study 11 patients (18%) had ruptured chordae: 9 (22% of 41 patients) had active IE complicating previously anatomically normal mitral valves and 8 of them had clinical and morphologic evidence of mitral regurgitation; 2 patients (10% of 21 patients) had active IE complicating previously anatomically abnormal valves: 1 of them had preexisting mitral stenosis and no evidence of mitral regurgitation; the other patient had convincing evidence of regurgitation.

The other anatomic finding suggesting the presence of mitral regurgitation (at some time) is the presence of a perforation in a valve leaflet or actual tears or major indentations of a leaflet. In the present study 7 patients had a perforation in the anterior mitral leaflet and all of them had infection on a previously anatomically normal valve. At necropsy in 2 of the 7 patients the perforation was filled with vegetative material so that no regurgitation was occurring through the cuspal "perforation" shortly before death. At least 5 of these 7 patients, however, had clinical evidence of mitral regurgitation.

It is less difficult to determine if a mitral valve, which had previously been anatomically normal, was made incompetent by vegetations than when vegetations are superimposed on mitral leaflets that had previously been abnormal. In the present study 21 patients (34%) had previously abnormal mitral valves: rheumatic in 8, prolapse in 3, hypertrophic cardiomyopathy in 1, and mitral annular calcium in 9. Of the 8 rheumatic patients, 5 had preexisting mitral stenosis and the vegetations in them did not appear to cause mitral regurgitation, but they may have worsened the mitral stenosis because of the orifice space occupied by the vegetation.[3] Although 3 other patients had rheumatic heart disease as evidenced by diffuse fibrosis of the valve leaflets, none of them had clinical evidence of valvular dysfunction before the active IE. Of the 3 patients with prolapse, 2 were believed to have had some mitral regurgitation before the onset of active IE which did not appear to worsen the regurgitation. In the 1 patient with hypertrophic cardiomyopathy, it was not possible to determine if the preexisting mitral regurgitation was worsened by the mitral vegetations. And finally, active IE complicating mitral annular calcium did not cause chordal rupture or leaflet perforation in any patient, and none of these 9 patients were considered to have significant mitral regurgitation either before or after the active IE.

Acknowledgment: We wish to thank Vivian Norman and Rodger Marks for manuscript preparation, Michael Spencer for photography, and Leslie Berry for artwork preparation.

1. Andriole VT, Kravetz HM, Roberts WC, Utz JP. Candida endocarditis: clinical and pathologic studies. *Am J Med* 1962;32:251–285.
2. Roberts WC, Braunwald E, Morrow AG. Acute severe mitral regurgitation secondary to ruptured chordae tendineae: clinical, hemodynamic and pathologic considerations. *Circulation* 1966;33:58–70.
3. Roberts WC, Ewy GA, Glancy DL, Marcus FI. Valvular stenosis produced by active infective endocarditis. *Circulation* 1967;36:449–451.
4. Roberts WC, Buchbinder NA. Left-sided valvular active infective endocarditis: a study of forty-five necropsy patients. *Am J Med* 1972;53:20–35.
5. Buchbinder NA, Roberts WC. Alcoholism: an important but unemphasized factor predisposing to infective endocarditis. *Arch Intern Med* 1973;132:689–692.
6. Arnett EN, Roberts WC. Valve ring abscess in active infective endocarditis: frequency, location, and clues to clinical diagnosis from the study of 95 necropsy

cases. *Circulation* 1976;54:140–145.
7. Arnett EN, Roberts WC. Active infective endocarditis: a clinicopathologic analysis of 137 necropsy patients. *Curr Probl Cardiol* 1976;1:1–76.
8. Andy JJ, Sheikh MU, Ali N, Barnes BO, Fox LM, Curry CL, Roberts WC. Echocardiographic observations in opiate addicts with active infective endocarditis: frequency of involvement of the various valves and comparison of echocardiographic features of right- and left-sided cardiac valve endocarditis. *Am J Cardiol* 1977;40:17–23.
9. Roberts WC. Characteristics and consequences of infective endocarditis (active or healed or both) learned from morphologic studies. In: Rahimtoola SH, ed. Infective Endocarditis. New York: Grune & Stratton, 1978:55–123.
10. Sheikh MU, Covarrubias EA, Ali N, Lee WR, Sheikh NM, Roberts WC. M-mode echocardiographic observations during and after healing of active bacterial endocarditis limited to the mitral valve. *Am Heart J* 1981;101:37–45.
11. Dressler FA, Roberts WC. Infective endocarditis in opiate addicts: analysis of 80 cases studied at necropsy. *Am J Cardiol* 1989;63:1240–1257.
12. Roberts WC, Oluwole BO, Fernicola DJ. Comparison of active infective endocarditis involving a previously stenotic versus a previously nonstenotic aortic valve. *Am J Cardiol* 1993;71:1082–1088.
13. Roberts WC. Morphologic aspects of cardiac valve dysfunction. *Am Heart J* 1992;123:1610–1632.
14. Dollar AL, Roberts WC. Morphologic comparison of patients with mitral valve prolapse who died suddenly with patients who died from severe valvular dysfunction or other conditions. *J Am Coll Cardiol* 1991;17:921–931.
15. Roberts CS, Roberts WC. Morphologic features. In: Zipes DP, Rowlands DJ eds. Progress in Cardiology (2/2), Philadelphia: Lea & Febiger 1989:3–32.
16. Roberts WC, Waller BF. Effect of chronic hypercalcemia on the heart. An analysis of 18 necropsy patients. *Am J Med* 1981;71:371–384.
17. Silver MA, Roberts WC. Active infective endocarditis complicating idiopathic dilated cardiomyopathy. *Am J Cardiol* 1983;52:651–652.

Frequency of Ring Abscess and Cuspal Infection in Active Infective Endocarditis Involving Bioprosthetic Valves

Daniel J. Fernicola, MD,* and William C. Roberts, MD†

When active infective endocarditis (IE) involves a bioprosthetic valve, the infective process may involve only the cusps or sewing ring or both. We studied 34 patients with infected bioprostheses to determine whether the infection involved the cusps or ring, or both, because these locations could affect prognosis. In the 5 patients in whom active IE began <60 days after operation, the infection involved the cusps only in 2, the ring only in 2, and both in 1. The 29 patients in whom signs and symptoms of active IE appeared >60 days after valve replacement were subdivided into 3 categories based on the valve or valves replaced. In the 16 patients with isolated aortic valve replacement, the infection involved the cusps only in 6, the ring only in 4, and both in 6. In the 6 patients with isolated mitral valve replacement, the infection involved the cusps only in 2, the ring only in 1, and both in 3. In the remaining 7 patients, 15 native valves were replaced with bioprostheses, and 10 of them were infected. The infection involved the cusps only in 7, and both the cusps and ring in 3.

Of all 34 patients, 13 had operative excision of the infected bioprosthesis: 1 died within 60 days of the bioprosthetic excision, and 1 was lost to follow-up; of the remaining 11 patients, 4 died late (1.5, 3, 5 and 14 years), and the other 7 are alive 5 to 10 years after bioprosthetic excision (all in New York Heart Association functional class I or II). Thus, although infection limited to the bioprosthetic cusps may reasonably allow a better outlook, reoperation with infection involving the annular ring (8 of 13 reoperation patients) does not prevent successful outcome.

(Am J Cardiol 1993;72:314–323)

From the Pathology Branch, National Heart, Lung, and Blood Institute, National Institutes of Health, Bethesda, Maryland. Manuscript received February 5, 1993; revised manuscript received and accepted March 3, 1993.

*Current address: Division of Cardiology, Department of Medicine, Georgetown University Medical Center, Washington, D.C. 20058.

†Current address: Baylor Cardiovascular Institute, Baylor University Medical Center, 3500 Gaston Avenue, Dallas, Texas 75246.

When active infective endocarditis (IE) involves mechanical prostheses, the infective material is always located in the sewing ring (i.e., the site of attachment of the prosthesis).[1–3] When active IE involves a bioprosthesis, the infection may involve only the bioprosthetic cusps or sewing ring, or both. If the infection involves exclusively the cusps, reoperation should eliminate the infection in most patients. If, however, the infection involves the sewing ring, reoperation may not eliminate the infection, and therefore prognosis would be different. We examined 34 patients who had active IE after replacement of ≥1 cardiac valve with a bioprosthesis to determine anatomically the exact location of the infective material.

METHODS

Inclusion and exclusion criteria: Records from the Pathology Branch of the National Heart, Lung, and Blood Institute were searched for patients who had active IE after replacement of ≥1 cardiac valve with a bioprosthesis. Patients were included in this study if they had undergone replacement of ≥1 cardiac valve with a porcine, bovine or parietal pericardial bioprosthesis (mounted on a stent), and subsequently had ≥1 episode of active IE, and either died and an autopsy was performed, or the infected bioprosthesis was excised and examined by us. Patients were excluded from this study if a native cardiac valve was replaced with a homograft or if vegetations were present on a native cardiac valve that was excised and replaced with a bioprosthesis. If a patient, however, had active IE on a native cardiac valve and the infection healed before operative excision, the patient was not excluded from this study.

Division of patients: Of 34 patients, 13 (38%) underwent operative excision of the infected bioprosthesis. One of the 13 patients died within 24 hours of reoperation and his heart was examined at necropsy. A second patient died 5 years after operative excision of the infected bioprosthesis and her heart was examined at autopsy. Of these 13 patients, 5 had the second operation at the Clinical Center of the National Institutes of Health, and 8 had the second operation at Georgetown University Medical Center. These 13 patients are among 160 whose operatively excised bioprostheses are in the collection of the Pathology Branch of the National Heart, Lung, and Blood Institute.

The remaining 21 patients (61%) never had the infected bioprosthesis operatively excised, and they were studied at necropsy. The necropsy was performed at the Clinical Center of the National Institutes of Health in 4 patients, at Georgetown University Medical Center in 3, at the Washington Hospital Center, Washington, D.C., in 2, at the District of Columbia Veterans Administration Hospital in 2, and 1 at 10 different medical centers in 1 each.

Period of study: Of the 34 patients, 6 were studied in the decade 1971 to 1980, 27 from 1981 to 1990, and 1 in 1991.

Examiners of the hearts and infected bioprostheses: All 22 hearts with infected bioprostheses were examined initially by WCR, and 19 were subsequently examined by DJF. Operatively excised infected bioprostheses in the other 13 patients were examined initially by WCR and all were examined subsequently by DJF. Photographs of infected bioprostheses were available in 20 of the 22 necropsied hearts with infected bioprostheses and in all 13 patients with operatively excised infected bioprostheses.

Statistical analysis: Data were analyzed using the Stat View 512+ statistical software package. Categoric comparisons were obtained with 2-tailed chi-squared analysis. Numeric comparisons were obtained using a 2-tailed, unpaired *t* test. Statistical significance was defined as $p < 0.05$.

RESULTS

Specific clinical and necropsy findings in each of the 34 patients are listed in Table I and illustrated in Figures 1 to 13. Patients were divided into 2 major groups. One group included 5 patients whose interval from valve replacement to onset of signs or symptoms, or both, of bioprosthetic endocarditis was <60 days (range 12 to 32, mean 20) (early infection). The interval from signs or symptoms, or both, of bioprosthetic endocarditis to death or operative excision of the infected bioprosthesis ranged from 6 to 108 days (mean 43), and that between the first valve replacement to death (n = 4) or operative excision of the infected bioprosthesis ranged from 36 to 120 days (mean 65). It is presumed that the infection in each of these 5 patients was initiated at the first valve replacement or shortly thereafter. Five of the 6 bioprostheses in these 5 patients were infected; the infection was limited to the cusps in 1 patient and to the ring only in 2, and it involved both the cusps and ring in 2.

The other major group included the 29 patients in whom the interval from valve replacement to onset of

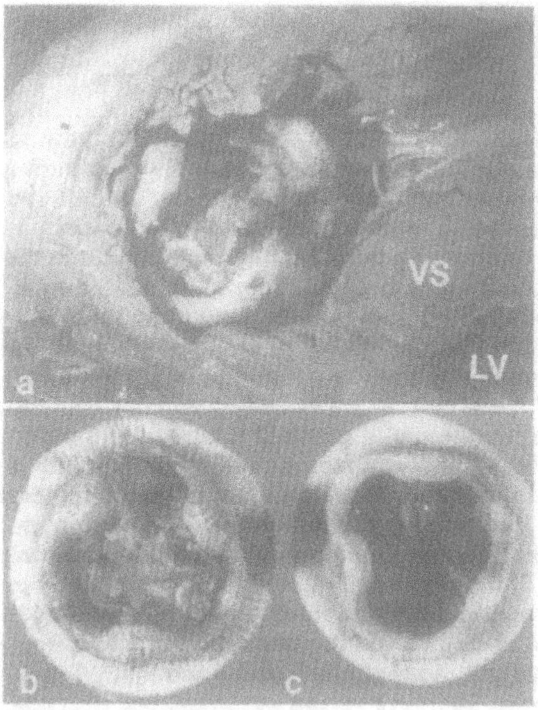

FIGURE 1. Patient 5; Table I. *Candida albicans* bioprosthetic valve endocarditis in a 63-year-old white woman (NIH #A86-79) who had had mitral and tricuspid valve replacements 36 days before death. *a*, a view of the ventricular aspect of the bioprosthetic valve in the tricuspid position. The infected material fills each of the 3 bioprosthetic sinuses. *b*, excised bioprosthesis from the tricuspid position. *c*, excised bioprosthesis from the mitral position, which is free of infection. LV = left ventricular cavity; VS = ventricular septum.

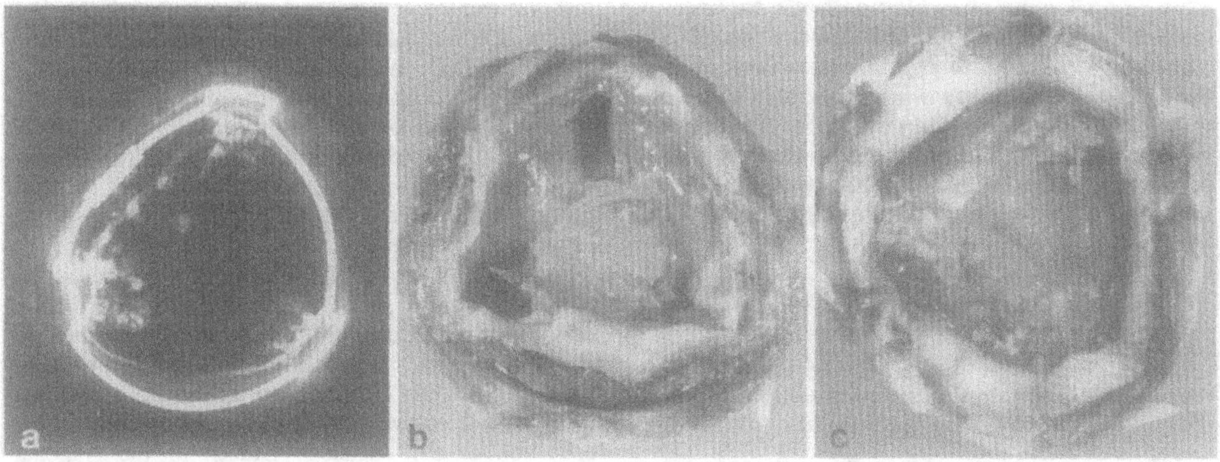

FIGURE 2. Patient 6. Alpha streptococcus bioprosthetic valve endocarditis in a 20-year-old man (GT #81S-4273) who had undergone aortic valve replacement 48 months earlier. *a*, radiograph of the excised bioprosthesis. Calcific deposits are present at the lateral attachments of each of the cusps. *b*, ventricular aspect of the excised bioprosthesis. The cusps are torn. *c*, aortic aspect of the excised bioprosthesis.

TABLE I Clinical and Morphologic Features of Patients with Infective Endocarditis Involving a Bioprosthetic Valve

No.	Age (years) at VR/or BPE or @Death	Sex	Necropsy and/or Surgery	BPV Type	BPV Location	Interval VR to S/S of BPE	Interval 1st VR to Death/2d VR	Bioprosthetic Dysfunction During Active IE			Infecting Organism
								Stenosis	Regurgitation	CHB	
Early Infection (onset signs and symptoms of bioprosthetic endocarditis <60 days after mitral valve replacement)											
1	63	M	N	H	A	21 days	43 days	0	0	0	*Staphylococcus aureus*
2	78	F	N	CE	A	32 days	39 days	0	+	+	*Aspergillus fumigatus*
3	61	M	S	H	Mi	14 days	89 days	0	+	0	*Staphylococcus epidermidis*
4	66	F	N	H	Mi	12 days	120 days	0	0	0	*Staphylococcus aureus*[2]
5	63	F	N	H	Mi[3]	20 days	36 days	0	0	0	*Candida albicans*
			N	H	T			+	0	0	
Total	63[4]	2M/3F				20 days[4]	43 days[4]	1	2	1	
Late Infection (onset signs and symptoms of bioprosthetic endocarditis >60 days after initial valve replacement)											
6	20	M	S	CE	A	47 months	48 months	0	+	0	Alpha streptococcus
7	31	M	S	H	A	56 months	72 months	+	+	0	Negative
8	72	M	S	H	A	120 months	121 months	+	+	+	Alpha streptococcus
9	73	M	S	CE	A	32 months	34 months	0	+	0	Peptostreptococcus[5]
10	74	M	S	CE	A	36 months	37 months	0	+	0	Alpha streptococcus
11	18	M	N	CE	A	15 months	17 months	+	0	0	Alpha streptococcus
12	29	M	N	CE	A	3 months	3 months	0	+[6]	—	—[7]
13	53	M	N	P	A	30 months	31 months	+	–	0	Group D Streptococcus
14	58	M	N	CE	A	3 months	4 months	0	+	+	*Staphylococcus epidermidis*
15	58	M	N	CE	A	7 months	8 months	0	+	0	—
16	64	M	N	CE	A	3 months	9 months	0	+	0	Alpha streptococcus
17	65	M	N	P	A	4 months	6 months	—	+	0	*Staphylococcus epidermidis*
18	70	M	N	B	A	60 months	61 months	+	+	+	*Staphylococcus aureus*
19	70	M	N	P	A	5 months	9 months	0	+	0	Alpha streptococcus
20	78	M	N	CE	A	25 months	25 months	+	0	0	—[11]
21	89	M	N	B	A	36 months	38 months	0	0	0	Alpha streptococcus
Subtotal	65[4]	16M/0F				28 months[4]	28 months[4]	6	12	3	
22	54	F	S[13]	H	Mi	26 months	27 months	0	+	0	Negative[14]
23	62	F	S	CE	Mi	108 months	144 months	+	0	0	Alpha streptococcus
24	63	F	S	H	Mi	36 months	84 months	0	+	0	Staphylococcus species
25	66	F	S	CE	Mi	48 months	49 months	0	0[15]	0	*Staphylococcus aureus*
26	59	F	N	B	Mi	84 months	84 months	0	+	0	*Staphylococcus aureus*
27	82	M	N	P	Mi	3 months	3 months	0	+	0	Beta streptococcus
Subtotal	63[4]	1M/5F				42 months[4]	66 months[4]	1	4	0	
28	30	F	S	H	Mi	4 months	44 months	0	0	0	Alpha streptococcus
			S	H	T[3]				0	0	
29	72	F	S	H	Mi	94 months	96 months	0	+	0	Streptococcal specie
			S	H	T[3]				+		
30	29	M[18]	N	H	Mi	8 months	8 months	0	0	0	*Staphylococcus aureus*
			N	H	T			+	0		
31	53	F	N	H	Mi	108 months	110 months	0	+	0	Alpha streptococcus
			N	H	T[3]			0	0		
32	58	M	S[21]	H	Mi	12 months	125 months	0	+	0	Negative[14]
			S	H	A[3]			0	0		
33	67	M	N	H	Mi	9 months	9 months	0	0	+	*Staphylococcus aureus*
			N	H	A[3]			0	0		
34	58	M	N	H	Mi	36 months[23]	37 months	0	+	0	Alpha streptococcus
			N	H	A			0	+		
			N		T			0	+		
Subtotal	58[4]	4M/3F				65 months[4]	44 months[4]	2	7	1	
Totals	62[4]	21M/8F				30 months[4]	37 months[4]	9	23	4	

[1]Mediastinal infection; [2]pseudomonas aeruginosa grown from sternal wound and blood 1 week before death; [3]bioprosthesis not infected; [4]median; [5]actinobacillus grown from blood cultures; [6]valve dehiscence; [7]died before arrival at hospital; [8]necrosis limited to papillary muscle; [9]coronary artery embolus; [10]central line infection; [11]culture not obtained; diagnosis of endocarditis unsuspected; [12]pneumonia; [13]necropsy 5 years after replacement of infected bioprosthesis; [14]received antibiotics before blood cultures; [15]indication for operation was persistent bacteremia despite antibiotics; [16]central line placement; [17]dental abscesses; [18]Löffler's fibroblastic parietal endocarditis; [19]cellulitis 1 month before death; [20]percutaneous liver biopsy; [21]patient died 24 hours after surgery; [22]ring abscess extended into the sewing ring of the bioprosthesis in the aortic position; [23]this fatal episode of endocarditis was preceded by 2 episodes of endocarditis 12 and 24 months after valve replacement.

A = aortic; AS = aortic stenosis; B = bovine; BPE = bioprosthetic endocarditis; BPV = bioprosthetic valve; Ca^{2} = calcium; CE = Carpentier-Edwards; CHD = complete heart block; CHF = congestive heart failure; F = female; Fi = fibrosis; H = Hancock; HA = habitual alcoholism; HW = heart weight; IE = infective endocarditis; IVDA = intravenous drug abuse; LV = left ventricular; M = male; Mi = mitral; MS = mitral stenosis; N = necropsy; Ne = necrosis; P = porcine; S = surgery; S/S = signs and symptoms; SE = systemic emboli; T = tricuspid; VR = valve replacement.

TABLE I (Cont'd)

No.	Location of Infective Material		Bioprosthesis			Gross Features of Heart at Necropsy				During BPE			Native Valve Before VR		Predisposing Factors to IE			Other Operative Procedure	IE Before VR
							LV												
	Cusp	Ring	Ca^{2+} (0–4+)	Tears	Perforations	HW (g)	Fi	Ne	Myocardial Abscess	CHF	SE	Noncardiac Infection	MS	AS	IVDA	HA	Dental Procedure		
Early Infection (onset signs and symptoms of bioprosthetic endocarditis < 60 days after mitral valve replacement)																			
1	0	+	0	0	0	760	0	0	0	+	+	+[1]	0	0	0	0	0	0	+
2	+	+	0	+	+	—	0	0	0	0	0	0	0	0	0	0	0	0	–
3	0	+	0	0	0	—	—	—	—	+	0	0	+	0	0	0	0	0	0
4	+	0	0	0	0	560	0	0	0	+	+	+[1]	+	0	0	0	0	0	0
5	0	0	0	0	0	370	0	0	0	+	0	+	+	0	0	0	0	0	0
	+	0	0	0	0														
Total	3	3	0	1	1	560[4]	0	0	0	4	2	3	3	0	0	0	0	0	1
Late Infection (onset signs and sumptoms of bioprosthetic endocarditis > 60 days after initial valve replacement)																			
6	+	0	4+	+	0	—	—	—	—	+	0	0	0	+	0	0	0	0	0
7	+	+	3+	0	0	—	—	—	—	0	0	0	0	0	0	0	+	0	0
8	+	+	0	0	+	—	—	—	—	+	0	0	0	+	0	0	+	0	0
9	+	0	0	+	0	—	—	—	—	+	0	0	0	+	0	0	+	0	+
10	0	+	0	0	0	—	—	—	—	+	0	0	0	+	0	0	0	0	0
11	+	0	3+	0	0	630	0	0	0	—	—	—	0	+	0	0	+	0	0
12	+	+	0	+	+	650	0	+[8]	0	+	0	0	0	0	0	0	—	—	+
13	+	0	0	0	0	—	0	+[9]	0	+	+[9]	0	0	+	+	0	0	0	0
14	0	+	0	0	0	560	0	0	+	+	0	0	0	+	0	0	0	0	0
15	+	+	0	+	0	675	+	0	0	+	0	0	0	+	0	0	—	—	0
16	0	+	0	0	0	515	0	+[9]	0	0	+[9]	0	0	+	0	0	0	0	0
17	+	+	—	—	—	510	+	0	0	+	—	—	+	+	0	0	0	0	0
18	+	+	0	0	0	790	0	0	0	0	0	+[10]	0	+	0	0	0	0	0
19	+	0	1+	0	+	630	+	0	0	0	0	0	0	+	0	0	0	0	0
20	+	0	0	0	0	525	+	0	0	0	+	+[12]	+	+	0	0	0	0	0
21	0	+	0	0	0	650	0	0	0	0	0	0	0	+	0	0	+	0	0
Subtotal	11	10	4	4	3	630[4]	4	3	1	9	3	2	2	4	1	0	5	0	2
22	0	+	0	0	0	550	0	0	0	+	0	0	+	0	0	0	0	0	0
23	+	+	4+	0	0	—	—	—	—	—	—	—	+	0	0	0	—	—	0
24	+	+	0	+	+	—	—	—	—	—	—	—	+	0	0	0	0	0	0
25	+	+	0	0	0	—	—	—	—	0	0	0	—	—	0	0	0	+[16]	0
26	+	0	2+	+	0	535	0	0	0	+	+	0	+	0	0	0	0	0	0
27	+	0	0	0	0	540	0	0	0	+	0	0	0	0	0	0	0	0	0
Subtotal	5	4	2	2	1	540[4]	0	0	0	3	1	0	4	0	0	0	0	1	0
28	+	0	0	0	0	—	—	—	—	0	+	+[17]	0	0	+	0	+	0	+
	0	0	0	0	+														
29	+	0	0	0	0	—	—	—	—	+	0	0	+	0	0	0	0	0	0
	0	0	0	0	0														
30	+	0	0	0	0	470	0	0	0	+	0	+[19]	0	0	0	0	0	0	0
	+	0	0	0	0														
31	+	0	2+	+	+	720	0	0	0	+	0	0	+	0	0	0	0	+[20]	0
	0	0	2+	0	0														
32	+	+[22]	0	+	0	675	0	0	0	+	+	+	+	+	0	0	0	0	0
	0	0	1+	0	0														
33	+	+	0	0	0	540	+	+[9]	0	0	+[9]	0	0	0	0	+	0	0	+
	0	0	0	0	0														
34	+	0	0	+	0	650	0	0	0	+	0	0	0	0	0	0	0	0	+
	+	+	0	+	0														
	+	0	0	0	0														
Subtotal	10	3	3	4	2	650[4]	1	1	0	5	3	3	3	1	1	1	1	1	3
Totals	26	17	9	10	6	595[4]	5	4	1	17	7	5	9	5	2	1	6	2	6

signs and symptoms of bioprosthetic endocarditis was >60 days (range 3 to 120 months, mean 36) (late infection); the interval from the first valve replacement to the replacement of a bioprosthesis (n = 12) ranged from 27 to 144 months (mean 73), and that from the first valve replacement to death (n = 17) ranged from 3 to 110 months (mean 28). Two of the 12 patients who had operative excision of an infected bioprosthesis subsequently died, and an autopsy was performed; patient 22 (Table I) died 5 years after successful excision of the infected bioprosthesis, and patient 32 (Table I) died 1 day after operative excision of the infected bioprosthesis.

The 29 patients in whom ≥1 bioprosthesis became infected late also were subdivided into 3 groups: 1 group consisted of 16 patients with isolated aortic valve replacement with a bioprosthesis; 1 consisted of 6 patients with isolated mitral valve replacement, and 1 consisted of 7 patients in whom ≥2 cardiac valves were replaced.

Of the 29 patients with infection late, 24 had evidence of active IE involving ≥1 bioprosthesis, and the active nature of the bioprosthetic endocarditis was confirmed by morphologic study of the operatively excised bioprosthesis or from necropsy study of the bioprosthesis. The other 5 patients (nos. 7, 16, 23, 24 and 28; Table

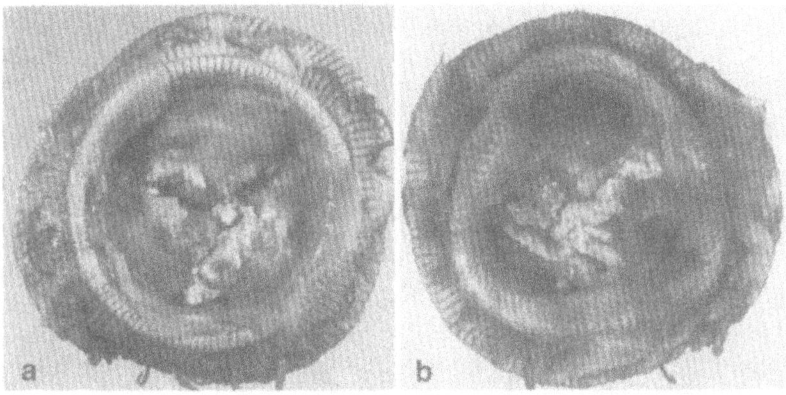

FIGURE 3. Patient 7. Bioprosthetic valve endocarditis in a 31-year-old man (GT #83S-4176) 56 months after aortic valve replacement. Signs and symptoms of active infective endocarditis occurred after dental work, despite prophylaxis. *a*, ventricular aspect of the bioprosthesis. *b*, aortic aspect of the bioprosthesis. Infective material is present on both sides of the cusps.

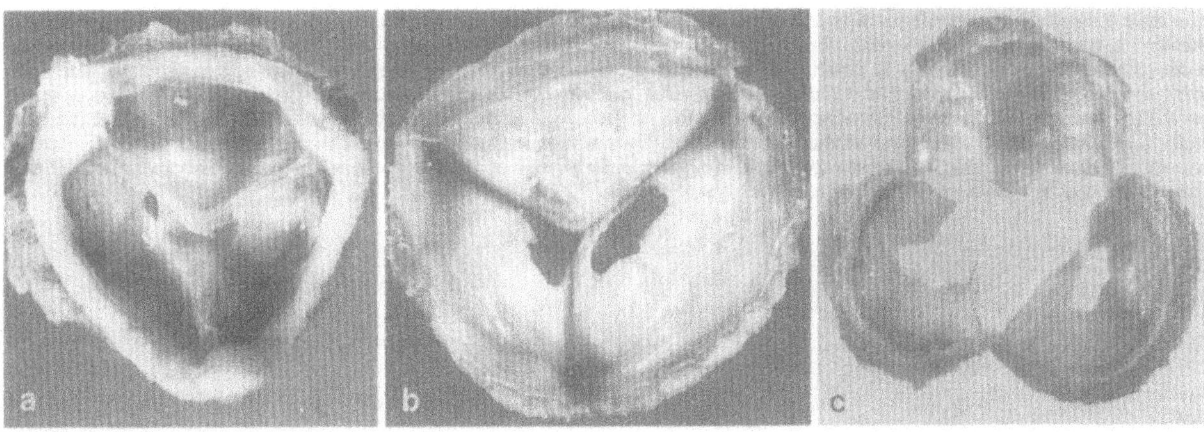

FIGURE 4. Patient 9. Alpha streptococcus bioprosthetic valve endocarditis in a 73-year-old man (GT# 82S-7589). This bioprosthesis was excised 34 months after aortic valve replacement. The patient received nearly 7 weeks of antibiotics before the second valve replacement. *a*, aortic aspect of the bioprosthetic valve. *b*, ventricular aspect of the bioprosthetic valve, showing an indentation and perforation of the cusp. *c*, cusps have been removed from the stent and laid flat, better showing the indentation and perforation.

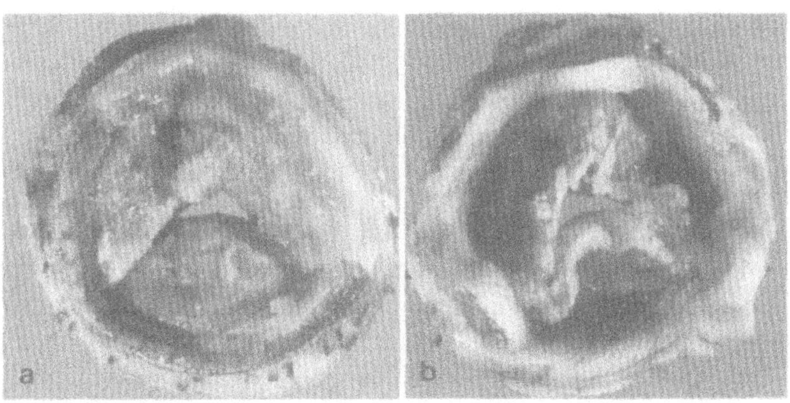

FIGURE 5. Patient 11. Alpha streptococcus bioprosthetic valve endocarditis in an 18-year-old white man (Jewish Hospital #83A-88) who died 17 months after aortic valve replacement. Signs and symptoms of bioprosthetic endocarditis appeared 15 months after operation. The patient died 2 days after completing a 6-week course of antibiotics. *a*, ventricular aspect of the excised bioprosthesis showing diffusely thickened cusps. *b*, aortic aspect showing the degree of cuspal thickening.

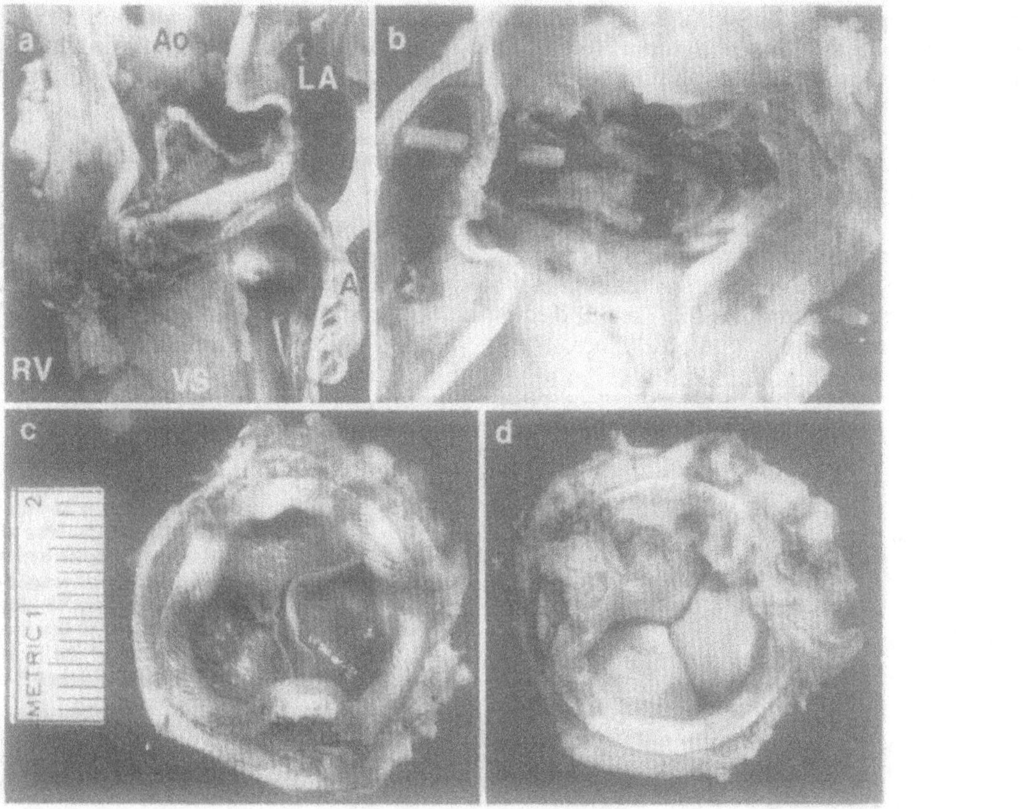

FIGURE 6. Patient 14. *Staphylococcus epidermidis* bioprosthetic valve endocarditis in a 58-year-old man (DCGH# 87A-113) who died 4 months after aortic valve replacement. Syncope due to ventricular tachycardia appeared 1 month before death. Substernal chest pain and conduction disturbances, including left bundle branch block and complete heart block, appeared 3 days before death. On the day of death, 3 of 3 blood cultures were positive for *Staphylococcus epidermidis*. An aortogram showed an aorto–left ventricular fistula (paravalvular leak) and an aorto–right atrial-right ventricular fistula. *a*, opened aorta (Ao) and left ventricular outflow tract, showing the ring abscess in the ventricular septum (VS) and left atrial (LA) wall. *b*, opened aorta after removal of the bioprosthesis. The probe is in the fistula between aorta and right atrium. *c*, aortic aspect of the bioprosthesis. The cusps are normal. *d*, ventricular aspect of the bioprosthesis showing infective material at the sewing ring. A = anterior mitral leaflet; RV = right ventricle.

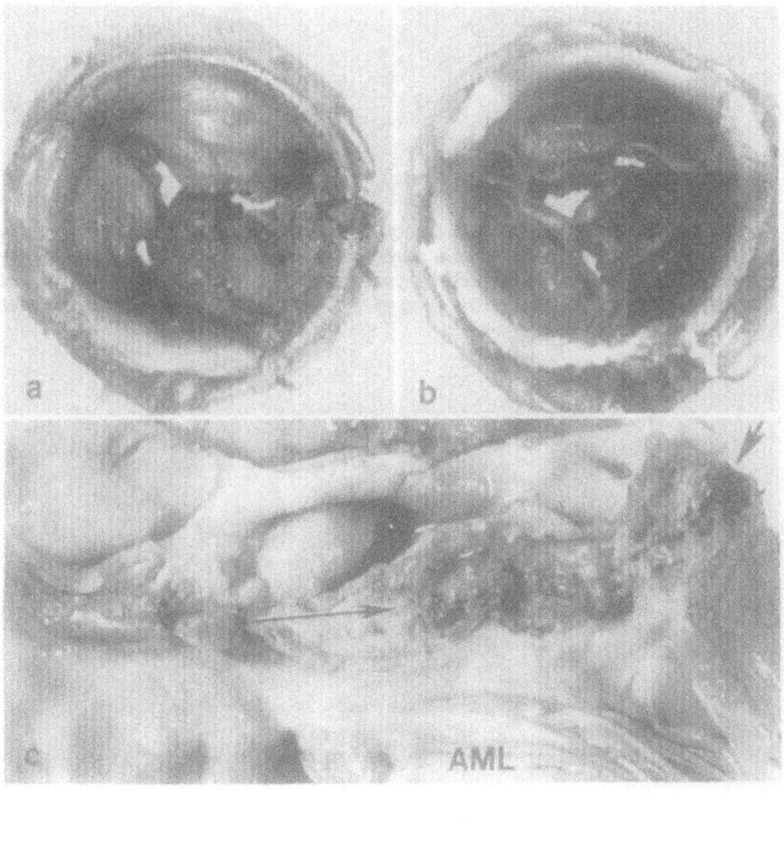

FIGURE 7. Patient 15. Bioprosthetic valve endocarditis in a 58-year-old man (Martinsburgh VAH) who had aortic valve replacement 8 months before death. Congestive heart failure appeared as the first symptom of bioprosthetic endocarditis 1 month before death. *a*, ventricular aspect of the bioprosthesis. Infective material is present on each cusp. *b*, aortic aspect of the bioprosthesis. Infective material extends into the orifice. *c*, a ring abscess *(between arrows)* is present. AML = anterior mitral leaflet.

I) had unequivocal clinical evidence of active infection involving a bioprosthesis, but operative excision of the involved bioprosthesis was not performed until 6 to 48 months (mean 27) after the onset of signs or symptoms, or both, of active bioprosthetic endocarditis. Examination of the operatively excised bioprostheses in 2 of the 5 patients (nos. 24 and 28) disclosed perforations in 2 of the 3 bioprosthetic cusps, a finding typical of healed IE[4]; each of the other 3 patients had parabasilar leaks, with parabasilar aneurysm, from disruption of the bioprosthetic ring from the native valve annulus due to the infection, which had healed. The paraannular aneurysms are indicative of previous IE.[5] None of the 5 patients at any time had evidence of active IE of a native cardiac

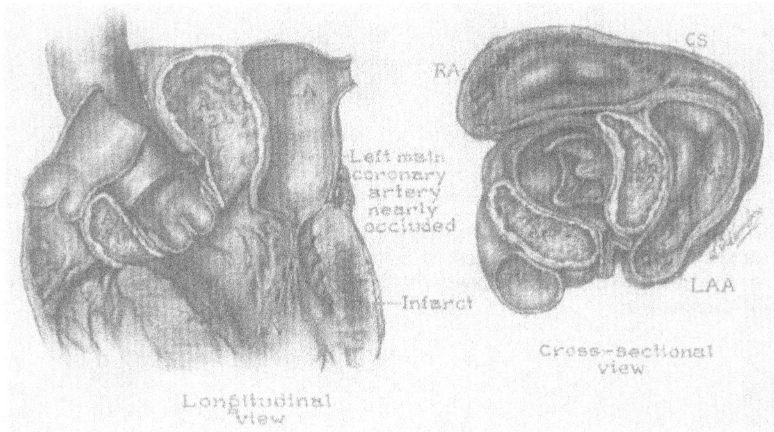

FIGURE 8. Patient 16. Drawing of the heart of a 64-year-old man (GT# 83A-106) who underwent aortic valve replacement 10 months before death. Before death, the active infective endocarditis had healed. Alpha streptococcus bioprosthetic valve endocarditis occurred 3 months after operation and was treated with antibiotics. An acute myocardial infarction occurred 5 months later, and the patient died during cardiac catheterization. The 2 aneurysms (An) were the result of a ring abscess that had healed; neither were of functional significance despite their large size, and neither contained thrombus. Only trace aortic regurgitation was present by aortogram. CS = coronary sinus; LA = left atrium; LAA = left atrial appendage; PV = pulmonic valve; RA = right atrium; RV = right ventricle.

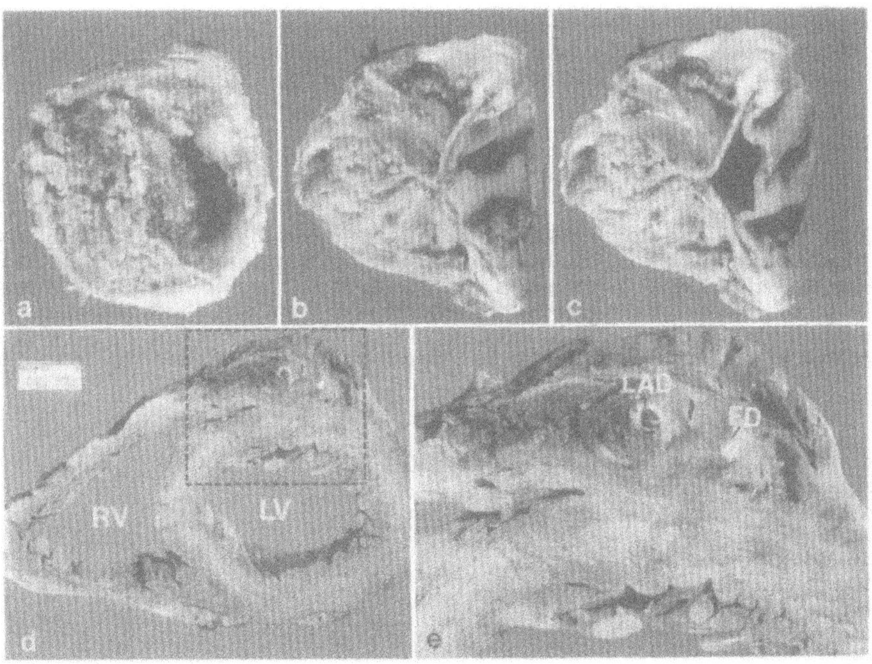

FIGURE 9. Patient 18. *Staphylococcus aureus* bioprosthetic endocarditis in a 70-year-old man (GT# 87A-134) who died 5 years after aortic valve replacement. Signs and symptoms of active infective endocarditis appeared 40 days before death. A series of 5 echocardiograms obtained in the last 33 days of life did not demonstrate a "vegetation" on the bioprosthesis. Despite large doses of antibiotics, bacteremia persisted. The patient had an anterior wall myocardial infarction 9 days before death. *a*, bioprosthesis from the ventricular aspect. The vegetative material occludes >75% of the orifice. *b*, excised bioprosthesis in ventricular "diastole." *c*, in ventricular "systole," the mobility is greatly impaired. *d*, a transverse section of the heart showing biventricular dilatation and extension of the ring abscess along the course of the left anterior descending (LAD) and first diagonal (FD) coronary arteries. *e*, close-up of the LAD and FD. Both are surrounded by necrotic tissue from the ring abscess. The LAD is >75% occluded in cross-sectional area by an embolus. The FD is 100% occluded in cross-sectional area by atherosclerotic plaque. LV = left ventricle; RV = right ventricle.

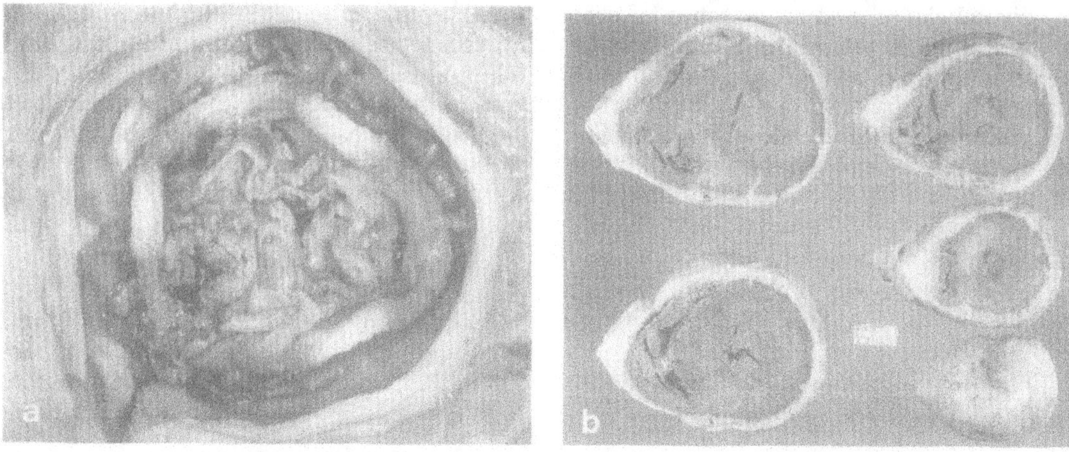

FIGURE 10. Patient 20. Undiagnosed bioprosthetic endocarditis in a 78-year-old man (NNMC# A88-068) who died 25 months after aortic valve replacement. The patient was hospitalized 2 days before death with fever, malaise and dyspnea. Large vegetations are present on the cusps of the bioprosthesis *(a)*. There was no left ventricular necrosis or fibrosis, and the ventricular cavities are not dilated *(b)*.

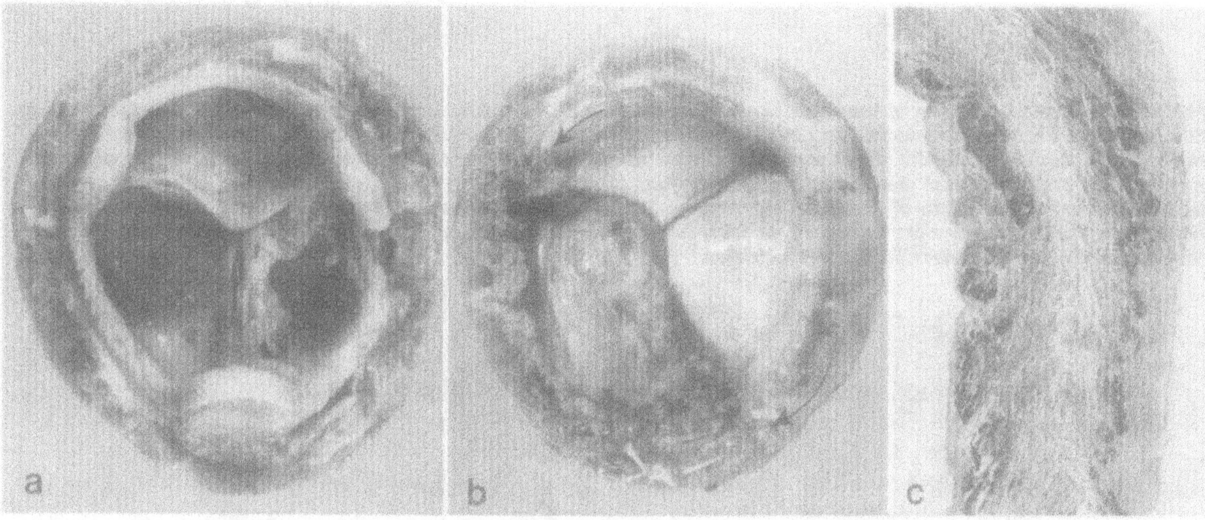

FIGURE 11. Patient 25. *Staphylococcus aureus* bioprosthetic valve endocarditis in a 66-year-old woman (GT# 84S-4958). Signs and symptoms of bioprosthetic endocarditis appeared 44 months after valve replacement. A central line was inserted for dehydration before the onset of signs and symptoms of bioprosthetic endocarditis. Although the bioprosthetic valve functioned normally, it was removed because of persistent bacteremia. *a*, ventricular aspect of the bioprosthetic valve. A vegetation is present on 1 cusp. *b*, atrial aspect. Infective material extends into the sewing ring *(arrows)*. *c*, microscopic section through vegetation and cusp. Colonies of organisms are present (hematoxylin-eosin ×54; reduced by 27%).

FIGURE 12. Patient 26. *Staphylococcus aureus* bioprosthetic endocarditis in a 59-year-old woman (FSH# 84A87) who had undergone mitral valve replacement 7 years before death. Less than a year before death, there was a 10 mm Hg gradient across the bioprosthesis and trace regurgitation. One day before death, signs and symptoms of bioprosthetic endocarditis appeared. The patient died from severe bradycardia without complete heart block. *a*, bioprosthesis from the left atrial aspect. Vegetative material is present on all cusps. *b*, ventricular aspect of the bioprosthesis. Two stents are visible, and 1 cusp has torn at both stents. Calcific deposits limit the mobility of each cusp.

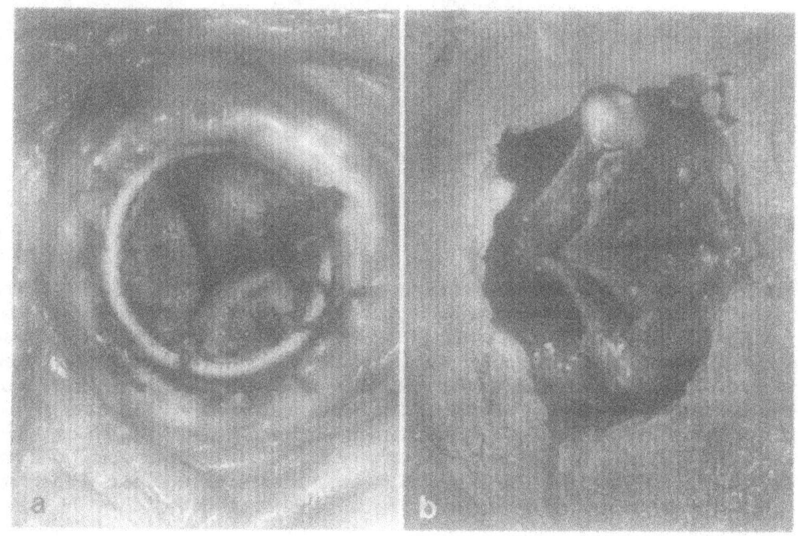

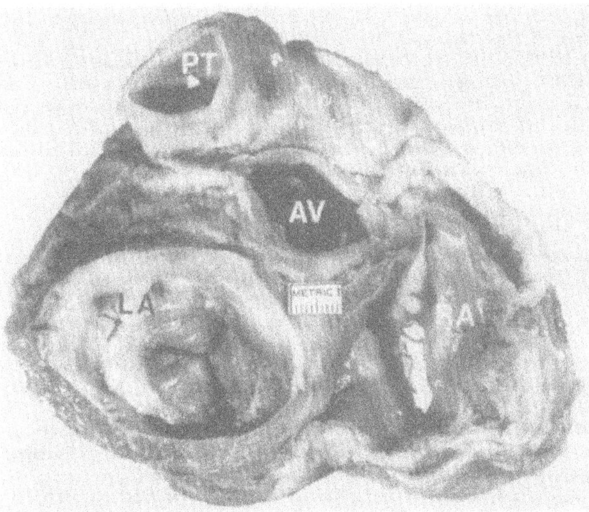

FIGURE 13. Patient 33. ***Staphylococcus aureus*** **bioprosthetic endocarditis in a 67-year-old alcoholic man (DCGH# 85A-18) who had undergone aortic and mitral valve replacement 8 months before death. His first symptom was an acute anterior myocardial infarction from a coronary artery embolus. He died that day after developing complete heart block. Shown here is a view of the base of the heart after removal of the left (LA) and right (RA) atriums. Approximately 50% of the circumference of the sewing ring of the bioprosthesis in the mitral position is involved by the ring abscess. The fibrous covering of the sewing ring is denuded, exposing the cloth-covered sewing ring. Portions of the bioprosthesis in the aortic position (AV) are visible. PT = pulmonary trunk.**

valve (i.e., at the time of operation and replacement with a bioprosthesis).

Location of the infection in the late infection group: Of the 22 patients with isolated aortic valve (n = 16) or mitral (n = 6) replacement, the infection involved the valvular cusps only in 8 (36%), the ring only in 6 (27%), and both the cusps and ring in 8 (36%). Thus, the bioprosthetic ring was involved in 14 patients (64%) and the cusps only in 8 (36%). Of the 7 patients with multiple valve replacement, a total of 15 valves were replaced with bioprostheses: of the 7 bioprostheses in the mitral position, all were infected (cusps only in 5, and cusps and ring in 2); of the 3 bioprostheses in the aortic valve position, 1 was infected (cusps and ring); of the 5 bioprostheses in the tricuspid valve position, 2 were infected (cusps only).

Thus, of the 29 patients with late infection, a total of 37 valves were replaced with bioprostheses: of the 19 bioprostheses in the aortic valve position, 17 were infected (cusps only in 6, ring only in 4, and both in 7); of the 13 bioprostheses in the mitral position, all were infected (cusps only in 7, ring only in 1, and both in 5); of the 5 bioprostheses in the tricuspid valve position, 2 were infected (cusps only). Thus, in the 29 patients with late infection, 37 bioprostheses were inserted: 32 were infected (cusps only in 15 [47%], ring only in 5 [16%], and both in 12 [37%]) and 5 were not. Of the latter 5 bioprostheses, 3 had been in the tricuspid valve position and 2 in the aortic valve position.

Of the 13 patients in whom the infected bioprosthesis was excised, follow-up information was available in 12. Of these 12 patients, 7 are alive and well at present (New York Heart Association functional classes I and II) 5 to 10 years (mean 7) after excision of the infected bioprosthesis. In these 7 patients, the infective material was located on the cusp only in 2, and on both the cusp and ring in 5. One of the latter 5 patients had a parabasilar leak. The remaining 5 patients are dead. One patient died <24 hours after reoperation for active bioprosthetic endocarditis, including an abscess at the junction of the aorta and left atrium. The other 4 patients had operative excision of the infected bioprosthesis (n = 3) or after healing of the bioprosthetic infection (n = 1); 1 died from a noncardiac cause (cancer of the lung) 1.5 years after reoperation, 1, an opiate addict, died from active bioprosthetic endocarditis 3 years after the first infective bioprosthesis was excised, 1 died shortly after pericardiectomy for constriction 5 years after excision of the infected bioprosthesis, and 1 died of pneumonia 14 years after excision of the infected bioprosthesis. The latter patient had a parabasilar bioprosthetic communication.

DISCUSSION

In this study, the location of the infective material was sought in the 13 patients who had operative excision of a presently (n = 9) or previously (n = 4) infected valvular bioprosthesis and in the 21 who were studied at necropsy with a presently (n = 20) or previously (n = 1) infected valvular bioprosthesis. Five of the total 34 patients (15%) developed clinical evidence of active IE within 60 days of replacement of a native cardiac valve with a bioprosthesis, and 29 patients (85%) developed evidence of bioprosthetic endocarditis at later periods. Of the 43 bioprostheses in the 34 patients, 37 were sites of infection: the infection involved the bioprosthetic cusps only in 17 (46%), the sewing ring only in 8 (21%), and both the cusps and sewing ring in 12 (33%). No significant differences were noted in the location of infection based on the specific organism causing infection. Of the 13 patients having operative excision, 9 had active infection at the time, and operative survival and outcome were similar in the 4 in whom the infection was limited to the cusps and in the 5 in whom the sewing ring was involved with (n = 2) or without (n = 3) involvement of the valve cups.

Although a number of previous publications described infection of a bioprosthesis,[6–12] we found only 2 reports that provided data on individual patients with an infected bioprosthesis.[8,11] The study by Bortolotti et al[8] included 9 patients (10 bioprostheses), and that by Nùñez et al[10] included 13 patients (16 bioprostheses) with presently or previously infected bioprosthetic valves: 9 developed infection early (<60 days) and 13 at later periods. Of the 30 bioprostheses in the 22 patients, 24 were sites of infection: the infection involved the bioprosthetic cusps only in 16 (66%), the sewing ring only in 2 (8%), and both in 4 (16%). It is unclear why so few of our 34 patients had the bioprosthetic infection limited to the bioprosthetic cusps and why so many of the previously reported cases had the infection limited to the cusps. In contrast to our study, however, where only 1 of 13 patients having operative excision of the bioprosthesis died early (<60 days), ≥7 of the 22 previously reported patients having operative excision of the bioprosthesis died early.

Acknowledgment: We wish to thank Vivian Norman and Linda Raley for assistance with manuscript preparation, and Michael Spencer for photography of gross specimens.

1. Cohn LH, Roberts WC, Rockoff SD, Morrow AG. Bacterial endocarditis following aortic valve replacement. Clinical and pathologic correlations. *Circulation* 1966;33:209–217.
2. Arnett EN, Roberts WC. Prosthetic valve endocarditis: clinicopathologic analysis of 22 necropsy patients with comparison of observations in 74 necropsy patients with active infective endocarditis involving natural left-sided cardiac valves. *Am J Cardiol* 1976;38:281–292.
3. Arnett EN, Roberts WC. Valve ring abscess in active infective endocarditis. Frequency, location, and clues to clinical diagnosis from the study of 95 necropsy patients. *Circulation* 1976;54:140–145.
4. Buchbinder NA, Roberts WC. Healed left-sided infection: a clinicopathologic study of 59 patients. *Am J Cardiol* 1977;40:876–888.
5. McManus BM, Katz NM, Blackbourne BD, Gottdiener JS, Wallace RB, Roberts WC. Acquired cor triatriatum (left ventricular false aneurysm): complication of active infective endocarditis of the aortic valve with ring abscess treated by valve replacement. *Am Heart J* 1982;104:312–314.
6. Magilligan DJ, Quinn EL, Davila JC. Bacteremia, endocarditis, and the Hancock valve. *Ann Thorac Surg* 1977;24:508–519.
7. Ferrans VJ, Boyce SW, Billingham ME, Spray TL, Roberts WC. Infection of glutaraldehyde-preserved procine valve heterografts. *Am J Cardiol* 1979;43: 1123–1136.
8. Bortolotti U, Thiene G, Milano A, Panizzon G, Valente M, Gallucci V. Pathological study of infective endocarditis on Hancock porcine bioprosthesis. *J Thorac Cardiovasc Surg* 1981;81:934–942.
9. Arnett EN, Roberts WC. Pathology of active infective endocarditis: a necropsy analysis of 192 patients. *Thorac Cardiovasc Surg* 1982;30:327–335.
10. Nùñez L, de la Llana R, Aguado GM, Iglesias A, Larrea JL, Celemin D. Bioprosthetic valve endocarditis: indicators for surgical intervention. *Ann Thorac Surg* 1983;35:262–270.
11. Glazier JJ, Verwilghen J, Donaldson RM, Ross DN. Treatment of complicated prosthetic aortic valve endocarditis with anular abscess formation by homograft aortic root replacement. *J Am Coll Cardiol* 1991;71:1177–1182.
12. Gagliardi C, Di Tommaso L, Mastroroberto P, Stassano P, Spampinato N. Bioprosthetic valve endocarditis: factors affecting bad outcome. *J Cardiovasc Surg* 1991;32:800–806.

Infective endocarditis superimposed on a massively calcified severely stenotic congenitally bicuspid aortic valve

Syed Sarmast, MD, Jeffrey M. Schussler, MD, Jong M. Ko, BA, and William C. Roberts, MD

We describe a 55-year-old man who presented with a stroke resulting from active infective endocarditis (IE) involving a heavily calcified bicuspid aortic valve. The case highlights the infrequency of IE involving a heavily calcified valve, the inability of the infection to penetrate the calcific deposits, and the ability of the infection to spread to the adjacent soft tissues, leading to ring abscess and its multiple complications.

The aortic valve is the most common site for one or more vegetations to form in infective endocarditis (IE) (1). Since the introduction of corticosteroids and the increased frequency of immunotherapy and intravenous drug addiction, infection involving the aortic valve has most commonly involved a previously structurally normal valve. The next most common aortic valve to be involved by IE was a congenitally malformed bicuspid aortic valve that had functioned normally or had only mild dysfunction (2). IE involving a previously calcified valve is unusual and particularly so when the aortic valve is massively calcified. The present report was prompted by study of a patient who developed IE on a previously heavily calcified, severely stenotic aortic valve.

CASE DESCRIPTION

A 55-year-old white man, on chronic hemodialysis for end-stage renal disease believed to be secondary to diabetes mellitus, was hospitalized because of the sudden onset of confusion. Diabetes mellitus was diagnosed when he was 43 years old (2001), requiring insulin therapy by age 49. Systemic hypertension was diagnosed at age 50. He had a sedentary lifestyle and was obese (body mass index 35 kg/m^2). Twelve months earlier, hemodialysis had been initiated; 7 months earlier, a malfunctioning right arm arteriovenous fistula had been repaired; and 1 month earlier, he presented with fever, nausea, vomiting, and abdominal pain. Methicillin-resistant *Staphylococcus aureus* bacteremia related to a right internal jugular PermaCath infection was diagnosed. During that admission, a grade 2/6 precordial systolic ejection murmur was heard. Echocardiography revealed a calcified stenotic bicuspid aortic valve with trace aortic regurgitation, and a small mobile mass attached to the aortic valve was seen. An aortic root abscess also was seen. He was discharged home to receive intravenous vancomycin for 6 weeks and then returned because of confusion. Repeat blood cultures again grew *Staphylococcus aureus*. He was treated with daptomycin.

On July 31, 2010, the aortic valve (bioprosthesis) and proximal portion of the ascending aorta were replaced (the latter was a homograft), the paravalvular abscess was debrided, and the coronary ostial sites were implanted into the homograft. The excised stenotic and infected aortic valve weighed 8.36 g and was congenitally bicuspid *(Figure 1)*. Culture of the excised valve grew methicillin-resistant *Staphylococcus aureus*. The patient's early postoperative course was complicated by episodes of paroxysmal atrial fibrillation and nonsustained ventricular tachycardia.

One month following the operation, the patient was back at home and continuing his hemodialysis treatments 3 times a week. A successful renal transplant was performed on September 13, 2012, and hemodialysis was discontinued. As of October 2013, he remains active and exercises 30 minutes a day at least 3 times a week. He is currently unemployed and on disability.

DISCUSSION

The patient described herein with end-stage renal disease requiring chronic hemodialysis had a heavily calcified stenotic congenitally bicuspid aortic valve and developed superimposed IE initiated as a result of infection at the percutaneous dialysis entry site. The infection, unable to grow well in the calcified valve, rapidly spread to the adjoining soft tissue, producing a ring abscess.

The unusual feature of the present patient is the development of IE on a massively calcified aortic valve. The normal aortic valve weighs about 0.4 g. Thus, the valve in the present patient (8.36 g) was 20 times heavier than normal, and most of that excessive weight was the result of the calcific deposits, not the superimposed vegetative material. Roberts and Ko (3) initially reported weights of operatively excised stenotic aortic valves in 2003 and from January 1998 to August 2013 had

From the Division of Cardiology, Department of Internal Medicine, Baylor University Medical Center at Dallas and the Jack and Jane Hamilton Heart and Vascular Hospital, Dallas, Texas.

Corresponding author: Syed Sarmast, MD, Baylor Heart and Vascular Hospital, 621 N. Hall Street, Dallas, TX 75226 (e-mail: Syed.Sarmast@BaylorHealth.edu).

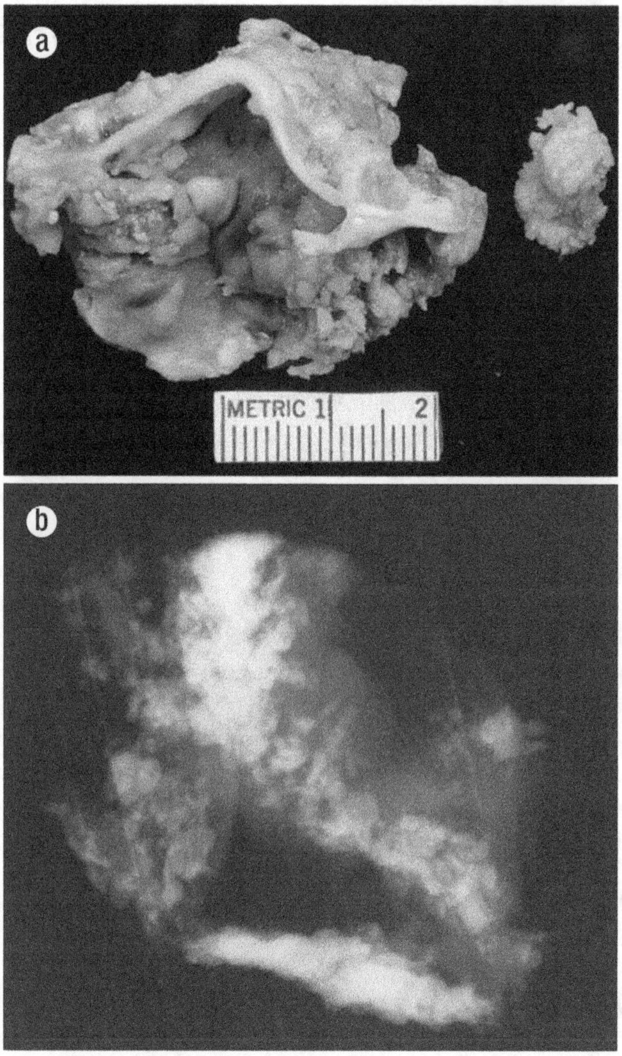

Figure 1. (a) Photograph of the operatively excised stenotic aortic valve and **(b)** radiograph of the valve in the patient described.

weighed 1726 stenotic aortic valves: only 12 (0.7%) weighed >8 g, and none of the other 11 patients had IE. Indeed, the lighter the aortic valve, the greater the likelihood of its being complicated by IE (2).

IE involving a stenotic aortic valve is far less common than IE involving a nonstenotic aortic valve. Fernicola and Roberts (4) studied at necropsy 96 patients with active IE involving the aortic valve: 25 (26%) had underlying stenosis and 71 (74%) had an underlying nonstenotic valve. Of the 25 with underlying stenosis, 21 (84%) had a ring abscess and 10 (40%) had an underlying congenitally bicuspid valve; of the 71 with a nonstenotic aortic valve, 37 (52%) had a ring abscess ($P = 0.005$) and 21 (30%), a congenitally bicuspid valve (ns).

The patient described had two reasons for having a heavily calcified aortic valve: 1) the underlying bicuspid condition (2), and 2) the presence of end-stage renal disease with chronic hemodialysis (5).

1. Arnett EN, Roberts WC. Pathology of active infective endocarditis: a necropsy analysis of 192 patients. *Thorac Cardiovasc Surg* 1982;30(6):327–335.
2. Roberts WC, Vowels TJ, Ko JM. Natural history of adults with congenitally malformed aortic valves (unicuspid or bicuspid). *Medicine (Baltimore)* 2012;91(6):287–308.
3. Roberts WC, Ko JM. Weights of operatively-excised stenotic unicuspid, bicuspid, and tricuspid aortic valves and their relation to age, sex, body mass index, and presence or absence of concomitant coronary artery bypass grafting. *Am J Cardiol* 2003;92(9):1057–1065.
4. Roberts WC, Oluwole BO, Fernicola DJ. Comparison of active infective endocarditis involving a previously stenotic versus a previously nonstenotic aortic valve. *Am J Cardiol* 1993;71(12):1082–1088.
5. Roberts WC, Taylor MA, Shirani J. Cardiac findings at necropsy in patients with chronic kidney disease maintained on chronic hemodialysis. *Medicine (Baltimore)* 2012;91(3):165–178.

www.ingramcontent.com/pod-product-compliance
Lightning Source LLC
LaVergne TN
LVHW062139200926
848484LV00007B/1832